EMERGENCY MEDICAL RESPONDER

A SKILLS APPROACH

FOURTH CANADIAN EDITION

EMERGENCY MEDICAL RESPONDER

A SKILLS APPROACH

FOURTH CANADIAN EDITION

Daniel Limmer, EMT–P
Paramedic, Kennebunk Fire-Rescue, Kennebunk, Maine
Adjunct Faculty, Southern Maine Technical College, South Portland, Maine

Keith J. Karren, Ph. D.
Professor, Department of Health Sciences, Brigham Young University, Provo, Utah

Brent Q. Hafen, Ph. D
Late of Brigham Young University

John Mackay, EMTP-III, ACP(S)
Winnipeg Fire Paramedic Service, Manitoba

Michelle Mackay, BA
Editor, Paramedic Network News

PEARSON

Toronto

Senior Acquisitions Editor: Lisa Rahn
Marketing Manager: Jenna Wulff
Program Manager: Madhu Ranadive
Developmental Editor: Eleanor MacKay
Project Manager: Rachel Thompson
Production Services: Aptara®, Inc.
Permissions Project Manager: Marnie Lamb
Photo Permissions Research: Rebecca O'Malley
Text Permissions Research: Sam Bingenheimer
Art Director: Zeneth Denchik
Cover and Interior Designer: Anthony Leung
Cover Image: SuperStock/Alamy

10 9 8 7 6 5 4 3 2 1 [CK]

Library and Archives Canada Cataloguing in Publication

Karren, Keith J., author
Emergency medical responder: a skills approach/Daniel Limmer, EMT-P Paramedic, Kennebunk Fire-Rescue, Kennebunk, Maine, Adjunct Faculty, Southern Maine Technical College, South Portland, Maine, Keith J. Karren, Ph.D., Professor, Department of Health Sciences, Brigham Young University, Provo, Utah, Brent Q. Hafen, Ph.D., Late of Brigham Young University, John Mackay, EMTP-III, PCP, Winnipeg Fire Paramedic Service, Manitoba, Michelle Mackay, BA, Editor, Paramedic Network News.—Fourth Canadian edition.

Includes index.
Revision of: Emergency medical responder : a skills approach/Daniel Limmer … [et al.].—3rd Canadian ed.—Toronto : Pearson Canada, [2009], c2010.

ISBN 978-0-13-289257-5 (pbk.)

1. Medical emergencies—Textbooks.   2. Emergency medical services—Textbooks.   3. Transport of sick and wounded—Textbooks.   4. Emergency medical technicians—Textbooks.   I. Hafen, Brent Q., author   II. Limmer, Daniel, author   III. Mackay, John, author   IV. Mackay, Michelle (Editor), author   V. Title.

RC86.7.E64 2013   616.02'5   C2013-907078-8

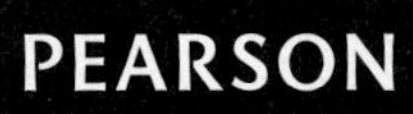

ISBN 978-0-13-289257-5

To those in EMS who have given their lives in the line of duty and to those who continue to toil.

Patient Assessment Plan

SCENE ASSESSMENT

ASSESS PERSONAL SAFETY INCLUDING:

- BSI Precautions • Scene Safety

IDENTIFY MECHANISM OF INJURY / NATURE OF ILLNESS
DETERMINE NECESSARY RESOURCES INCLUDING:

- Number of Patients • Hazardous Materials • Special Rescue Needs

PRIMARY ASSESSMENT

FORM A GENERAL IMPRESSION
ASSESS LEVEL OF CONSCIOUSNESS
ASSESS AIRWAY, BREATHING, AND CIRCULATION
UPDATE EMS

SECONDARY ASSESSMENT

USE DOTS TO EXAMINE:

- Head • Neck • Chest • Abdomen • Pelvis • Extremities

ASSESS VITAL SIGNS

PATIENT HISTORY

GATHER A SAMPLE HISTORY:

- Signs and Symptoms • Allergies • Medications • Pertinent Past History
- Last Oral Intake • Events

ONGOING ASSESSMENT

REPEAT THE PRIMARY ASSESSMENT
REPEAT THE SECONDARY ASSESSMENT, INCLUDING VITAL SIGNS
REASSESS TREATMENT AND INTERVENTIONS
CALM AND REASSURE THE PATIENT

HAND-OFF REPORT

INCLUDES:

- Patient Age and Sex • Chief Complaint • Level of Consciousness • Airway, Breathing, and Circulation Status • Secondary Assessment Findings • SAMPLE History • Treatment/Interventions

Brief Contents

Contents

Preface

We have revised *Emergency Medical Responder: A Skills Approach*, Fourth Canadian Edition, extensively to meet faculty needs and to conform to the National Occupational Competency Profiles and Curriculum Blueprints of the Paramedic Association of Canada (PAC). The fourth edition, like the first three, has been adapted for the exclusive use of the Canadian emergency medical responder (EMR).

An EMR may be a member of any of the three emergency services—ambulance, fire, or police—or may be a specially trained private citizen or public employee. Around the world, the field of emergency medical services (EMS) changes constantly. This book, written specifically for Canadians, will help students learn and adapt to the contemporary practice of pre-hospital care.

PAC NATIONAL OCCUPATIONAL COMPETENCY PROFILES AND CURRICULUM BLUEPRINTS

The Paramedic Association of Canada began in the mid-1990s as a grassroots movement of practitioners across Canada. The goal of the organization was to create national standards—the National Occupational Competency Profiles and Curriculum Blueprints—that would help unify a previously fragmented profession. This initiative was accomplished after years of investigation and consensus building with the country's pre-hospital care stakeholders. These standards for EMRs are now widely accepted across Canada.

Accordingly, we present a list of the specific Paramedic Association of Canada's National Occupational Competency Profiles. These appear at the end of each chapter before the review questions (look for the acronym NOCP). Before each competency is a General Competency number and the degree of competency. Please refer to the legend below to understand the degree of competency required as an EMR.

X Practitioner must demonstrate a basic awareness of this competency, but no understanding or practical exposure is required.

A Practitioner must demonstrate an academic understanding of this competency.

S Practitioner must demonstrate this competency in a *simulated setting* (including skill stations and/or scenario practice). It is assumed that in competency areas 4 and 5, all items that require this degree of competency will be performed on a human subject where legally and ethically acceptable.

Note: This textbook does not include the national competencies that are not applicable to the EMR. For a list of the General Competencies, please refer to the Appendix, pages 494–518.

APPROACH AND ORGANIZATION

The organization of *Emergency Medical Responder*, Fourth Canadian Edition, follows the needs of EMR training curricula as identified by the Paramedic Association of Canada.

Part 1 introduces the EMS system; addresses personal, legal, and ethical issues; and acquaints the EMR with human anatomy as a learning base for all patient assessment and treatment (as outlined in the Patient Assessment Plan). For this edition, we expanded the coverage of "diseases of concern" and increased the emphasis on the use of personal protective equipment and body substance isolation. Chapter 5 introduces the EMR to pharmaceuticals as they pertain to EMR patient assessment.

Parts 2 through 6 of the new edition detail all assessments, including scene, primary, and secondary ones, as well as treatment and reporting pertaining to trauma or medical calls. Most notably, we updated this edition to reflect the fundamental shift in CPR standards from A-B-C to C-A-B. While Airway, Breathing, and Circulation remain crucial for assessment and treatment of patients with a pulse, the emphasis on prompt cardiac compressions for a pulseless patient is well supported by current medical research. Additionally, this revision required careful reworking of all chapters with CPR content. Pertinent changes were made to Chapters 7, 8, and 9, as well as to chapters including patient assessment and pediatrics.

This edition presents the five links of the "Chain of Survival" for adults and children as identified by the Heart and Stroke Foundation of Canada and in accordance with CPR standards. The links have been increased from four to five by the Heart and Stroke Foundation. The chain includes the same information but with some altered wording for each link as well as the new addition of the importance of early post cardiac arrest care. This chain continues to emphasize the importance of immediate activation by EMS, chest compressions, defibrillation, advanced life support, and post cardiac arrest care.

We expanded discussion on the treatment and care of bariatric patients in various chapters, as EMRs now encounter these patients more often.

FEATURES OF THE FOURTH CANADIAN EDITION

The Fourth Canadian Edition of *Emergency Medical Responder: A Skills Approach* includes several features to help students grasp the material.

Learning Objectives—Each chapter begins with a general objective list of competencies as they relate to each facet of the text. These learning objectives reflect the National Occupational Competency Profiles.

Case Studies—Each chapter contains one detailed scenario that describes scene safety, patient assessment, and patient care from the perspective of an on-scene emergency medical responder. Each case study walks students through all the relevant steps of the patient assessment plan. The Case Study Follow-up appears toward the end of the chapter, after the EMR Focus.

TIP Boxes—These highlighted flags appear periodically throughout the text to cue readers to important considerations during assessment and treatment. This edition showcases numerous new TIP boxes. The tips originate from longtime practitioners who offer the advice as a "trick of the trade" or "word to the wise."

EMR Focus—This feature reduces the chapter to the most salient points and insights that will be most important to students in the field.

NOCPs—Relevant Paramedic Association of Canada National Occupational Competency Profiles appear at the end of each chapter prior to the review questions.

Review Questions—Placed at the end of each chapter, review questions help students remember and retain key points through practice. The fourth edition features more questions than previous versions.

Appendix—The expanded index features the most current Paramedic Association of Canada National Occupational Competency Profiles. The appendix includes both the general and specific competencies for each area.

NEW TO THE FOURTH CANADIAN EDITION

- Chapter 2 captures updated material regarding transmittable diseases that are of concern for EMRs, as well as enhanced recommendations for cleaning activities and dealing with exposure.
- Chapter 6 offers more information on lifting and positioning techniques, including the HAINES position.
- Chapter 18 discusses the use of the Taser by Canadian police services and handling the removal of Taser darts.
- Chapter 19 updates the EMR approach to the control of bleeding.
- Chapter 20 incorporates the use of a cravat roll to stabilize an impaled object and expands coverage of the application of eye dressings.
- Chapter 34 discusses special rescue situations, including elevator rescues, and covers procedures for handling bariatric patients.
- All chapters and the Appendix capture current Paramedic Association of Canada National Occupational Competency Profiles.
- 150+ new photos reflect current standards and procedures.

SUPPLEMENTS

Supplements for Instructors

The following instructor supplements can be downloaded from a password-protected section of Pearson Canada's online catalogue. Navigate to your book's catalogue page to view a list of those supplements that are available. Ask your local Pearson sales representative for details and access.

Instructor's Manual This manual provides an at-a-glance summary of the learning objectives for each chapter, a list of resources and equipment that may be required to teach the material in the chapter, and background information that gives an overview of the chapter content. It also offers teaching suggestions, including warm-up activities, tips and strategies, a lesson outline, and a summary and review section that provides answers to the end-of-chapter review questions and offers suggestions for homework assignments.

MyTest The MyTest from Pearson Education Canada is a powerful assessment generation program that helps instructors easily create and print quizzes, tests, exams, and homework or practice handouts. Questions and tests can all be authored online, allowing instructors ultimate flexibility and the ability to efficiently manage assessments at any time, from anywhere. MyTest for *Emergency Medical Responder: A Skills Approach,* Fourth Canadian Edition, includes over 700 questions in a variety of formats, including true/false, multiple choice, and completion exercises.

Test Item File This test bank is a Microsoft Word version of the MyTest, which includes the same type and number of questions.

PowerPoints PowerPoint presentations offer an introduction and overview of the key concepts presented in each chapter.

Image Library The Image Library is a bank of most figures and selected photos from the Fourth Canadian Edition, which can be incorporated into your lecture presentations.

CourseSmart for Instructors

CourseSmart goes beyond traditional expectations—providing instant, online access to the textbooks and course materials. Faculty can save time with a digital eTextbook that provides the ability to search for the most relevant content at the very moment needed. Whether it's evaluating textbooks or creating lecture notes to help students with difficult concepts, CourseSmart can make life a little easier. Visit www.coursesmart.com.

Supplements for Students

Workbook A chapter-by-chapter study guide, the workbook includes summaries of key ideas, a comprehensive review of content using different question formats (and answer key), and case studies that test the students' analytical skills.

PEARSON CUSTOM LIBRARY

For enrollments of at least 25 students, you can create your own textbook by choosing the chapters that best suit your own course needs. To begin building your custom text, visit www.pearsoncustomlibrary.com. You may also work with your Pearson Canada Sales Representative to create your ideal text—publishing your own original content or mixing and matching Pearson content. Contact your local Pearson Representative to get started.

Acknowledgments

The authors wish to thank the authors of Brady *First Responder: A Skills Approach*, from which the first edition of this text originated. While much work was required to adapt the text to the needs of Canadian readers, the source material was, and continues to be, invaluable.

Thank you to the staff and management of both SMART EMS and the Winnipeg Fire Paramedic Service, including staff from Winnipeg EMS and the Winnipeg Fire Department, for their willingness to help recreate photo material for the text.

Thanks go to Dr. Claude Murphy and Dr. Ian Reid for their friendship and photogenic qualities during our photo sessions.

And of course, thanks to our sons, Ian Mackay and Orrin Mackay, who offered technical assistance with hardware and software as well as a high degree of patience during photo sessions … even as models.

A sincere, albeit insufficient, thank you goes to the staff of Pearson Canada, who are always available to offer assistance. You were never impatient and always encouraging when work was overwhelming. It has been a pleasure to work virtually with Eleanor MacKay and Don Thompson, as well as Lisa Rahn who was parachuted in late in the project to help us wrap it up! Eleanor never seemed alarmed by stumbling blocks and was always calm, understanding, and very positive.

Most of all, we are thankful to God from whom all blessings and opportunities are provided. It is such a privilege to be part of such an important text for Emergency Medical Responder students, including the many dedicated folks at St. John Ambulance who have answered the call to be "Good Samaritans."

Finally, this book would not be complete without the valuable contribution of the following reviewers, who, as key EMS players in Canada, found the time to provide much advice and feedback while the EMR manuscript was being considered for the fourth edition:

Josephine Hall, St. John Ambulance

Richard Hepditch, Conestoga College and Waterloo Fire Rescue

John Jacob, Justice Institute of British Columbia

Jodie Marshall, Justice Institute of British Columbia

John Pulkrabek, Northern Alberta Institute of Technology

Notices

Notice on Care Procedures

The material in this book contains the most current information available at the time of publication. However, national, provincial, and local guidelines concerning clinical practices, including, without limitations, those governing infection control and universal precautions, change rapidly. The reader should note, therefore, that new regulations may require changes in some procedures.

It is the responsibility of the reader to familiarize himself or herself with the policies and procedures set by national, provincial, and local agencies as well as the institution or agency where he or she is employed. The authors and publisher of this book have taken care to make certain that these procedures reflect currently accepted clinical practice; however, the recommendations cannot be considered absolute. The authors and the publisher disclaim any liability, loss, or risk resulting directly or indirectly from the suggested procedures and theory, from any undetected errors, or from the reader's misunderstanding of the text. It is the reader's responsibility to stay informed of any new changes or recommendations made by any national, provincial, or local agency as well as by his or her employing institution or agency.

Notice on Drugs and Drug Dosages

Every effort has been made to ensure that the administration and usage of drugs and/or dosages presented in this book are in accordance with nationally accepted standards. It is the responsibility of the reader to be familiar with the drugs used in his or her system, as well as the dosages specified by his or her medical director. The drugs presented in this book should only be administered by direct verbal or accepted order of a licensed physician.

CHAPTER

1

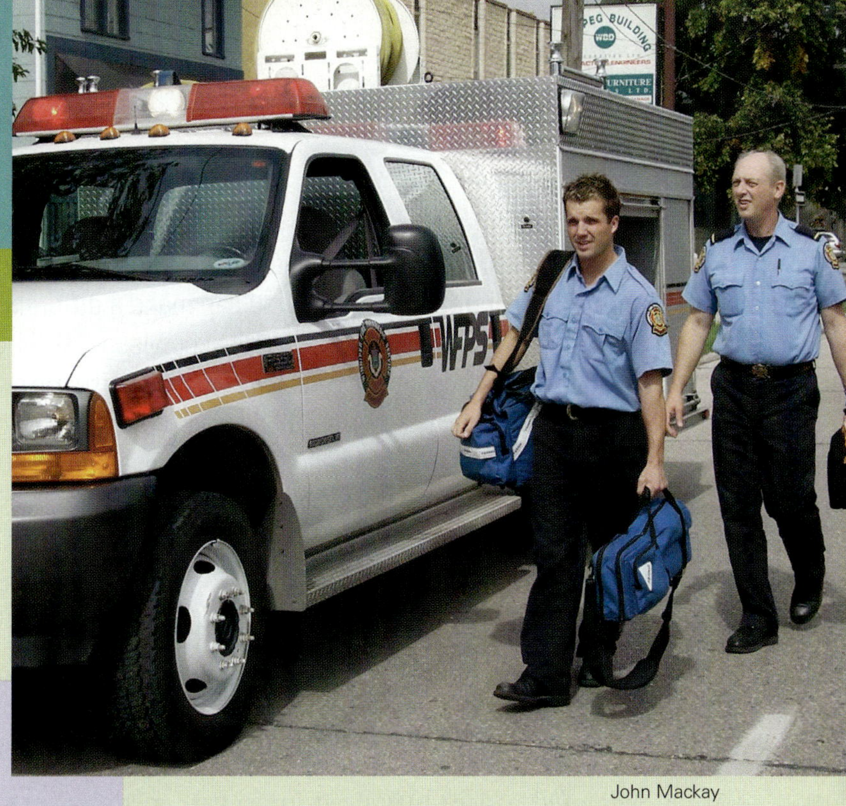

John Mackay

Introduction to the Emergency Medical Services System

OBJECTIVES

1. Describe the components of the emergency medical services (EMS) system and the two public methods by which it can be accessed.

2. Differentiate the roles and responsibilities of the emergency medical responder (EMR) from those of the three other pre-hospital emergency care providers.

3. List six responsibilities of an EMR in accordance with the standards of an EMS professional.

4. Explain why non-discrimination is important when caring for a patient.

5. Discuss the two types of medical control and the EMR's relation to them.

6. State the specific statutes and regulations of the EMS system in your province.

INTRODUCTION

You are about to join a vitally important profession. Every year, thousands of people in Canada die or are permanently injured because they did not receive emergency care in time. As an **emergency medical responder (EMR),** you can make a difference.

This course will help you gain the knowledge, skills, and attitudes you need. To begin, your instructor will describe what you can expect in the course. He or she will inform you of required immunizations and physical exams and will outline your provincial and local certification requirements. Your instructor will also explain the implications of harassment in the classroom environment.

SECTION 1
EMERGENCY MEDICAL SERVICES (EMS)

An ill or injured patient may need immediate medical care to prevent permanent disability or death. Too often, those who arrive first at the emergency scene are not trained to give proper care. As a result, patients who might have been saved die.

The first 60 minutes following an accident are known as the golden hour. Appropriate interventions during this time can make a difference between life and death.

In general, the **emergency medical services (EMS) system** is a network of resources linked together for one purpose—to provide emergency care and transport to victims of sudden illness or

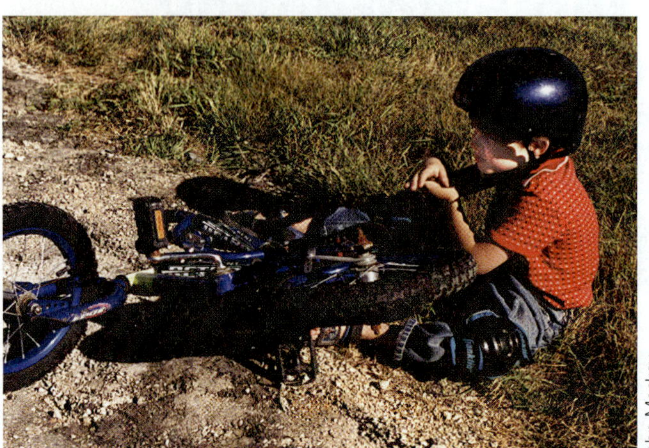

Figure 1–1a Patient.

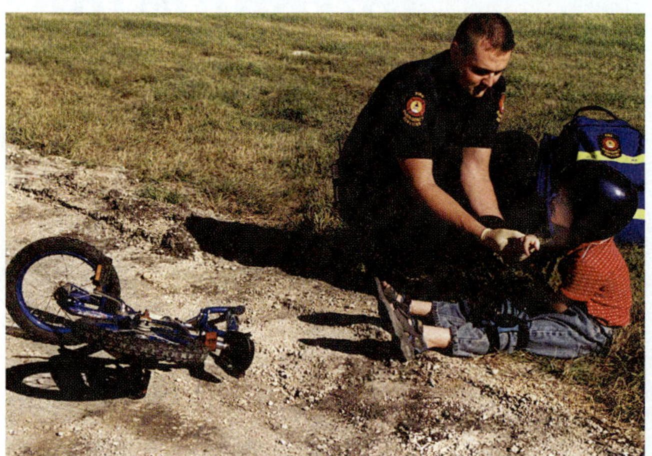

Figure 1–1b Emergency medical responder.

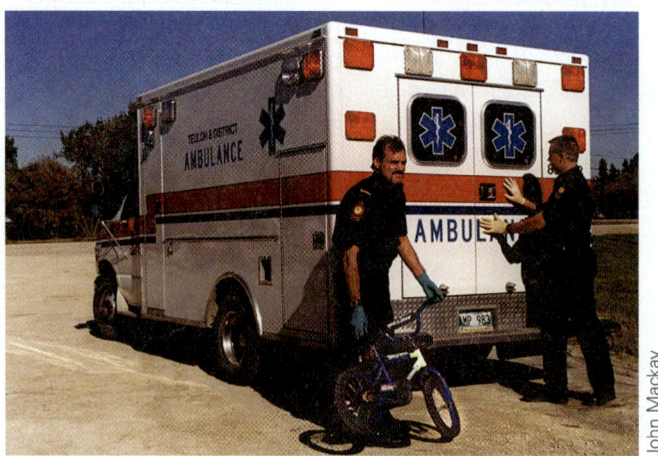

Figure 1–1c Paramedics.

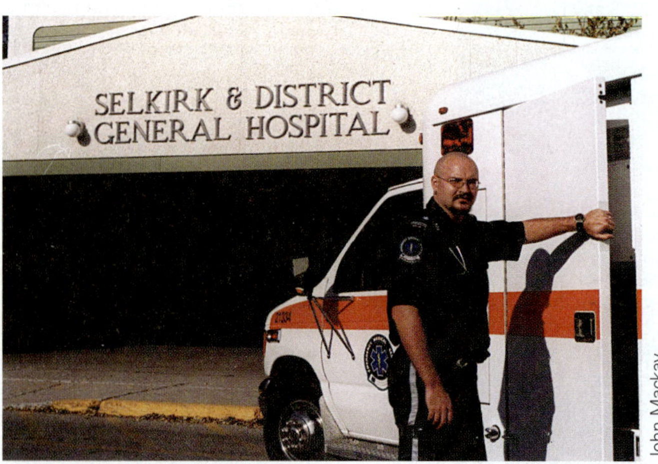

Figure 1–1d Hospital emergency department staff.

CASE STUDY

Dispatch

We were dispatched to a woman with chest pain at 426 Clifford Street. I had not been on many calls, but my partner had been on hundreds. I felt very nervous, especially with the lights and siren on.

Scene Assessment

When we approached the scene, my partner turned off the lights and siren. We grabbed protective gloves and, when we saw it was safe, we left our rig. We both kept alert for signs of danger as we approached the house.

Primary Assessment

Inside the house, we saw our patient sitting on a chair. Our general impression was that she was pale and sweaty. I also remember thinking that she looked really sick. Almost immediately, we began to assess her ABCs—airway, breathing, and circulation.

My partner gave me a look which let me know that he believed the patient could be in serious condition. I radioed the dispatcher to update the incoming paramedic unit. My partner administered oxygen to the patient while keeping her and her husband calm.

> You will encounter a wide range of calls as an EMR. Some may be medical calls such as this one. Others may involve trauma (injury). Is the patient's condition new or pre-existing? What events or circumstances led to your being called to the emergency? At the end of this chapter, you will learn how these EMRs handled their patient's emergency.

injury (Figure 1–1). For example, when an emergency occurs, a citizen at the scene recognizes it and calls for help. If the citizen has dialed 9-1-1 or another emergency number, he or she will receive patient care instructions from an EMS dispatcher. When the EMRs arrive, they will assess the situation and take over care of the patient. When necessary, they inform dispatch of the need for additional EMS resources. Usually, EMS rescuers with higher levels of training are called to the scene. They continue the care and transport the patient to the hospital. There, patient care is transferred to emergency department personnel and, finally, to the in-hospital care system.

Classic Components of EMS

Each province in Canada has control of its own EMS system. Canada's EMS systems can vary from province to province and even from city to city or town to town. (Some of the provincial information provided in this text may apply to territories as well.) The Paramedic Association of Canada (PAC), along with the former Human Resources Development Canada (HRDC), has developed national competency profiles and a blueprint curriculum that define a national scope of practice for emergency care. There are 10 classic components of any EMS system:

1. *Regulation and policy.* Each province must have laws, regulations, policies, and procedures that govern its EMS system. Each province is also required to provide leadership to local jurisdictions.
2. *Resources management.* Each province must have central control of EMS resources so that all patients have equal access to acceptable emergency care.
3. *Human resources and training.* All personnel who staff ambulances and transport patients

must be trained to a minimum level as determined by the province.

4. *Transportation*. Patients must be safely and reliably transported by ground or air ambulance.

5. *Facilities*. Every seriously ill or injured patient must be delivered in a timely manner to an appropriate medical facility.

6. *Communications*. A system for public access to the EMS system must be in place. Communication among dispatchers, ambulance crews, and hospitals must also be possible.

7. *Public information and education*. EMS personnel should participate in programs designed to educate the public. The programs are to focus on injury prevention and how to properly access the EMS system.

8. *Medical control*. Each EMS system must have a physician as its medical director.

9. *Trauma systems*. Each province must develop a system of specialized care for trauma patients, including one or more trauma centres and rehabilitation programs. It must also develop systems for assigning and transporting patients to those facilities.

10. *Evaluation*. Each province must have a quality improvement system in place for continuous evaluation and upgrading of its EMS system.

Access to EMS

There are two general systems by which the public can access the EMS system: 9-1-1 and non-9-1-1. Often called the universal number, 9-1-1 is used in many areas to access police, fire, rescue, and ambulance services. Generally, calls are received at a **public safety answering point (PSAP)**. There, a dispatcher decides which resource is to be activated and alerts the appropriate service (Figure 1–2).

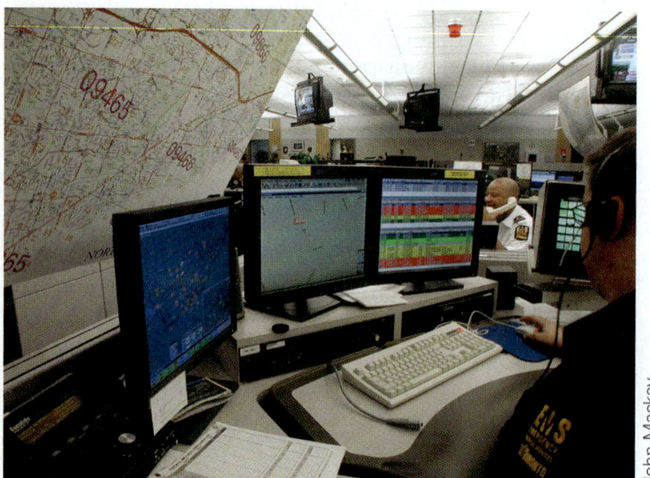

Figure 1–2 The emergency medical dispatcher (EMD) is an important member of the EMS team.

There are two main benefits of a universal number. First, the PSAP is generally staffed by trained technicians known as emergency medical dispatchers (EMDs). Sometimes trained as EMRs themselves, the EMDs may offer medical advice over the phone while the patient waits for rescuers to arrive. This is referred to as **emergency medical dispatching**. The second benefit of a universal number is that it minimizes delay. Callers do not have to look up a number since 9-1-1 is easily remembered by even the youngest caller.

With **enhanced 9-1-1**, or E-9-1-1, the EMS dispatcher is able to see the caller's street address and phone number on a computer screen. This information is valuable when a patient becomes unconscious before conveying an address. Roadway, location, and caller-specific hazards may also be recorded and updated with E-9-1-1 dispatch information.

In areas not served by 9-1-1, callers dial either a dispatch centre or the specific service they need (police, EMS, fire, etc.). Probably the most serious drawback of a non-9-1-1 system is the delay in reaching the appropriate services.

Levels of Training

Although some provinces and individual services may use unique titles, there are four nationally recognized levels of emergency medical services training: **emergency medical responder (EMR)**, **primary care paramedic (PCP)**, **advanced care paramedic (ACP)**, and **critical care paramedic (CCP)**:

1. *EMR* (Figure 1–3). The EMR is the first person on the scene with emergency training. He or she may be a police officer, firefighter, truck driver, school teacher, industrial health officer, or community volunteer. Training includes the following:
   - Airway care and suctioning
   - Patient assessment
   - Cardiopulmonary resuscitation (CPR)
   - Bleeding control
   - Stabilization of injuries to the spine and extremities
   - Care for medical and trauma emergencies
   - Use of a limited amount of equipment
   - Assisting other EMS providers
   - Other skills and procedures as permitted by local or provincial regulations

2. *PCP* (Figure 1–4). The PCP can do everything that the EMR does, as well as administer symptomatic relief drugs and perform pulse oximetry, blood glucose testing, defibrillation, complex immobilization procedures, and patient restraint, as well as staff and drive ambulances.

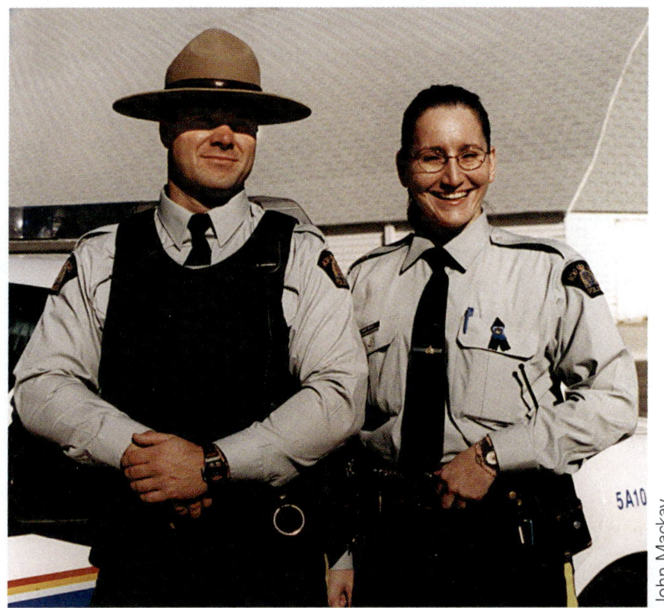

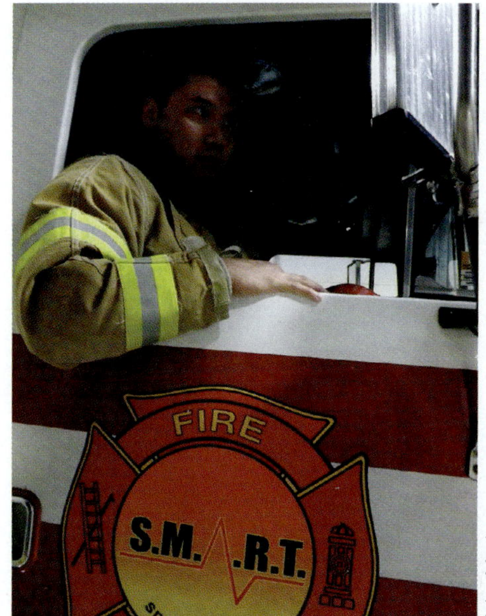

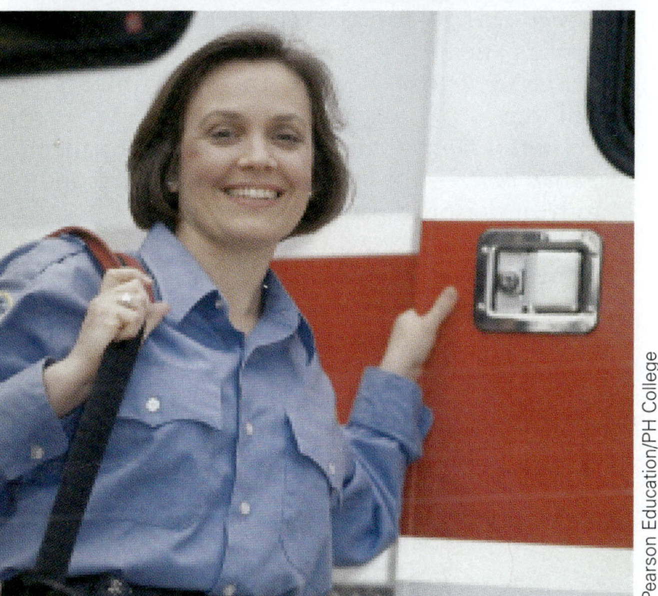

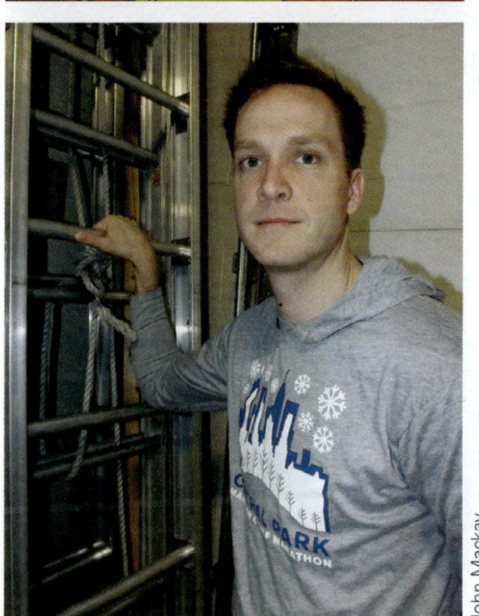

Figure 1–3 EMRs may be police officers, firefighters, educators, truck drivers, industrial workers, or community volunteers.

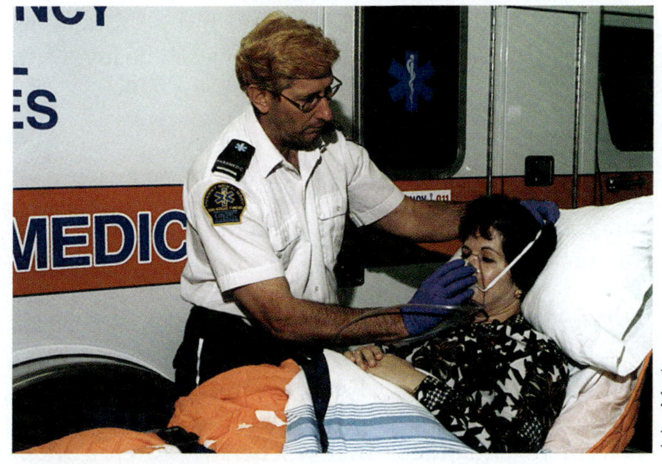

Figure 1–4 Primary care paramedic (PCP).

3. *ACP* (Figure 1–5). The ACP can do everything that an EMR and PCP can do, as well as perform a number of advanced techniques and administer many medications.

4. *CCP* (Figure 1–6). The CCP has the most advanced EMS training. He or she can do everything that those at the three previous levels do, plus administer more medications and perform more advanced techniques.

As an EMR, the aeromedical transport staff you encounter may be PCPs, ACPs, CCPs, nurses, or physicians.

Note that responsibilities for each level may vary from province to province. However, the minimum

pre ¿ out of Hospi

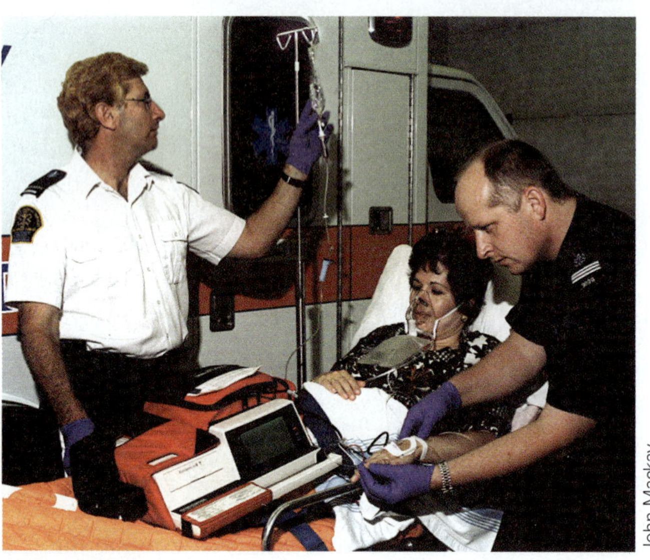

Figure 1–5 Advanced care paramedic (ACP).

Figure 1–6 Critical care paramedic (CCP).

certification guidelines are published by PAC. The guidelines can be accessed on the PAC website (http://paramedic.ca/nocp). The PAC National Occupational Competency Profiles (NOCPs) were formed in July 2001 and updated in October 2011. (Competencies pertaining to each chapter are found just before the review questions at the end of each chapter. A more comprehensive list of EMR-specific competencies can be found in the appendix that follows Chapter 34.) Although individual services and educational institutions may exceed training at the identified levels, in the future, registration with PAC will be important for the portability of licensure and the maintenance of an appropriate practitioner standard of care. You can contact PAC (http://paramedic.ca) to find your local

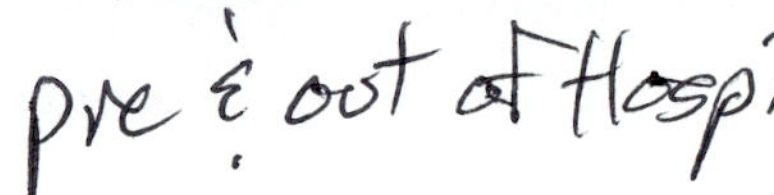

professional association and get further information about all the levels of training for Canadian medics.

In-Hospital Care System

EMRs and paramedics provide **pre-hospital care**, or emergency medical treatment, before and during transport to a medical facility. In some areas, the term **out-of-hospital care** is preferred. It reflects a trend toward providing care on the scene with or without transport to a hospital. (Your instructor will provide information on how these terms apply to your EMS system.)

Specialized facilities to which some patients may be taken include the following:

- *Trauma centre*—for injury treatment that may exceed that of a general hospital
- *Burn centre*—for treatment of burns, often including long-term care and rehabilitation
- *Stroke centre*—for assessment and treatment of stroke patients
- *Pediatric centre*—for treatment of infants and children
- *Perinatal centre*—for high-risk pregnant patients
- *Poison centre*—for information and advice on how to treat poisoned patients

The most familiar destination for an EMS patient is the local hospital emergency department. There, a staff of physicians, nurses, and other allied health professionals stabilize the patient and prepare him or her for further care elsewhere in the hospital.

SECTION 2
THE EMR

As an EMR, you may be called to emergencies where you are the only trained rescuer on the scene. At other times, specialized rescue teams and fire personnel, as well as law enforcement personnel, may all be involved.

Your Role

After ensuring your personal safety, your primary concern as an EMR is your patient. Generally, your role includes the following:

- *Protect your safety and the safety of your crew, the patient, and bystanders.* This is your first and most important priority. Remember that you cannot help the patient if you are injured. You also do not want to endanger other rescuers by forcing them to rescue you. Once scene safety is ensured, the patient's needs become your primary concern.

- *Gain access to the patient.* In some emergencies, you may need to move one patient in order to gain access to a more critically injured one. At other times you may require the assistance of other agencies to help you reach your patient.
- *Assess the patient to identify life-threatening problems.* Always perform a primary assessment to help you identify threats to life. Such problems may include a blocked airway, heart attack, or severe bleeding.
- *Alert additional EMS resources.* In cases where a patient needs medical care or transport to a medical facility, you must remain with the patient until other EMS personnel take over.
- *Provide care based on assessment findings.* While you are waiting for EMS resources to arrive, you must provide patient care based on the needs you identify during patient assessment.
- *Assist other EMS personnel.* When requested, assist other EMS personnel with patient care. This may include accompanying them during transport and assisting with lifting and handling at the hospital.
- *Participate in record keeping and data collection as required.* You may be required by provincial law or your local EMS system to document your calls, especially if a patient refuses care.
- *Act as a liaison for other public safety workers.* These may include local, provincial, or federal law enforcement personnel, fire department personnel, other EMS providers, and other community support agencies.

Your Responsibilities

The responsibilities of an EMR vary from one province to another. However, they always include ensuring scene safety and maintaining a professional attitude and appearance and up-to-date skills. Specifically, you should do the following:

- *Guard your personal health and safety.* Drive safely at all times. Use a seat belt whenever you drive or ride in a vehicle. Remove yourself from such hazards as gas leaks, fires, chemical spills, and so on, and follow the directions of specialized rescuers at those scenes. Never enter a crime scene or an angry crowd until it has been controlled by the police. Locate or create a safe area in which you can care for patients. Stay away from high-traffic areas. Re-direct traffic as needed. Always wear the proper personal protective equipment, including, when appropriate, a hard hat and leather gloves. (See Chapter 2 for more details.)
- *Maintain a caring attitude.* Often, you will arrive at an emergency scene to find the patient, family, and bystanders in a state of panic or pandemo-

nium. These can be normal reactions. Reassure and comfort them. Identify yourself, assure them that you will begin to stabilize the patient, and let them know that more help is on the way.

- *Maintain your own composure.* Many calls will be routine and patient care will be simple. However, some calls will involve life-threatening or emotionally charged problems. In those cases, it is critical that you stay calm so that you can get an accurate picture of the scene and properly establish your priorities. Rather than trying to do everything yourself, delegate tasks as appropriate.
- *Keep your appearance neat, clean, and professional.* Excellent personal grooming and a crisp, clean appearance help instill confidence in patients. Being clean also helps protect your patients from contamination from dirty hands or soiled clothing. Respond to every call in complete uniform or other appropriate clothing. Project a positive image. Remember that you are on a medical team. Your appearance can send the message that you are competent and trustworthy. Promoting awareness of the EMS system and profession is your responsibility.
- *Maintain up-to-date knowledge and skills.* New research often shows us better ways of doing things. Take every opportunity to continue your education, including participating in quality assurance programs and refresher courses offered through your local EMS system.
- *Maintain current knowledge of local, provincial, and national issues affecting the EMS system.* Attend conferences and read professional journals dedicated to EMS issues.

You will be expected to accept and uphold the responsibilities of an EMR in accordance with the standards of an EMS professional. As an EMR, you will come into contact with people of different genders, ages, cultures, and socioeconomic backgrounds. It is your responsibility to meet the standard of care for all your patients. The Canada Health Act states that all people should have equal access to health care. Discriminating against or stereotyping patients may interfere with your ability to properly assess them.

Medical Director

A formal relationship exists between a community's EMS providers and the physician who is responsible for out-of-hospital emergency medical care. This physician is often referred to as the system **medical director**. He or she is legally responsible for the clinical and patient care aspects of an EMS system.

Every EMS system *must* have a medical director. He or she must provide guidance to and medical oversight of all emergency care and rescue personnel. The medical director is also responsible for reviewing and improving the quality of care in an EMS system.

Direct and Indirect Medical Control

Two basic types of medical control are **direct medical control** and **indirect medical control**. Direct medical control occurs when the medical director or another physician directs an EMS rescuer at the scene of an emergency. This may be done via telephone, radio, or in person. This usually occurs when an EMS rescuer asks for help with the care of a patient. Note that direct medical control is also called "online," "base station," "immediate," or "concurrent." Medical control may also be exercised through a paramedic medical supervisor as an extension of the medical director.

Indirect medical control may also be called "offline," "retrospective," or "prospective." It includes such things as system design and quality management. Through indirect medical control, **protocols** spell out the accepted practice for EMRs in your area. They tell you things like whether or not you can give oxygen to a patient or how to respond to a family who refuses your help. They also tell you how to document each call, participate in reviews, gather feedback, and maintain your skills.

The EMR

In general, EMRs are the designated agents of the medical director. If this holds true for your area, the care you render by law may be considered an extension of the medical director's authority. Your instructor will tell you what the law is in your area.

EMR FOCUS

As an EMR, you play a vital role in the emergency medical care of patients experiencing an illness or injury. Perhaps the most important reason your role is so crucial is that you are responsible for the first few minutes with the patient. The EMS system depends on your action during this time to set the foundation for the remainder of the call.

It is during this time that correcting a breathing problem or stopping bleeding can actually save a life.

You will also help non-critical patients when you prevent further injury, perform the proper assessments, gather the medical history, and prepare for the arrival of the paramedics. While your scope of practice is clearly defined by the service for which you work, you may at times be asked to assist other health care personnel while they perform their duties both in and out of the hospital.

CASE STUDY FOLLOW-UP

At the beginning of this chapter, you read that EMRs were caring for a patient with chest pain. To see how the chapter material applies to this emergency, read the following. It describes how the call was completed.

PATIENT HISTORY

The woman told us she was 67 years old and her name was Paula McMaster. She said that she'd had a heavy feeling in her chest for about two hours. It radiated to her left shoulder. The pain had come on while she was watching TV. The patient told us that she had had high blood pressure for many years. She had had two heart attacks over the past five years. She took blood pressure medication and a pill for diabetes. She denied having any allergies. Her last meal was about two hours before, when she had a sandwich and coffee.

SECONDARY ASSESSMENT

The patient denied any injury such as a fall or car crash. Because of this, we did not perform a hands-on, head-to-toe exam. We did check her chest, shoulders, and arms for pain. We took her vital signs and found that her pulse was 96, weak, and irregular. Her respirations were 20 and laboured. Blood pressure was 100/56. Listening to her chest, we heard adequate air entering on both lungs.

According to protocol we administered oxygen and made sure the paramedics were on the way.

ONGOING ASSESSMENT

We remained concerned because the patient was pale and sweaty, with some difficulty breathing. We verified that the patient was still alert and breathing adequately. Oxygen continued to flow through a non-rebreather mask. We made sure the patient was as comfortable as she could be and tried to reassure her and her husband. We finished taking another set of vitals just as the ambulance pulled up.

TRANSFER OF CARE

Since my partner had responsibility for patient care during this call, he gave the paramedics the hand-off report:

"We have a 67-year-old female patient, Mrs. McMaster. She began having heaviness in the chest and left shoulder about two hours ago while watching TV. She is pale and sweaty with some laboured breathing. Her vital signs are: blood pressure 100/56; pulse 96, weak, and irregular; and respirations 20 and laboured. She has a history of heart attack, high blood pressure, and diabetes. We tried to make her comfortable and gave her oxygen by non-rebreather mask."

After we made sure the paramedics didn't need us any longer, we radioed dispatch to say we were available for our next call and headed back to headquarters.

> It takes all the resources of an EMS system working together to help a patient survive an illness or injury. As an EMR, you are a valuable part of that system.

NOCPs

1.1 c Dress appropriately and maintain personal hygiene **A**
   d Maintain appropriate personal interaction with patients **A**
   f Participate in quality assurance and enhancement programs **A**
   g Promote awareness of EMS system and profession **A**
   h Participate in professional association **A**
   j Function as patient advocate **A**
1.2 a Develop personal plan for continuing personal development **X**

1.3 a Comply with scope of practice **S**
1.5 a Work collaboratively with a partner **S**
1.6 b Practise effective problem solving **S**
   c Delegate tasks appropriately **S**
2.4 a Employ empathy and compassion while providing care **S**
   d Act in a confident manner **S**
8.1 d Utilize community support agencies as appropriate **A**
8.2 a Work collaboratively with other emergency response agencies **A**

REVIEW QUESTIONS

Page references where answers may be found or supported are provided at the end of each question.

SECTION 1

1. What is the purpose of the EMS system? (p. 2)
2. What is the typical sequence of events from the time an emergency occurs and EMS is activated to the time the patient is transferred to the in-hospital care system? (pp. 2–3)
3. What are five of the ten classic components of an EMS system? (pp. 3–4)
4. What are two basic ways to access the EMS system? (pp. 3–4)
5. How many nationally recognized levels of training are offered in the EMS system? Briefly describe each one. (p. 4)
6. What certification level(s) might you find when encountering aeromedical staff? (p. 5)
7. What are three types of medical facility to which an EMS patient may be taken? (p. 6)

SECTION 2

8. What roles do EMRs fill at the scene of an emergency? (pp. 6–7)
9. What are the EMR's responsibilities? (p. 7)

SECTION 3

10. What are the two types of medical control? Describe each one. (p. 8)
11. An on-scene medical supervisor represents which kind of medical control? (p. 8)

2

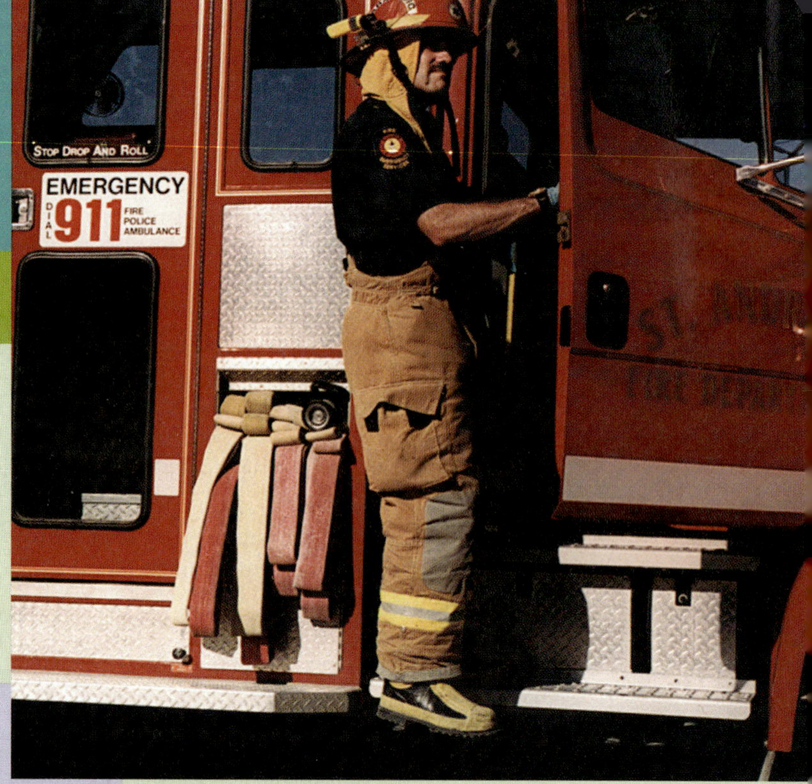

John Mackay

The Well-Being of the Emergency Medical Responder

OBJECTIVES

1. Identify reactions that may be experienced by the EMR, a patient, or a patient's family during or after a critical incident. Describe how these emotions may manifest themselves and how you as an EMR can respond to them.

2. Describe ways to show care and compassion and display empathy for dying patients and their families.

3. Recognize signs and symptoms of stress and explain strategies for dealing with its impact on you and your family.

4. List proper cleanup and contaminated waste disposal methods.

5. Describe the need for scene safety and which personal precautions should be taken in a variety of emergency situations.

INTRODUCTION

As a rescuer, your safety always comes first. It comes before that of the patient and before that of any bystander at the scene. The reason is simple: if you are injured, you lose the ability to help those who need you. Instead of providing emergency care, you end up needing it yourself.

Many elements make up rescuer safety. Most basic training programs teach how to react safely to a variety of environmental threats, such as fire and flood. But the most common threats to a rescuer are likely to be something simple, such as oncoming traffic.

This chapter outlines the basic steps you should take to maintain your well-being. It includes how to anticipate and handle the emotional aspects of emergencies and how to protect yourself against infection. It also introduces scene safety.

SECTION 1
EMOTIONAL ASPECTS OF EMERGENCY MEDICAL CARE

Stress is any change in the body's internal balance. It occurs when outside demands are greater than the body's resources. High-stress situations include incidents with multiple patients, injury to an infant or child, death of a patient, an amputation, violence, abuse, and injury or death of a co-worker.

A rescuer's emotional responses to high stress may include crying, panicking, or speaking in an abnormal tone. Physical responses to high stress may include weakness, nausea, vomiting, or fainting. You can help avoid these reactions by using the following techniques:

- Remind yourself that the patient desperately needs you and your skills. You must be in control to give the best care.
- Close your eyes and take several long, deep breaths. Focus on counting each breath. When you feel more in control, return to giving emergency care.
- Change your thought patterns. Hum very quietly or mentally sing a peaceful song.
- Eat properly to maintain your blood sugar. Low blood sugar can contribute to fainting.

Death and Dying

Death and dying are inherent parts of emergency medical care. When your patient is dying, you must care for his or her emotional needs as well as treat the injury or illness. If the patient dies suddenly, you will need to help the family or bystanders deal with their grief.

The Grieving Process

Dying patients, and those close to them, experience five general stages. These stages make up the grieving process. Each person progresses through the stages at his or her own pace and in his or her own way.

Patients with non-fatal emergencies may also go through a grieving process. For example, a patient who loses both legs in a factory accident will grieve the loss of his or her limbs.

As an EMR, you will not witness all five stages during emergency care. A critically injured patient, for example, who is aware that death is imminent, may just be beginning the process. A terminally ill patient, who is more prepared, may be at the final acceptance stage. The key is to accept all emotions as real and necessary. Respond accordingly.

The five stages of the grieving process occur as follows:

1. *Denial ("Not me!")*. At first, the patient may refuse to accept the idea that death is near. This refusal creates a buffer between the shock of approaching death and the need to deal with the illness or injury. Families of dying patients are often at the denial stage.
2. *Anger ("Why me?")*. Watch out. You may be the target of this anger, but remember that it is a normal part of the grieving process. Do not take it personally. Be tolerant, and try to understand. Use your best listening and communication skills.
3. *Bargaining ("Okay, but first let me . . .")*. In the patient's mind, a bargain, or agreement of sorts, will postpone death. For example, a patient may mentally determine that if he is allowed to live, he will patch up a long-standing break with his parents.
4. *Depression ("Okay, but I haven't . . .")*. As reality sets in, the patient may become silent, distant, withdrawn, and sad. The patient is usually

CASE STUDY

Dispatch

My partner and I are community volunteers. We were on the 3-to-12 shift, and it was just about time to quit when dispatch called. There was a person bleeding at 1433 Magnolia.

We got into our unit. It was my partner's turn to drive. I got out the town map and located the residence. On the way, I mentally went over the procedures for body substance isolation and bleeding control.

Scene Assessment

We arrived at the patient's house in about four minutes. We approached carefully. Without any more information than "a person bleeding," we had to be ready for anything. When we got to the door, we waited a second and listened.

Men were yelling, and I heard glass breaking. Loud thumps and scuffling made it obvious that people were fighting in there.

> Caution will help you recognize potential dangers at an emergency scene, but is violence the only kind of danger you may face? What precautions would you take in the situation described above? Consider your answer as you read Chapter 2.

thinking about those he or she is leaving behind and all the things that will be left undone.

5. *Acceptance ("Okay, I am not afraid.").* Finally, though not happy about it, the patient may appear to accept the fact that he or she is dying. At this stage, the family usually needs more support than the patient does.

Dealing with the Dying Patient

It is one of your jobs to help a patient and his or her family through the grieving process. Keep in mind that different individuals may progress through the stages of grief at different rates. Whatever stage they are in, their needs include dignity, respect, sharing, communication, privacy, and control. You must be diplomatic and use tact and discretion. To help reduce their emotional burden, consider the following:

- *Do everything possible to maintain the patient's dignity.* Avoid negative statements about the patient's condition. Even an unconscious patient may hear what you say and sense the fear in your words. Talk to the patient as if he or she were fully alert. Explain the care you are providing.

- *Show the greatest possible respect for the patient.* Do this especially when death is imminent. Family members will be extra sensitive at this time. Even attitudes and unspoken messages are perceived. Therefore, explain what you are doing. Assure family members that you are making every possible effort to help the patient. It is important for them to know with certainty that you never simply gave up.

- *Communicate.* Help the patient become oriented to the surroundings. If necessary, explain several times what happened and where. Explain who you are and what you and others are planning. Without interrupting care, communicate the same message to the family. Explain any procedure you need to carry out. Answer their questions. Do not guess—report only what you know to be true.

- *Allow family members to express rage, anger, and despair.* They should be able to scream, cry, or vent grief, but in a way that is not dangerous to you or others. Be tolerant. If they vent their anger at you, do not get angry or hostile.

- *Listen with empathy.* Many dying people want messages delivered to survivors. Take notes. Assure the patient that you will do whatever you can to honour his or her requests. Then follow through on your promise. If possible, stay with the family to listen to their concerns and answer their questions.

- *Do not give false assurances, but allow for some hope.* Be honest, but tactful. If the patient asks if he or she is dying, do not confirm it. Patients who do most poorly are often the ones who feel hopeless. Instead, say something like, "We are doing everything we can. We need you to help us by not giving up." If the patient insists that death is imminent, say, "That might be possible, but we can still try the best we can, can't we?"
- *Use a gentle tone of voice.* Be kind to both the patient and the family. Explain the scope of the injury, the medical care you are giving, and, when necessary, the suspected cause of death to the best of your ability. Do so as gently and kindly as you can in words they will understand.
- *Let the patient know that everything that can be done will be done.* Emphasize that you are not going to give up. Say that you are doing everything possible and that you will see that the patient gets to a hospital as quickly as possible for further care.
- *Use a reassuring touch, if appropriate.* In addition, if family members want to touch or hold the body after death, and local protocol allows, arrange for it. Do what you can to improve the appearance of the body. If the body is mutilated, warn the family first. Tell them you covered the badly injured parts. Note that at a possible crime scene, you should *never* clean the patient or remove any blood from the patient or the scene.
- *Do what you can to comfort the family.* Arrange for them to briefly see or talk to the patient. However, do not interrupt your emergency care or delay transport. If the patient is deceased, and the family asks you to pray with them, do so. Stay with the family until the medical examiner or coroner arrives, unless police or paramedics take over and release you from the scene.

Stress Management

Many EMRs expose themselves to a great deal of stress in order to meet the needs of their patients. They feel completely responsible for everything that happens at the scene, even things clearly out of their control. Some become so involved that their self-image is actually based on job performance.

Chronic stress at work, plus emotionally charged emergency environments, can lead to a state of exhaustion and irritability. Beware—that state can markedly decrease your effectiveness. Even some of the very best EMS workers have had to leave the system because of it.

Recognize Warning Signs

One of the best ways to manage chronic stress and prevent burnout is to be aware of the warning signs. The earlier they are spotted, the easier they are to remedy. The warning signs include the following (Figure 2–1):

- Irritability with co-workers, patients, family, and friends

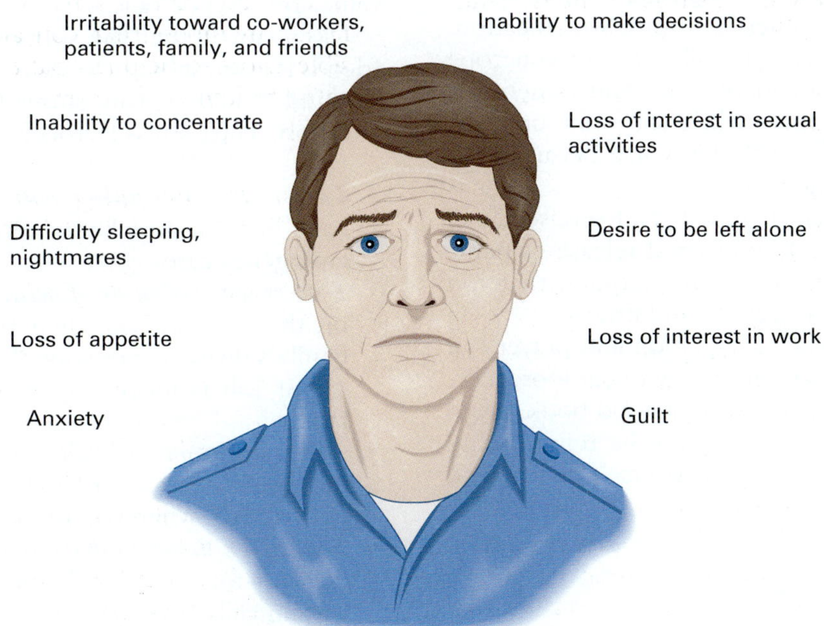

Figure 2–1 The warning signs of stress.

- Inability to concentrate
- Difficulty sleeping or nightmares
- Anxiety
- Inability to make decisions
- Guilt
- Loss of appetite
- Loss of sexual desire
- Self-isolation
- Loss of interest in work

In addition, the following general signs and symptoms have been identified with stress:

- *Cognitive*—confusion, inability to make judgments or decisions, loss of motivation, memory problems, loss of objectivity
- *Psychological*—depression, excessive anger, negativism, hostility, defensiveness, mood swings, feelings of worthlessness
- *Physical*—constant exhaustion, headaches, stomach problems, dizziness, pounding heart
- *Behavioural*—overeating, increased use of drugs or alcohol, grinding teeth, hyperactivity, lack of energy
- *Social*—frequent arguments, decreased ability to relate to patients

Make Lifestyle Changes

Certain lifestyle changes can be helpful in dealing with chronic stress. One change you can make is to your diet. Certain foods, such as sugar, caffeine, and alcohol, aggravate the body's response to stress, so you may want to limit your intake of these. Avoid fatty foods, and eat more low-fat carbohydrates. While at work, eat often but in small amounts.

Avoid alcohol and other kinds of self-medication. Reaching for a drink or pills will not help you cope with stress; in fact, they increase it. And remember, problems will still be there when you wake up from your stupor. They may even be worse because you did not act on them right away.

Exercise more often (Figure 2–2). Exercise has all kinds of benefits, including physical release of pent-up emotions. A long career in EMS requires that you maintain good physical strength and fitness.

Finally, learn to relax. Meditation and prayer can be helpful. You may also want to try to cut loose a little bit: watch a funny movie, read a good book, or go dancing or to a concert. Music can be rejuvenating whether you play an instrument yourself or listen to something you enjoy.

Keep Balance in Your Life

One way to balance work, recreation, health, and family is to assess your priorities. Take a few minutes

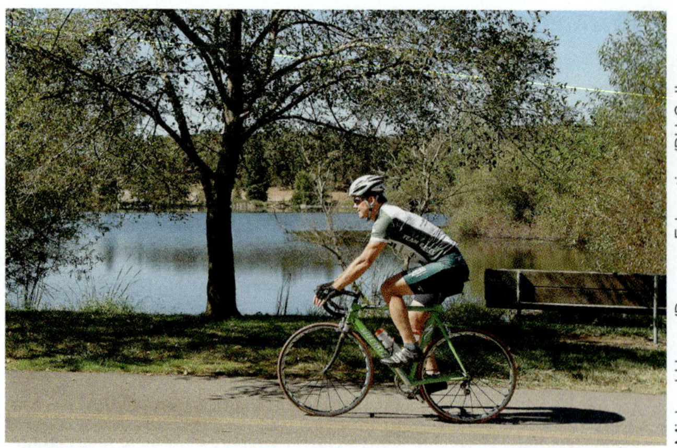

Figure 2–2 As an EMR, you must safeguard your own health.

to list all your activities on paper. Write "1" beside your first priority. Write "2" beside your second, and so on. Then perform them in the order you assigned. If you have a spouse, keep in mind that when your family does not rank high on the list, there may be additional stress created by their feelings of being left out. Your spouse should be your biggest supporter, if you maintain balance.

Be sure to share your worries with someone else. Talk to someone you trust and respect. It can help relieve stress and help you discover alternatives. A good confidante listens well and asks questions that help you explore your ideas honestly.

Still another way to help keep balance in your life is to accept the fact that you will sometimes make mistakes. Admit to yourself that no person is right all the time. Understand that a mistake does not reduce your value. You do not have to be perfect to do a good job.

Remember that the support of your family and friends is essential to helping you manage stress. Keep in mind that they, too, suffer from stress related to your job. Their stress factors include the following:

- *Lack of understanding your job.* Families typically have little, if any, knowledge about pre-hospital emergency care.
- *Fear of separation or of being ignored.* Long hours on the job can take their toll and increase your family's distress over your absences. You may hear, "Your job is more important to you than your family!"
- *Worry about on-call situations.* Stress at home may increase because your family may focus on the danger you face when you respond to emergency calls.
- *Frustrated desire to share your pain.* It may be too difficult for you to talk about what happened on certain calls. Even though your family and friends understand that, they may still feel frustrated by their inability to help and support you.

You can help keep balance in your life by changing your work environment if at all possible. Request work shifts that allow for more time to relax with family and friends. Ask for a rotation of duty to an assignment that is less stressful. Take periodic breaks to exercise and to support and encourage co-workers.

Seek Professional Help

Mental health professionals, social workers, and clergy can help you realize that your reactions are normal. They can also help you mobilize your best coping strategies and suggest more effective ways to deal with stress.

Critical Incident Stress Debriefing (CISD)

A critical incident is any event that causes unusually strong emotions that interfere with your ability to function either during the incident or later. This type of stress requires aggressive and immediate management, including:

- Pre-incident stress education
- On-scene peer support
- One-on-one support
- Disaster support services
- Follow-up services
- Spouse and family support
- Community outreach programs
- Other general health and welfare initiatives, such as wellness programs

In addition, a system has been developed to help rescuers cope with critical incident stress. It is called critical incident stress debriefing (CISD). CISD combines a team of peer counsellors with mental health professionals (Figure 2–3). It is successful because it helps rescuers vent their feelings quickly. The non-threatening environment also encourages rescuers to feel free to air their concerns and reactions.

CISD includes anyone involved in an incident—police, firefighters, EMS personnel, dispatchers, doctors, and so on. In some cases, it may also include their families. After mass casualty incidents, such as earthquakes or explosions, a number of CISD meetings may be needed.

There are two basic CISD techniques: defusing and debriefing.

Defusing

Much shorter and less formal than a debriefing, a defusing is usually held within hours of the critical

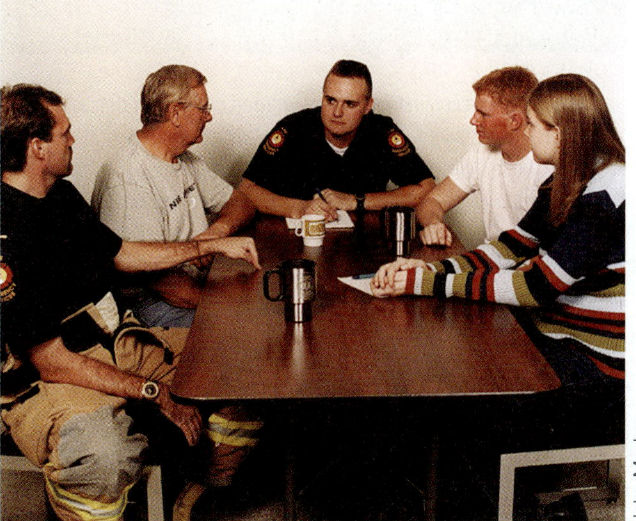

Figure 2–3 The critical incident stress debriefing (CISD) helps rescuers deal with particularly stressful incidents.

incident. It is attended only by those most directly involved and lasts about 30 to 45 minutes. A defusing gives rescuers a chance to vent their feelings and get information they may need before a larger group meets. It may either eliminate the need for a formal debriefing, or it may enhance a later debriefing.

Debriefing

Ideally, a debriefing is held within 24 to 72 hours of a critical incident. It is not an investigation or an interrogation. Everything that is said at a debriefing is confidential. Rescuers are urged to explore any physical, mental, or emotional symptoms they are experiencing. CISD counsellors and mental health professionals then evaluate the information and offer suggestions on how to cope with the stress resulting from the incident.

Accessing CISD

Generally, your agency or organization will organize a CISD. Consider attending if you have been involved in the following:

- Serious injury or death of a rescuer in the line of duty
- Multiple-casualty incident
- Suicide of an emergency worker
- An event that attracts media attention
- Injury or death of someone you know
- Any disaster

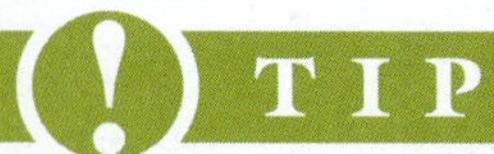

Although long recommended as a preferred method for debriefing after critical incidents, CISD has come under scrutiny in recent years. Those disavowing the approach maintain that it is forced on EMS personnel who may not be ready immediately to talk about calls that affect them. Advocates, however, claim that CISD is a tried-and-true method aimed at relieving emotional pressure. It is up to each individual to decide if or when he or she requires peer support.

Also consider accessing CISD after any event that has an unusual impact on you. That may include an incident in which injury or death of a person was caused by a rescuer, such as when an ambulance collides with a car. The death of a patient, child abuse or neglect, an event that threatens your life, or one that has distressing sights, sounds, or smells may all be cause for accessing CISD. Not addressing the stress that a critical incident can cause may lead to post-traumatic stress disorder (PTSD), which can inhibit your effectiveness at your job and affect you for years.

Ask your instructor about the CISD programs available through your EMS system.

SECTION 2
PREVENTING DISEASE TRANSMISSION

As an EMR, you will come into contact with patients who may have an infectious disease. If you are worried about catching their illness, you are justified.

However, don't despair. The following section will explain how diseases are transmitted and describe the ones of most concern to EMS personnel. It will also outline proven ways for you to protect yourself.

How Diseases Are Transmitted

Diseases are caused by pathogens, which are microorganisms such as bacteria and viruses. An infectious disease is one that spreads from one person to another (Figure 2–4). It can spread *directly* through blood-to-blood contact (blood-borne transmission), contact with open wounds or exposed tissues, and contact with the mucous membranes of the eyes, nose, and mouth. An infectious disease can also spread *indirectly* by way of a contaminated object, such as a needle, or by way of infected droplets breathed into the respiratory tract (airborne transmission).

Some pathogens are transmitted easily, such as the viruses that cause the common cold. Others need specific routes of transmission. The tuberculosis bacterium, for example, is transmitted by droplets from the cough or sneeze of an infected patient. Poor nutrition, poor hygiene, crowded or unsanitary living conditions, and stress make infection from any disease more likely.

In order to protect yourself, you must *always* make use of the appropriate personal protective equipment (PPE). That includes using a barrier device, such as a pocket face mask, *every time* you ventilate a patient (Figure 2–5). Make sure the ventilating device has a one-way valve that prevents fluid from backing up.

Diseases of Concern

As an EMR, you may be exposed to infectious diseases whenever you treat a patient. Outbreaks of

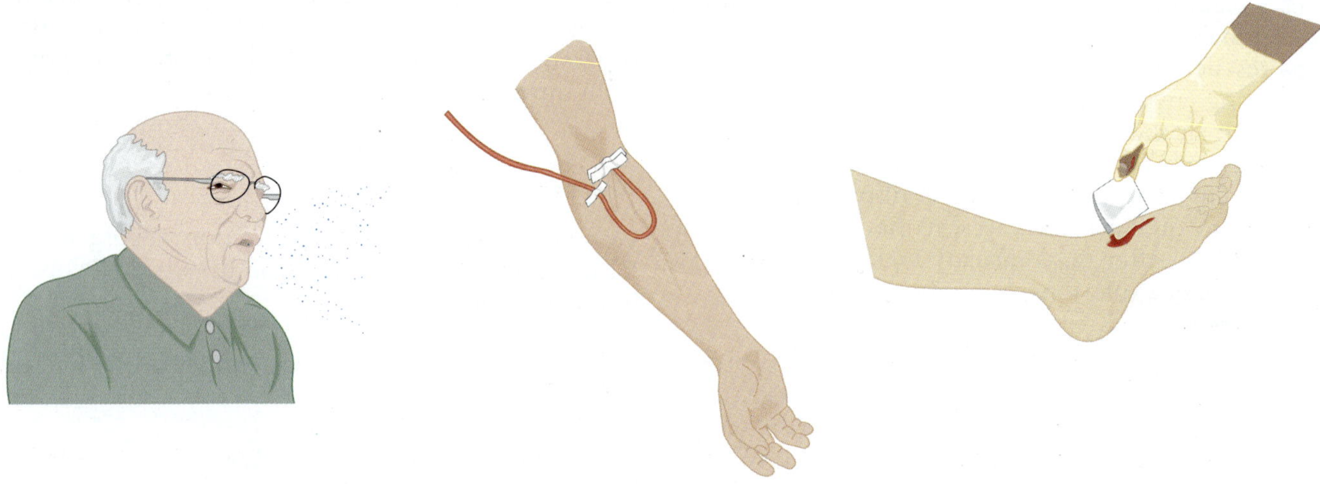

Figure 2–4 How infectious diseases can spread.

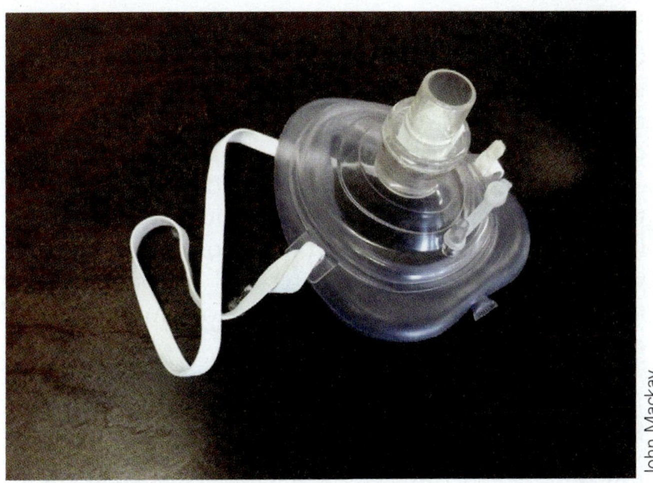

Figure 2–5 A pocket face mask with one-way valve and carrying case.

severe acute respiratory syndrome (SARS), Asian flu, influenza, meningitis, and necrotizing fasciitis (flesh-eating disease) have all been seen in Canada. The three diseases that have historically presented the most ongoing concern are described below.

Hepatitis B and C

Hepatitis B virus (HBV) is a virus that directly affects the liver. It can cause hepatitis B, a serious disease that can last for months. Hepatitis B (hep B) is contracted through blood and body fluids. A major source of the virus is the "chronic carrier." This person can carry the virus for years. He or she usually has no signs or symptoms and is often unaware of being ill. When signs and symptoms do appear, they may include the following:

- Fatigue
- Nausea
- Loss of appetite
- Abdominal pain
- Headache
- Fever
- Yellowish colour of the skin and whites of the eyes

If you suspect that you have been exposed to HBV, report the incident to your supervisor. Immediately contact a physician or your local public health agency for care, which may include an injection of hepatitis B immunoglobulin (HBIG). HBIG is a preparation containing antibodies that attack the HBV. You may also receive a hep B vaccination if you have not already had one.

Hep C is similar to hep B, but can cause liver failure. There is neither a vaccine nor a cure for hep C.

Note that the most effective way to deal with hepatitis is prevention. Medical authorities strongly recommend getting the hep B vaccine.

Tuberculosis

Tuberculosis (TB) was at one time nearly eradicated, but it is back. In fact, researchers are worried because new drug-resistant strains are developing. The pathogen that causes TB is found in the lungs and other tissues of the infected patient. You can be infected from droplets in a patient's cough or from infected sputum. The main signs and symptoms of TB include the following:

- Fever
- Cough
- Night sweats
- Weight loss

The Canadian Centre for Occupational Health and Safety (CCOHS) recommends all isolation precautions when treating a patient with TB, including a protective respiratory device (Figure 2–6) and negative ventilation of an enclosed space to the outside. Masks should be supplemented with protective eyewear. Employ universal precautions whenever you suspect TB, and use approved artificial respiration equipment that can be properly cleaned or discarded after use.

Acquired Immune Deficiency Syndrome (AIDS)

Simply stated, the human immunodeficiency virus (HIV) knocks out the body's ability to fight infection. HIV infection leads to acquired immune deficiency syndrome (AIDS). People with AIDS get infections caused by viruses, bacteria, fungi, and parasites. These are serious illnesses that do not occur (or occur only mildly) among people with healthy

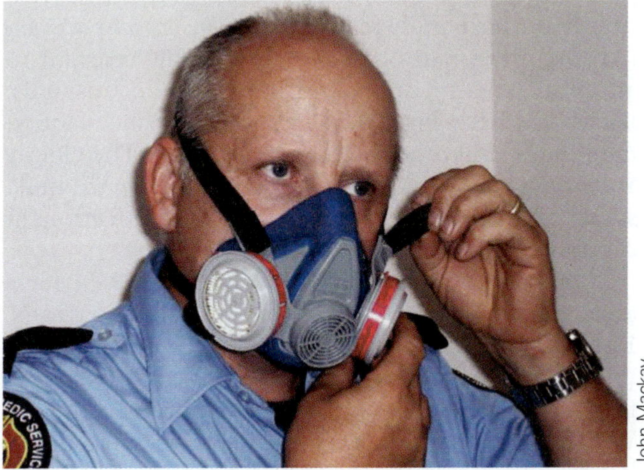

Figure 2-6 An appropriate respirator mask should be worn when you suspect a patient of having a respiratory infection. An N-95 mask should be properly fitted and retested annually.

immune systems. These illnesses involve many organs of the body, causing a wide array of signs and symptoms. Fortunately, AIDS is not spread through casual contact. It cannot be spread by touching intact skin, coughing, sneezing, sharing eating utensils, or other indirect ways. *Transmission requires intimate contact with the body fluids of infected persons.* Infection may occur through the following:

- Sexual contact involving the exchange of semen, saliva, blood, urine, or feces
- Infected needles
- Infected blood or blood products
- Mother-to-child transmission during pregnancy, birth, or breastfeeding

Not everyone infected with HIV develops AIDS. However, people who carry HIV are still able to spread the infection to others. So, because any patient could be infected with HIV, or any other disease, follow all the precautions described below at all times and with all patients.

Other Diseases of Concern

SARS gained notoriety in 2003 when approximately 8000 people contracted the virus that causes it. Of those victims, slightly less than 10 percent died. SARS is spread by body fluids and droplets, and symptoms can include high fever, headache, body aches, diarrhea, dry cough, and often pneumonia.

Other diseases spread by viruses or bacteria found in oral and nasal droplets or body secretions include meningitis, pneumonia, influenza, and whooping cough (pertussis).

Staphylococcal (staph) skin infections are acquired by contact with open wounds, sores, or contaminated objects. Methicillin-resistant *Staphylococcus aureus* (MRSA) is a strain of staph that is highly resistant to antibiotic treatment. Found frequently in hospitals, it has also been known to lurk in ambulances, nursing homes, and other health care facilities. The elderly and those with weakened immune systems are most susceptible to the skin, tissue, and lung infections it can cause.

Vancomycin-resistant *Enterococci* (VRE) have also achieved notoriety in health care settings. Enterococcus is a bacterium that lives in the digestive tract of most humans. It is transmitted from hand to hand and by contact with contaminated surfaces. While this bacterium can live in and on our bodies, it only becomes a concern when it infects the bloodstream through a wound or sore. Some strains of Enterococci have developed resistance to antibiotics and can therefore pose a serious problem for a person who is already combating an illness or injury.

Necrotizing fasciitis, or flesh-eating disease, is a rare but well-known disease that is most commonly caused by *Streptococcus pyogenes,* which also causes other infections such as strep throat. Flesh-eating disease can also be caused by other bacteria, including staph.

Clostridium difficile, or C. diff, is a bacterium that is found virtually everywhere and can be acquired in a health care setting. C. diff becomes problematic when it flourishes in the intestinal tracts of people taking antibiotics. Diarrhea and serious inflammation of the colon can result.

Body Substance Isolation

For many years, guidelines have required EMS personnel to take steps to protect themselves against diseases transmitted through blood. This is known as taking universal precautions. Health Canada and the Laboratory Centre for Disease Control (LCDC) have published guidelines that set a new standard. That standard requires the responder to assume that all blood and body fluids are infectious. EMS personnel must practise a strict form of infection control with all patients. This is called **body substance isolation (BSI)**. With BSI precautions, it is possible to take care of all patients safely, even those with infectious diseases. BSI precautions include handwashing; proper cleaning, disinfection, or sterilization of equipment; and use of PPE.

Handwashing

Handwashing is the single most important thing you can do to prevent the spread of infection. Most contaminants can be removed from the skin with 10 to 15 seconds of vigorous lathering and scrubbing with plain soap.

Always wash your hands after caring for a patient, *even if you were wearing gloves.* For maximum protection, begin by removing all jewellery from your hands and arms. Then lather up and rub together all surfaces of your hands. Pay attention to creases, crevices, and the areas between your fingers. Use a brush to scrub under and around your fingernails (Figure 2–7a). It is a good idea for you to keep your nails short and unpainted. If your hands are visibly soiled, spend more time washing them. Wash your wrists and forearms as well. Rinse thoroughly under a stream of water and dry well. Use a disposable towel if possible.

If you do not have access to soap and running water, you can use a foam or liquid washing agent. As soon as you can, wash your hands again using the procedure described above. Anti-microbial hand lotions will destroy over 99 percent of microorganisms and

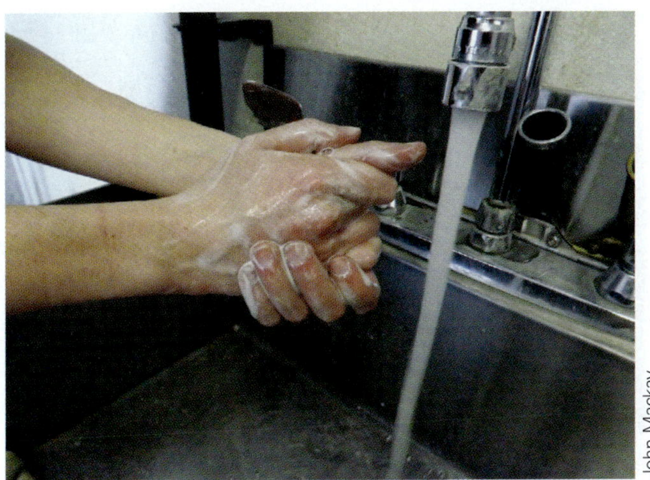

Figure 2–7a The first line of protection against infectious disease is handwashing.

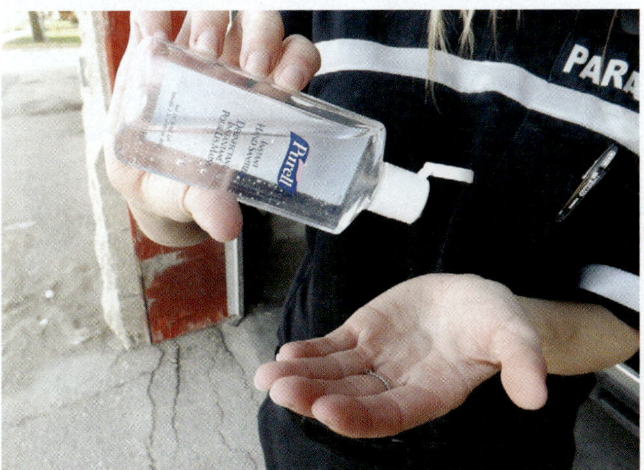

Figure 2–7b Anti-microbial hand lotion can offer extended protection.

continue to offer protection for four to six hours after application. Portable dispensing pumps may be offered to patients for use as well when appropriate (Figure 2–7b). Anti-microbial hand lotions, in effect, offer an invisible barrier of protection before personal protective equipment is used.

Cleaning Equipment

Cleaning, *disinfecting*, and *sterilizing* are related terms. Cleaning is simply the process of washing a soiled object with soap and water. Disinfecting is cleaning plus the use of a chemical, either alcohol or bleach, to kill many of the microorganisms on an object. Sterilizing is a process in which a chemical or other substance, such as superheated steam, kills all the microorganisms on an object.

Generally, disinfecting is used for items that come into contact with the patient's intact skin. Items that come into contact with open wounds or mucous membranes should be sterilized.

Whenever possible, use disposable equipment. *Never reuse disposable items.* Instead, place them in a plastic bag that is clearly labelled "infectious waste" (Figure 2–8). Then seal the bag. Disposable items used with patients who have HBV or HIV should be double bagged.

After each use, clean non-disposable equipment. Wash off all blood, mucus, tissue, and other residue. Be sure to wear a good pair of utility gloves and other appropriate PPE while doing so. Then disinfect or sterilize the equipment as per local protocols.

Wash the items that do not normally touch the patient. Rinse them with clear water and dry thoroughly. Clean the walls or window coverings in an ambulance or rescue vehicle when they get soiled. Then use a hospital-grade disinfectant or a solution of household bleach and water to clean up any blood or body fluids.

Writing utensils, clipboards, computers, and radios may become contaminated if you have used them while wearing exposed personal protective

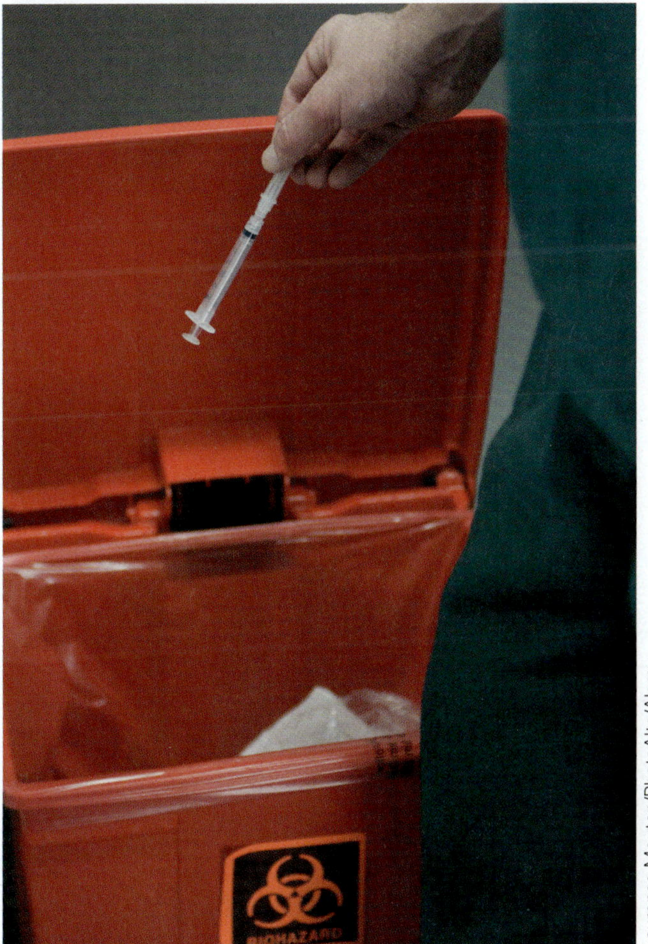

Figure 2–8 Be sure to discard contaminated items properly.

equipment. Remove dirty gloves before using such items and don clean ones again before touching the patient. Your vehicle's interior seats, handles, radios, and medical bags should also be cleaned as necessary.

If your clothes get soiled with body fluids, remove, bag, and label them. Wash them in hot, soapy water for at least 25 minutes. Then, if possible, take a shower and rinse thoroughly.

Personal Protective Equipment (PPE)

Always use PPE as a barrier against infection. Such items will keep you from coming into contact with a patient's blood or body fluids. PPE includes eye protection, gloves, gowns, and masks (Figure 2–9):

- *Eye protection.* Use eye shields to prevent blood and body fluids from splashing into your eyes. Several types are available. Clear plastic shields cover the eyes or the whole face. Safety glasses have side shields. If you wear prescription glasses, attach removable side shields. Form-fitting goggles are also available, but are not required.
- *Gloves* (Figure 2-10). Wear high-quality vinyl or latex gloves whenever you care for a patient. Never

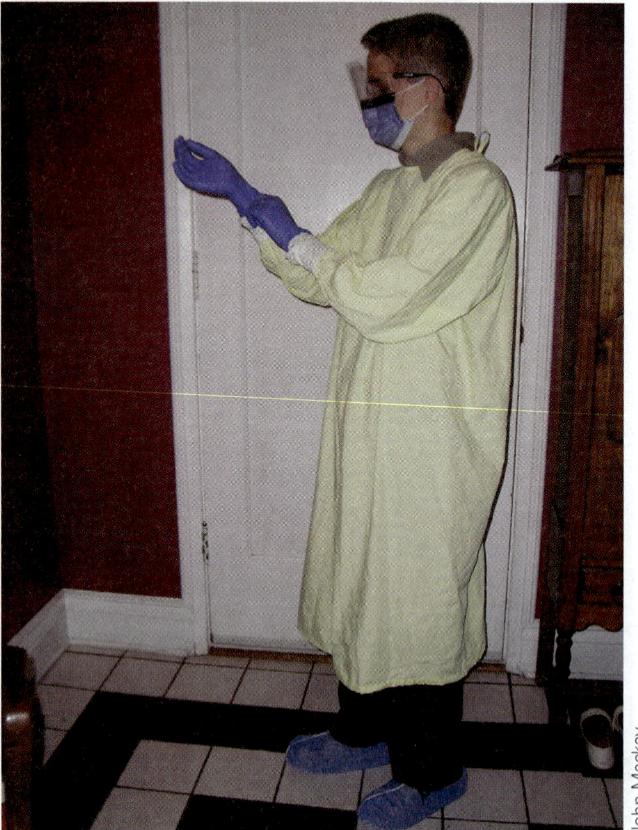

Figure 2–9 Personal protective equipment (PPE) includes safety glasses or goggles, face mask or shield, gown or apron, gloves, cap, and shoe coverings.

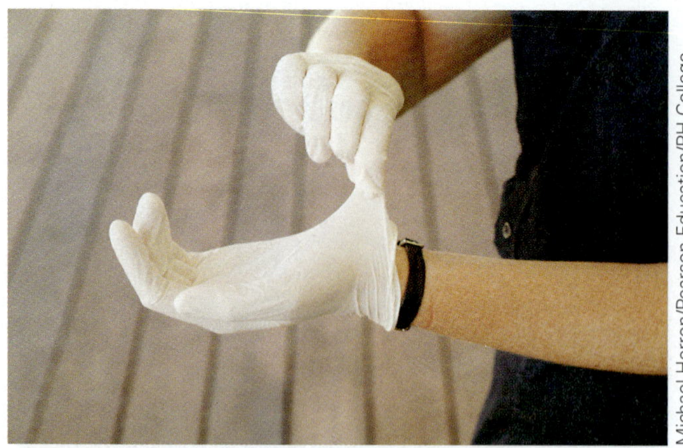

Figure 2–10a Wear protective gloves whenever you care for a patient.

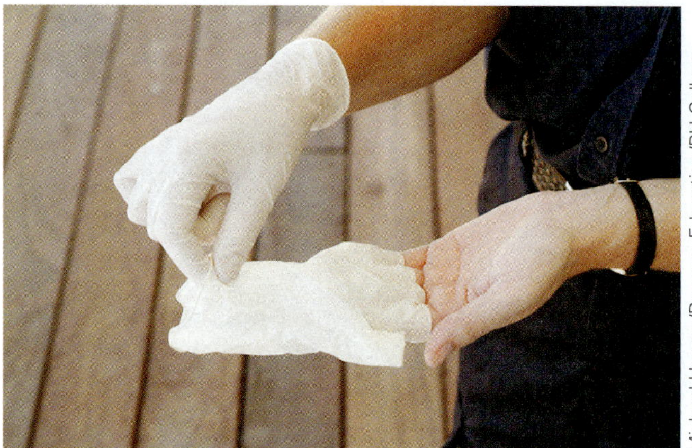

Figure 2–10b Never touch the contaminated outer side of gloves when removing them prior to handwashing.

reuse them. Put on a new pair for each patient to avoid exposing one patient to another's infection. Soiled gloves must be replaced as soon as it is practical to do so. If a glove tears accidentally, remove it as soon as you can do so safely. Then wash your hands and replace the torn glove with a new one. If disposable medical gloves are unavailable, you can improvise with the use of rubber dishwashing gloves, leather work gloves, or plastic bags. These substitutes decrease your dexterity, but offer a barrier for personal protection.
- *Gowns.* Wear a gown when there might be significant splashing of blood or body fluids. Generally, you will need a gown during childbirth or treatment of a major injury. Whenever possible, use a disposable gown. It is also recommended that you change your clothes if the gown gets soiled.
- *Masks.* Wear a disposable, surgical-type face mask to protect yourself against possible splatter of blood or body fluids. Eye protection is recommended for use while dealing with suspected TB patients.

Use PPE yourself and be sure to remind other EMS personnel at the scene to wear it. Make gloves and other PPE available to others who arrive to help. When PPE is contaminated during a call, make every reasonable effort to change the soiled items. This will help prevent **cross contamination**, in which disease or infection can be transferred by a responder wearing exposed equipment for a prolonged period of time.

Another approach to consider for personal protection is to use reverse isolation techniques with the patient. An immune-compromised patient is already ill or very susceptible to catching a disease from others. These patients can use PPE in order to prevent contamination from the environment or persons attending to them. When a patient wears a protective mask or is covered in a sheet that is not fluid permeable, this barrier can provide protection to both the patient and the EMR who is attending to them.

Immunizations

Before you start active duty, have a physician make sure you are adequately protected against common infectious diseases. The following immunizations are recommended for active duty EMRs:

- Tetanus prophylaxis (every 10 years)
- Hepatitis B vaccine
- Influenza vaccine (every year)
- Polio vaccine
- Measles, mumps, rubella (MMR) vaccine

Because some immunizations offer only partial protection, have your physician verify your immune status against measles, mumps, and rubella. Remember, *always* practise BSI precautions—even after being vaccinated.

Have a tuberculin tine test done at least once every year while you are on duty. It will tell you if you have been exposed to TB. Your agency's Occupational Health and Safety representative or your physician can advise you about what to do if you have been exposed.

Reporting Exposures

In general, report any suspected exposure to blood or body fluids. Report the incident as soon as possible to your supervisor and to medical control. Report the exposure especially if the patient is HIV positive, has hepatitis B or C, or is in a high-risk category for infection. Include in your report the date and time of the suspected exposure, the type and amount of body fluid involved, the precautions you were using, and details of the incident. Exposure report forms should be provided by your organization. Occupational Health and

Safety personnel, the Workers' Compensation Board (WCB), and department management will all play a role in any follow-up that needs to take place subsequent to an exposure. As an EMR, you need to be a good custodian of your own health care and make sure your incident receives all necessary attention. Several provinces are attempting to legislate a Blood Samples Act that would compel patients who may have infected emergency workers to provide blood samples for disease analysis. Provincial laws vary. Be sure to follow all local protocols.

SECTION 3
SCENE SAFETY

Be very sure to protect yourself at scenes involving hazardous materials (HazMat), car crashes, or violence (Figure 2–11). It is imperative that you do not fall victim to the same problems that affect your patients.

As you approach a scene, turn off your lights and siren to avoid broadcasting your arrival. Take a good look at the neighbourhood. If possible, do not park directly in front of the call address. This is so you can assess the scene unnoticed and save a place for an ambulance to park.

Then decide whether it is safe to approach the patient. If any of the following exist on the scene, you may need to call for help:

- Motor vehicle or airplane crashes
- Presence of toxic substances or low levels of oxygen
- Crime scenes
- Presence of a weapon of any kind
- Possible drug or alcohol use
- Arguing, threats, violent behaviour, broken glass, overturned furniture
- Unstable surfaces, such as water and ice

While each emergency scene is unique, a general rule applies to all. *If the scene is unsafe, make it safe before you enter.* Otherwise, wait for help to arrive. Specialized personnel will have the training, equipment, and protective gear needed to enter an unstable scene safely. Chapters 30 through 34 address many other environments and situations that you may encounter.

Once a scene is secure, take measures to protect the patient from hazards. These include fire, structural instability, gasoline leaks, chemical spills, oncoming traffic, and extremes in temperature. Bystanders should also be protected from illness and injury.

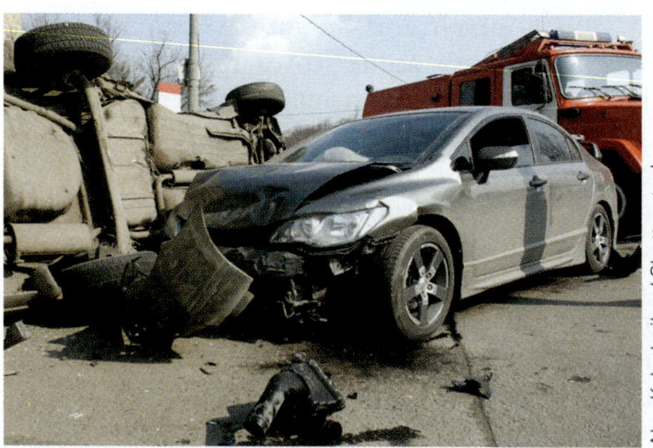

Hazardous materials.

Motor vehicle crash.

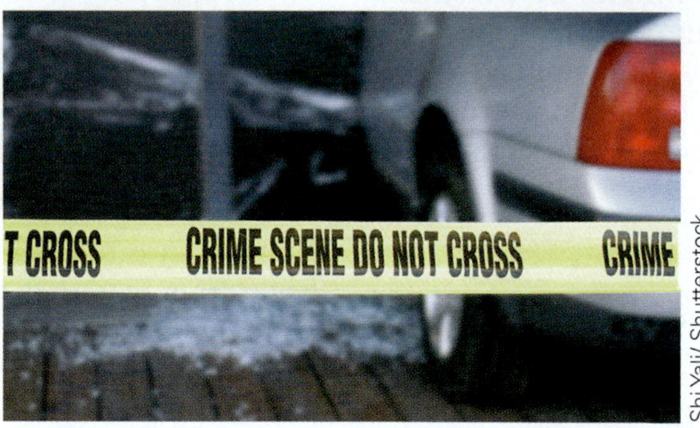

Crime scene.

Figure 2–11 Always be alert to potential hazards as you approach an emergency scene.

Hazardous Materials

Do not enter a scene involving hazardous materials. Call a specialized team of rescuers to secure the scene first. Provide emergency care only after the scene is safe and patient contamination is limited. In general, rescuers should wear protective clothing, such as a self-contained breathing apparatus (SCBA) (Figure 2–12) and a HazMat suit (Figure 2–13). Check with your instructor about the availability of training for HazMat situations. Also, learn how to access your local HazMat team. (Hazardous materials are discussed in more detail in Chapter 30.)

Motor Vehicle Crashes

Some car crashes lead to situations that threaten the lives of both patients and rescuers. Examples of such life-threatening situations are:

- Downed power lines or other potential sources of electrocution
- Fire or the potential for fire, such as leaking gasoline
- Explosion or the potential for explosion
- Hazardous materials
- Oncoming traffic

When there is life-threatening danger on the scene, call for specially trained personnel before you

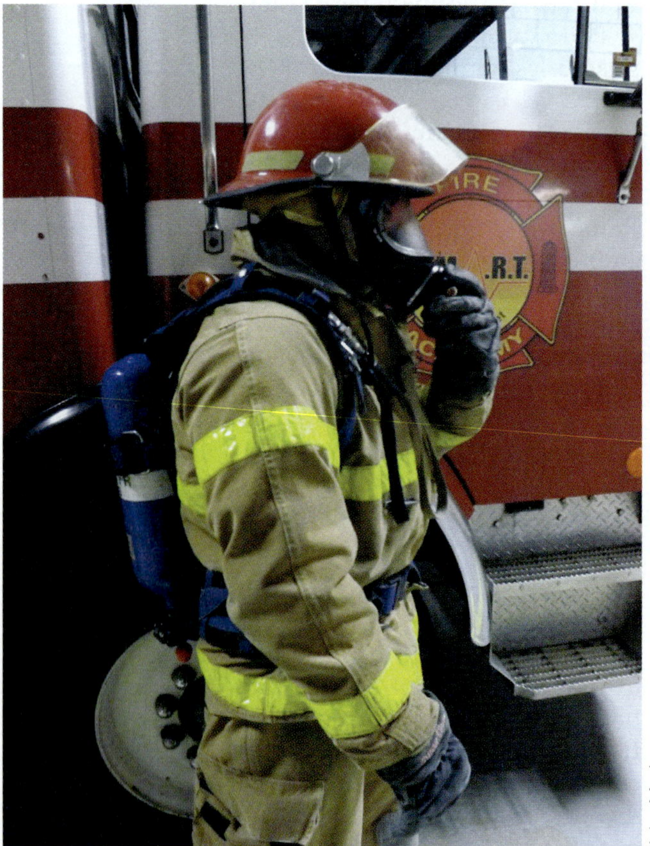

Figure 2–12 Self-contained breathing apparatus (SCBA).

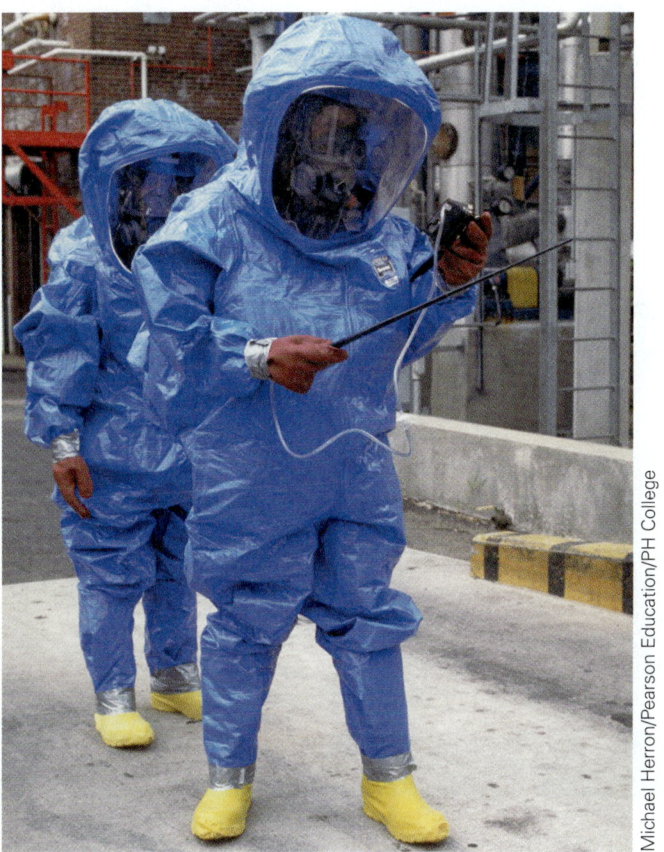

Figure 2–13 Typical hazardous materials (HazMat) protective suit.

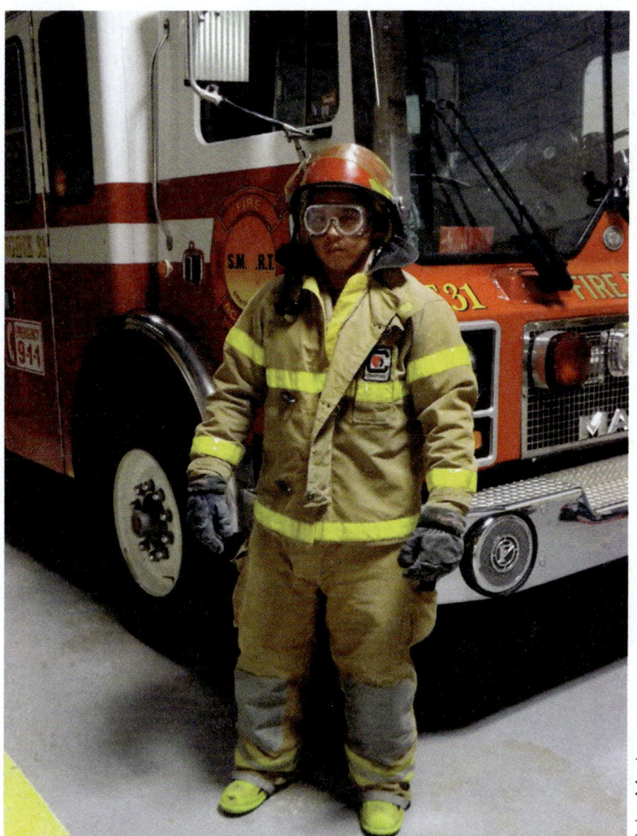

Figure 2–14 Turnout gear, plus helmet, eyewear, puncture-proof gloves, and boots.

enter it. Also, call for special teams when a complex or extensive rescue is needed. Once a scene is safe, make sure you are wearing the proper PPE before you enter the scene. The equipment may include turnout gear, puncture-proof gloves, helmet, and eye protection (Figure 2–14). Follow local protocols.

Many traffic accidents occur in the dark or in bad weather. Therefore, be sure to wear reflective clothing. Depending on the scene, you might also consider waterproof boots and slip-resistant gloves in wet weather. Wear gloves, a warm hat, and long underwear in cold weather. An impact-resistant helmet with reflective tape and a chin strap is also useful to protect against falling debris.

Violence

You may face unexpected violence from a patient, bystander, or the perpetrator of a crime. If you suspect potential violence, *call law enforcement before you enter the scene.* Never enter the scene to give patient care until it has been adequately controlled by the police. (Chapter 10 briefly discusses some additional principles for safely entering a potentially violent scene.)

Always call for law enforcement in cases of domestic disputes, street or gang fights, bar fights, or potential suicide. Call them for any type of crime scene and for scenes that involve angry family or bystanders.

No matter where you work, consider using body armour (Figure 2–15). It is made of Kevlar or other synthetic materials that resist penetration by bullets. The amount of protection the armour offers depends on the tightness of the weave and the number of layers. Contemporary designs can also reduce knife or shank

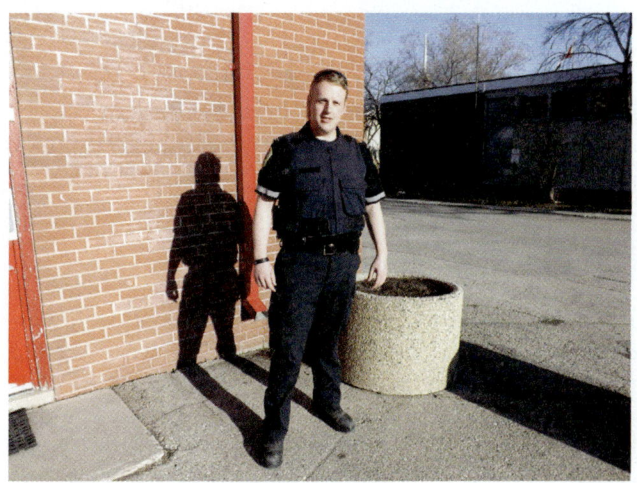

Figure 2-15 Body armour.

penetration. Although it will protect you, body armour will not make you invincible. You are still vulnerable in the areas that are not covered. You can still be killed by the blunt force of a bullet even if it does not penetrate the armour. Never take chances you normally would avoid just because you are wearing armour.

If you need to treat patients at a crime scene, you must preserve the evidence needed for investigation and prosecution. A general rule is to avoid disturbing the scene unless absolutely necessary for medical care. Preservation of evidence will be discussed further in Chapter 3.

EMR FOCUS

Television has led us to believe that it is okay to rush into calls without regard for our own well-being. This is not true. TV is not real life. The fact is that if you become ill or injured, you will not be able to help your patient.

One of the most important factors to be considered within the first 10 minutes of a call is your own personal safety. Practise BSI precautions on every call.

Always remain alert for violence, hazardous materials, and other unsafe conditions.

It is understandable that all you want to do so early in your career is to focus on information about illness and injury. However, do not underestimate the importance of the information in this chapter. Just to make sure you realize how important it is, there will be reminders in every chapter of this book.

CASE STUDY FOLLOW-UP

At the beginning of this chapter, you read that EMRs were at a violent and potentially dangerous scene. To see how the chapter skills apply to this emergency, read the following. It describes how the call was completed.

SCENE ASSESSMENT *(Continued)*

My partner and I looked at each other. We returned to our vehicle and immediately called the police. I'm glad we did because otherwise we would have been right in the middle of a fight.

We moved our vehicle out of sight and waited. When the police arrived, we reported what we knew, and they went in. After a few minutes, they radioed to tell us the scene was secure. We still approached it very cautiously.

The officers told us that two brothers had been in a fist fight. One of the brothers said his hands went through a window. Both brothers appeared to be intoxicated.

PRIMARY ASSESSMENT

After we put on eye protection and gloves, we introduced ourselves to Mike, the brother who needed medical help. He seemed calm. Mike had moderate bleeding from his right forearm. His airway and breathing were good. He denied any other injuries or falls.

SECONDARY ASSESSMENT

Even though Mike denied other injuries, we decided to do a physical exam anyway. Sometimes people get into fights and get so excited that they don't know they're hurt. Since there were two of us, my partner controlled the bleeding while I checked Mike's head, neck, chest, abdomen, and extremities.

While we were waiting for an ambulance, Mike's brother became loud and abusive to the police. We had the patient walk outside with us to get away from the potential danger. Then we checked his pulse and respirations.

PATIENT HISTORY

Mike admitted to drinking six or eight cans of beer before the fight started. He told us that he had asthma but wasn't feeling any respiratory distress or problems. He owned an asthma inhaler but didn't have it with him then. He continued to deny any injuries other than the cut to his forearm.

ONGOING ASSESSMENT

We checked Mike's airway and breathing. They were okay. Mike didn't have any changes in mental status. The bleeding was controlled and the bandages were secure. We didn't get to recheck the vitals before the ambulance arrived.

TRANSFER OF CARE

We advised the paramedics as follows:

"The patient's name is Mike. He's a 22-year-old male who has sustained a laceration to his right forearm from it going through a window. The wound has been dressed and bandaged. The bleeding was moderate and was easily controlled. Mike had been drinking but has been alert and oriented throughout the call. His airway and breathing are good. He denies any other injuries. He has a history of asthma and uses an inhaler. The secondary assessment was negative for injuries anywhere other than his arm. His pulse is 88, strong, and regular. His respirations are 18 and adequate. We were about to recheck his vitals as you pulled up."

> Your safety and well-being are your top priorities. Without them, you cannot be an effective EMR. Throughout this textbook, you will find reminders about taking BSI and other safety precautions. Take note of them.

NOCPs

2.4 c Recognize and react appropriately to persons exhibiting emotional reactions **A**

 f Exhibit diplomacy, tact, and discretion **S**

3.1 a Maintain balance in personal lifestyle **X**

 b Develop and maintain an appropriate support system **X**

 c Manage personal stress **X**

 d Practise effective strategies to improve physical and mental health related to career **X**

 e Exhibit physical strength and fitness consistent with the requirements of professional practice **S**

3.3 b Address potential occupational hazards **S**

 f Practise infection control techniques **S**

 g Clean and disinfect equipment **S**

 h Clean and disinfect work environment **A**

6.1 m Provide care to patient experiencing terminal illness **S**

8.1 c Work collaboratively with other members of the health care community **A**

REVIEW QUESTIONS

Page references where answers may be found or supported are provided at the end of each question.

SECTION 1

1. What are the four techniques you can use to avoid such responses as nausea or fainting in an emergency situation? (p. 11)

2. What are the five stages of the grieving process? (pp. 11–12)

3. In addition to providing medical care, what can you do to help a dying patient? (pp. 12–13)

4. What are five signs of chronic stress and burnout? (pp. 13–14)

5. What are some of the negative feelings an EMR's family may have about the EMR's job? (p. 14)

6. Give three examples of situations that may cause stress during critical incidents. (p. 15)

7. What is critical incident stress debriefing (CISD)? (p. 15)

8. How does debriefing differ from defusing? (p. 15)

SECTION 2

9. How does an infectious disease spread from person to person? (p. 16)

10. What are the differences between cleaning, disinfecting, and sterilizing? (p. 19)

11. What equipment is needed to take BSI precautions? (pp. 20–21)

12. List five immunizations that should be kept up to date by an EMR. (p. 21)

SECTION 3

13. What rule applies to all unsafe emergency scenes? (p. 21)

3

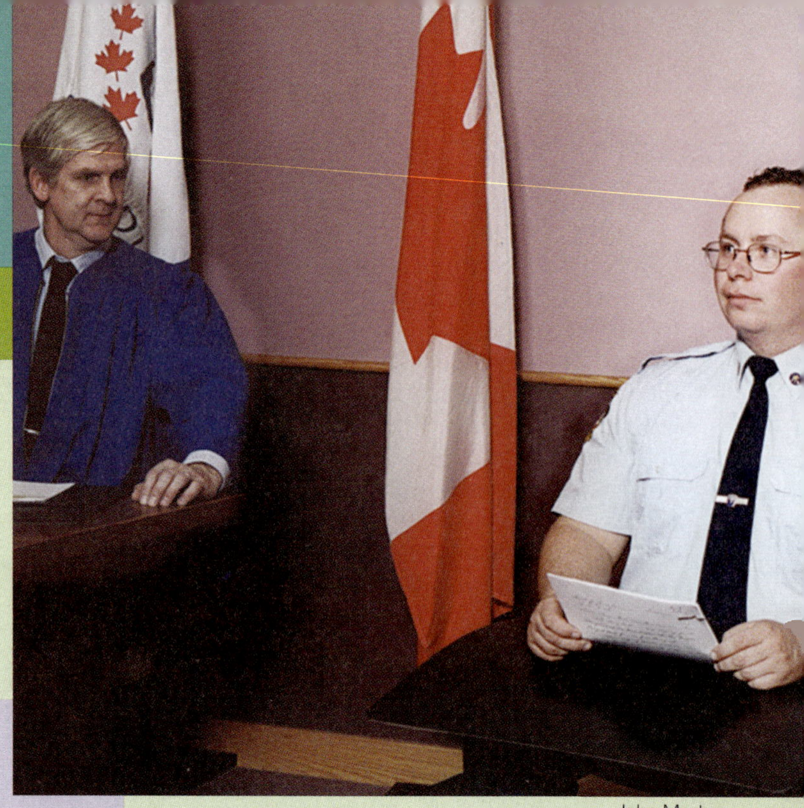

John Mackay

Legal and Ethical Issues

OBJECTIVES

1. Define the EMR scope of practice as it relates to patient consent, treatment of minors, patient transport, and do not resuscitate orders.

2. Discuss the legal issues that pertain to the EMR's duties.

3. List the actions that an EMR should take to assist in the preservation of a crime scene, and state at what point police involvement is necessary.

4. Discuss issues concerning the fundamental components of special documentation.

INTRODUCTION

Legal and ethical issues must be clearly understood by the EMR because they apply both on and off duty. You may already have some questions. For example, should you stop to treat an accident victim when you are off duty? Should patient information be released to a lawyer over the phone? May a child be treated without a parent's or guardian's consent?

This chapter will help you answer these questions. It will describe your scope of practice and what it means to have a duty to act. It will define patient consent and explain advance directives. It will also give you an overview of various other legal issues that will affect you in the field.

SECTION 1
SCOPE OF PRACTICE

Emergency care has changed a lot since its early days. One improvement has been in the quality of EMS training. People have come to expect a competent EMR—one who understands and accepts his or her responsibilities to patients and to the public.

Legal Duties

Each province defines an EMR's scope of practice, or actions that are legally allowed. All EMRs are to provide for the well-being of their patients as outlined in their scope of practice. For example, providing CPR when needed is within your scope of practice. However, stitching up a deep wound is not. Therefore, for you, it is illegal.

Provincial law is enhanced by your local medical director. In fact, your legal right to act as an EMR depends on medical control. Provincial law is further enhanced by the EMR National Curriculum established by PAC and HRDC.

When providing medical care, you should do the following:

- Follow **standing orders** and protocols as approved by the medical director.
- Consult a medical director via phone or radio any time there is a question about the scope of practice.
- Communicate clearly and completely with the medical director.
- Follow the orders the medical director gives.

Ethical Responsibilities

A code of ethics is a list of rules for ideal conduct. Basically, if you place the welfare of a patient above all else during emergency care, you will rarely do anything unethical.

Your ethical responsibilities are as follows:

- Make the physical and emotional needs of the patient a priority. Serve those needs with respect for human dignity and with no regard to nationality, race, gender, creed, or status.
- Practise your skills to the point of mastery. Show respect for the competence of other medical workers.
- Continue your education and take refresher courses. Stay on top of changes in EMS. Help define and uphold professional standards.
- Critically review your performance. Seek ways to improve response time, patient outcome, and communication.
- Report with honesty. Hold in confidence all information obtained in the course of your work unless required by law to share it.
- Work in harmony with other EMRs, paramedics, and other members of the health care team.

SECTION 2
PATIENT CONSENT AND REFUSAL

Patient Competence

A competent adult is one who is lucid and able to make an informed decision about medical care. He or she understands your questions and understands the implications of decisions made about medical care. A patient must be competent in order to legitimately refuse treatment. Therefore, you must determine competence in every adult you need to treat.

CASE STUDY

Dispatch

Our EMR unit was dispatched to a child who had fallen. I remember thinking how calls involving kids bother me. I hoped we could help this child.

Scene Assessment

We arrived to find the patient sitting up and crying. It appeared that he had fallen from his bike when it hit a tree. The bike's front tire was flat, the front end was bent in, and there were several yards of obvious skid marks. The patient had been wearing a helmet.

A police officer was kneeling and quietly talking to the boy. The officer motioned us to approach. He said, "A dog jumped onto the path. Amar did his best to avoid hitting it, but then that darn tree got in the way."

We introduced ourselves to the patient. He said he was nine years old. While my partner began a primary assessment, I spoke to the police officer to see if contact had been made with the boy's parents.

> Why are they looking for the child's parents? Can't they just treat the child's injuries? These questions revolve around the issue of consent, one of many legal and ethical issues you will face as an EMR. As you read Chapter 3, consider how you might answer these questions.

Generally, consider an adult incompetent if he or she fulfills any of the following criteria:

- Is under the influence of alcohol or drugs
- Has an altered mental status
- Has a serious illness or injury that could affect judgment
- Has a mental illness or has an intellectual disability

Patient Consent

By law, you must get a patient's consent, or permission, before you can provide emergency care. In order for that consent to be valid, the patient must be competent and the consent must be informed. It is your responsibility, therefore, to fully explain the care you plan to give as well as the related risks.

There are two general types of consent: **expressed consent** and **implied consent.**

Expressed Consent

Expressed consent may consist of verbal consent, a nod, or an affirming gesture from a competent adult. To get it, you must explain your plan for emergency care *in terms that the patient can understand.* Be sure to also include the risks. In other words, the patient needs a clear idea of all the factors that would affect a reasonable person's decision to either accept or refuse treatment.

You must get a conscious, competent adult's expressed consent before you render treatment. To do so, first tell the patient who you are. Identify your level of training and then carefully explain your plan for emergency care. Make sure you identify both the benefits and the risks. To be sure the patient understands, question him or her briefly.

Implied Consent

In an emergency when an unconscious patient is at risk of death, disability, or deterioration of condition, the law assumes that he or she would agree to care. This is called implied consent. It applies when you assume that a patient who cannot consent to life-saving care would do so if he or she were able to.

Implied consent also applies to a patient who refuses care but who then becomes unconscious and to a patient who is not competent to refuse care.

Minors and Incompetent Adults

Depending on provincial law, a **minor** is usually any person under the age of 18 years. A parent or legal guardian must give consent before you can treat a minor. The same is true for an incompetent adult. However, if a life-threatening condition exists and the parent or guardian is not available, provide emergency care under the principle of implied consent.

An **emancipated minor** is one who is married, pregnant, a parent, a member of the armed forces, or financially independent and living away from home with the permission of the court. You do not need the consent of a parent or legal guardian to treat this patient. You only need the patient's consent.

Advance Directives

An **advance directive**, advance care plan, or health care directive (HCD) is written in advance of an emergency. Such directives express a patient's desire regarding the rendering or withholding of treat-ment options. It must be signed by the patient. A "living will" or a **do not resuscitate (DNR) order** is a doctor- and family-mediated form (Figure 3–1). It documents the wish of the chronically or terminally ill patient not to be resuscitated. It allows the EMR to legally withhold resuscitation.

There may be a time when you are called to treat a terminally ill patient. The patient may ask you to let him or her die if his or her heart or lungs stop working. Legally, if the patient is competent, he or she has the right to make this request.

When you are given an advance directive, you must determine to the best of your ability if it is valid. Usually,

---

PREHOSPITAL DO NOT RESUSCITATE ORDERS

<u>ATTENDING PHYSICIAN</u>

In completing this prehospital DNR form, please check Part A if no intervention by pre-hospital personnel is indicated. Please check Part A and options from Part B if specific interventions by prehospital personnel are indicated. To give a valid prehospital DNR order, this form must be completed by the patient's attending physician and must be provided to prehospital personnel.

A) ______________**Do Not Resuscitate (DNR):**
No Cardiopulmonary Resuscitation or Advanced Cardiac Life Support may be performed by prehospital personnel

B) ______________**Modified Support:**
Prehospital personnel may administer the following checked options:
______________Oxygen administration
______________Full airway support: intubation, airways, bag/valve/mask
______________Venipuncture: IV crystalloids and/or blood draw
______________External cardiac pacing
______________Cardiopulmonary resuscitation
______________Cardiac defibrillator
______________Pneumatic anti-shock garment
______________Ventilator
______________ACLS meds
______________Other interventions/medications (physician specify)
____

Prehospital personnel are informed that (print patient name)____________________________
should receive no resuscitation (DNR) or should receive Modified Support as indicated. This directive is medically appropriate and is further documented by a physician's order and a progress note on the patient's permanent medical record. Informed consent from the capacitated patient or the incapacitated patient's legitimate surrogate is documented on the patient's permanent medical record. The DNR order is in full force and effect as of the date indicated below.

______________________________   ______________________________

Attending Physician's Signature

______________________________   ______________________________

Print Attending Physician's Name   Print Patient's Name and Location
                                          (Home Address or Health Care Facility)

____

Attending Physician's Telephone

______________________________   ______________________________

Date   Expiration Date (6 Mos from Signature)

Figure 3–1 Example of an EMS do not resuscitate (DNR) order.

it is accompanied by a doctor's written instructions. Check to see that it is written clearly and concisely. It should also be typed or written legibly on professional letterhead. Phrases like "no heroics" or "no extraordinary treatment" are *not* clear enough to be legal.

In many areas, a standard form is used for a DNR order. The document must be physically present when needed. The EMR may not simply take a person's word that the order exists.

By its very nature, a DNR order is best suited to a hospital or nursing home. There, all personnel know the patient and his or her physician. If the DNR order is needed, it must be found and verified quickly. However, in the field, there may be a problem. In the time it takes to verify a DNR order, precious life-saving moments can be lost.

There are varying degrees of DNR orders. For example, one order may explain that a patient allows all medical care except long-term life support. Another might say that the patient specifically does not allow the use of a mechanical artificial ventilation.

If you are ever in doubt about the validity of an advance directive, you must begin full resuscitation immediately. However, always consult your medical director or the hospital emergency department physician before you decide to follow or put aside a DNR order.

Be sure to review all provincial laws and local protocols on this issue.

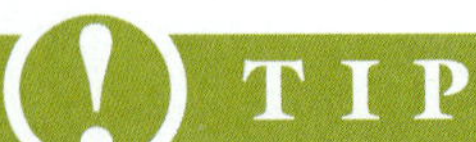

If a written DNR order is not in your hand, you cannot assume it exists. You are not on solid legal ground if you withhold care based on someone else's word alone.

Patient Refusal

Competent adults have the right to refuse treatment for themselves or their children. Under the law, such adults must first be informed of the treatment, fully understand it, and completely comprehend the risks involved in refusing it. They may refuse verbally, by pulling away, shaking their head, gesturing, or pushing you away.

Competent adults have the right to withdraw from treatment after it has started. This is true for patients who initially give consent but then change their mind. It is also true for patients who at first were unconscious but then wake up and ask you to stop.

A patient's legal refusal of treatment or transport must follow the rules of expressed consent; that is, the patient must be mentally competent and of legal age. The patient must also be informed of all the risks *in terms he or she can fully understand*. When in doubt, always err in favour of providing care.

Make every reasonable effort to persuade the patient, parent, or guardian to give consent for care. If he or she still refuses, insist that additional EMS personnel evaluate the patient.

Complete and accurate records are key to protecting yourself from liability. So before you leave the scene, do the following:

- *Try again to persuade the patient to accept treatment or transport.* Tell him or her clearly why it is essential. Be especially clear when you explain what could happen if he or she refuses care. Write down what you tell the patient. Then have the patient read it aloud to see if he or she understands.
- *Be sure the patient is able to make a rational, informed decision.* Note that a patient who is seriously ill or injured may only appear to be competent. Such a patient may be emotionally, intellectually, or physically impaired and may not be able to absorb all the information you give.
- *Obtain medical direction as required by local protocol.*
- *Have the patient sign a refusal or "release from liability" form* (Figures 3–2 and 3–3). It must be signed by the patient and a witness. If the patient refuses to sign, indicate that on the form and have

<table>
<tr><td>

RELEASE FROM RESPONSIBILITY WHEN PATIENT REFUSES SERVICE

This is to certify that I, _______________________________________, am refusing the service(s) of the Emergency Response Service and its staff and absolve the Service, its staff, and the consulting health care facility (if applicable) of any and all responsibility from any ill effects or adverse outcomes which may result from this action.

Signed_______________________________   Witness _______________________________

Relationship (if patient is a minor or under Order of Supervision) _______________________________

</td></tr>
</table>

Figure 3–2 Example of a patient refusal form.

EMS PATIENT REFUSAL CHECKLIST

PATIENT NAME: ____ AGE: ___________________

LOCATION OF CALL: ____ DATE: __________________

AGENCY INCIDENT #: _________________________________ AGENCY CODE: ___________________

NAME OF PERSON FILLING OUT FORM: ____

I.   ASSESSMENT OF PATIENT (Circle appropriate response for each item)

1.	Oriented to:	Person?	Yes	No
		Place?	Yes	No
		Time?	Yes	No
		Situation?	Yes	No
2.	Altered level of consciousness?		Yes	No
3.	Head injury?		Yes	No
4.	Alcohol or drug ingestion by exam or history?		Yes	No

II.   PATIENT INFORMED (Circle appropriate response for each item)

Yes	No	Medical treatment/evaluation needed
Yes	No	Ambulance transport needed
Yes	No	Further harm could result without medical treatment/evaluation
Yes	No	Transport by means other than ambulance could be hazardous in light of patient's illness/injury
Yes	No	Patient provided with Refusal Information Sheet
Yes	No	Patient accepted Refusal Information Sheet

III.   DISPOSITION

_______ Refused all EMS services

_______ Refused field treatment, but accepted transport

_______ Refused transport, but accepted field treatment

_______ Refused transport to recommended facility

_______ Patient transported by private vehicle to ____

_______ Released in care or custody of self

_______ Released in care or custody of relative or friend

Name: ____________________________ Relationship: ________________________________

_______ Released in custody of law enforcement agency

Agency: ____________________________ Officer: ___________________________________

_______ Released in custody of other agency

Agency: ____________________________ Officer: ___________________________________

IV.   COMMENTS: ____

____

____

Figure 3-3   Example of a patient refusal checklist.

a witness sign it. Many areas use official documents for patients to sign. Check local protocols.

- *Before you leave, encourage the patient to seek help if certain symptoms develop.* Be specific. Avoid using terms the patient may not understand. For example, you might tell a patient to go to the hospital emergency department "if you get a burning pain in your stomach" or "if you start having shortness of breath." Then document the fact that you gave such advice.
- *Advise the patient to immediately call EMS again if he or she changes his or her mind.*

SECTION 3
OTHER LEGAL ASPECTS OF EMERGENCY CARE

Common Assault

There are several types of assault named in the Criminal Code of Canada. Common assault, assault causing bodily harm, and aggravated assault are just three. While the Criminal Code may have slight variations from province to province, common assault is the most likely of the assault charges an EMR might face from patients who claim they were mishandled or did not want to be touched. This criminal charge may be hard to prove since it is unlikely that a plaintiff could prove that the EMR had intent to mishandle or inappropriately touch the patient. Nevertheless, the EMR should remain cautious in light of the possibility of civil litigation. Whenever possible, obtain consent before touching a patient's clothing or body.

Abandonment and Negligence

Simply stated, **abandonment** means you stopped providing care to a patient without making sure that the same or better care would be continued. Under the law, once you start giving emergency care to a patient, you must continue until another equally trained or higher trained health care professional takes over.

Negligence is defined as carelessness, inattention, disregard, inadvertence, or oversight that was accidental but avoidable. You may be charged with negligence if your care deviates from the accepted **standard of care** and results in further injury to the patient. Standard of care is defined as the care that would be expected to be provided to the same patient under the same conditions by another EMR who had received the same training. (This is referred to as the "reasonable person" test.)

To establish negligence, the court must decide that all four of the following are true:

1. *The EMR had a duty to act.* The concept known as **duty to act** refers to your contractual or legal obligation to provide care. This means that while you are on duty you must care for a patient who needs it and consents to it.
2. *There was a breach of duty.* A **breach of duty** exists when an EMR either fails to act or fails to act appropriately. This means that the EMR violated the standard of care reasonably expected of an EMR.
3. *The patient was injured physically or psychologically.*
4. *The EMR caused the injury.* It must be proven that the EMR's breach of duty is what caused or contributed to the patient's injury.

Your duty to act also means that you must render care to a patient to the best of your ability. You must follow accepted guidelines for care and act as any other prudent EMR would in the same situation.

In some cases, a duty to act refers to an implied contractual or legal obligation. For example, a patient may call for EMS. The dispatcher confirms that help will be sent. All EMS members who respond—including EMRs—then have a legal obligation to provide treatment to the patient.

In most provinces, you do not have a duty to act when you are off duty or driving an emergency vehicle outside your company's service area. (Check your provincial laws.) However, you may feel a certain moral or ethical obligation to help. In such cases, take extra steps to protect yourself against legal risk. Carefully document all aspects of the call, including the treatment you give and a patient's refusal of care.

In general, your best defence against negligence is to have a professional attitude, to provide a consistently high standard of care, and to correctly and completely document the care you provide.

Confidentiality

A patient's history, condition, and emergency care are confidential. To release this information, you must have a written form signed by the patient or a parent or legal guardian. Never release any patient information on request unless you are authorized to do so in writing.

By law, you are allowed to release information without a patient's or a parent's or guardian's permission only if one of the following applies:

- Another health care provider needs it in order to continue medical care.
- You are required by legal subpoena to provide it in court (Figure 3–4).

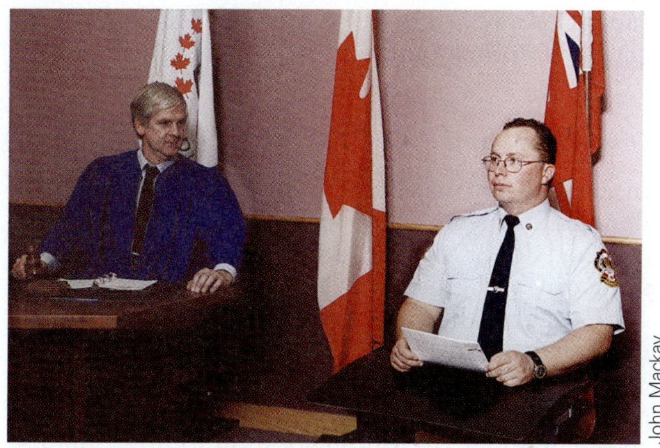

Figure 3–4 EMRs may be asked to testify in court.

Volunteer Service Acts

Most provinces and territories have common laws that govern the responsibility of emergency services personnel. While off duty, you may not be legally required to stop and assist at a scene, but there is a recognized duty to assist according to your level of certification when you do render help. Be sure to learn local laws that relate specifically to your level of care.

Generally, these laws protect an EMR from liability for acts performed in good faith unless those acts are grossly negligent. Under these laws, the person suing must prove that emergency care was markedly below the standard of care.

If you are sued and the case goes to court, a tort proceeding will be held. This is a civil court action, not a criminal one. It determines whether or not the natural rights of an individual have been violated. In a tort proceeding, it must be proven that you are guilty of gross negligence.

Volunteer Service Acts do not prevent you from being sued. However, they may give you some protection against losing the lawsuit if you have performed according to the standard of care for an EMR. So, while on or off duty, your best defence against lawsuits is prevention. Always render care to the best of your ability. Do no more or less than your scope of care allows. If you keep your patient's best interests in mind, you will seldom, if ever, go wrong.

Preservation of Evidence

Whenever an EMR is called to a **potential crime scene**, dispatch should also notify the police. In general, a potential crime scene is any scene that may require police support. That includes a potential or actual suicide, homicide, any death outside a hospital (whether expected or not), drug overdose, domestic dispute, abuse, hit-and-run, riot, robbery, or any scene involving gunfire or a weapon.

Your first concern should always be your own safety. *If you suspect that a crime is in progress or a criminal is active at the scene, do not try to provide care to any patient.* Wait until the police arrive and tell you that the scene is safe. Once the scene is safe, your priority is patient care.

When on the scene, do not disturb any item that may be evidence. Basic guidelines include the following:

- Observe and document anything unusual at the scene.
- Touch only what you need to touch.
- Never wipe away blood. It can be used as evidence.
- Move only what you need to move to protect the patient and provide emergency care.
- Do not use the telephone unless the police give you permission to do so. They may wish to find out who the last caller was.
- Move the patient only if he or she is in danger or must be moved in order for you to provide emergency care.
- If possible, do not cut through holes in the patient's clothing. They may have been caused by bullets or stabbing.
- Do not cut through any knot in a rope or tie. Knots are often used as evidence.
- If the crime is a rape, do not wash the patient or allow the patient to wash. Ask him or her not to change clothing, use the bathroom, or take anything by mouth. Doing any of these things could destroy evidence.

Special Documentation

In general, physicians must report suspected child, elder, and spouse abuse. Some provinces require others—such as teachers and EMS workers—to report such abuse as well. Related provincial laws often grant immunity from liability for libel or slander as long as the report is made in good faith.

EMS personnel may be required to report an injury that may be the result of a crime. That includes gunshot wounds, knife wounds, and poisonings. Your province may also want you to report any injury that you suspect was caused by sexual assault.

In some areas, EMS workers must report all suspected infectious disease exposure. That includes exposure to TB, hepatitis B, and AIDS. Other situations to report may include use of restraints on a patient, attempted suicides, and dog bites. Learn your local and provincial requirements.

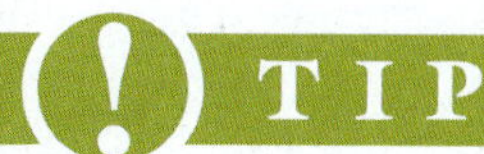

Even though patient privacy must be respected, become familiar with provincial laws regarding incident reporting.

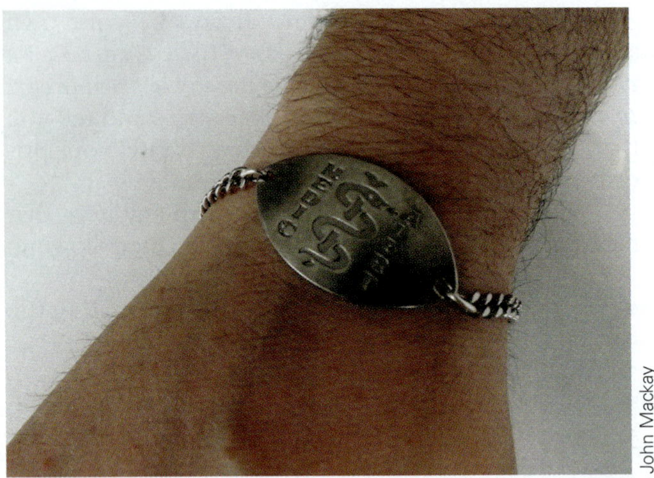

Figure 3–5 A medical identification tag.

Special Situations

Medical Identification Tags

Some patients may wear a medical identification tag (Figure 3–5) or carry a medical identification card. Such tags may be found on a bracelet or necklace. The card may be carried in a wallet. They identify a specific medical condition, such as an allergy, epilepsy, or diabetes. Look for them whenever you examine a patient. Many list a phone number you can call for detailed information.

Organ Donation

In general, organs can be donated only if there is a signed document giving permission to harvest them. A signed donor card, including those that accompany some driver's licences, is a legal document.

Patients who are about to die (or who have recently died) are potential organ donors. A potential organ donor should be treated the same as any other patient. Remember, the person is a patient first and an organ donor last. So, in addition to providing the appropriate emergency medical care, you can do the following:

- *Identify the patient as a potential donor.* The hospital staff and the patient's family must make the ultimate decision.
- *Communicate with medical control.* You can begin the organ retrieval process by alerting the paramedics who take over patient care. They will in turn alert the hospital emergency staff.
- *Provide life-saving emergency care such as CPR.* It will help maintain vital organs. This is best accomplished by treating every patient equally well.

EMR FOCUS

Legal issues are a large part of the first few minutes of a call. For example, it is during this time that you must obtain consent from your patient. You may also be faced with legal documents such as DNR orders.

Consider this scenario: You walk into a house and find a patient lying on a couch. The relative who meets you says, "I think he's dead. He's had cancer and we got this paper from his doctor so he can die in peace." Picture the situation. You have a patient who needs CPR and a relative who presents you with some type of form. Every second you spend trying to figure out what it is and what to do about it is time you could be using to help the patient.

This does not have to happen to you. Learn the regulations that affect your duties as an EMR well *before* you find yourself in a situation like this.

CASE STUDY FOLLOW-UP

At the beginning of this chapter, you read about a nine-year-old patient who had fallen from his bike. To see how the chapter information applies to this emergency, read the following. It describes how the call was completed.

PRIMARY ASSESSMENT

My partner confirmed that the patient's **ABCs—airway, breathing, and circulation**—were adequate. There was no obvious external bleeding. Our initial impression was that of a nine-year-old boy who had hit a tree with his bike. He complained of pain in his arm.

Just then, Amar's mother arrived on the scene. She gave consent for his care, and my partner continued his assessment.

SECONDARY ASSESSMENT

The mother's presence calmed the boy. We checked Amar carefully. We examined his head, neck, chest, abdomen, and extremities. The only sign of injury was to his arm. He wasn't thrown from the bike, so we did not suspect spinal injuries. His pulse was 88, strong, and regular, and his respirations were 18 and adequate. My partner manually stabilized the arm to prevent further injury. I spoke to Amar's mother about his medical history.

PATIENT HISTORY

I was told that Amar was basically healthy. He had had a heart murmur since birth, but no related problems or complications. He takes no medication. He had a full lunch consisting of rice and fish. He has no allergies.

ONGOING ASSESSMENT

Amar continued to be conscious. He responded to his mother well, which is an important sign in a child. He was wondering if he was going to have a cast on his arm for his friends to sign. His ABCs were still fine. His pulse, respirations, skin colour, and temperature were unchanged.

TRANSFER OF CARE

We introduced Amar and his mother to the paramedics who would be taking him to the hospital. We told the paramedics that Amar had hit a tree with his bicycle and fallen. We went on with our report:

> "He is complaining of pain to his right arm, which we are now stabilizing. He was wearing a helmet. He is not complaining of neck or back problems. Amar never lost consciousness and has no other complaints. His pulse is 88 and respirations, 18. He had rice and fish for lunch. He has a heart murmur but no problems with it. No meds, no allergies."

The paramedics thanked us and took over care. My partner was asked to stay since Amar felt comfortable with him. I manually stabilized Amar's arm while the paramedic applied a splint. Amar's mother thanked us as she got into the ambulance with her son.

Amar did indeed need a cast for his broken arm, but it was expected to heal completely. While this might not have been a critical emergency, just by stabilizing Amar's arm we prevented further injury and problems that could have stayed with him his whole life.

> Consent is one of many legal and ethical issues you will face as an EMR. Learn the laws related to you and your EMS system.

NOCPs

1.1 a Maintain patient dignity **S**
    b Reflect professionalism through use of appropriate language **S**
    d Maintain appropriate personal interaction with patients **A**
    e Maintain patient confidentiality **A**
    h Participate in professional associations **A**
    i Behave ethically **A**

1.2 a Develop personal plan for continuing professional development **X**
    b Self-evaluate and set goals for improvement, as related to professional practice **X**

1.3 a Comply with scope of practice **S**
    b Recognize the rights of the patient and the implications on the role of the provider **A**
    c Include all pertinent and required information on reports and medical records **S**

1.4 a Function within relevant legislation, policies, and procedures **A**

1.5 a Work collaboratively with a partner **S**
    b Accept and deliver constructive feedback **S**

1.6 a Employ reasonable and prudent judgment **S**

2.1 d Provide information to patient about their situation and how they will be cared for **S**

2.4 b Employ empathy and compassion while providing care **S**

6.2 c Provide care for geriatric patient **A**

REVIEW QUESTIONS

Page references where answers may be found or supported are provided at the end of each question.

SECTION 1

1. What is an EMR's scope of practice? (p. 27)

SECTION 2

2. Explain the difference between expressed and implied consent. (p. 28)
3. What is an advance care plan? (p. 29)
4. What is a DNR order? What should an EMR do if presented with one? (pp. 29–30)
5. How should you handle a patient's refusal of treatment? (pp. 30–32)

SECTION 3

6. What must happen in order for an EMR to be liable for abandonment or negligence? (p. 32)
7. What does it mean for an EMR to have a duty to act? (p. 32)
8. Under what conditions may an EMR release confidential patient information? (p. 32)
9. What are some ways an EMR can help preserve evidence at a crime scene? (p. 33)
10. What are the situations an EMR may be required to report to police or hospital staff? (pp. 33–34)

CHAPTER 4

The Human Body

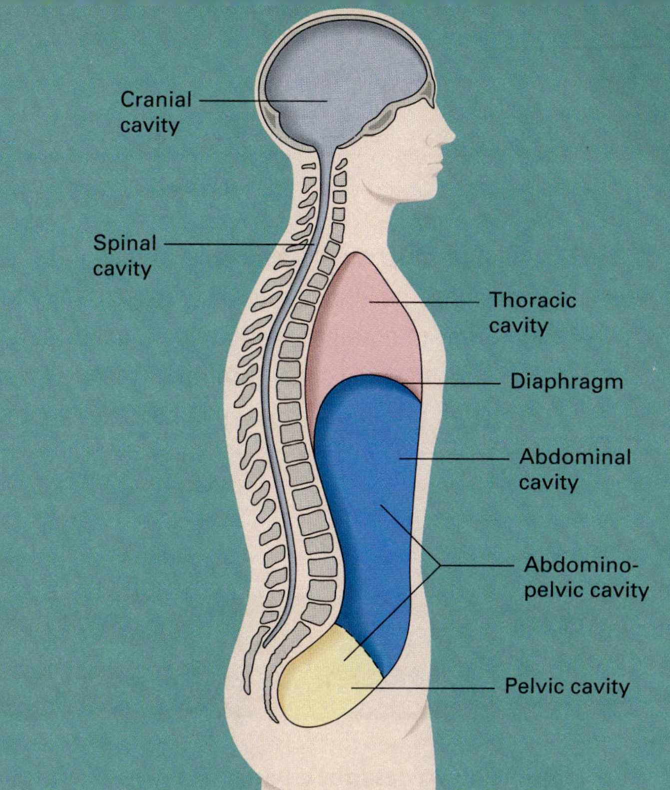

OBJECTIVES

1. Explain the four terms of position and the twelve terms of anatomical direction and location.
2. Describe the three main body cavities and identify the organs they contain.
3. Describe the anatomy and function of the major body systems, including the musculoskeletal, respiratory, circulatory, nervous, skin, digestive, urinary, endocrine, and reproductive systems.

INTRODUCTION

As an EMR, you must be able to recognize illness and injury and know how to care for them. You must also be able to quickly and accurately tell other medical personnel about a patient's problem. In order to do all this, you need a solid foundation in basic knowledge of the human body. In this chapter, you will study **anatomy** (the structure of the body) and **physiology** (how the body works). You will also be introduced to common anatomical terms.

SECTION 1
ANATOMICAL TERMS

It is important to describe a patient's position and the anatomical direction and location of injuries to other EMS personnel. Using correct terms will help you communicate the extent of a patient's injury quickly and accurately.

Terms of position include the following (Figure 4–1):

- **Anatomical position**. In this position, a patient's body stands erect with arms down at the sides, palms facing you. "Right" and "left" refer to the patient's right and left.
- **Supine position**. The patient is lying face up on his or her back.
- **Prone position**. The patient is lying face down on his or her stomach.
- **Lateral recumbent position**. The patient is lying on the left or right side. This is also known as the

HAINES position and is similar to the **recovery position**. These will be discussed in Chapter 7.

Terms of anatomical direction and location are as follows:

- **Superior** means toward, or closer to, the head. **Inferior** means toward, or closer to, the feet.
- **Anterior** is toward the front. **Posterior** is toward the back.
- **Medial** means toward the midline, or centre, of the body. **Lateral** refers to the left or right of the midline.
- **Proximal** means closer to or near the point of reference. **Distal** is distant or farther away from the point of reference. The point of reference is usually the torso. For example, a wound of the forearm is proximal to the wrist because the wound is closer to the torso than the wrist is. That same wound is distal to the elbow because it is farther away from the torso than the elbow is.
- **Superficial** is near the surface. **Deep** is remote, or far from the surface.
- **Internal** means inside. **External** means outside.

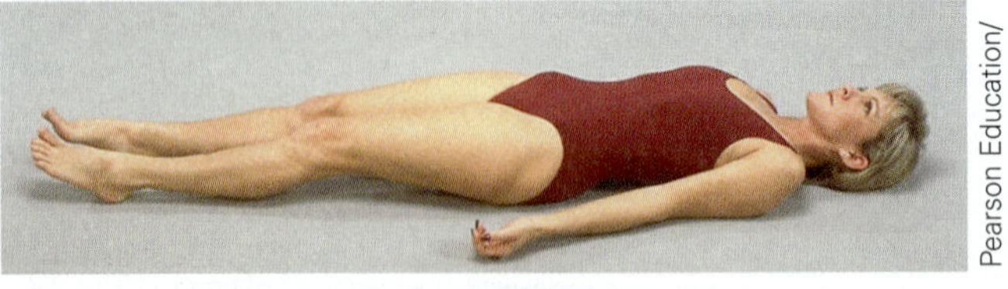

Figure 4–1a Supine position.

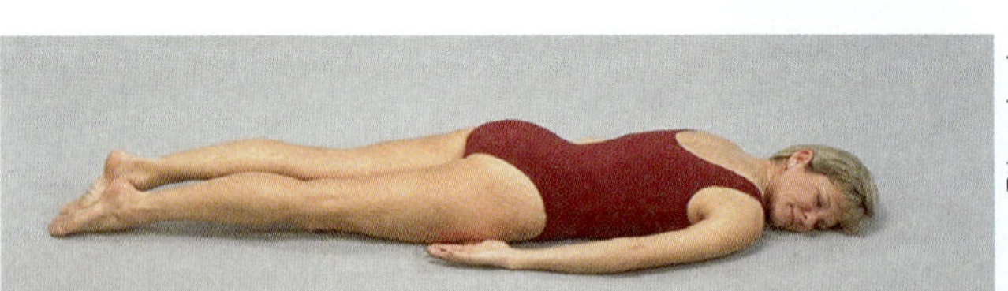

Figure 4–1b Prone position.

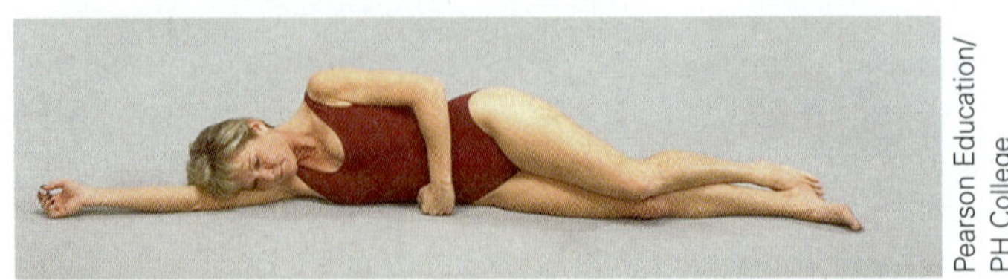

Figure 4–1c Right lateral recumbent position.

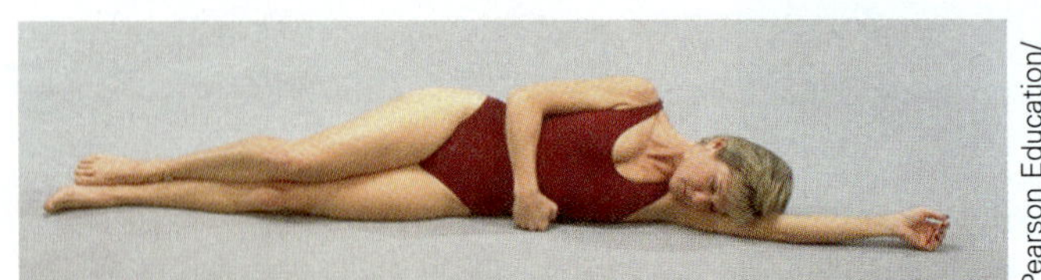

Figure 4–1d Left lateral recumbent position.

CASE ST...

Dispatch

My first-res... son injured." A woman had missed a ste... leg.

Scene Ass...

We scanned ... sure there were no prob-lems. The pa... ental note to check with the patient abou... a step or two or down the whole flight?

Primary A...

The woman w... out or injuring her head or spine. She ha... eeding. She told us that her left shin bone...

Secondary ...

We conducted ... other than to the left lower leg. It was de... ing. We manually stabi-lized the leg t... ulse and found it to be 88, strong, and re... deep, and her blood pres-sure was 110/8... a pulse, movement, and sensation below...

...the basic anatomy and physiology ...man body is key to this course. It is the foundation on which you will build all your skills. Consider the patient in this Case Study as you read Chapter 4. How would you communicate her condition to the responding paramedics?

Anatomical regions and **topographic anatomy** are the internal and external landmarks of the body (Figures 4–2 and 4–3). During assessment of a patient, refer to these landmarks. They will help make the description of a patient's condition clear to others, particularly when you use a radio.

The organs of the body are located in certain body cavities (Figure 4–4 on p. 41). The main body cavities include the following:

- **Thoracic cavity** (also called the chest cavity). The lungs and heart are found here. The **diaphragm**—a muscle that moves up and down during respiration—separates this cavity from the abdomen.
- **Abdominal cavity**. It contains organs of digestion and excretion, including the stomach, intestines, liver, gallbladder, spleen, pancreas, and kidneys.
- **Pelvic cavity**. It is bounded by the lower part of the spine, the hip bones, and the pubis. It protects the lower abdomen, including the bladder, rectum, and internal female reproductive organs.

Think of the abdomen as being divided into four parts or quadrants. Health care workers often refer to it that way. The quadrants are formed by imaginary lines. One line is drawn horizontally through the navel. The other line is drawn vertically through the midline of the body (Figure 4–5 on p. 42).

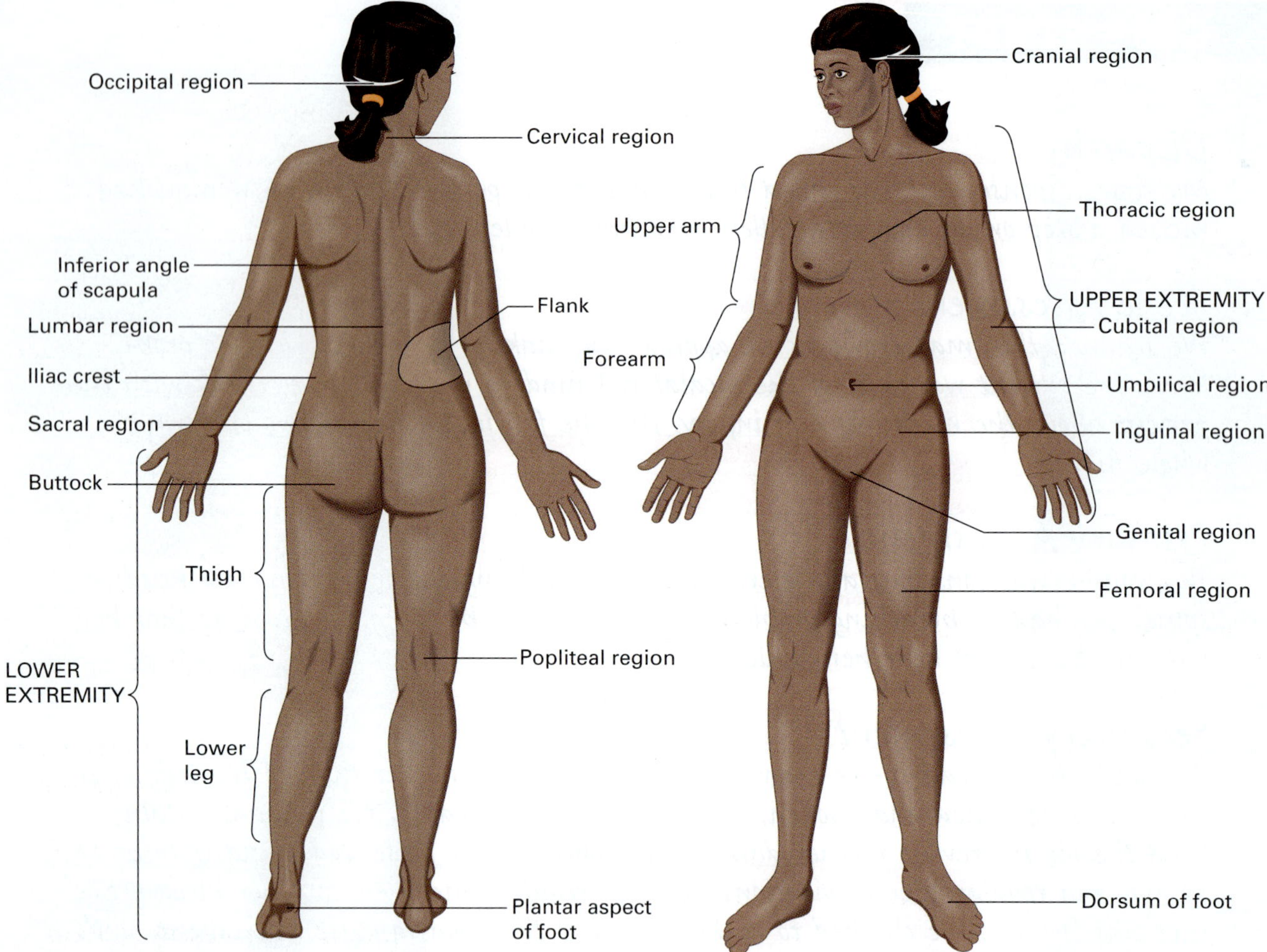

Figure 4–2 Anatomical regions.

SECTION 2
BODY SYSTEMS

The Musculoskeletal System

The **musculoskeletal system** is made up of the skeleton and muscles. Each helps give the body shape and protects internal organs. The muscles also provide for movement.

The Skeleton

The human body is shaped by its bony framework (Figure 4–6 on p. 43). Bone is composed of living cells and nonliving matter. The nonliving matter contains calcium compounds that help make bones hard and rigid. Without bones, the body would collapse.

The adult skeleton has 206 bones. It must be strong to support and protect, jointed to permit motion, and flexible to withstand stress. It is held together mainly by **ligaments**, **tendons**, and layers of muscle. Ligaments connect bone to bone. Tendons connect muscle to bone. Bone ends fit into each other at joints. The three kinds of joints are immovable (like the skull), slightly movable (like the spine), and freely movable (like the hip) (Figure 4–7 on p. 44).

The major areas of the skeleton include the following:

- The **skull** has a number of broad, flat bones that form a hollow shell. The top (including the forehead), back, and sides of the shell make up the **cranium**. It houses and protects the brain. There are several small bones of the face. They give shape to the face and permit the jaw to move. The major features of the face are the nose, ears, eyes, cheeks, mouth, and jowls.
- The **spinal column** houses and protects the spinal cord. The spinal column is the central supportive bony structure of the body. It consists of 33 bones known as **vertebrae**. The spine is divided into five

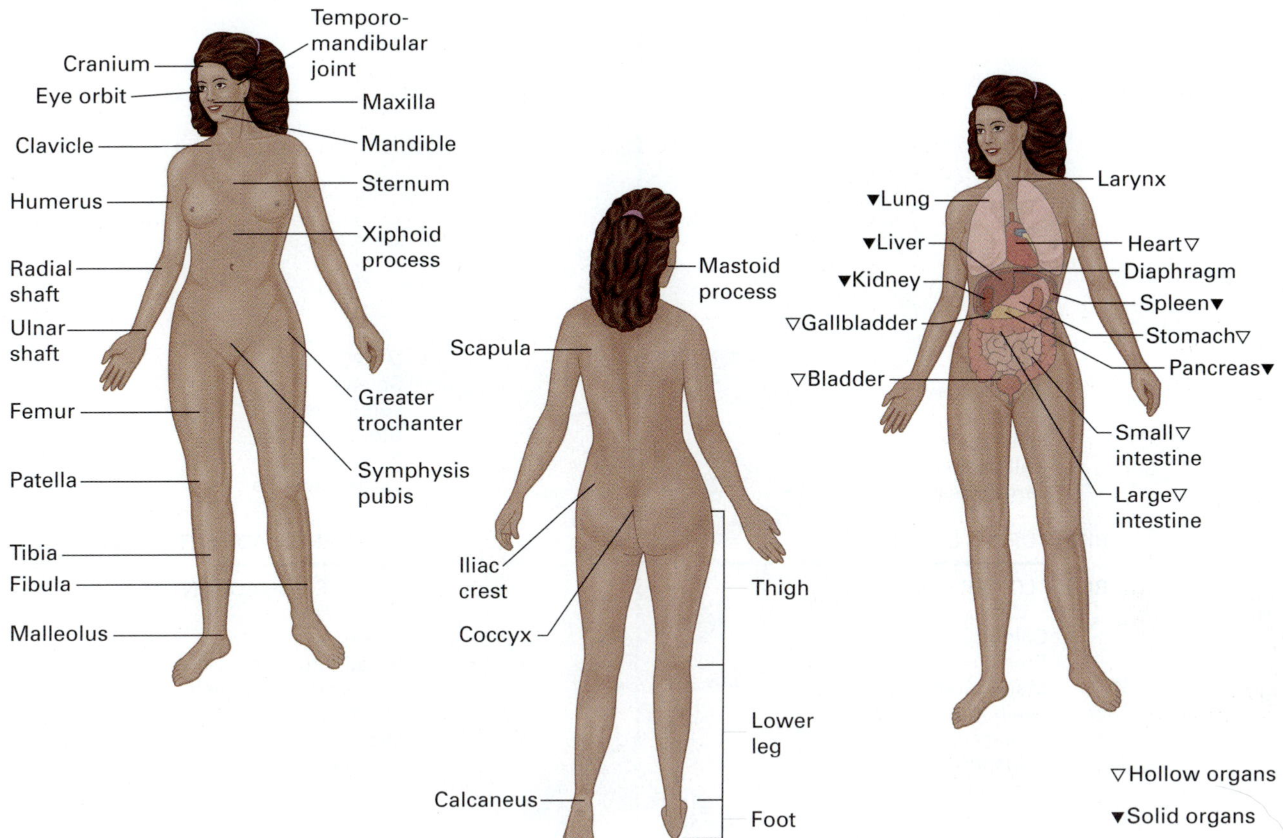

Figure 4–3 Topographic anatomy.

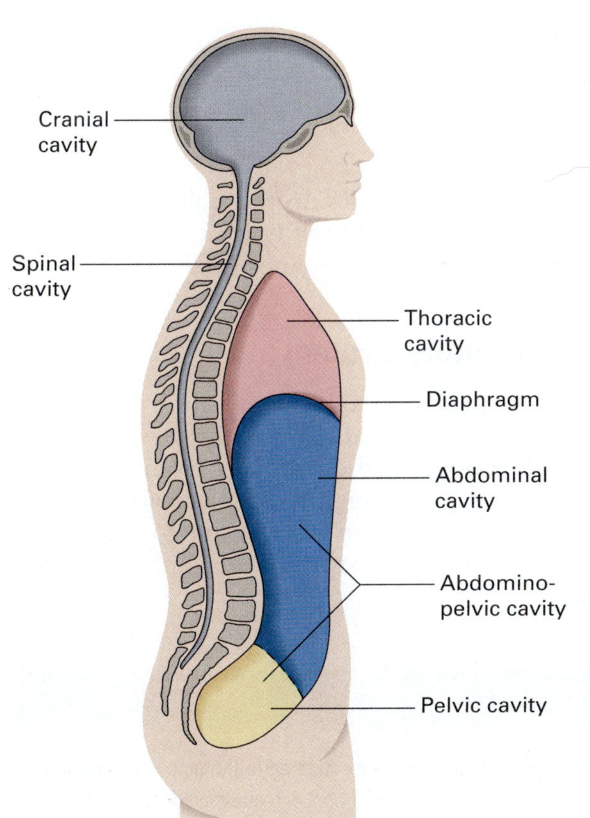

Figure 4–4 Main body cavities.

sections: the **cervical spine** (the neck, formed by seven vertebrae), the **thoracic spine** (the upper back, formed by 12 vertebrae), the **lumbar spine** (the lower back, formed by five vertebrae), the **sacrum** (the lower part of the spine, formed by five fused vertebrae), and the **coccyx** (the tail bone, formed by four fused vertebrae).

- The **thorax**, or rib cage, protects the heart and lungs—vital organs of the body. They are enclosed by 12 pairs of ribs that are attached at the back to the spine. The top 10 are also attached in the front to the **sternum**, or breastbone. The lowest portion of the sternum is called the **xiphoid process**.
- The **pelvis**, or hip bones, consists of the **ilium**, **pubis**, and **ischium**. Iliac crests form the "wings" of the pelvis. The pubis is the anterior portion of the pelvis. The ischium is in the posterior portion.
- The **shoulder girdle** consists of the **clavicle** (the collarbone) and the **scapula** (shoulder blade).
- The upper **extremities** extend from the shoulders to the fingertips. The upper arm (shoulder to elbow) has one bone known as the **humerus**. The bones in the forearm (elbow to wrist) are the **radius** and **ulna**. The lower extremities extend from the hips to the toes. The bone in the thigh, or upper leg, is known as the **femur**. The bones in the lower leg are the **tibia** and **fibula**. The knee cap is called the **patella**.

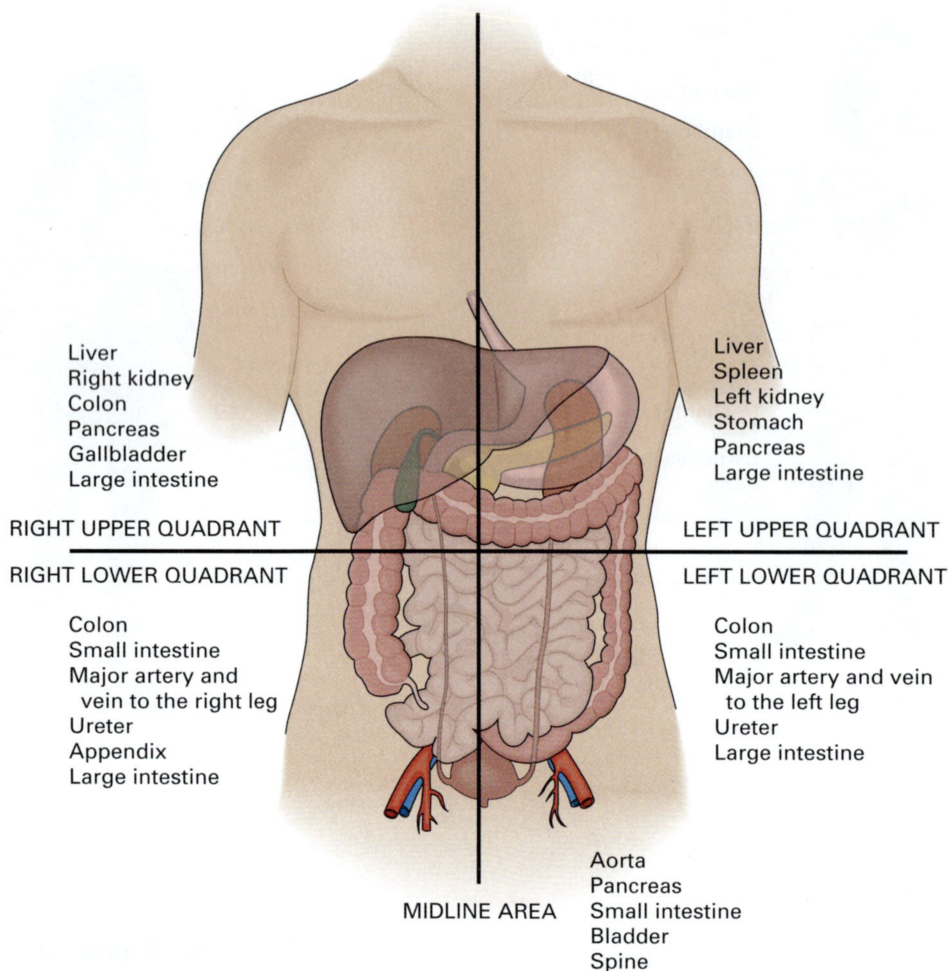

Figure 4–5 The abdominal area in quadrants.

The Muscles

Movement of the body depends on the work performed by the muscles. Muscles have the ability to contract (become shorter and thicker) when stimulated by a nerve impulse. Each muscle is made up of long threadlike cells called fibres, which are closely packed or bundled. Overlapping bundles are bound by connective tissue (Figure 4–8 on p. 45).

There are three basic kinds of muscle (Figure 4–9 on p. 46):

- **Skeletal muscle**, or **voluntary muscle**, makes possible all deliberate acts such as walking and chewing. It helps shape the body and forms its walls. In the trunk, this type of muscle is broad, flat, and expanded. In the extremities, it is long and round.
- **Smooth muscle**, or **involuntary muscle**, is made of longer fibres. It is found in the walls of tubelike organs, ducts, and blood vessels. It also forms much of the intestinal wall. A person has little or no control over this type of muscle.
- **Cardiac muscle** makes up the walls of the heart. It is able to stimulate itself to contract, even when disconnected from the brain.

The Respiratory System

The body depends on a constant supply of oxygen. The **respiratory system** delivers this oxygen to the lungs and removes carbon dioxide from the lungs. The body may get enough nutrition from a meal to last several weeks. It can store water to last several days. However, it can store oxygen for only a few minutes.

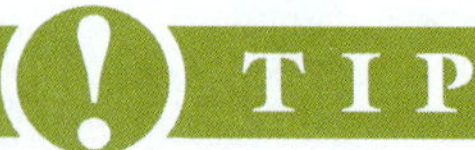

If you consider what you have learned in thoracic anatomy, you may be more effective when applying chest compressions to a cardiac arrest victim.

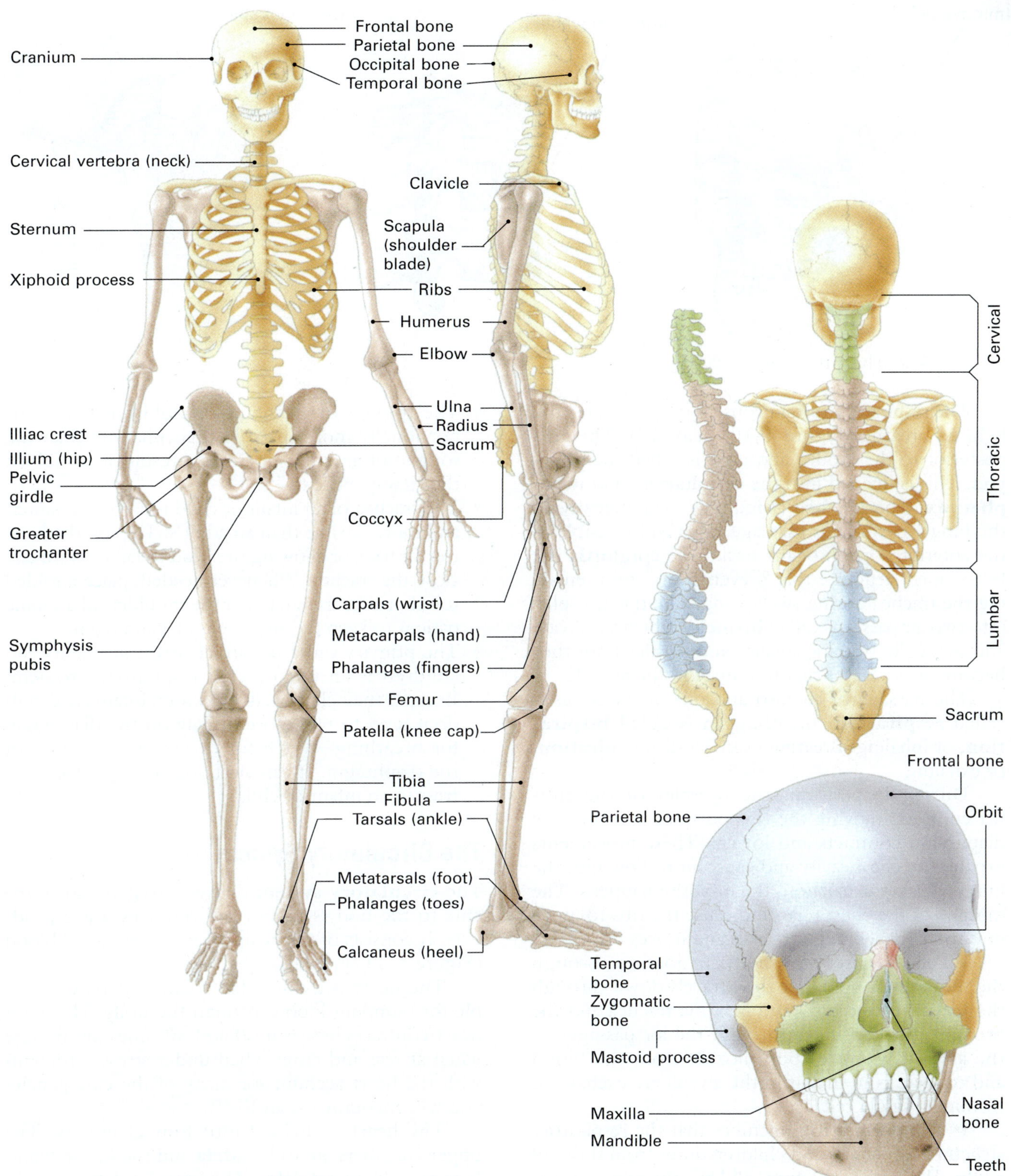

Figure 4–6 The skeletal system.

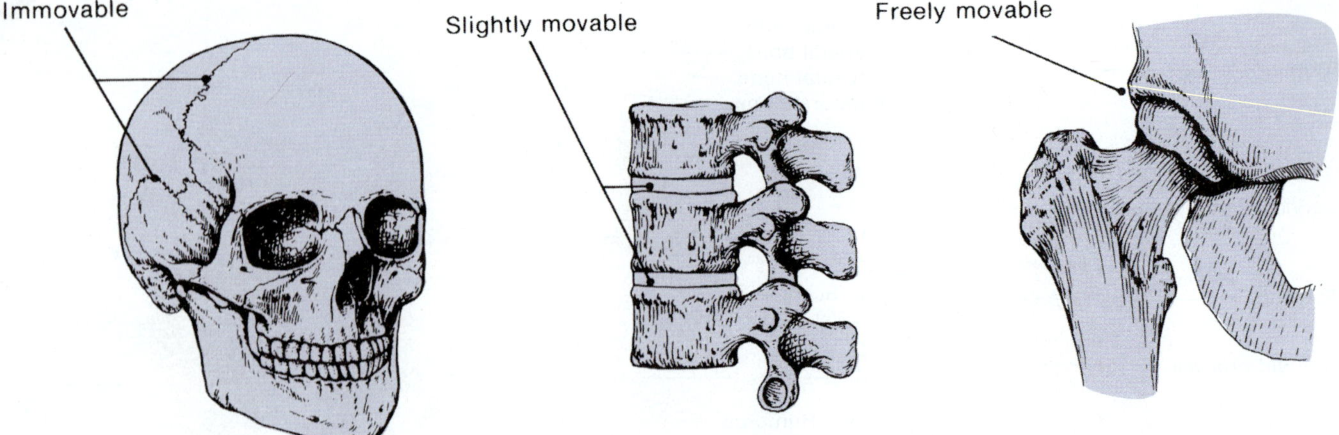

Figure 4–7 Three types of joints.

The respiratory system consists of the organs that help us breathe (Figure 4–10 on p. 47). The area posterior to the mouth and nose is called the **pharynx**. This is divided into the **oropharynx** and **nasopharynx**. The **trachea** (windpipe) is the airway to the lungs. It contains cartilage rings and is visible in the anterior portion of the neck. The **epiglottis** is a leaf-shaped structure that prevents food from entering the trachea during swallowing. The trachea splits into two air passages called **bronchi**, which subdivide and gradually become smaller and smaller until they become bronchioles that terminate in the **alveoli**.

The passage of air into and out of the lungs is called **respiration**. Breathing in is called **inspiration**, or inhaling. Breathing out is called **expiration**, or exhaling.

During inspiration, the muscles of the thorax contract, moving the ribs outward and up. The diaphragm contracts and lowers. These movements expand the chest cavity and cause air to flow into the lungs. During exhalation, the opposite happens. The muscles of the chest relax and cause the ribs to move inward. The diaphragm relaxes and moves up.

When air enters the body, it does so through the mouth and nose. Air then travels down through the **larynx** (voice box) and into the trachea and the bronchi. Air continues through the air passages to the alveoli, where carbon dioxide from the blood and oxygen from the air in the alveoli are exchanged through a single cell layer.

It is important to remember that the respiratory structures of infants and children differ from those of adults. While the structures all have the same names, they are smaller or less developed in infants and children. These differences are very important:

- All structures, including, for example, the mouth and nose, are more easily obstructed by small objects, blood, or swelling. Pay extra attention to an infant or child to be sure the airway stays open.

- The tongue of an infant or child takes up proportionally more space in their pharynx than the tongue of an adult does. As a result, it can block the airway more easily.
- The trachea of an infant or child is narrower, softer, and more flexible than an adult's. Tipping the head too far back or allowing the head to fall forward can close the trachea. Whenever needed, place a folded towel or similar item under the shoulders of a supine patient to keep the airway aligned and open.
- The primary cause of cardiac arrest in infants and children is an uncorrected respiratory problem. Because their chest walls are softer, infants and children tend to rely more heavily on the diaphragm for breathing. Watch for excessive movement of the diaphragm. It can alert you to respiratory distress in an infant or child.

The Circulatory System

The **circulatory system** delivers oxygen and nutrients to the body's tissues and removes waste products. It consists of the heart, blood vessels, and blood (Figure 4–11 on p. 48).

The heart is a muscular organ that is responsible for pumping blood through the body. The adult heart contracts between 60 and 80 times per minute when at rest and faster when under stress. Problems with the heart account for many of the emergencies you will encounter as an EMR.

The heart is divided into four chambers. The upper chambers are called **atria** and the lower chambers are called **ventricles**. The heart has left and right sides, each of which has an atrium and a ventricle. The right side of the heart receives deoxygenated blood from the body and pumps it to the lungs. The left side of the heart receives oxygenated blood from the lungs and pumps it to the body.

When the heart pumps blood from the left ventricle, blood enters the arteries. This pumping action

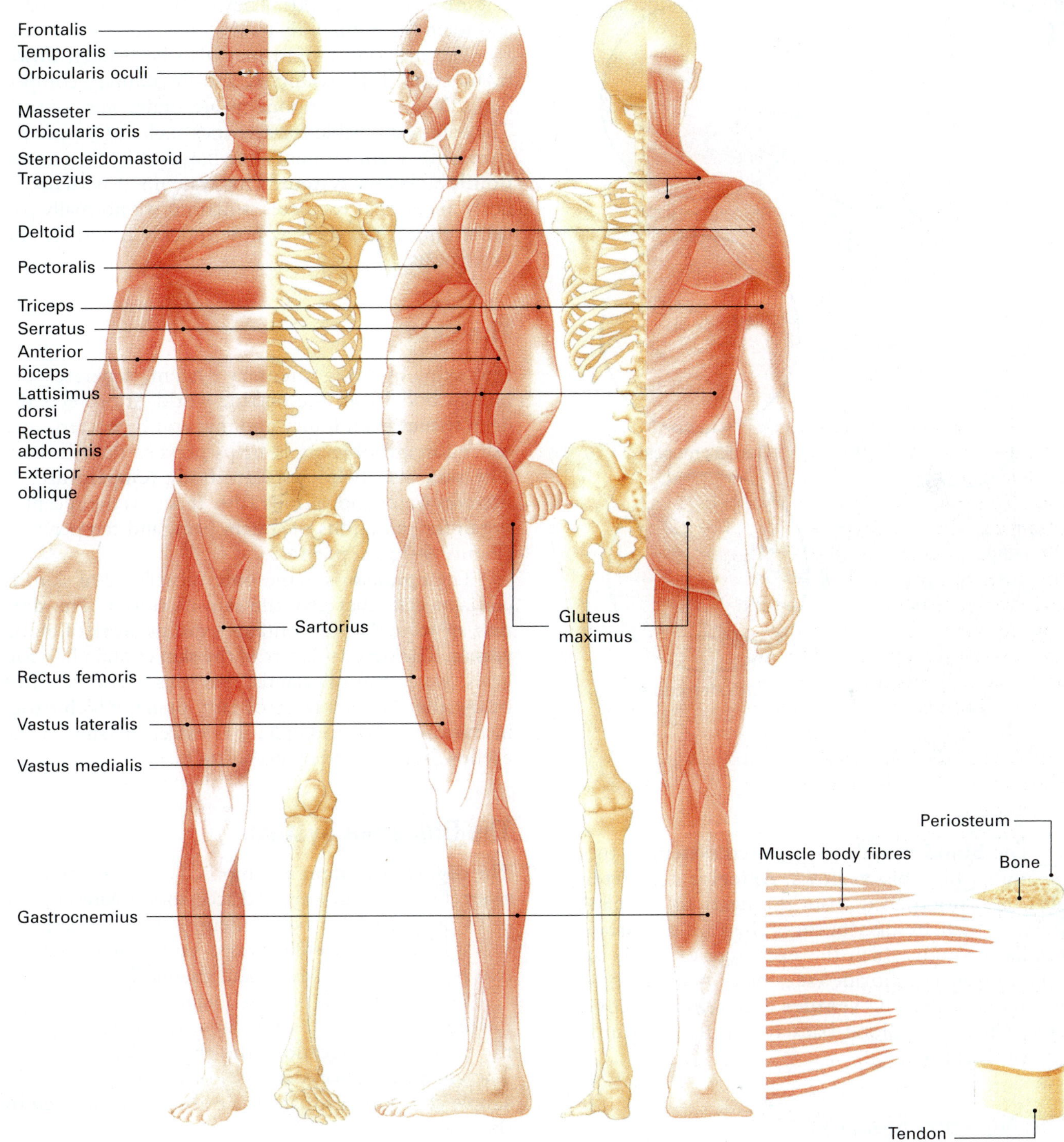

Figure 4–8 The muscular system.

causes a wave of pressure that can be felt as a **pulse** when you depress a patient's artery between your finger and a hard surface such as bone. There are many points where a pulse can be felt in the body. The most common are as follows:

- The **carotid pulse point**, felt on either side of the neck
- The **brachial pulse point**, felt on the inside of the arm between the elbow and the shoulder
- The **radial pulse point**, felt on the inside of the wrist
- The **femoral pulse point**, felt in the area of the groin in the crease between the abdomen and thigh

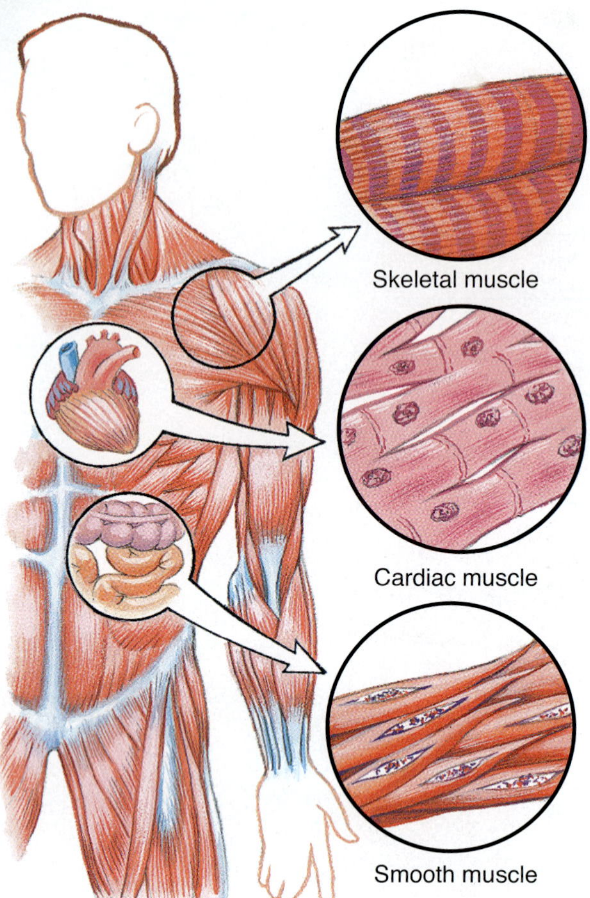

Figure 4–9 Three types of muscle.

The **blood vessels** are a closed system of tubes through which blood flows. **Arteries** and **arterioles** take blood away from the heart to the **capillaries**, which are distributors. They are the smallest vessels through which the exchange of fluid, oxygen, and carbon dioxide takes place between blood and tissue cells. The **venules** and **veins** are collectors. They carry blood back to the heart from the rest of the body.

The Nervous System

The **nervous system** is composed of the brain, the spinal cord, and nerves. It has two major functions: communication and control. It allows a person to be aware of and react to the environment. It coordinates the body's responses to stimuli and keeps body systems working together.

The nervous system has two main parts: the **central nervous system (CNS)** and the **peripheral nervous system**. The central nervous system consists of the brain and spinal cord (Figure 4–12a on p. 49). The peripheral nervous system consists of the nerves

(Figure 4–12b on p. 50). They carry information back and forth from the body to the spinal cord and brain.

The nervous system may also be broken down by function or by voluntary and involuntary components. Voluntary components are under our control. They are responsible for activities such as movement. Involuntary components are handled by the **autonomic nervous system**. This system is a network of nerve tissue that regulates functions we normally pay no attention to, such as how quickly or slowly the heart beats.

The Skin

The skin, or integumentary system, separates the human body from the outside world. It protects the deep tissues from injury and invasion by bacteria and other foreign objects. It helps prevent dehydration. The skin also helps regulate body temperature. It excretes water and various salts. It acts as the receptor organ for sensations of touch, pain, and temperature (Figure 4–13 on p. 51).

The **epidermis** is the outermost layer of skin. It contains cells that give the skin its colour. The **dermis**, or second layer, contains a vast network of blood vessels. The deepest layers of the skin contain hair follicles, sweat and oil glands, and sensory nerves. Just below the skin is a layer of fatty tissue, which varies in thickness. For example, it is extremely thin in the eyelids, but thick over the buttocks.

The Digestive System

The **digestive system** is composed of the **alimentary tract** (food passageway) and accessory organs (Figure 4–14 on p. 51). Its main functions are to ingest and digest food and get rid of waste. Digestion consists of two processes: mechanical and chemical.

The mechanical process includes chewing, swallowing, the rhythmic movement of matter through the tract, and defecation (the elimination of waste). The chemical process consists of breaking food into simple components that can be absorbed and used by the body.

Except for the mouth and **esophagus**, the organs of this system are in the abdomen. They include the stomach, pancreas, liver, gallbladder, small intestine, and large intestine.

The Urinary System

The **urinary system** filters the blood and excretes waste from the body. It consists of two kidneys, two ureters, the urinary bladder, and the urethra (Figure 4–15 on p. 52). The ureters take urine from the

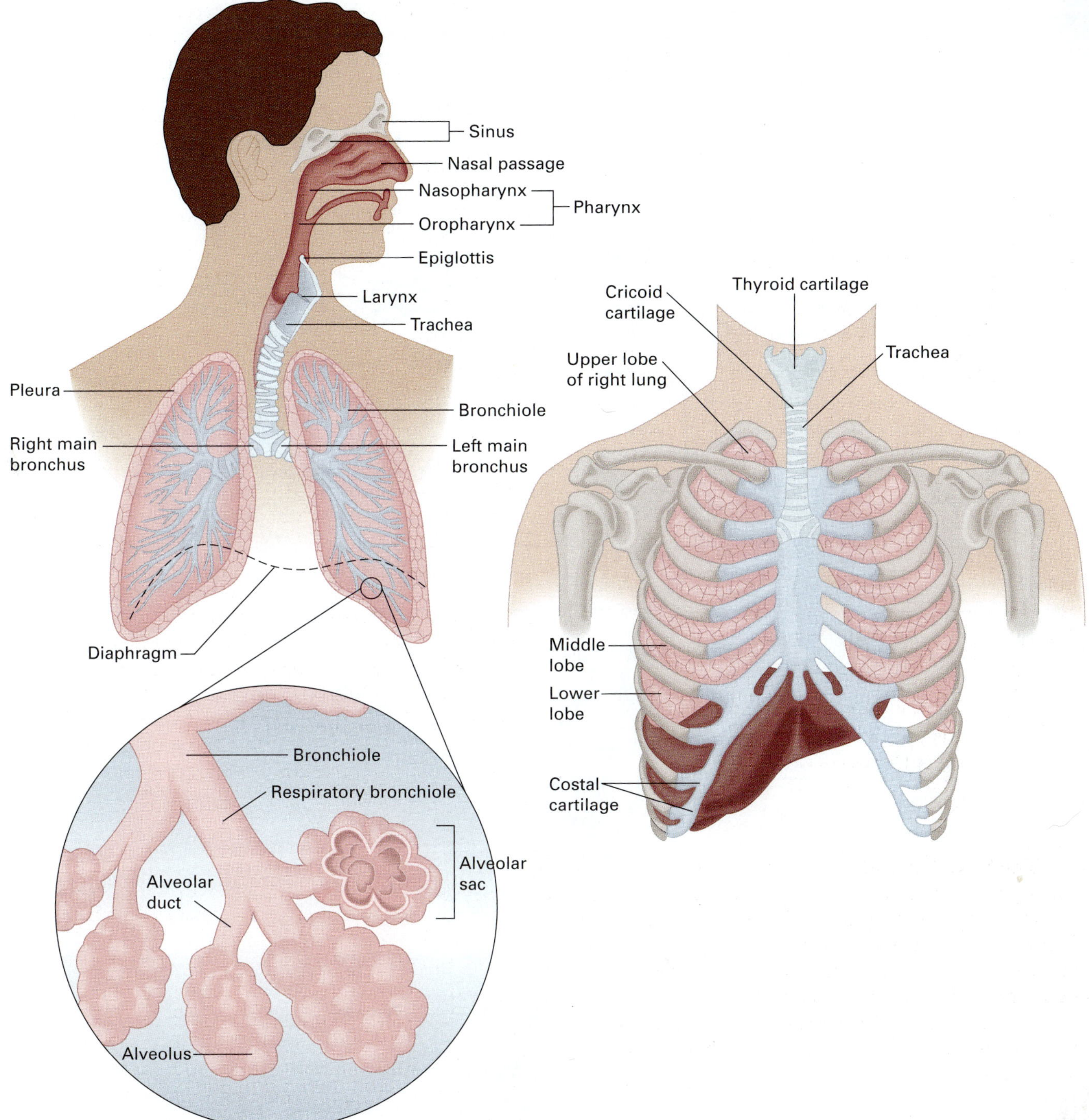

Figure 4–10 The respiratory system.

kidneys to the bladder. The bladder stores urine until it is passed through the urethra and excreted from the body.

The urinary system helps the body maintain the delicate balance of water and chemicals needed for survival. During the process of urine formation, wastes are removed and useful products are returned to the blood.

The Endocrine System

The **endocrine system** is made up of endocrine glands, which regulate the body by secreting hormones directly into the bloodstream. They affect physical strength, mental ability, stature, reproduction, hair growth, voice pitch, and behaviour. How people think, feel, and sometimes act can depend largely on these tiny secretions.

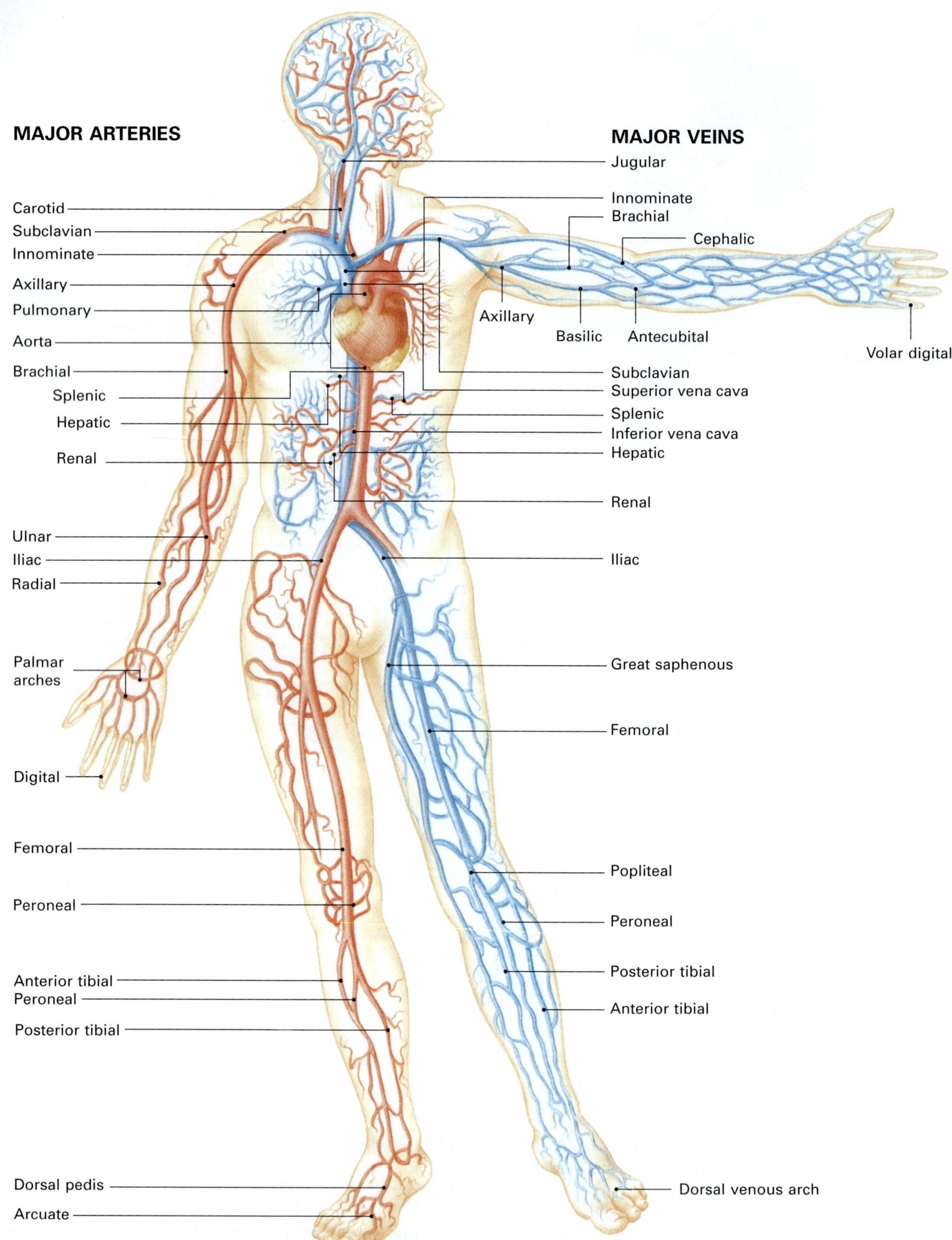

Figure 4–11 The circulatory system.

THE BRAIN

DIVISIONS OF THE SPINAL CORD

THE SPINAL CORD

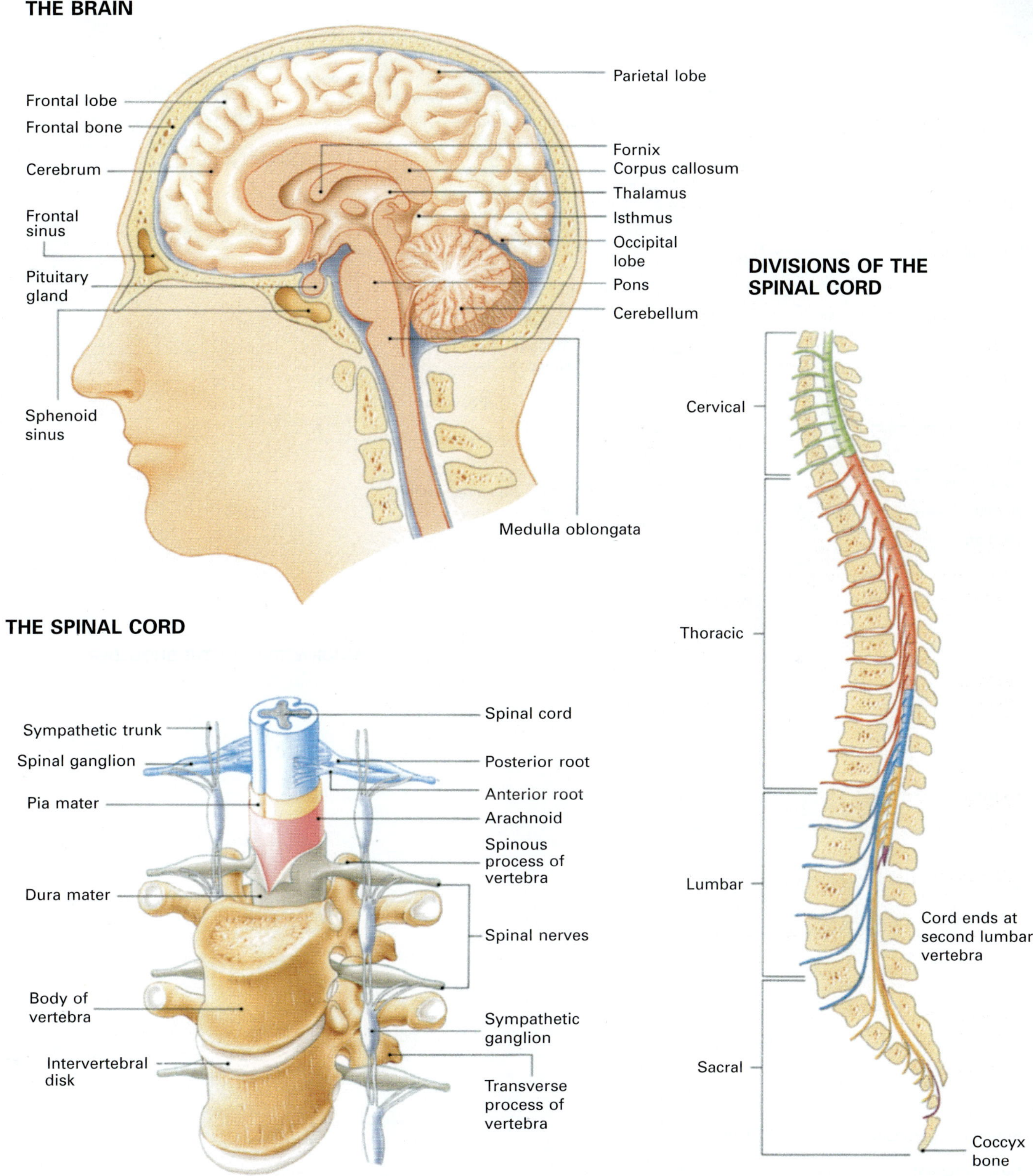

Figure 4–12a The central nervous system.

Each gland produces one or more hormones. The glands include the thyroid, parathyroids, adrenals, ovaries, testes, islets of Langerhans, and the pituitary.

The pancreas, while considered part of the digestive system, also functions within the endocrine system. It secretes insulin and glucagon, which are very important for maintaining blood sugar levels.

The Reproductive System

The **reproductive system** of the male includes two testes, a duct system, accessory glands, and the penis. The reproductive system of the female consists of two ovaries, two fallopian tubes, the uterus, vagina, and external genitals (Figure 4–16 on p. 52).

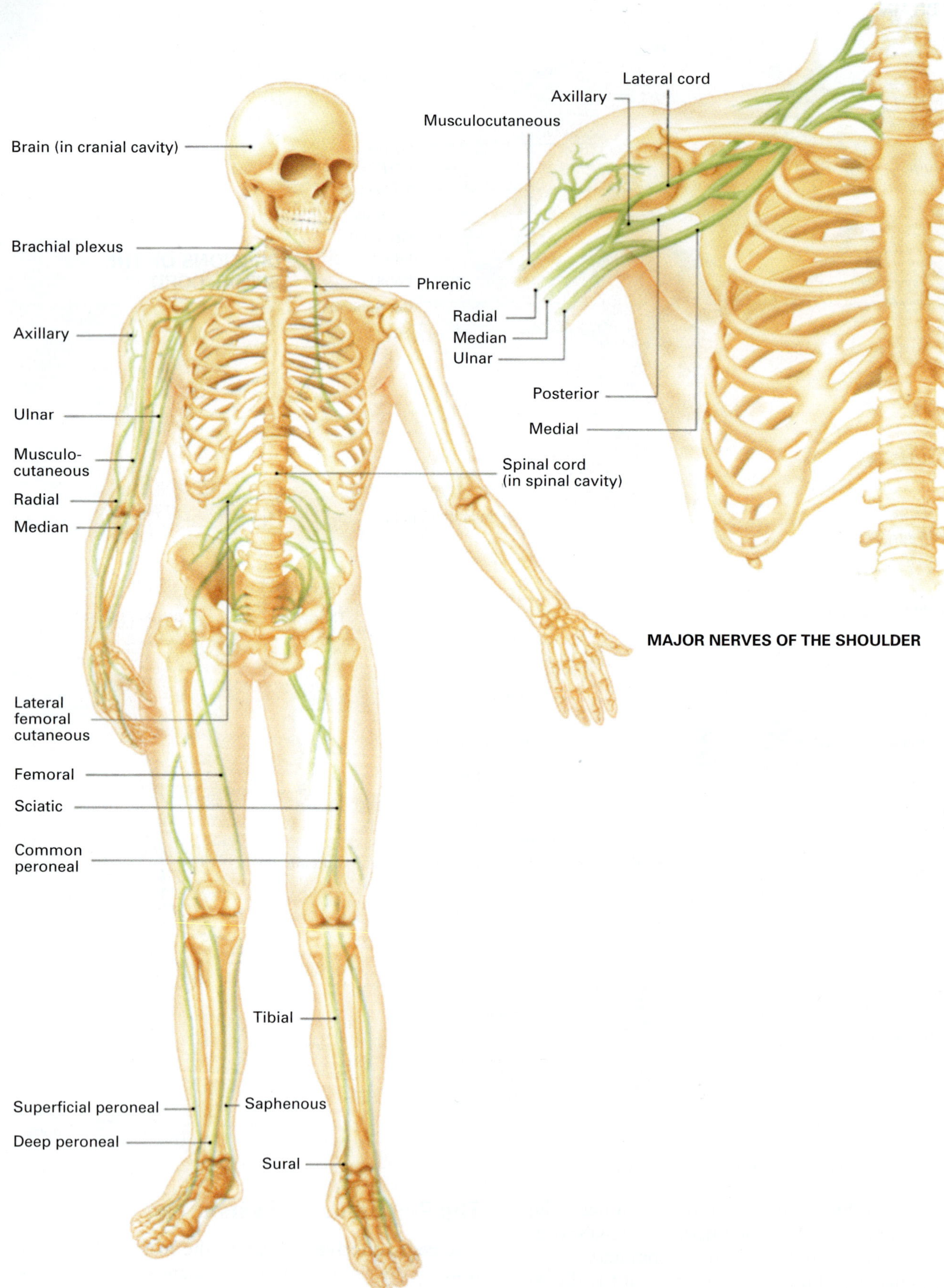

Figure 4-12b   The peripheral nervous system.

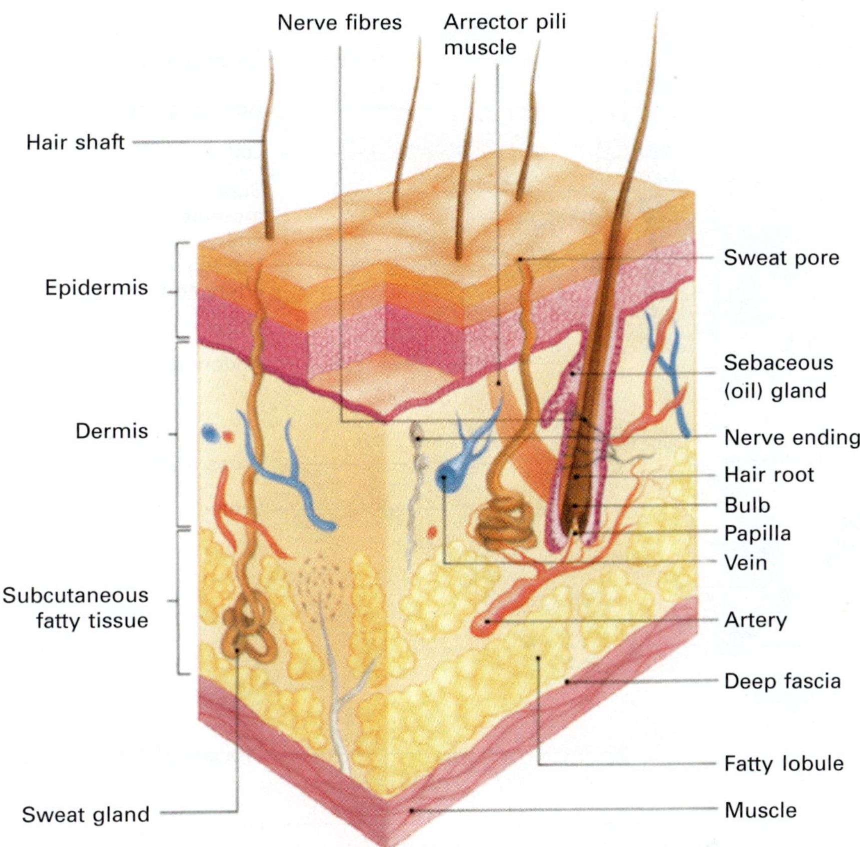

Figure 4–13 Structure of skin.

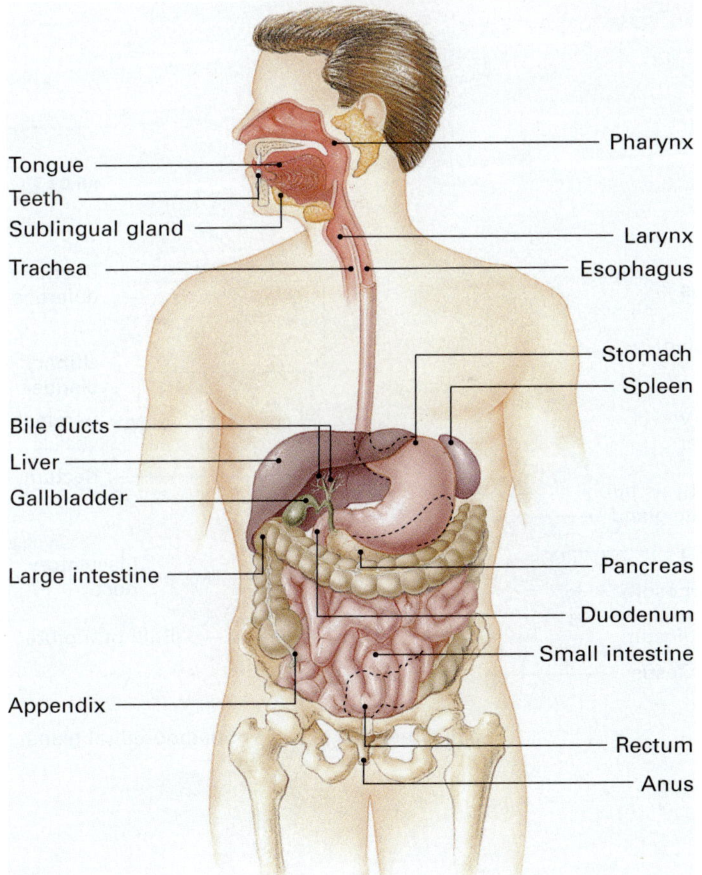

Figure 4–14 The digestive system.

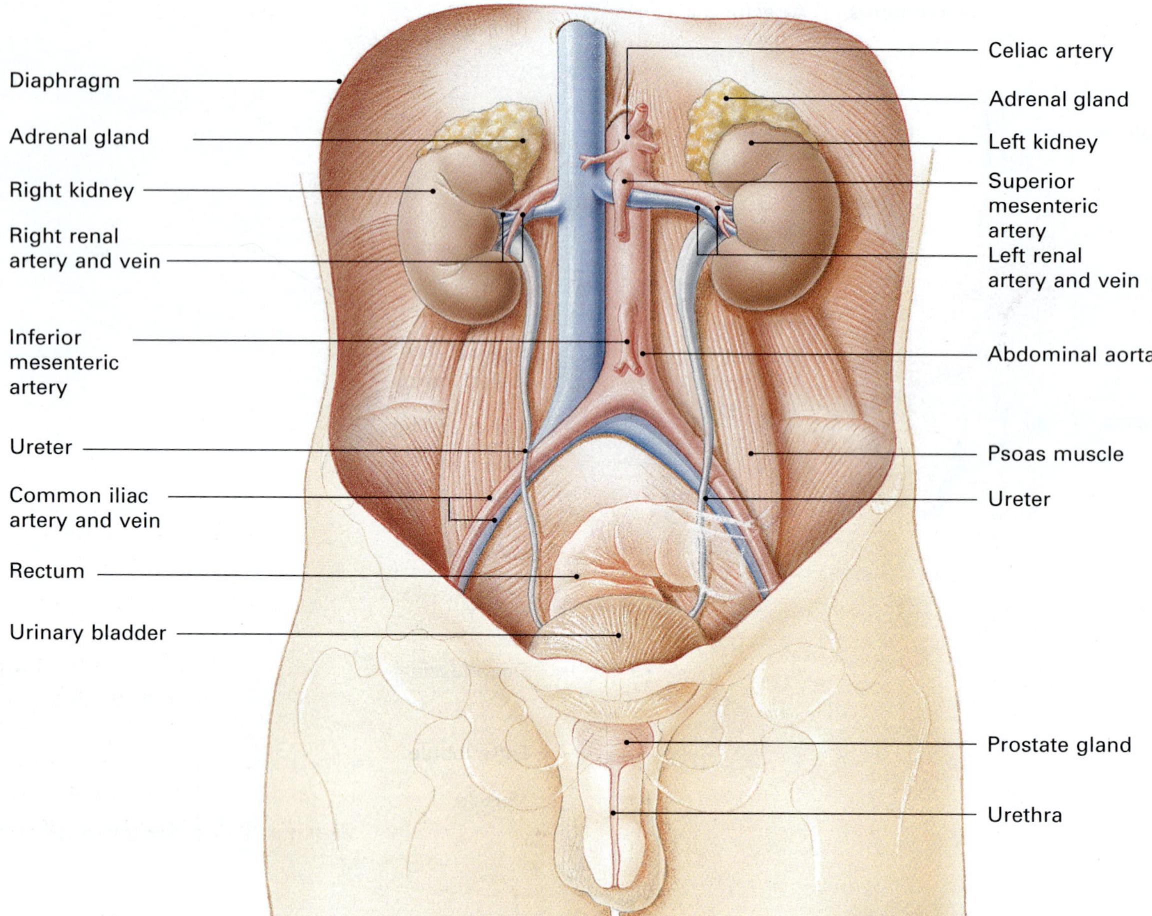

Figure 4–15 The urinary system.

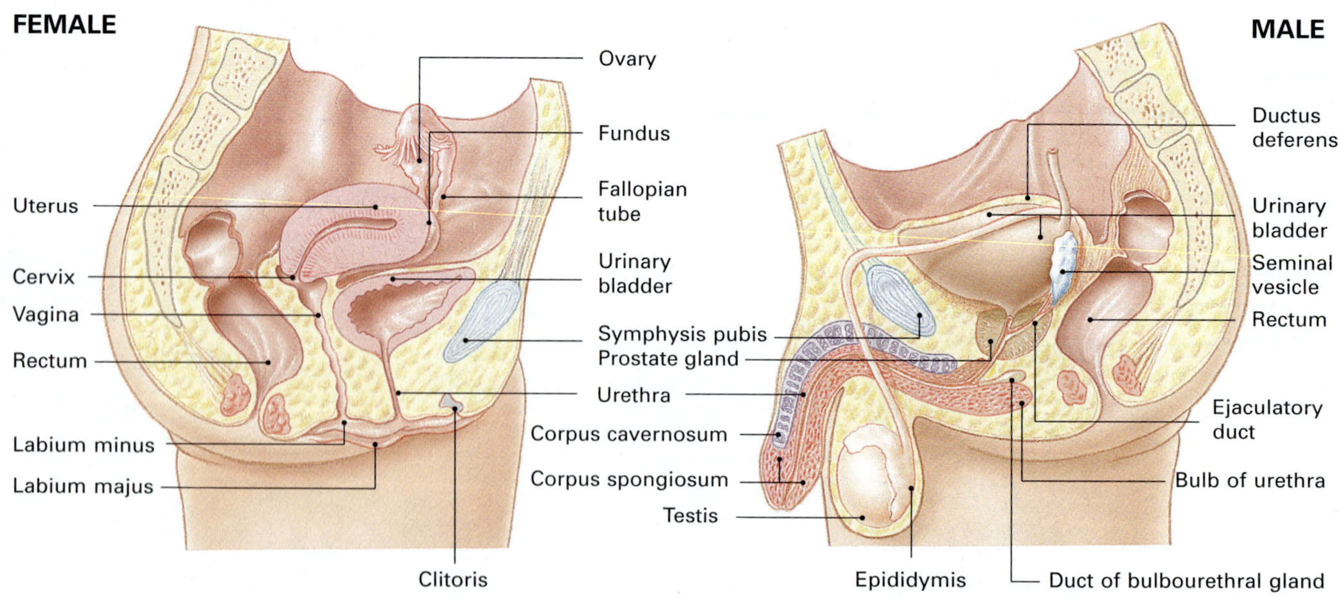

Figure 4–16 The reproductive system.

EMR FOCUS

Consider these important tasks: opening an airway, examining a patient for the ability to move a part of his or her body, and updating incoming EMS personnel via radio. Each task requires knowledge of the human body.

To open an airway or examine a patient for breathing, you must know how the body breathes and how to recognize when it is not doing so adequately. To examine for injuries to the spine or certain bones, you may wish to check for the patient's ability to wiggle his or her fingers and toes. Your knowledge of the human body will let you know why that is important. When reporting a patient's condition, you must be able to describe it accurately to the incoming paramedics. It is your knowledge of the body that will make this possible.

CASE STUDY FOLLOW-UP

At the beginning of this chapter, you read that EMRs were providing emergency care to a patient who "hurt her left leg." To see how the chapter information applies to this emergency, read the following. It describes how the call was completed.

PATIENT HISTORY

I asked the patient to describe what happened. She said she missed a step as she was getting off the escalator. She didn't fall the entire flight. She said she felt a twisting and then a sudden pain in her lower left leg. She denied allergies. She told us that she didn't take any medications or have any medical problems. She had eaten a burger for lunch at the mall's food court.

ONGOING ASSESSMENT

We rechecked the pulse, movement, and sensation below the injury. They were all present and the same as the first time we checked. We rechecked her vital signs. Pulse was 84, strong, and regular. Respirations were 16, regular, and deep. Blood pressure was 114/78. We made sure she was comfortable and continued to monitor her carefully.

TRANSFER OF CARE

When the paramedics arrived, my partner gave them the hand-off report:

"This is Ellen Levine. She is 43 years old. She was getting off the escalator and missed a step. She felt a twisting in her left lower leg. She never lost consciousness and denies any other injury from the fall. She has pain, swelling, and deformity in the distal third of her tib/fib. There is adequate pulse, motor function, and sensation distal to the injury. The remainder of the physical exam was negative. We've held manual stabilization on the injured leg. Ellen's vital signs are pulse 84, strong, and regular; respirations 16 and adequate; blood pressure 114/78."

While the paramedics immobilized the patient's leg in a splint, we helped keep onlookers from invading her privacy. It wasn't long before the paramedics and the patient were ready to head for the ambulance. We walked with them to make sure the way was clear. At the ambulance, we helped get the stretcher loaded.

It was an eventful night. We were glad that the patient turned out to be okay.

It is of the utmost importance that you have basic knowledge of the human body. It is just as important for you to be able to use that knowledge to communicate a patient's condition to other health care professionals. Learn the language. Speak it and write it every chance you get. You will need it throughout this course and in the field.

NOCPs

6.1 Utilize differential diagnosis skills, decision making skills, and psychomotor skills in providing care to patients.

REVIEW QUESTIONS

Page references where answers may be found or supported are provided at the end of each question.

SECTION 1

1. How does a patient appear when he or she is in the anatomical position? Lateral recumbent position? Supine? Prone? (p. 38)

2. What are the definitions of the terms *anterior, medial, distal, superficial,* and *external?* (p. 38)

SECTION 2

3. What is the anatomy and function of the musculoskeletal system? Give a brief description. (pp. 40–42)

4. What is the anatomy and function of the respiratory system? Give a brief description. (pp. 42, 44)

5. What is the anatomy and function of the circulatory system? Give a brief description. (pp. 44–46)

6. State three functions of the integumentary system. (p. 46)

7. Which system does not function properly in a person with diabetes? (pp. 47–49)

5

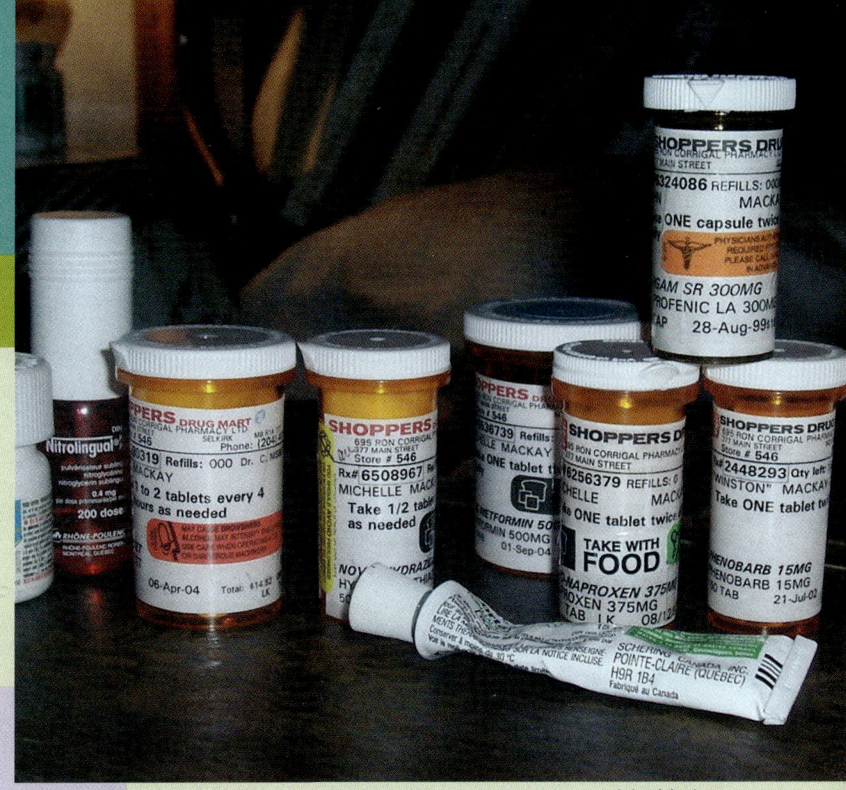

John Mackay

Pharmaceuticals

OBJECTIVES

1. List the four different ways to name a drug.
2. Differentiate among the different classes of medication.
3. Describe at least four routes of drug administration.
4. Explain how basic knowledge of pharmaceuticals can help you perform your duties as an EMR, and explain how you can identify a drug.

INTRODUCTION

There are many different patient medications that you, as an EMR, will encounter while assessing a scene. Many of these will show up very often since, as you will learn, there are a number of common medical conditions associated with specific groups within the population.

While your patient and bystanders may not always be able to convey a concise medical history, the medications you do discover can alert you to your patient's pre-existing conditions. This chapter will introduce you to common classes of medications, what the medications are used for, and how they might be administered.

SECTION 1
DRUG NAMES AND CLASSIFICATION

As an EMR, you need not become a pharmacist in order to be able to deduce a patient's medical history. Familiarizing yourself with popular drug classes as you read this chapter and as you encounter them in your practice will better equip you to understand a patient's medical condition.

Drug Names

There are four different ways to name a drug (Table 5–1). The **chemical name** describes the chemical and molecular structure of a drug. The **official name** can be found in the **Compendium of Pharmaceuticals and Specialties (CPS)**, which is used by hospital staff and pharmacists across Canada (Figure 5–1). As an EMR, you will most often use the **generic name**, which is a non-proprietary name, or the **brand name**, which is a proprietary name given by the manufacturer and most readily identified by consumers. Brand names are capitalized; generic names are not.

Whereas paramedics and hospital staff can perform tests to discover the cause of a patient's condition, you, as the EMR, can learn a lot about a patient from the medications you find at a call. As you read this chapter, and as you become acquainted with common medications during your practice, you will see that much can be learned by reading labels.

Drug Classifications

Depending on its use, a drug is categorized into one of several broad groups, called its **classification**. Table 5–2 lists several drug classifications, including some of the most common generic and brand names that you will encounter in your practice. In the first column, generic names are listed first, and brand names are given in parentheses. Note the complications that can arise if a patient takes an **overdose (OD)**.

Understanding classifications of pharmaceuticals can help you paint a clearer picture of a patient's current condition. A patient, recently prescribed a pain control medication, who is now lethargic or confused, may be sensitive to that medication. Elderly patients who appear dehydrated may not be drinking

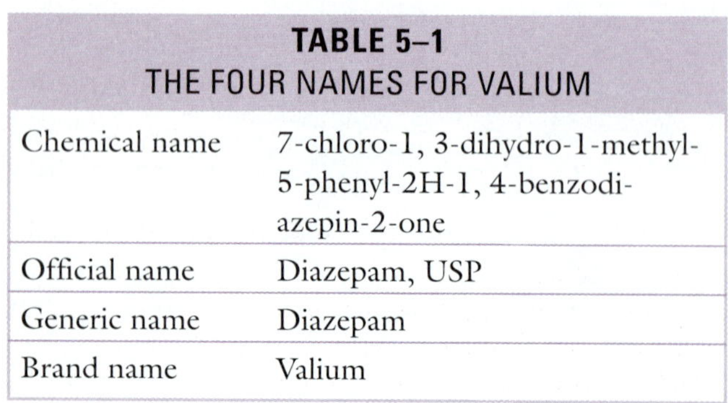

TABLE 5–1
THE FOUR NAMES FOR VALIUM

Chemical name	7-chloro-1, 3-dihydro-1-methyl-5-phenyl-2H-1, 4-benzodi-azepin-2-one
Official name	Diazepam, USP
Generic name	Diazepam
Brand name	Valium

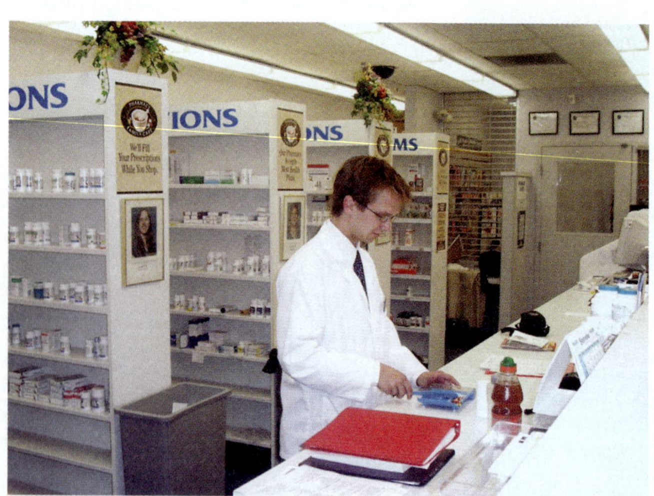

Figure 5–1 A pharmacist.

CASE STUDY

Dispatch

Our EMR unit was dispatched for a confused patient with an unknown medical history.

Scene Assessment

The caretaker of the apartment building to which we were dispatched met us at the front door and informed us that our patient was a woman of "40 something" who had moved into the complex two weeks before. The caretaker, Gus, had scheduled maintenance on the patient's air conditioner that morning, but he had to let himself in when there was no reply at her door. After putting on our gloves, we entered and found Mrs. Frankeweiller lying dishevelled with a cushion and quilt on the floor of her living room, between the couch and the coffee table. The rest of the apartment was clean and tidy, but the patient's clothes were soiled with urine and vomit.

Primary Assessment

The patient seemed to look right through us and could not respond intelligently through her snoring respirations. Her skin was pale and sweaty, and her radial pulse was notably fast. Seeing that she was too conscious for us to insert an oral airway, we applied a non-rebreather mask and notified the paramedics as we continued our assessment.

> There are numerous causes of altered mental status and different types of abnormal respirations. Are snoring respirations indicative of airway compromise? How might they differ from an airway obstruction, and what might be their relation to an altered level of consciousness? These will be discussed in later chapters.

or eating enough, or they may have recently increased their dosage of water pills.

Counting the number of pills in a bottle can be very helpful when determining if the patient has been adhering to the recommended daily dosage. The label will tell you how much medication was originally in the bottle. Based on the current date, if you calculate the number of pills that should be left in the bottle if taken properly, you may be able to determine if the medication has been ignored or taken in excess. This is particularly helpful when you are called to a potential overdose.

SECTION 2
DRUG ADMINISTRATION AND DRUG FORMS

The most common medication administered by EMRs and paramedics is supplemental oxygen. Some EMS systems may allow you to assist a patient with taking their own prescribed medication such as ASA or nitroglycerin. In order to avoid contamination or absorption,

TABLE 5–2
CLASSIFICATION OF COMMON MEDICATIONS

Medication	Uses	Conditions occurring with OD
Anti-inflammatories, Analgesics		
Acetaminophen (Tylenol)	Pain	Liver failure
Acetaminophen and oxycodone (ratio-Oxycocet, Percocet)	Pain	Liver failure, respiratory depression
Acetylsalicylic acid, ASA (Aspirin)	Pain, reducing clotting	Respiratory alkalosis, bleeding, arrhythmias, seizures, coma
Ibuprofen (Advil, Motrin)	Pain	Gastrointestinal bleeding
Antianxiety Drugs, Sedatives		
Diazepam (Valium)	Anxiety, seizures	Respiratory depression, depressed level of consciousness (LOC)
Triazolam (Halcion)	Sedative effect	Depressed LOC
Antibiotics		
Ciprofloxacin (Cipro)	Bacterial infections	Seizures, dysuria, weakness, skin discolouration
Erythromycin	Bacterial infections	Nausea, vomiting, abdominal pain, hearing loss
Penicillin (Pen-Vee)	Bacterial infections	Confusion, rash, dysuria, seizures
Tetracycline (Novo-Tetra)	Bacterial infections	Nausea, vomiting, diarrhea
Antimalarial Drugs		
Quinine (Apo-Quinine)	Malaria	Headache, nausea, vomiting, confusion, vision/hearing loss, sweating, irregular heart rate, fainting, death
Antihyperlipidemic Drugs		
Atorvastatin (Lipitor)	High cholesterol	No life-threatening conditions identified
Simvastatin (Zocor)	High cholesterol	No life-threatening conditions identified
Anticonvulsants		
Carbamazepine (Tegretol)	Epilepsy, seizure disorders	Respiratory depression, coma
Clonazepam (Rivotril)	Seizures	Depressed LOC, respiratory depression
Lorazepam (Ativan)	Seizures	Depressed LOC
Phenytoin (Dilantin)	Epilepsy, seizures	Arrhythmias, respiratory depression
Valproic acid (Depakene)	Epilepsy, seizures	Arrhythmias, coma
Antidepressants		
Amitriptyline (Elavil)	Depression	Cardiac arrest, seizures
Citalopram (Celexa)	Depression	Seizures
Doxepin (Sinequan)	Depression	Cardiac arrest, seizures
Paroxetine (Paxil)	Depression	Seizures
Sertraline (Zoloft)	Depression	Seizures
Venlafaxine (Effexor)	Depression	Seizures
Antihistamines		
Diphenhydramine (Benadryl)	Allergy symptoms	Confusion, seizures, fatigue, flushing, fever
Sympathomimetics		
Epinephrine (EpiPen)	Emergency treatment of severe allergic reaction	Tachycardia, headache, decreased vision

(continued)

Medication	Uses	Conditions occurring with OD
Antihypertensives, Diuretics ("water pills")		
Amlodipine (Norvasc)	Hypertension (HTN), congestive heart failure (CHF)	Hypotension, bradycardia
Captopril (Capoten)	HTN, CHF	Hypotension
Enalapril (Vasotec)	HTN	Hypotension
Furosemide (Lasix)	HTN, CHF	Hypotension, dehydration
Hydrochlorothiazide (Apo-Hydro)	HTN, CHF	Hypotension, dehydration
Labetalol (Trandate)	HTN	Hypotension, bradycardia
Lisinopril (Zestril)	HTN, CHF	Hypotension
Metoprolol (Lopressor)	Angina, HTN, arrhythmias	Hypotension, bradycardia
Nifedipine (Adalat)	HTN	Hypotension, bradycardia
Potassium chloride (Slow-K)	CHF	Electrolyte imbalance
Spironolactone (Aldactone)	HTN, CHF	Nausea, vomiting, diarrhea, gastric bleeding, drowsiness
Antidysrhythmics, Antianginals (cardiac medications)		
Amiodarone (Cordarone)	Severe tachycardia, V-tach/fib	CNS effects, hypotension, bradycardia
Digoxin (Lanoxin)	CHF, irregular heartbeat (A-fib)	Potential for cardiac complications
Diltiazem (Cardizem)	Angina, HTN, arrhythmias	Hypotension, bradycardia
Isosorbide dinitrate (Isordil)	Angina	Hypotension
Metoprolol (Lopressor)	Angina, HTN, arrhythmias	Hypotension, bradycardia
Nitroglycerin	Angina, CHF	Hypotension, headache, nausea
Anticoagulants		
Warfarin (Coumadin)	Blood thinning, reducing clotting	Bleeding, bruising
ASA (Aspirin)	Pain, reducing clotting	Respiratory alkalosis, bleeding, arrhythmias, seizures, coma
Bronchodilators		
Aminophylline	Severe asthma, chronic obstructive pulmonary disease (COPD)	Arrhythmias, seizures
Budesonide and formoterol (Symbicort)	Asthma, COPD	Chest pain, nausea, vomiting, insomnia, tremors, tachycardia, fainting, seizures
Fluticasone (Flovent)	Asthma, COPD	Tachycardia
Ipratropium (Atrovent)	Asthma, COPD	Tachycardia
Salbutamol (Ventolin)	Asthma, COPD	Tachycardia
Salmeterol and fluticasone (Advair)	Asthma, COPD	Tachycardia
Diabetic Drugs		
Glyburide (Diabeta)	Hyperglycemia	Hypoglycemia
Insulin (Humulin)	Regulation of blood sugar	Hypoglycemia
Metformin (Glucophage)	Regulation of blood sugar	Hypoglycemia, gastric upset
Thyroid Regulators		
Levothyroxine (Synthroid)	Low thyroid hormone	Chest pain, tremors, shortness of breath, leg cramps, confusion, vomiting, diarrhea, seizures

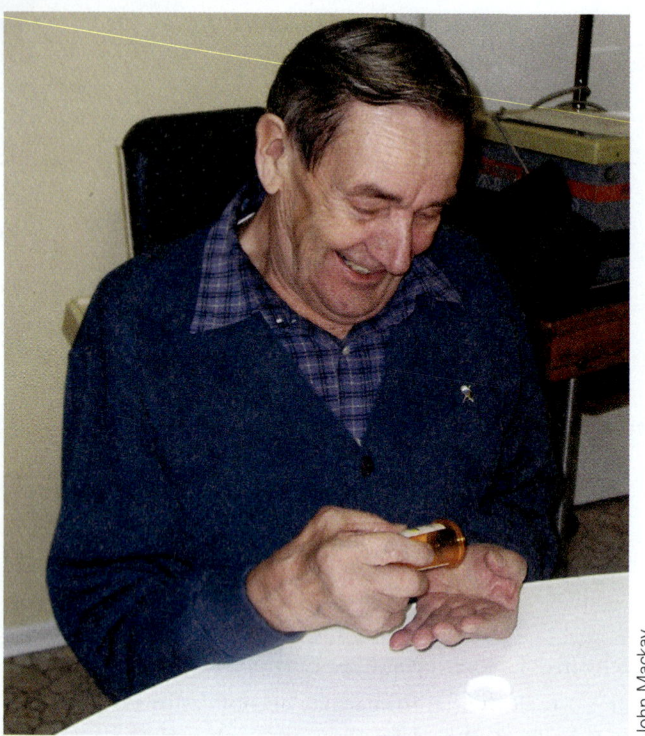

Figure 5–2 A patient taking medication.

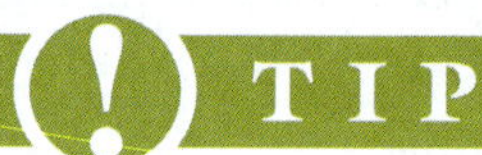

you should wear gloves and not touch the medication directly. Medication such as ASA can be collected in the cap of the container it is provided in and then dumped into the patient's hand for self-administration. Generally, a patient must be able to take the medication independently before you can assist him or her (Figure 5–2). Do not assist with medication administration unless warranted in your own local protocols.

Other than symptom-relief drugs like salbutamol, nitroglycerin, and epinephrine auto-injectors (EpiPens) (Figure 5–3), you should encourage patients to hold off taking prescription medications until paramedics arrive. Patients who are nauseated may vomit when trying to take oral medication.

> **TIP**
>
> As an EMR you will often witness paramedics administer symptom-relief drugs. These can include acetylsalicylic acid (ASA), nitroglycerin (commonly called "nitro"), salbutamol (Ventolin), oral glucose, and, of course, oxygen, the drug most often given for emergency patients.

Consider the five "rights" of drug administration as you inspect a patient's medication:

1. The right patient: The drug prescription was designated for this patient.
2. The right drug: Patients often store pills in bottles other than the original one!

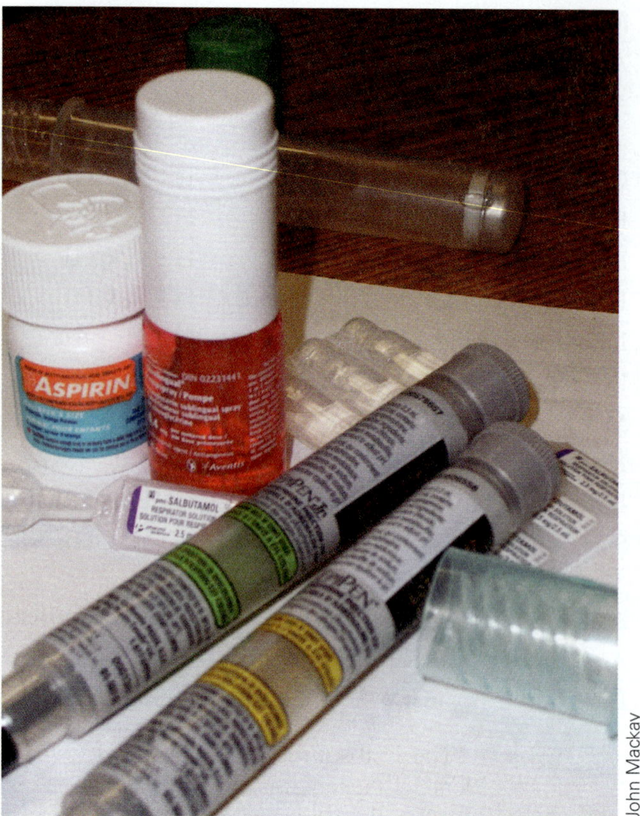

Figure 5–3 Symptom-relief medications.

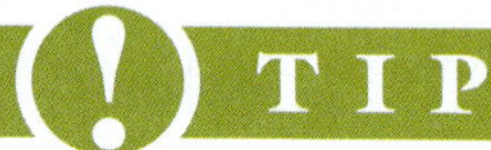

3. The right date and time: Expired drugs may be ineffective; medication should be taken at the prescribed time.
4. The right dosage: Taking too little or too much of a drug can adversely affect its effectiveness.
5. The right route: The right route is important in order for the drug to have the desired effect.

> **TIP**
>
> You should assess a patient's vital signs before he or she self-administers any medication. Nitroglycerin, for example, can dramatically lower the blood pressure of a patient who may already be suffering from hypotension.

The route by which a drug is administered will determine how quickly it is absorbed and utilized by the body. Having a basic understanding of the routes of administration and the forms that a drug comes in will allow you to better understand a patient's condition and, therefore, his or her medical history.

There are two main routes by which drugs are taken: **enteral** and **parenteral**. Enteral routes are those that involve the digestive tract, which begins at the mouth and ends at the rectum. The routes may be oral, nasogastric, orogastric, sublingual, buccal, or rectal. Parenteral routes are those that do not involve the digestive tract. These routes may be intravenous, endotracheal, umbilical, topical, intramuscular, nasal, or others. Some parenteral routes offer a faster method of delivery and absorption than enteral routes.

Enteral Routes

- *Oral.* Taking medication by mouth, or **PO (per os)**, is the most common method since it is a good way to self-administer drugs. Patients use this method for most of their everyday medications. Aside from ASA (Aspirin), which may be given by paramedics when a heart attack is suspected, very few drugs are given orally in emergency situations.
- *Nasogastric/orogastric (NG/OG).* This route delivers medication to the stomach through a tube that is already in place. It is an alternative to the oral route.
- *Sublingual (SL).* The below-the-tongue route can be used by the patient or the emergency worker since the capillaries in the mouth very quickly absorb medication. There is little potential for gastric upset because the drug is absorbed in the oral cavity. Nitro spray or tablets are taken this way for angina.
- *Buccal.* This route is similar to the sublingual one, with absorption occurring between the cheek and gums. Oral glucose paste or gel may be absorbed by the sublingual or buccal route.
- *Rectal.* This route is used when a patient is vomiting, unconscious, or very young and cannot cooperate with oral or intravenous administration. Diazepam (Valium) for seizures or dimenhydrinate (Gravol) for nausea may be given by emergency personnel through this route, and patients may use rectal suppositories or enemas for constipation. Small children may receive an acetaminophen (Tylenol) suppository to help control a high temperature if they are nauseated or cannot swallow pills.

Parenteral Routes

- *Intravenous (IV).* This route is most used during emergencies because it delivers the medication directly into the bloodstream. Epinephrine (also called adrenaline) for cardiac conditions, diazepam (Valium) for seizures, and dextrose (a sugar) for diabetes are routinely administered intravenously by paramedics.
- *Endotracheal (ET).* Paramedics may insert an endotracheal tube into a patient's trachea as a means of securing the airway. If an IV has not been established, some medications may be administered down the ET tube to be rapidly absorbed by the rich vasculature of the lungs.
- *Intraosseous (IO).* Young children have soft bones that are still developing. Periodically, this route may be used by inserting a needle into the marrow of a long bone (where blood cells originate). Fluid or medication may be given by this route because it dumps directly from the bone into the circulatory system. The IO has become more popular in adult resuscitation.
- *Umbilical.* In newborns, the umbilical vein or arteries can provide suitable IV access.
- *Intramuscular (IM).* Injection into muscular tissue is a slower route of administration than an IV injection but does allow the drug to pass into the capillaries. Paramedics or patients themselves may use an epinephrine auto-injector (EpiPen) to counteract the effects of an allergic reaction. This route, by allowing the drug to be absorbed more slowly, can benefit the patient for a longer period of time.
- *Subcutaneous (SC, SQ, or SubQ).* Medication injected just beneath the skin takes longer to absorb than an IM injection since there are fewer capillaries here than in muscle tissue.
- *Inhalation/nebulization.* Salbutamol (Ventolin) from puffers is self-administered by patients and is inhaled and absorbed by the lungs. The lungs also absorb the drug when PCPs or higher-level practitioners administer it through a nebulizer mask, which is set at 6 L/min (litres per minute).
- *Topical.* Medications in the form of a cream, gel, or ointment are applied to and absorbed directly through the skin.
- *Transdermal.* This route utilizes the skin as well. A nitro patch, for example, provides slow, continuous release of the drug through the skin.
- *Nasal.* Medication is absorbed directly into the nasal mucosa. Cocaine addicts and solvent sniffers are accustomed to this route; however, prescribed medications are just beginning to be offered this way.
- *Instillation.* Examples of medications delivered by this route are eye and ear drops and medications that can be directly applied into a wound. New trauma dressings that contain clotting agents can control bleeding when applied to a wound.

Drug Forms

Drugs may be categorized into two main forms: solids and liquids. Generally, solids are given orally. They include several forms. **Pills** are spherically shaped and sometimes coated to ease swallowing. **Powders**, although not very popular, can be mixed with a liquid and taken orally. **Tablets** are powders that have been compressed into a disk-like shape. **Suppositories** are bullet shaped and have a wax-like base that melts at body temperature when placed in the rectum or vagina. **Capsules** are gelatin containers that dissolve in the gastrointestinal tract, releasing the powders or small pills contained within them.

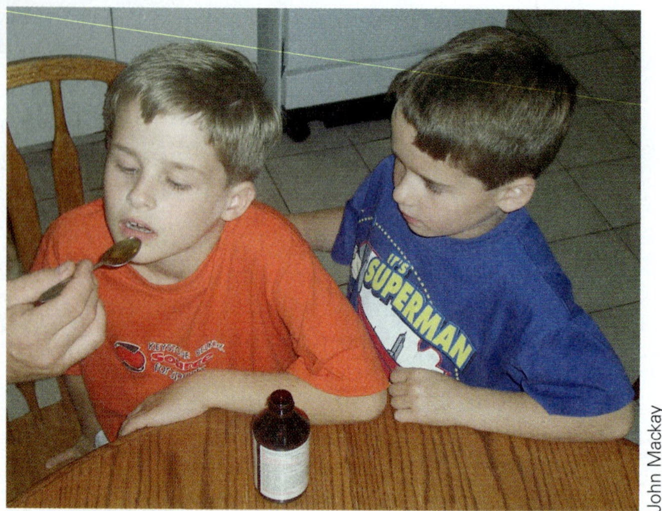

Figure 5–4 A child taking an elixir.

John Mackay

Liquid drugs are often composed of a solid drug (solute) that has been dissolved in a liquid base (solvent). They may be taken either enterally or parenterally and are supplied in several forms. **Solutions** generally use a water base but may be oil based. **Tinctures** are prepared by a process that uses alcohol to extract the drug. Some alcohol may remain in the end product. **Suspensions** are solutions in which the solute does not dissolve in the solvent but rather remains as minute particles suspended in the solvent. Shake suspensions well before using as the drug can settle out. **Emulsions** are drug suspensions in an oily solute or solvent. **Spirits** are solutions of volatile drugs dissolved in alcohol. **Elixirs** use alcohol and water as the solvent. Even though flavourings may be added to make them palatable, they still taste bad (Figure 5–4). **Syrups** are made from drugs dissolved in a thick sugar and water solution.

EMR FOCUS

Many common conditions are treated with several common medications. When you are unable to obtain a verbal history from anyone at a scene, the medications you discover can be as telling as physical evidence is to a crime scene investigator. You can interpret the clues immediately if you understand what different medications are used for. Reading the label is important—as important to you, the practitioner, as it is to the patient. If you are not sure what a particular medication is used for, you can ask the patient. You can also purchase a pocket drug reference guide at a medical bookstore.

CASE STUDY FOLLOW-UP

At the beginning of this chapter, you read that EMRs were on the scene with a female patient who displayed an altered mental status. To see how the chapter skills apply to this emergency, read the following. It describes how the call was completed.

PATIENT HISTORY

Mrs. Frankeweiller did not appear to have any family nearby and had kept mostly to herself since moving in, so there was no one who could convey her medical history to us. A glass of water and a full bottle of Tylenol were on the kitchen table. I asked my partner to check around for other medications. We found a bottle of Celexa and one of Dilantin in the cupboard above the sink, along with numerous vitamin bottles and a tub of betamethasone cream.

SECONDARY ASSESSMENT

I continued my assessment while speaking slowly and clearly to Mrs. Frankeweiller. My partner checked her vital signs. Her respirations were 22, and her pulse was 104. Her blood pressure was 132/90, and her skin was warm and drying up.

ONGOING ASSESSMENT

Mrs. Frankeweiller began to pull the oxygen mask off her face but then became more compliant as her level of consciousness seemed to improve. She still seemed somewhat confused, and she asked "What happened?" and "What are you doing here?" over and over again.

TRANSFER OF CARE

When the paramedics arrived, Mrs. Frankeweiller was alert enough to know that other people had entered the apartment. I conveyed to them the scenario we had discovered, the medications we had found, and her vital signs. Her snoring respirations cleared up as her level of consciousness improved. Having not smelled or seen evidence of alcohol, I suggested that she might have had a seizure. Her incontinence and the Dilantin were my best clues.

A paramedic agreed that a seizure was likely, but he also suggested that her antidepressant, Celexa, could have caused a seizure if she had OD'd. He checked her blood sugar to rule out a diabetic problem and said that there were a number of possible causes for her altered mental status, including stroke.

Mrs. Frankeweiller commented from the ambulance cot as they wheeled her away that she had epilepsy but had not had any seizures in the past six months. She said she had been overdoing it getting settled in her apartment and thought that maybe she had missed taking some of her pills.

Pharmacies can supply prescriptions in "bubble packs." These, as well as pill counters, can help you easily determine how compliant the patient has been with the instructions for his or her medication. Unfortunately, pills are often hoarded and sometimes stored in non-original bottles. Find all the medications you can when summoned to a patient's home, and do not hesitate to ask what they are being used for.

NOCPs

4.2 b Obtain patient's medication profile **S**

d Obtain information regarding patient's past medical history **S**

f Obtain information regarding incident through accurate and complete scene assessment **S**

REVIEW QUESTIONS

Page references where answers may be found or supported are provided at the end of each question.

SECTION 1

1. What is the CPS? (p. 56)

2. What is the difference between a brand name and a generic name of a medication? (p. 56)

3. Give a name of a drug used as a "water pill" and suggest what condition it might be used for. (p. 59)

SECTION 2

4. Which drug do EMRs and paramedics administer most frequently? (p. 57)

5. What precautions should be taken when inspecting a patient's medication? (p. 60)

6. How are most patients' medications administered? (p. 61)

7. What are two other ways in which a person might take his or her medication? (pp. 60–61)

8. Which routes of drug administration are most likely to be used by paramedics? (p. 61)

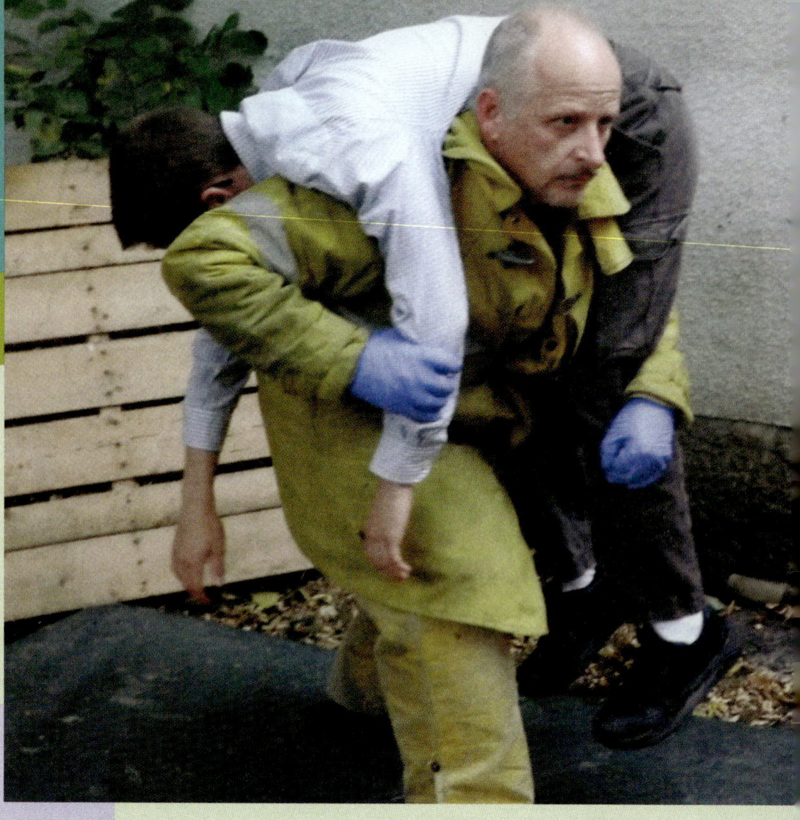

Lifting and Moving Patients

OBJECTIVES

1. Discuss body mechanics and the four principles that need to be followed when lifting or moving a patient.

2. Explain how good posture and physical fitness can contribute to your well-being as an EMS provider.

3. Describe the indications for both an emergency and a non-emergency move.

4. Describe and demonstrate five types of emergency moves, and discuss the devices you may use to move a patient.

INTRODUCTION

After receiving emergency care, a patient may need to be moved or transported. If this is done improperly, the patient may be injured further. It is your responsibility to see that the patient is not subjected to unnecessary pain or discomfort.

Each EMS system defines if and when EMRs may move patients. Generally, you may move only patients who are in immediate danger. You may position patients to prevent further injury. You also may assist other EMS workers in moving patients. Learn and follow your local protocols.

SECTION 1
BODY MECHANICS

Basic Principles

As an EMS worker, you may be asked to lift and carry either patients or heavy equipment. If you do it incorrectly, you could cause yourself injury, strain, and lifelong pain. With planning, good health, and skill, you can do your job with minimum risk to yourself.

Apply the principles of proper lifting and moving every day. Practise enough so that they become automatic. Make them a habit that increases your safety and performance, even in the most stressful emergency situations.

Body mechanics refers to the safest and most efficient methods of using your body to gain a mechanical advantage. It includes the following:

- *Use your legs to lift, not your back.* To move a heavy object, use the muscles of your legs, hips, and buttocks, plus the contracted muscles of your abdomen. These muscles let you safely generate a lot of power. Never use the muscles in your back to help you move or lift a heavy object.
- *Keep the weight of the object as close to your body as possible.* Try to reach only across a short distance to lift a heavy object (Figure 6–1). Back injury is much more likely to occur when you reach across a long distance to lift an object.
- *"Stack."* Visualize your shoulders stacked above your hips and your hips above your feet. Then move as a unit. If your shoulders, hips, and feet are not aligned, you could create twisting forces that can harm your lower back.
- *Reduce the height or distance you need to move the object.* Get closer to the object, or reposition it before you lift it. Lift in stages if you need to.

Apply the principles of body mechanics to lifting, carrying, moving, reaching, pushing, and pulling. The key to preventing injury during all these tasks is correct alignment of the spine. Keep a normal inward curve in the lower back. Keep the wrists and knees in normal alignment. Whenever possible, let the equipment do the lifting for you.

In an emergency, teamwork is essential. Just as a football coach positions players according to ability, rescuers should position themselves that way too. Doing so can help them use their abilities to ensure the best outcome in any emergency.

All members of a team should be trained in the proper techniques. Problems can occur when team members are greatly mismatched in strength. The stronger partner can be injured if the weaker one fails to lift. The weaker one can be injured if he or she tries to do too much. Ideally, partners in lifting and moving should have adequate and equal strength and height. Know your physical ability and limitations. Respect them. Consider the weight of the patient and what you are capable of lifting. Recognize when help is needed.

Team members also need to clearly and frequently communicate during a task. Use commands that are easy for team members to understand. Verbally coordinate each lift from beginning to end.

The Power Lift

The **power lift** is a technique that offers you the best defence against injury. It also protects the patient on a stretcher with a safe and stable move. It is especially useful for rescuers who have weak knees or thighs. Remember, when performing the power lift, keep your back locked and avoid bending at the waist (Figure 6–2). Follow these steps:

1. Place your feet a comfortable distance apart. For the average-sized person, this is usually about shoulder width. Taller rescuers might prefer a little wider stance.

CASE STUDY

Dispatch

My partner and I were returning from a call in our emergency medical response vehicle when we came upon the scene of a car crash. It really took us by surprise. At least when you are dispatched, you have time to prepare for what you might see.

Scene Assessment

We parked a safe distance away from the scene. As we were about to exit our vehicle, we saw smoke billowing out from under the hood of the car. The fire must have been fuelled by oil. We called the dispatcher to notify the fire department.

We had turnout gear on, so we carefully approached the car. A woman was in the driver's seat. She seemed dazed. The smoke was filling the car. The windshield was turning black. Then we saw flames. We were sure the passenger compartment would be on fire before long.

> Lifting and moving patients is an important responsibility. Many lifts and moves are routine, while others require quick thinking and skill. Consider this patient as you read Chapter 6. Is it within the EMRs' scope of care to move her? If so, how can they do it without causing further injury?

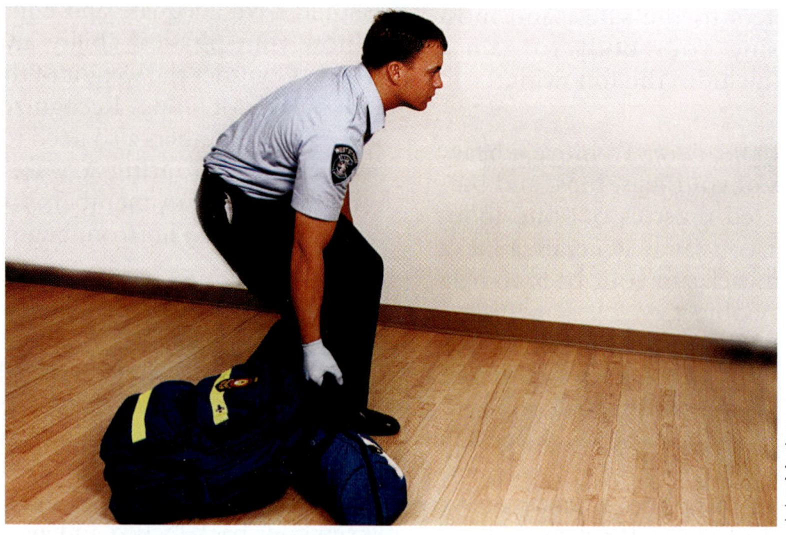

Figure 6–1 Keep weight close to the body as it is lifted.

POWER LIFT

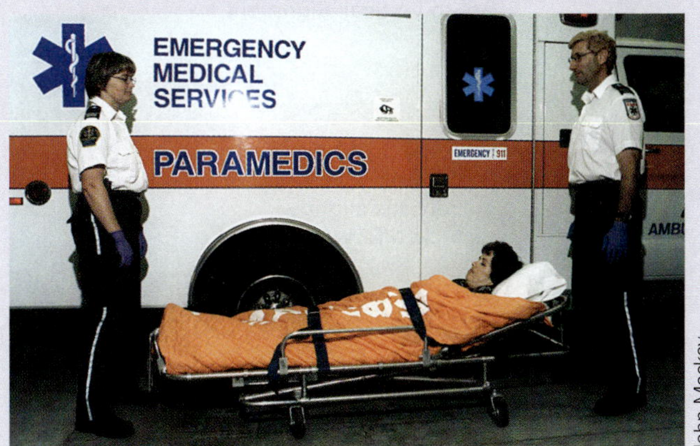

Figure 6–2a Get in position.

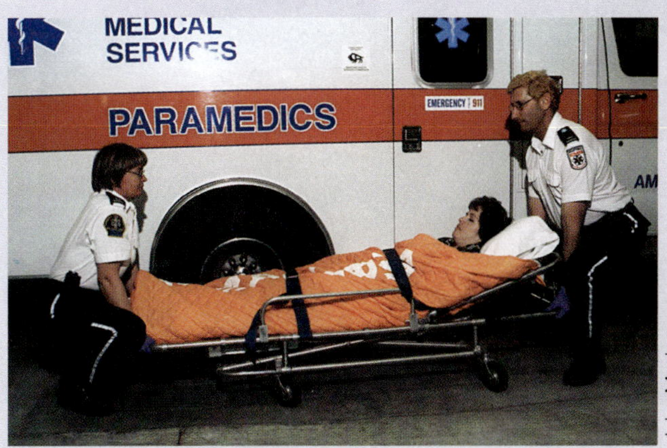

Figure 6–2b Lift in unison, keeping your back locked, knees bent, and feet flat.

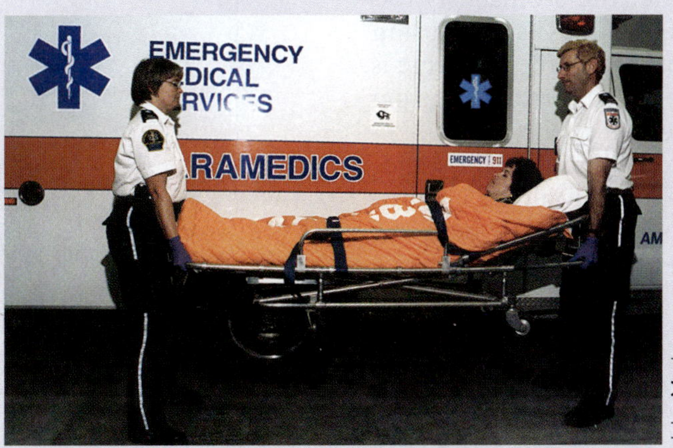

Figure 6–2c Stand straight, making sure your back remains locked.

2. Turn your feet slightly outward. Most people find that this helps them feel more comfortable and more stable.

3. Bend your knees to bring your centre of gravity closer to the object. As you bend your knees, you should feel as though you are sitting down, not falling forward.

4. Tighten the muscles of your back and abdomen to splint the vulnerable lower back. Your back should remain as straight as you can comfortably manage, with your head facing forward in a **neutral position**. This means that the head is not turned to the side, tilted forward, or tilted back.

5. Keep your feet flat with your weight evenly distributed and just forward of the heels.

6. Place your hands a comfortable distance from each other to provide balance to the object as it is lifted. This is usually at least 25 cm (centimetres).

7. Always use a **power grip** to get maximum force from your hands. Your palms and fingers should come in complete contact with the object, and all fingers should be bent at the same angle (Figure 6–3).

8. As the lifting begins, your back should remain locked as the force is driven through the heels and arches of your feet. Your upper body should come up before your hips do.

9. Reverse these steps to lower the object.

Posture and Fitness

Posture is a much overlooked part of body mechanics. When people spend a great deal of time sitting or standing, poor posture can easily tire the back and stomach muscles. This can only make back injury more likely.

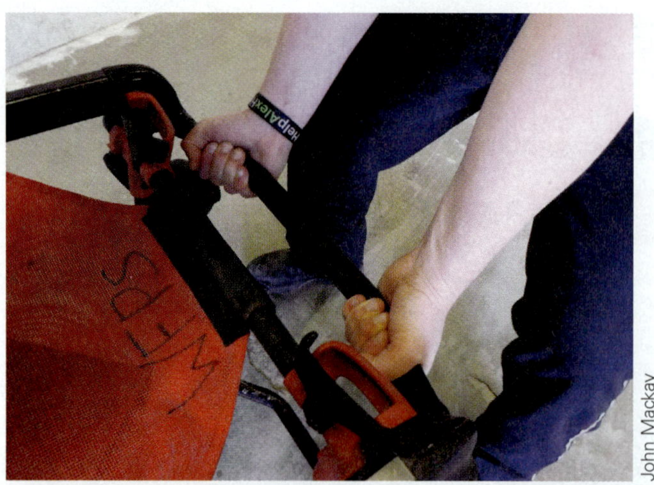

Figure 6–3 The power grip.

One extreme of poor posture is the swayback (Figure 6–4). In this example, the stomach is too far forward and the buttocks too far back, causing extreme stress on the lower back. Another extreme is the slouch. The shoulders are rolled forward, putting increased pressure on every region of the spine.

Be aware of your posture. While you are standing, your ears, shoulders, and hips should be in vertical alignment. Your knees should be slightly bent and your pelvis slightly tucked forward (Figure 6–5).

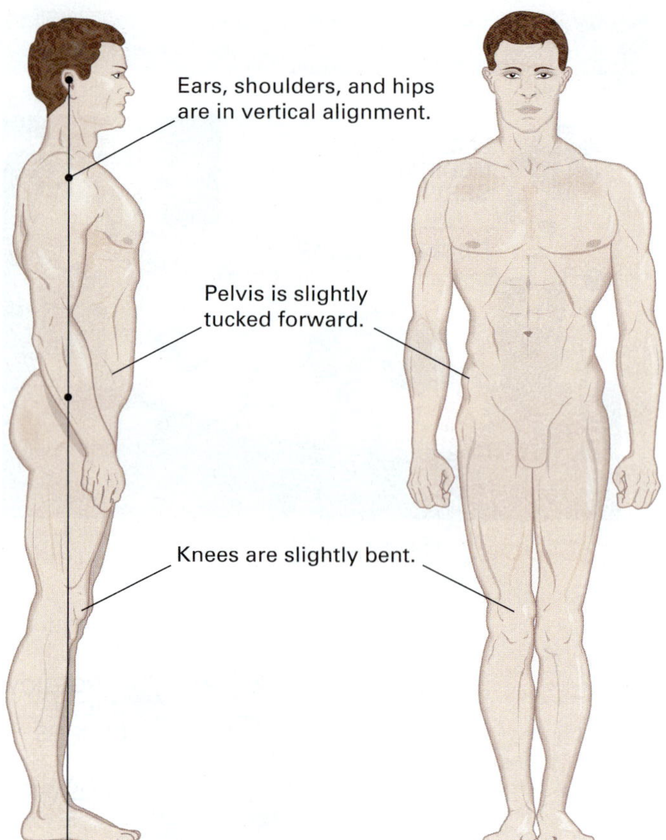

Figure 6–5 Proper standing position.

When you are sitting, your weight should be evenly distributed on both *ischia* (the lower portion of your pelvis) (Figure 6–6). Your ears, shoulders, and hips should be in vertical alignment. Your feet should be flat on the floor or crossed at the ankles. If possible, your lower back should be in contact with the support of the chair.

Finally, proper body mechanics will not protect you if you are not physically fit. Consider consulting a fitness coach or trainer. A proactive, well-balanced physical fitness program should include flexibility training, cardiovascular conditioning, strength training, and proper nutrition.

SECTION 2
PRINCIPLES OF MOVING PATIENTS

Emergency Moves

The top priority in emergency care is to maintain a patient's airway, breathing, and circulation. However, if the scene is unstable or poses an immediate threat, you may have to move the patient. Follow local protocols.

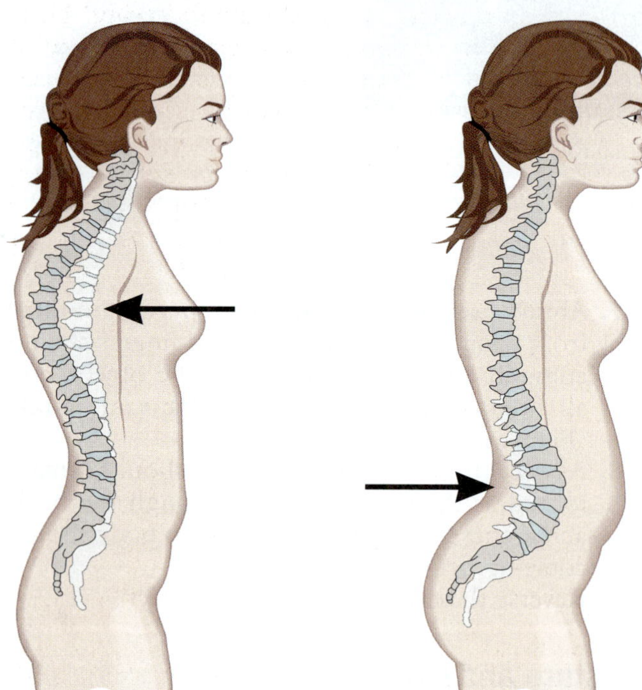

Figure 6–4 Slouch and swayback are extremes of poor posture.

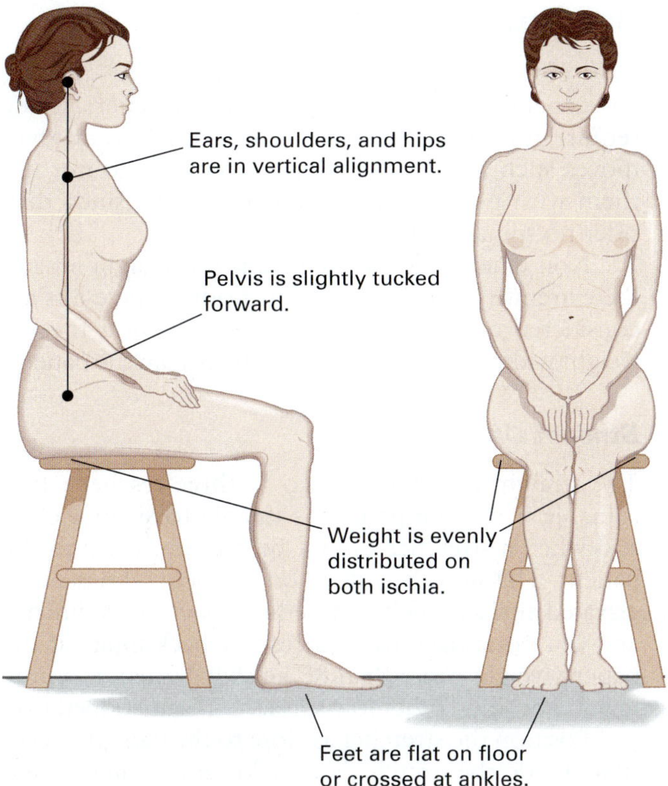

Figure 6–6 Proper sitting position.

In general, when there is no threat to life, provide emergency medical care and wait for the paramedics to move the patient. Make an **emergency move** only when there is an immediate danger to the patient. The following are conditions in which you may make an emergency move:

- *Fire or threat of fire.* Fire should always be considered a grave threat, not only to patients but also to rescuers.
- *Explosion or the threat of explosion.*
- *Inability to protect the patient from other hazards at the scene.* Examples of hazards include an unstable building, a rolled-over car, spilled gasoline or other hazardous materials, an unruly or hostile crowd, and extreme weather conditions.
- *Inability to gain access to other patients who need life-saving care.* For example, this may occur at the scene of a car crash involving two or more patients.
- *When life-saving care cannot be given because of the patient's location or position.* For example, a patient in cardiac arrest must be supine on a flat, hard surface in order for you to perform CPR properly. If that patient is sitting on a chair, an emergency move must be made in order for you to provide life-saving care.

The greatest danger in an emergency move is the possibility of worsening a spinal injury. To provide as much protection to the spine as possible, pull the patient in the direction of the long axis of the body.

It is impossible to move a patient from a vehicle quickly and protect the spine at the same time. Move the patient from the vehicle immediately only if one of the five conditions described above exists.

If the patient is on the floor or the ground, use one of the following emergency moves. However, be sure never to pull the patient's head away from the neck and shoulders. If there is time, you may wish to bind the patient's wrists together with a cravat or gauze. This will make the patient easier to move, and it will help protect the hands and arms from injury.

Shirt Drag

To perform a shirt drag, do the following. First, fasten the patient's hands or wrists loosely with a cravat or gauze to protect them during the move. Then, grasp the shoulders of the patient's shirt (not a T-shirt). Pull the shirt under the patient's head to form a support. Using the shoulders of the shirt, pull the patient toward you. Be careful not to strangle the patient. The pulling should engage the patient's armpits, not the neck (Figure 6–7).

Blanket Drag

To perform a blanket drag, do the following. First, spread a blanket alongside the patient. Gather half of it into lengthwise pleats. Roll the patient away from you onto his or her side, and tuck the pleated part of the blanket as far under him or her as you can. Then roll the patient back onto the centre of the blanket, preferably onto his or her back. Wrap the blanket securely around the patient. Grabbing the part of the blanket that is under the patient's head, drag the patient toward you (Figure 6–8).

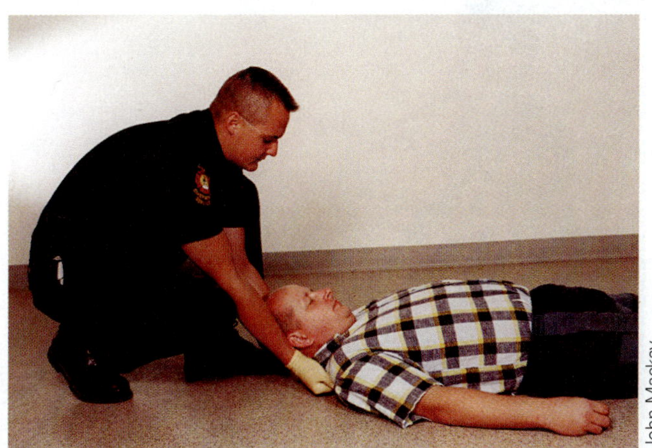

Figure 6–7 Shirt drag.

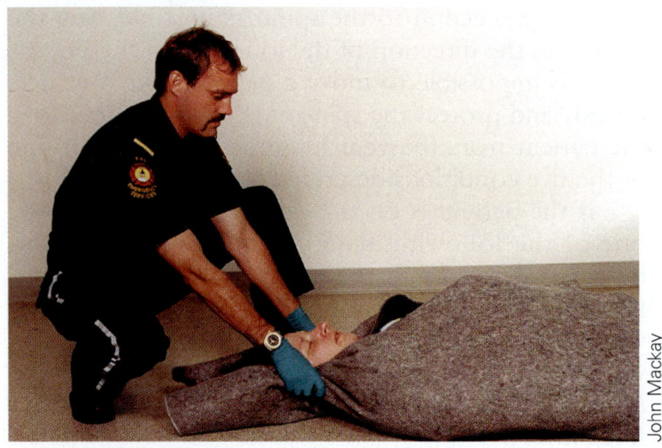

Figure 6–8 Blanket drag.

If you do not have a blanket, you can use a coat in the same way. A tarp with handles especially designed for lifting (Figure 6–14) will make a blanket drag easier but may not be as readily available as a sheet or blanket.

Shoulder and Forearm Drags

To perform a shoulder drag, do the following. First, stand at the patient's head. Then, slip your hands under the patient's armpits from the back (Figure 6–9). If you must drag the patient a long distance and need a better grip, then perform a forearm drag. Position yourself as you would in a shoulder drag. After you slip your hands under the patient's armpits, grasp the patient's forearms and drag the patient toward you. Use your own forearms as a support to keep the patient's head, neck, and spine in alignment.

Other Emergency Moves

Other emergency moves include the piggyback carry, one-rescuer crutch, cradle carry, firefighter's drag, and others (Figures 6–10 and 6–11).

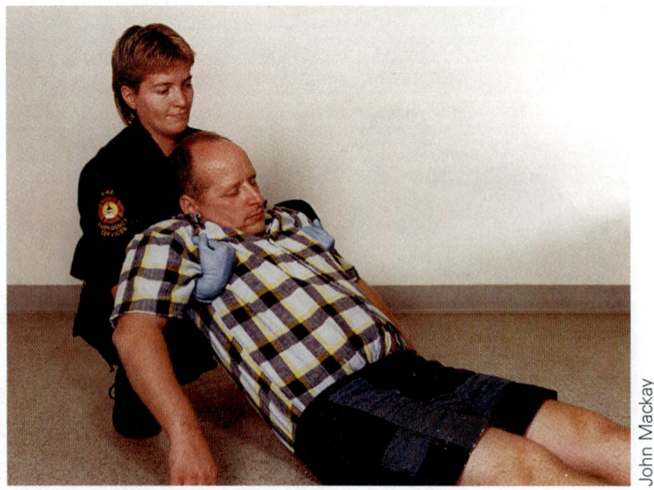

Figure 6–9 Shoulder drag.

Non-Emergency Moves

Non-emergency moves, or non-urgent moves, are generally performed with other rescuers. They require no equipment and may take less time than moves such as a blanket drag. However, do not use them with possible spinal injury patients since they offer no spinal protection.

Non-emergency moves include the straight lift and the extremity or fore and aft lift. Both of these lifts are considered **complete lifts** since rescuers bear the full weight without mechanical aid or help from the patient.

Straight Lift

The straight lift requires two or three rescuers. It is valuable when the patient is unable to sit in a chair and when a stretcher cannot be brought close to the patient. This lift is best done on a patient who is on an elevated surface, such as a bed or couch. It is difficult and can potentially cause a rescuer back injury if the patient weighs more than 85 kg (kilograms), is on the ground or some other low surface, or is uncooperative.

Position the stretcher as close to the patient as possible. Undo the stretcher straps, lower the railings, and clear any equipment off the mattress. Tell the patient what you are going to do. Warn him or her to remain still in order for you to preserve your balance. If possible, place the patient's arms on his or her chest.

To perform a straight lift, follow these steps (Figure 6–12 on p. 73):

1. Line up on one side of the patient. If at all possible, line up on the least injured side.
2. Kneel on one knee, preferably the same side for all rescuers.
3. Have the first rescuer cradle the patient's head by placing one arm under the neck and shoulder and the other arm under the patient's lower back.
4. Have the second rescuer place one arm under the patient's knees and the other arm above the buttocks.
5. If a third rescuer is available, have him or her place both arms under the patient's waist. The other two rescuers should slide their arms up to the middle of the back and down to the buttocks, as appropriate.
6. On signal, all rescuers lift the patient together to the level of their knees. Then, with a gentle rocking motion, together they roll the patient toward their chests until he or she is cradled in the bends of their elbows. The patient's head should be tucked in toward the first rescuer's chest.
7. On signal, the rescuers stand up and carry the patient to the stretcher.
8. To lower the patient onto the stretcher, the steps are reversed.

ONE-RESCUER MOVES

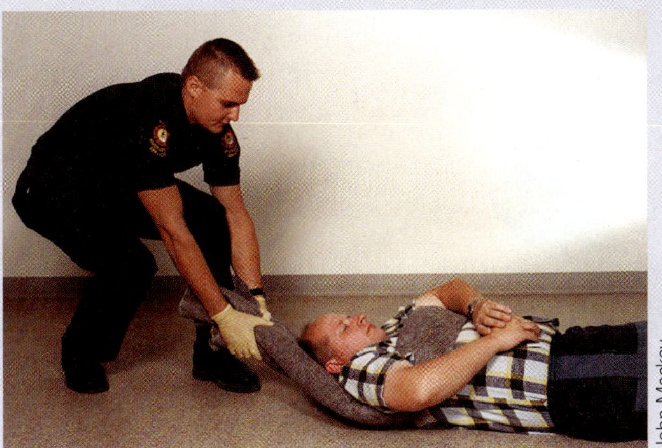

Figure 6–10a Sheet drag.

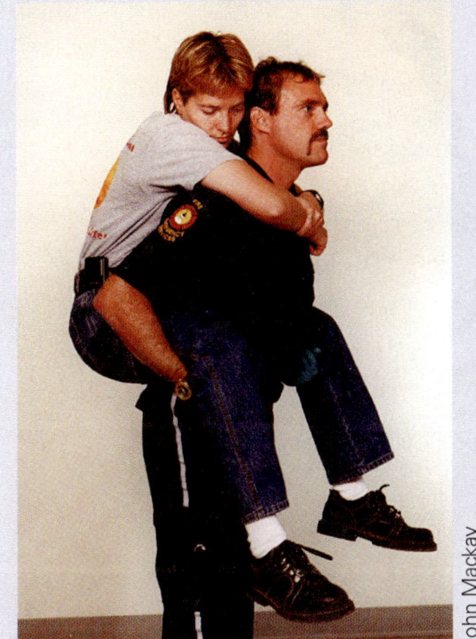

Figure 6–10b Piggyback carry.

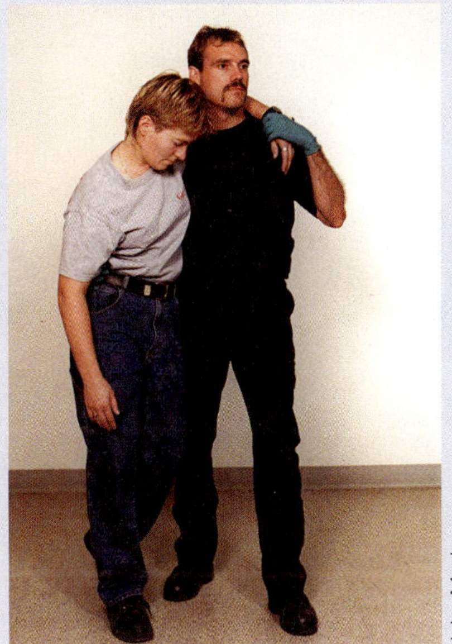

Figure 6–10c One-rescuer crutch.

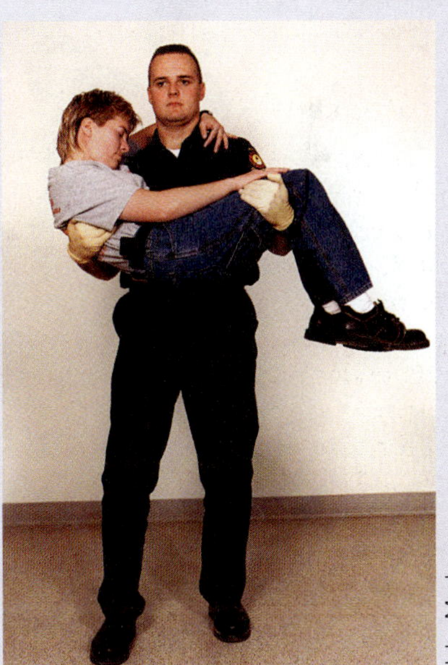

Figure 6–10d Cradle carry.

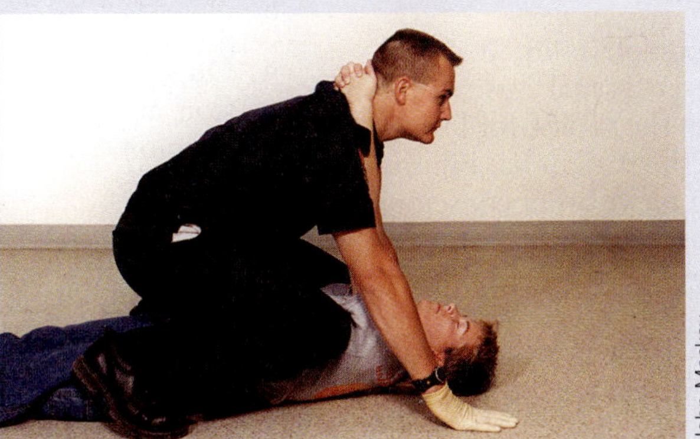

Figure 6–10e Firefighter's drag.

FIREFIGHTER'S CARRY

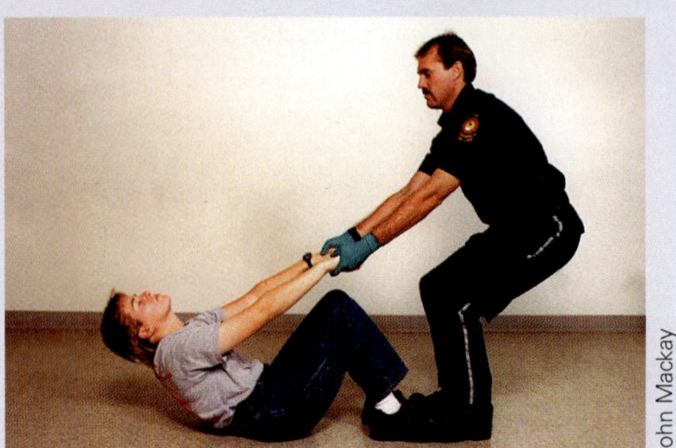

Figure 6–11a Grasp the patient's wrists.

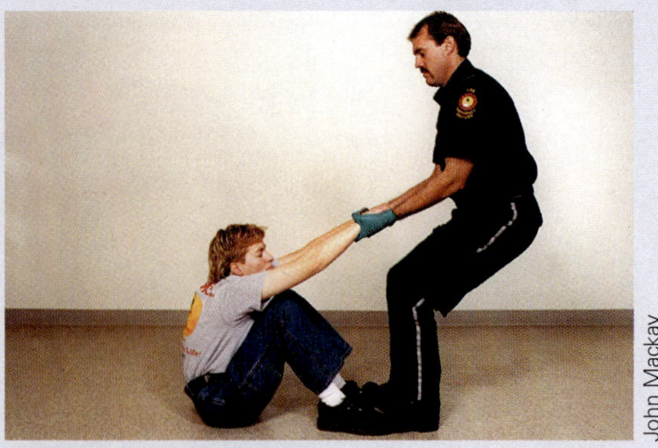

Figure 6–11b Stand on the patient's toes and pull.

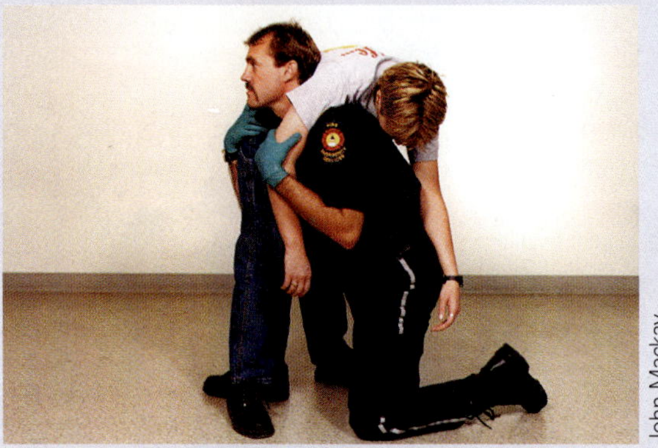

Figure 6–11c Pull the patient over one shoulder.

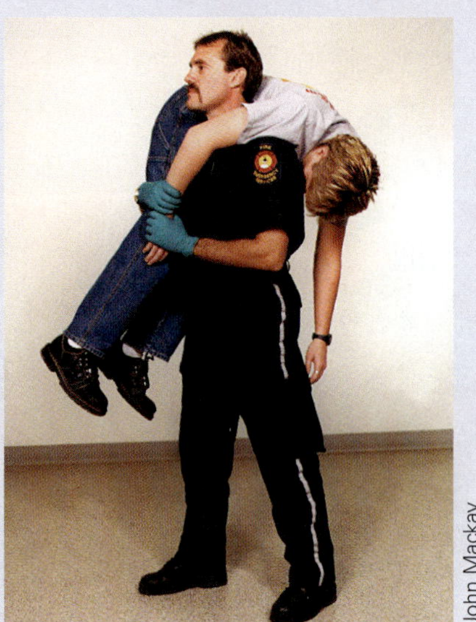

Figure 6–11d Pass an arm between the patient's legs and grasp the arm nearest you.

Extremity Lift (Fore and Aft Lift)

The extremity lift is another complete lift. It differs from the straight lift in that rescuers make use of the patient's extremities rather than the thorax for lifting. Do not use the extremity lift if the patient has injuries to arms or legs. Use this lift to move an unconscious patient from a chair to the floor. Two rescuers are needed to perform the lift (Figure 6–13 on p. 74):

1. One rescuer takes a crouching position at the patient's head. The second rescuer crouches by the patient's knees.
2. The rescuer at the head places one hand under each of the patient's arms, reaching through to grab the patient's wrists.
3. The second rescuer should slip his or her hands under the patient's knees.
4. On signal, both rescuers rise to a standing position and then move the patient to the desired location.

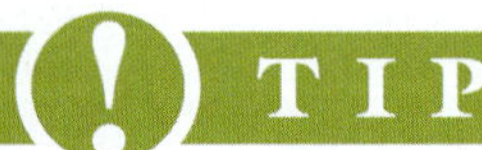

! T I P

Aside from back injuries, another potential danger is body fluid that a patient may be lying in as you attempt a move. A tarp specifically designed for lifting can minimize contact with contaminants and encourage you to lift with your legs instead of your back (Figure 6–14 on p. 75).

STRAIGHT LIFT

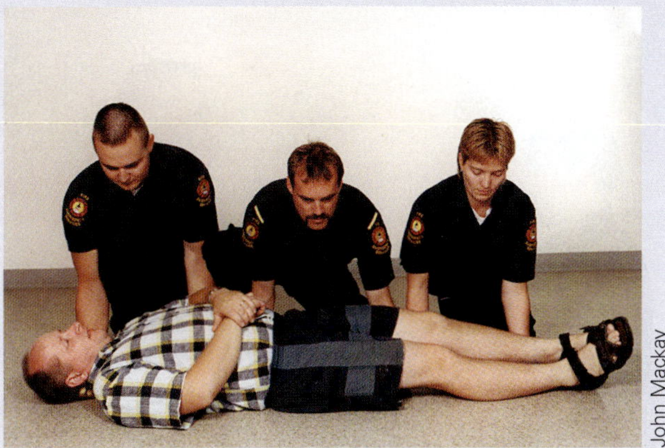

Figure 6–12a Kneel on one knee on the least injured side.

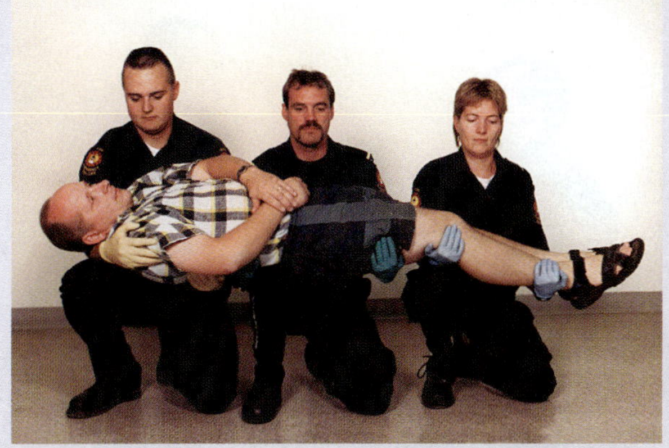

Figure 6–12b In unison, lift the patient to knee level.

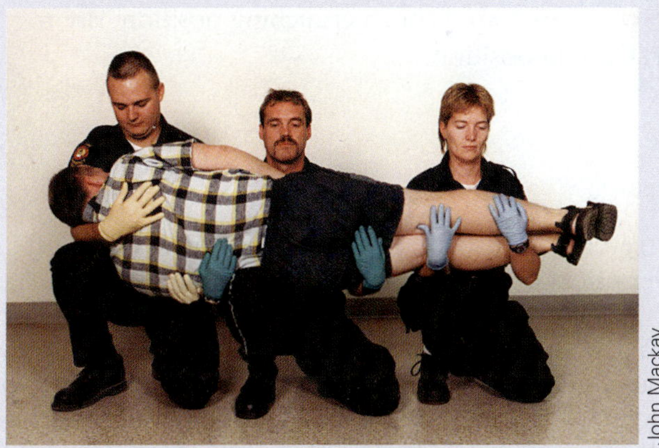

Figure 6–12c Slowly turn the patient toward you.

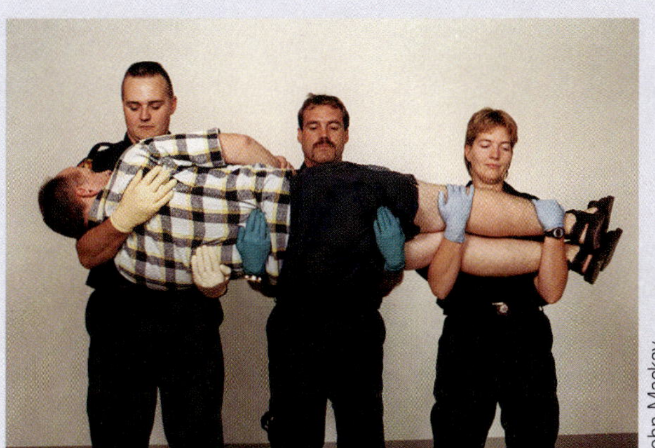

Figure 6–12d In unison, rise to a standing position.

Positioning the Patient

How you position a patient depends on the patient's condition. General guidelines include the following:

- An unconscious patient who is not injured should be placed in the recovery position. This is done by rolling the patient onto one side. The left side is preferable.
- Unless there is a life-threatening emergency, a patient who has been injured should not be moved. As necessary, the paramedics will evaluate, stabilize, and move the patient.
- A patient who shows signs of shock may be placed in the shock position. This is done by elevating the supine patient's legs 20 to 30 cm if this will not aggravate injuries to the legs or spine.
- A patient who has pain or breathing problems may get into any position that makes him or her more comfortable, unless injuries prevent it. Generally, a patient who has breathing difficulties will want to sit up. A patient with abdominal pain will want to lie on his or her side with knees drawn up.
- A conscious patient who is nauseated or vomiting should be allowed to remain in a position of comfort. However, you should always be positioned so that you can manage the patient's airway if needed.

EXTREMITY LIFT

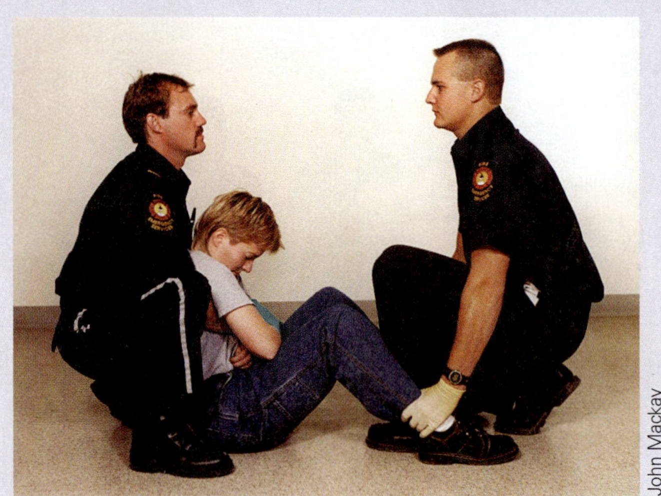

Figure 6–13a Get in position at the head and feet of the patient.

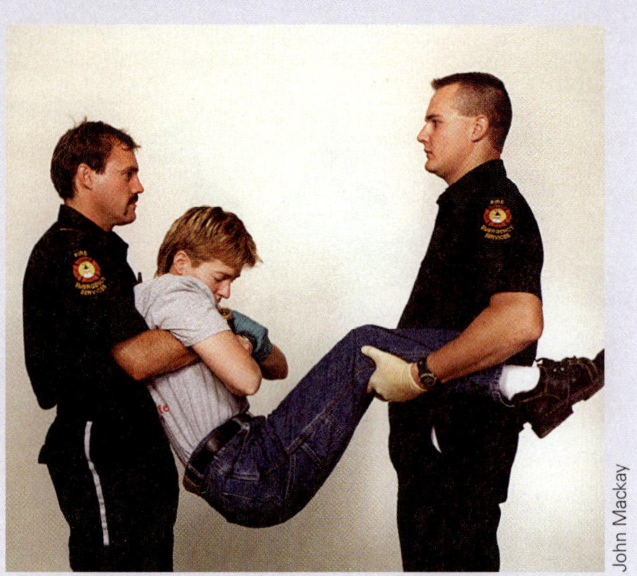

Figure 6–13b From a crouching position, rise to a standing position.

SECTION 3
EQUIPMENT

Become completely familiar with the equipment used to move patients in your EMS system. To decide which to use, base your decision on the patient's condition, the environment in which he or she is found, and the resources available. Generally, the best way to move a patient is the easiest way that will not cause injury or pain.

Let your equipment do the work whenever possible. Drag or slide the patient (not lift) whenever you can. If you must lift a patient, do it with a device designed for that purpose. As a rule, carry a patient only as far as absolutely necessary. Make sure you have adequate help. If you do not have it, get it. Never risk injuring yourself.

Typical equipment used in EMS includes various types of stretchers, the stair chair, the tarp, and backboards.

Stretchers

A standard stretcher, or cot, has wheeled legs. It also has a collapsible undercarriage that makes it possible to load it into an ambulance (Figure 6–15). This stretcher is also made with a power-assisted lift for very heavy (bariatric) patients (Figure 6–16).

A portable stretcher is lightweight, folds compactly, and is easy to clean. It does not have an undercarriage and wheels. It is comfortable to rest on, especially if the head is padded. It is valuable when there is not enough space for a standard stretcher or when there are many patients. There is a variety of styles (Figure 6–17 on p. 76). The most common, the No. 9 cot, has an aluminum frame with canvas fabric and is often used aboard air ambulances.

A scoop, or orthopedic, stretcher splits into two or four sections (Figure 6–18 on p. 76). Each section can be fitted around a patient who is lying on a relatively flat surface. It is used in confined areas where larger stretchers will not fit. Once secure in a scoop stretcher, the patient can be lifted and moved to a standard one. To operate a scoop stretcher, split it apart lengthwise. Carefully slide it under the patient from both sides. Then lock the brackets at each end and lift the patient.

A stretcher can also be improvised with a blanket, canvas, brattice cloth, or a strong sheet and two 2.5 m (metre) poles. To improvise a stretcher with two poles and a blanket, follow these steps (Figure 6–19 on p. 76):

1. Place one pole about 30 cm from the centre of the unfolded blanket.
2. Fold the short side of the blanket over the pole.

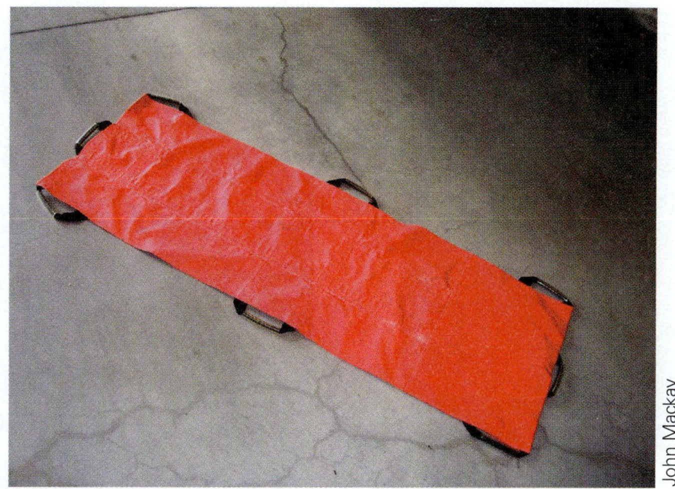

Figure 6–14a A tarp used to perform a complete lift and carry.

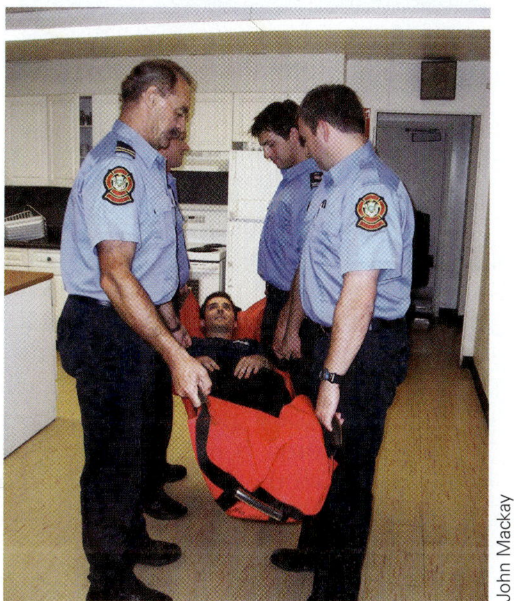

Figure 6–14b Straight lift with a tarp.

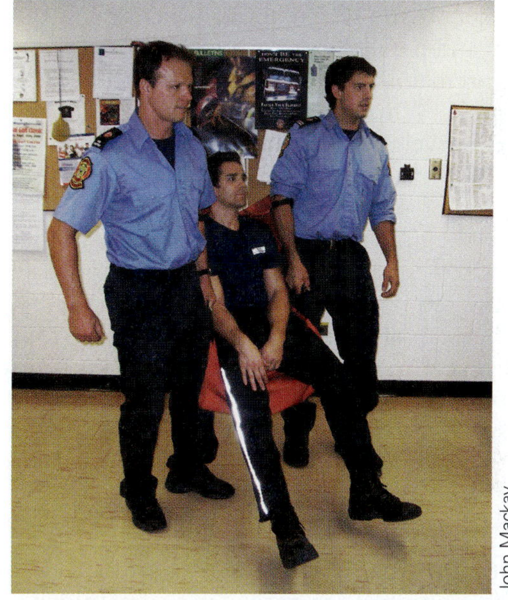

Figure 6–14c Chair lift with a tarp.

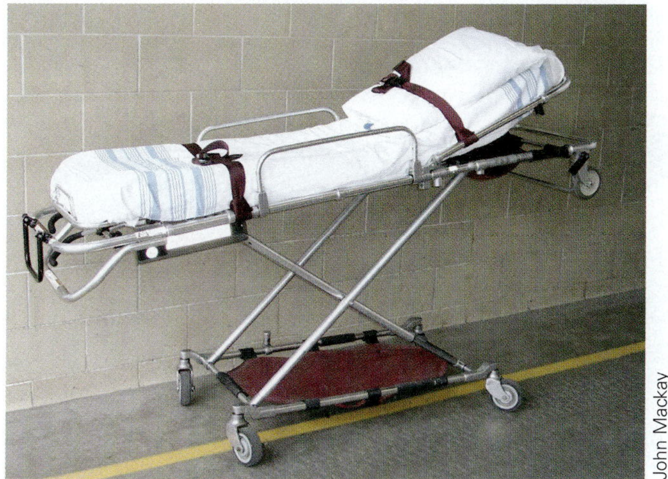

Figure 6–15 Standard stretcher.

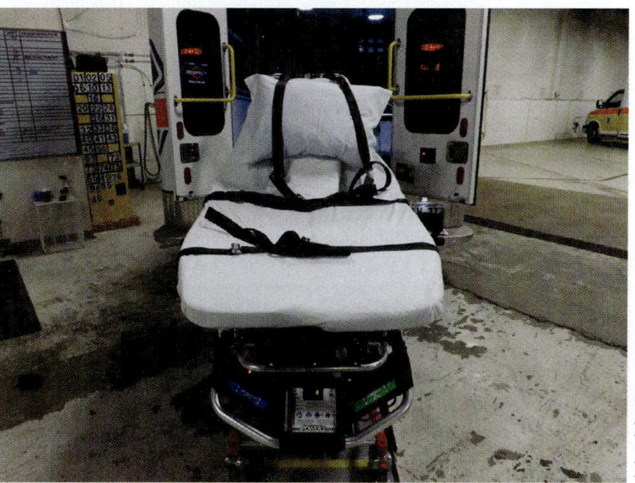

Figure 6–16 Power-assisted bariatric stretcher.

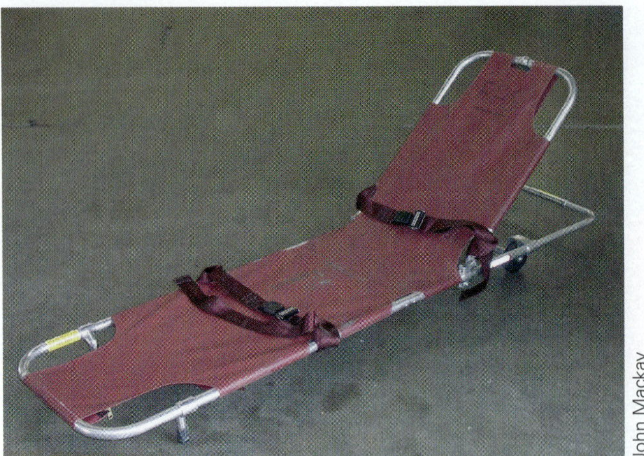

Figure 6–17 Portable ambulance stretcher.

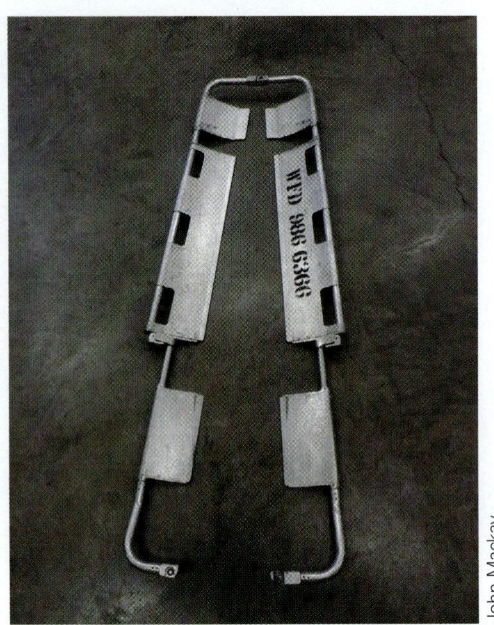

Figure 6–18 Scoop, or orthopedic, stretcher.

3. Place the second pole on top of the two folds of the blanket. It should be about 60 cm from the first pole and parallel to it.
4. Fold the remaining side of the blanket over the second pole. When the patient is placed on the blanket, the weight of the body secures the poles.

Cloth bags or sacks may be used as stretchers. Make holes in the bottoms of the bags or sacks so that the poles pass through them. Enough bags should be used to get the required length.

A stretcher can also be made from three or four coats or jackets. First, turn the sleeves inside out. Then, button the jacket with the sleeves inside the coat. Place a pole through each sleeve.

Stair Chairs

Moving patients up or down stairs dramatically increases the potential for rescuers to be injured.

The safest way to do it is with a stair chair (Figure 6–20a). A stair chair is a lightweight folding device. It has straps to secure the patient, wheeled legs, a grab bar below the patient's feet, and handles that extend behind the patient's shoulders.

When you use a stair chair (Figures 6–20b and 6–20c), make sure as many people as necessary are helping. A spotter is needed to help manoeuvre the stair chair down the stairs. He or she should continually tell how many stairs are left and what conditions are ahead. A spotter can also place a hand on the back of the rescuer who is moving backward to help steady him or her.

IMPROVISED STRETCHER

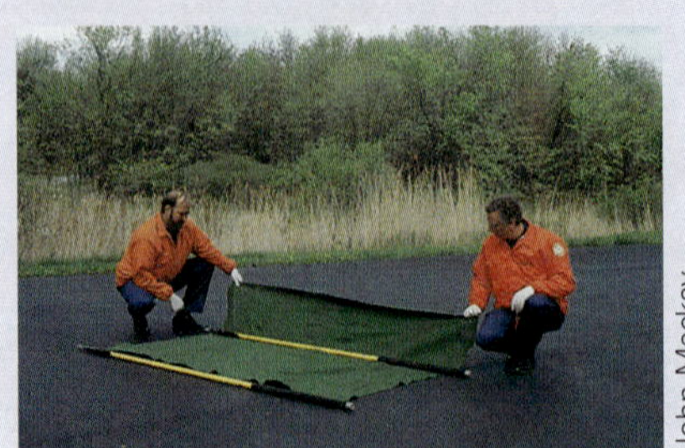

Figure 6–19a Fold the short side of the blanket over the first pole.

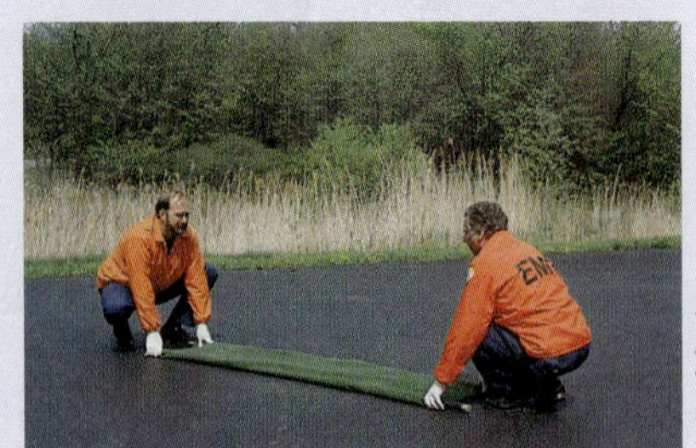

Figure 6–19b Fold the remaining side over the second pole.

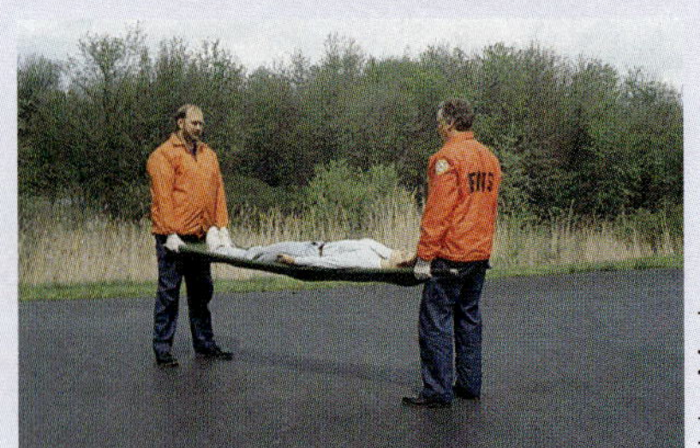

Figure 6–19c The weight of the patient should secure the poles.

USING A STAIR CHAIR

John Mackay

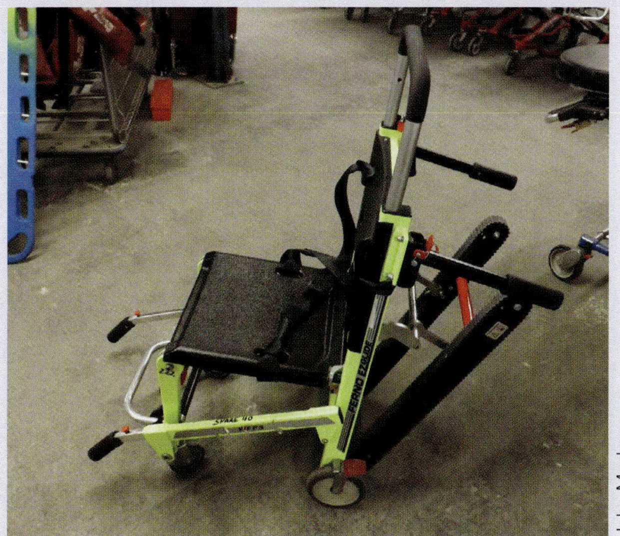

Figure 6–20a Stair chair.

John Mackay

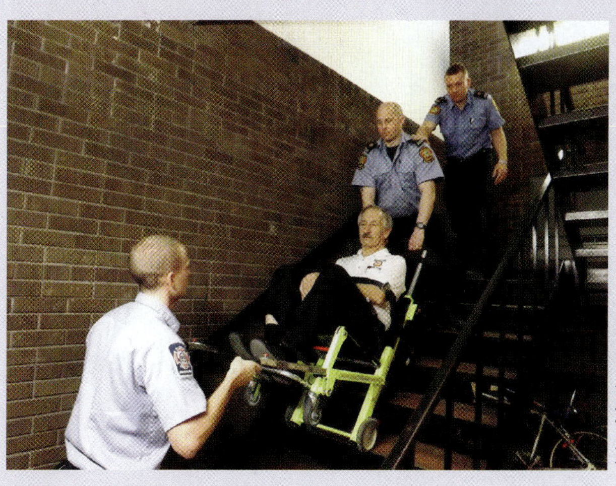

Figure 6–20b Moving a patient up steps with a third rescuer as spotter.

John Mackay

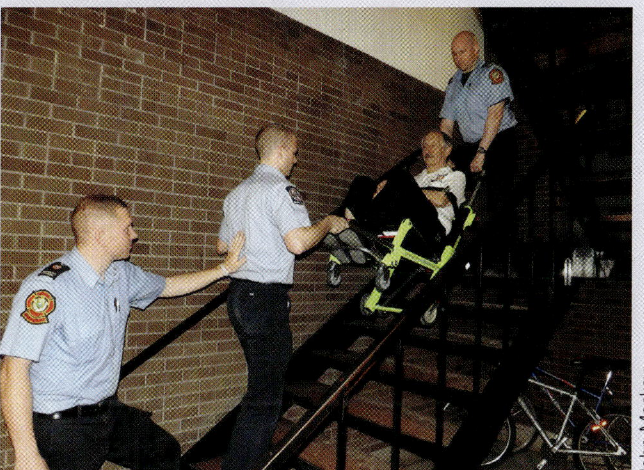

Figure 6–20c Moving a patient down steps with a third rescuer as spotter.

Rescuers carrying a patient in a stair chair should keep their backs in a locked position. They should flex at the hips instead of at the waist, bend at the knees, and keep the arms (and the weight of the chair) as close to their bodies as possible. Once off the stairs, the patient can be transferred to a conventional stretcher.

Stair chairs work well for patients in respiratory distress who need to be moved up or down stairs. The sitting position does not worsen the patient's breathing problems.

Backboards

There are both long and short backboards. A long backboard is approximately 2 m long, which means it can stabilize the patient's entire body (Figure 6–21). It is used for patients with suspected spinal injury who are lying down.

A short backboard is 1 to 1.25 m long and can stabilize the patient down to the hips (Figure 6–22). It is used to stabilize a patient with suspected spinal injuries who is in a sitting position.

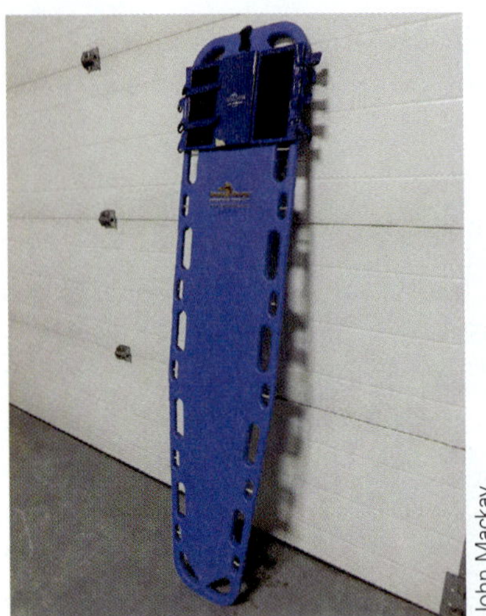

Figure 6–21 Traditional wooden long backboard.

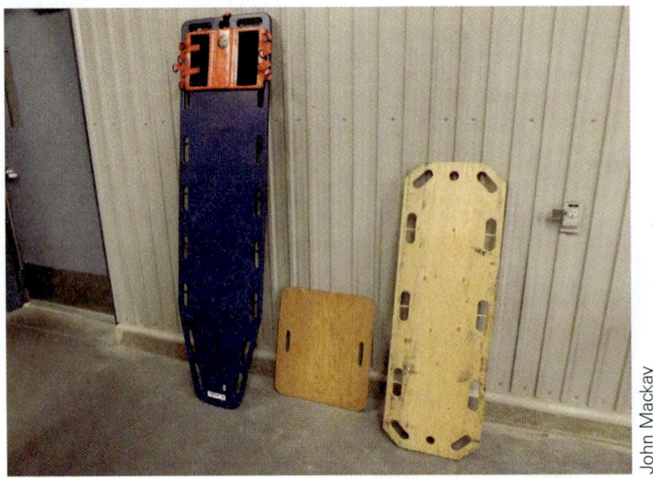

Figure 6–22 Short backboard.

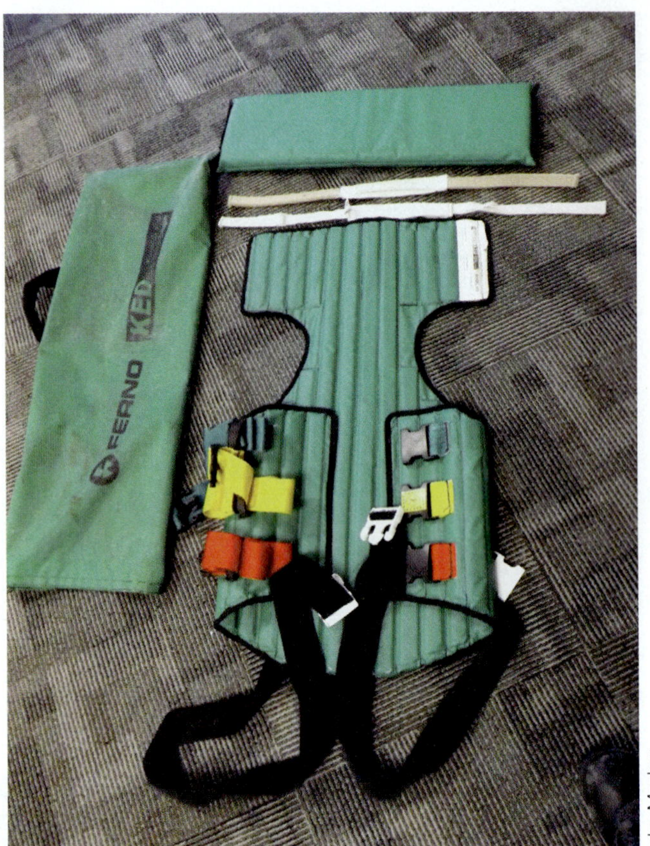

Figure 6–23 Vest-type immobilization device.

A vest-type immobilization device is also available (Figure 6–23). Both the long and short backboards feature handholds and straps. Most are made of synthetic material that will not absorb blood and are easy to clean (Figures 6–24 and 6–25). Regardless of whether you use a long or short backboard, always maintain manual support of the patient's head and neck in the normal, neutral position. Maintain that support until the patient is *fully* secured to the backboard.

Bariatric Equipment

Several devices are available to assist with patients who cannot otherwise be lifted or moved safely due to their size and weight.

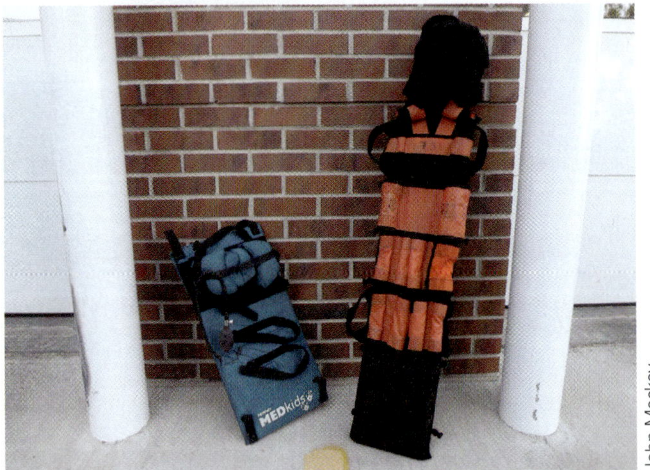

Figure 6–24 Synthetic short backboard with straps.

Large Body Surface (LBS) Bariatric Board

Motorized stretchers use electricity to lift an extremely obese patient. When a patient is too heavy to lift manually, he or she might also be larger than a standard size cot. An LBS board can be affixed to an electric stretcher to accommodate the oversized patient (Figure 6–26).

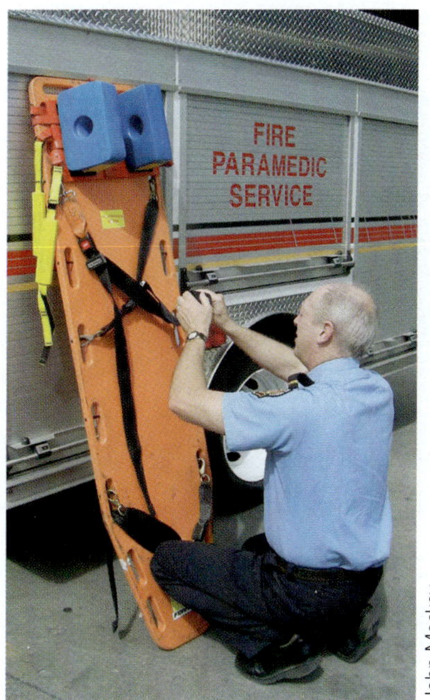

Figure 6–25 Long backboard with straps and head blocks.

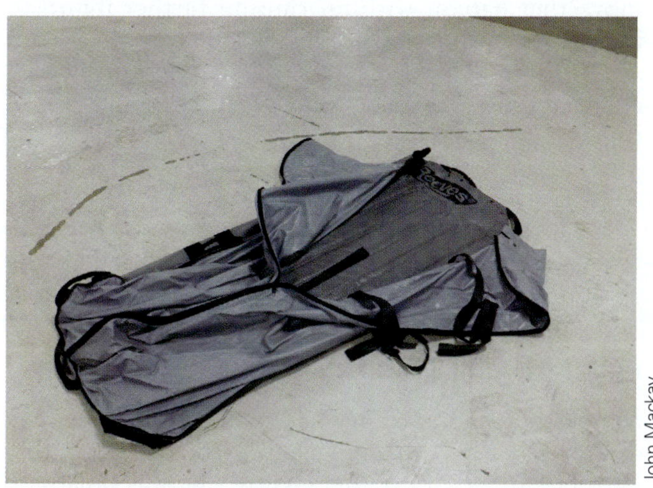

Figure 6–26 An LBS board.

Pneumatic Devices

Air-filled devices, like the HoverJack Rescue Mat, can be used to elevate a patient for transfer to an ambulance cot (Figure 6–27). Before inflating the device, the patient can be log-rolled back and forth to be positioned atop the mat. Once air is injected, the device can easily be slid horizontally around corners or even down stairs. Patients should always be secured to the device before inflating according to user instructions.

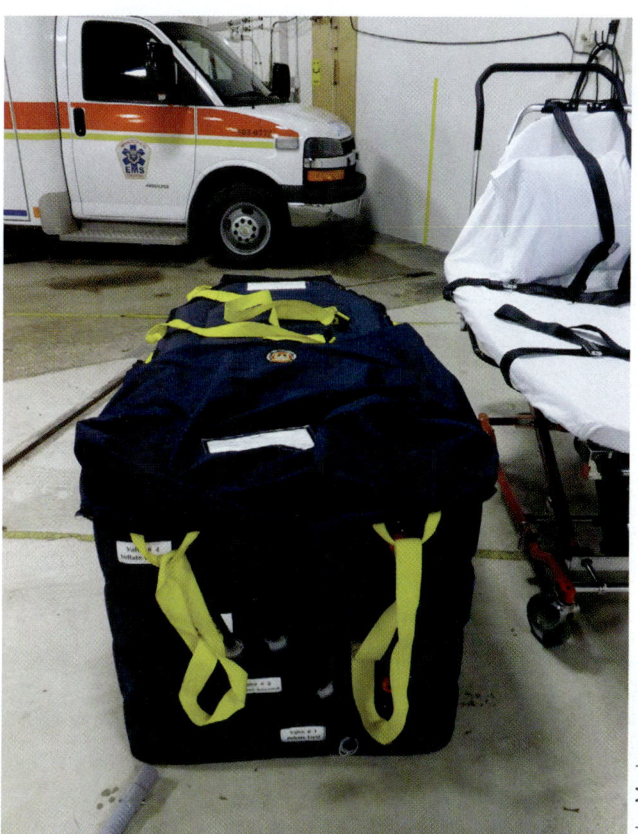

Figure 6–27 A pneumatic device that can be filled with air to help move a heavy patient.

Low Friction Devices

Synthetic flat sheet systems may be used for lateral transfers. Reducing friction allows rescuers to move a patient from surface to surface on the same horizontal plane (Figure 6–28).

Bariatric Tarp

A larger, reinforced tarp can be used by many hands to lighten the load on each individual when moving a larger patient (Figure 6–29). Tarps can also be used for rapid extrication and for patient removal from confined spaces.

T I P

A trick of the trade that can come in handy when moving, assessing, or treating a patient with long hair is to pull the hair up into a bun and secure it with an elastic.

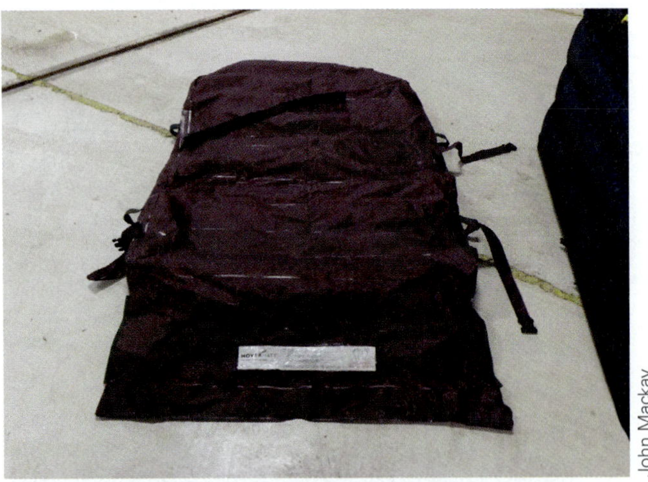

Figure 6–28 A low friction flat sheet used to help horizontal moves.

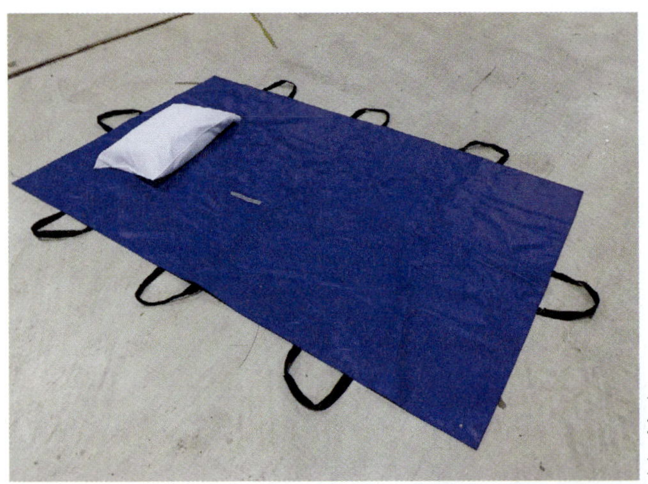

Figure 6–29 A bariatric tarp.

EMR FOCUS

You will find that most patients are in safe locations. Some have problems that would be worsened by movement. In most cases, a patient will not be moved until the paramedics arrive on the scene.

However, when moving a patient means the difference between life and death, your ability to do so safely and properly is key. For example, a patient in a burning vehicle must be moved. If you have a sound knowledge of the skills of lifting and moving, you can move that patient without causing further injury to the spine or other parts of his or her body.

Study and practise the skills presented in this chapter. You will use them more often than you think.

CASE STUDY FOLLOW-UP

At the beginning of this chapter, you read that the EMRs were at the scene of a collision. They were faced with a patient with unknown injuries and in serious danger from smoke and fire. To see how the chapter skills apply to this emergency, read the following. It describes how the call was completed.

SCENE ASSESSMENT *(Continued)*

We glanced at each other. We both knew the patient was in mortal danger and had to be moved immediately. While we were concerned about her possible injuries, we knew it was not possible to leave her in the smoke-filled, flaming car.

I grabbed her under her shoulders and began the move. I cradled her head in my arms to help minimize problems with her spine. My partner grabbed her legs. We moved her to a safe distance from the car and set her down carefully.

PRIMARY ASSESSMENT

My partner stabilized her head as I assessed her consciousness. She moaned when I spoke loudly. My partner kept an eye on her airway. She was breathing adequately and had no foreign material in her mouth, but that could change quickly. She had no signs of external bleeding.

Our general impression was that the woman was about 50 years old and in potentially serious condition. She may have injuries from the crash and from the smoke. We had oxygen available, so we applied a non-rebreather mask immediately.

We informed the incoming units of our suspicions so they could be prepared when they arrived on the scene.

SECONDARY ASSESSMENT

Based on the nature of the accident, any type of injury was possible. The patient was not alert and could not tell us what hurt. Palpations of her head and neck were negative for signs of injury. I palpated her chest and she groaned, indicating that she felt pain from an injury there. I listened to her chest and found unequal breathing sounds. They were diminished on the right, where she had the pain. She had some abrasions on her lower legs but no other injuries that I could find. As I finished the exam, my partner told me that her respirations were becoming inadequate. My partner began to assist them. I checked the patient's pulse, which was 112, regular, and weak. Her respirations were 28 and shallow.

PATIENT HISTORY

We didn't notice any medical information tags on the patient. She couldn't tell us anything about her condition, and no family members were present.

ONGOING ASSESSMENT

We continued to assist her respirations. They remained shallow and rapid. Her pulse increased slightly to 120 and remained weak. We concentrated on ventilating the patient until the paramedics arrived.

TRANSFER OF CARE

We told the paramedics about the situation we found on arrival. They agreed that the patient had to be moved fast. We told them the following:

"This is a female, about 50 years of age, involved in a motor vehicle crash. She responds only by moaning. We are currently assisting with ventilation because of inadequate breathing. We are stabilizing the spine because of the mechanism of injury. We noted pain in her chest while we palpated. Breath sounds on the right are diminished compared with the left. Her pulse increased from 112 to 120 and is weak. Her respirations are shallow and 28. We have no information on history. We'll give you a hand with the backboarding so that you can get off the scene quickly."

It turns out the patient suffered a collapsed lung in the crash. The smoke from the fire really didn't help. The paramedics told us that hospital staff corrected the lung problem right in the emergency department and the patient improved dramatically. She was expected to recover fully. Our actions at the scene were an important reason for her doing so well.

> When to move a patient is determined by the patient's condition and the environment in which he or she is found. How to move a patient is determined by considering the conditions, location, and resources available. Remember, in general, an EMR does not move a patient unless an emergency move must be made or the paramedics ask for assistance. When you do move a patient, be sure to follow the rules of good body mechanics.

NOCPs

3.2 a Practise safe biomechanics **S**
 b Transfer patient from various positions using applicable equipment and/or techniques **S**
 c Transfer patient using emergency evacuation techniques **S**
 d Secure patient safely to applicable equipment **S**

3.3 b Address potential occupational hazards **S**

6.2 f Provide care to bariatric patient **A**

REVIEW QUESTIONS

Page references where answers may be found or supported are provided at the end of each question.

SECTION 1

1. Why should you follow the principles of body mechanics? (p. 65)

SECTION 2

2. What are the five situations in which you should perform an emergency move of a patient? (p. 69)

3. When is it acceptable to not move a patient until the paramedics arrive? (p. 70)

4. How would you perform a shirt drag? (p. 69)

5. How would you perform a blanket drag? (p. 69)

6. How would you perform a straight lift? (pp. 70, 73)

7. How would you perform an extremity lift? (pp. 42, 74)

8. What is the preferred position for a patient who is unconscious? A patient who has difficulty breathing? A patient who is nauseated or vomiting? (p. 73)

SECTION 3

9. How is a stair chair used? (pp. 76–77)

10. How is a scoop stretcher used? (p. 74)

11. What are three common types of stretchers? (pp. 74, 76)

12. What are two common types of backboards? (pp. 77–78)

13. What are three main kinds of devices used to lift or move a bariatric patient? (pp. 78–79)

C H A P T E R

7

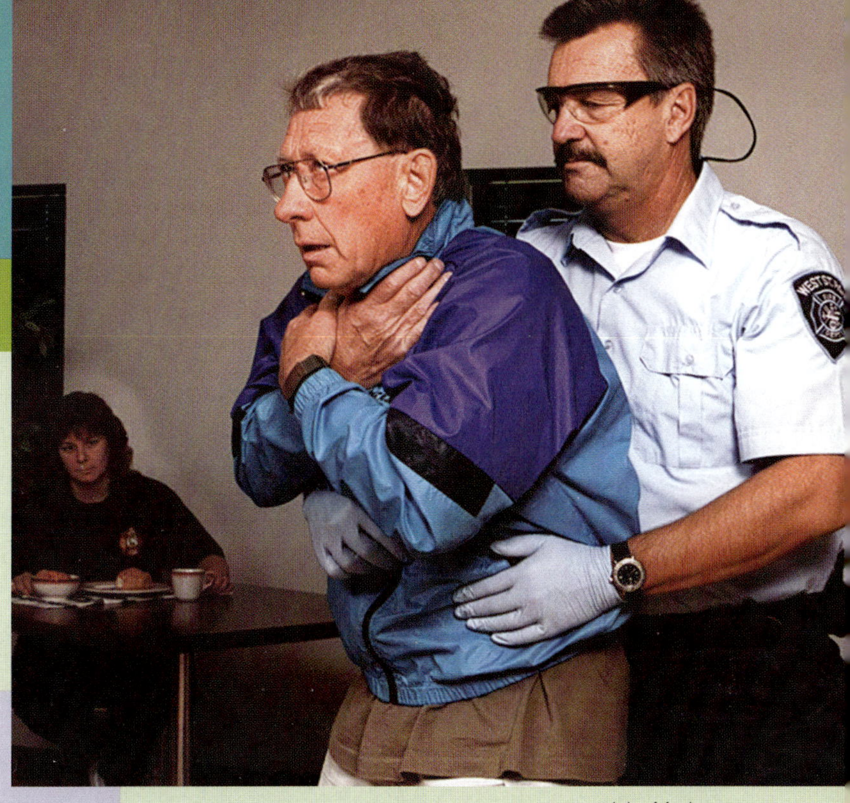
John Mackay

The Airway and Ventilation

O B J E C T I V E S

1. Use a diagram to label the major structures of the respiratory system.
2. Describe and demonstrate the steps in the head-tilt/chin-lift and jaw-thrust manoeuvres.
3. Explain how to use oropharyngeal and nasopharyngeal airway adjuncts.
4. State the importance of having a suction unit ready for immediate use when providing emergency medical care.
5. List the seven signs of inadequate breathing.
6. Describe and demonstrate how to ventilate a patient by mouth-to-mask, mouth-to-barrier device, mouth-to-stoma, and bag-valve-mask (BVM) ventilation and indicate the differences between ventilating an infant, child, and adult.
7. Describe the use of oxygen cylinders and delivery equipment.
8. Describe the special considerations for administering oxygen to patients with chronic obstructive pulmonary disease (COPD).
9. Explain how to clear a foreign body airway obstruction (FBAO).
10. Discuss how a mechanism of injury might affect the method used to open an airway.
11. Explain why basic life support ventilation and airway protective skills are second in priority only to pulse checks and cardiac compressions.

INTRODUCTION

The most important part of your job as an EMR involves a patient's airway. No matter what a patient's problem may be, you must first recognize whether or not they are breathing adequately. This can make the difference between life and death for a business executive who chokes on a piece of steak, a child who falls into a swimming pool, or an **unresponsive** patient whose tongue is blocking his or her airway. While the first "hands-on" skill you perform on a breathless and pulseless patient will be cardiac compressions (see Chapter 8), it is the recognition of inadequate breathing in an unresponsive patient that will cue you to begin basic life support techniques. The techniques discussed in this chapter should be employed only after the pulse has been assessed and cardiac compressions are initiated as necessary. Since most of your patients will have a pulse, it is imperative that you understand basic airway assessment and ventilation techniques, and their differing priorities in unresponsive versus pulseless patients.

SECTION 1
THE RESPIRATORY SYSTEM

The respiratory system supplies the body with the oxygen it needs. It also removes carbon dioxide. The body can store food for weeks and water for days, but it can store enough oxygen for only a few minutes. When oxygen is cut off, brain cells begin to die in about five minutes.

Anatomy of the Respiratory System

The major components of the respiratory system are the nose, mouth, pharynx (throat), epiglottis, trachea (windpipe), larynx (voice box), bronchi, lungs, and diaphragm (Figure 7–1 on p. 86). (You may also wish to review the diagrams of the respiratory system in Chapter 4.)

Nose and Mouth

Air normally enters the body through the nose or mouth. In the nose, it is warmed, moistened, and filtered as it flows over the damp, sticky mucous membrane.

Pharynx

From the back of the nose and mouth, the air enters the pharynx (throat), which is the passageway for both food and air. Air from the mouth enters through the oral portion of the pharynx, the oropharynx. Air from the nose enters through the nasal portion of the pharynx, the nasopharynx. At its lower end, the pharynx divides in two. One division is the esophagus, which leads to the stomach. The other is the trachea (windpipe), which leads to the lungs.

Trachea and Larynx

The trachea (windpipe) carries air from the nose and mouth to the lungs. Immediately above it is the larynx (voice box), or Adam's apple. The larynx can be easily felt with your fingertips at the front of the throat.

Epiglottis

The trachea is protected by a small, leaf-shaped flap called the epiglottis. Normally, this flap covers the entrance of the larynx during swallowing so that food and liquid cannot enter. However, with injury or illness, that reflex may not work properly. As a result, a patient could **aspirate** (inhale) liquid, including blood or vomit, into the trachea and lungs, causing suffocation.

Bronchi and Lungs

The lower end of the trachea divides into two tubes called bronchi. The bronchi lead to the lungs, which are two large, lobed organs that are the principal organs of respiration. Within the lungs, each bronchus divides into the smaller bronchioles, somewhat like the branches of a tree. At the ends of the bronchioles are thousands of tiny air sacs called alveoli. Each alveolus is enclosed in a network of capillaries and is responsible for the exchange of oxygen and carbon dioxide.

Diaphragm

The diaphragm is a powerful, dome-shaped muscle essential for breathing. It separates the thoracic cavity

CASE STUDY

Dispatch

Our EMR unit was dispatched to the home of an unconscious person.

Scene Assessment

We approached the house carefully as we always do. A man came to the door. He looked very concerned. He explained that his wife had slumped over in her chair minutes before. "She looks bad," he told us. "She's not breathing right. Please help her."

As we approached the patient, we asked her husband if she had had any falls or sustained any injuries. He assured us that she had not.

Primary Assessment

We already had our gloves and eyewear on when we reached the patient's side. She was unresponsive, with snoring respirations.

> The patient in this scenario requires immediate attention. No matter what the underlying reason for her condition, she will not survive without adequate respirations. Perhaps the most important part of her care will be that which she receives for her airway. Consider this patient as you read Chapter 7. What do you think the EMRs should do for her?

from the abdominal cavity. If it cannot contract effectively because of illness or injury, a patient will breathe inadequately and develop significant respiratory distress.

How Respiration Works

During inhalation, the diaphragm and the muscles between the ribs (intercostal muscles) contract. This increases the size of the thoracic cavity, making it possible for the lungs to expand. The diaphragm moves down slightly, flaring the lower portion of the rib cage, which then moves upward and outward. This decreases pressure in the chest and causes air to flow into the lungs (Figure 7–2 on p. 87).

In the lungs, gases pass through the thin walls of the alveoli and capillaries. Oxygen enters the alveoli during inhalation and passes through the capillary wall into the bloodstream. Carbon dioxide and other waste gases pass from the blood through the capillary wall into the alveoli so that they can be exhaled.

During exhalation, the diaphragm and the muscles between the ribs relax. This decreases the size of the thoracic cavity. The diaphragm moves up, the ribs move down and in, and air flows out of the lungs.

With some respiratory diseases, patients have difficulty moving air in and out of the lungs. They have to use additional muscles not only to draw air in but also to force air out. As a result, both inhalation and exhalation require a great deal of effort. Such patients tend to get exhausted quickly and will deteriorate rapidly.

Normal breathing occurs at a regular rate (Table 7–1). For adults, that is 12 to 20 breaths per minute. For children, it is 20 to 40 breaths per minute. For infants,

TABLE 7–1 NORMAL BREATHING RATES	
Patient	**Breathing Rate**
Infant	up to 60 breaths per minute
Child	20–40 breaths per minute
Adult	12–20 breaths per minute

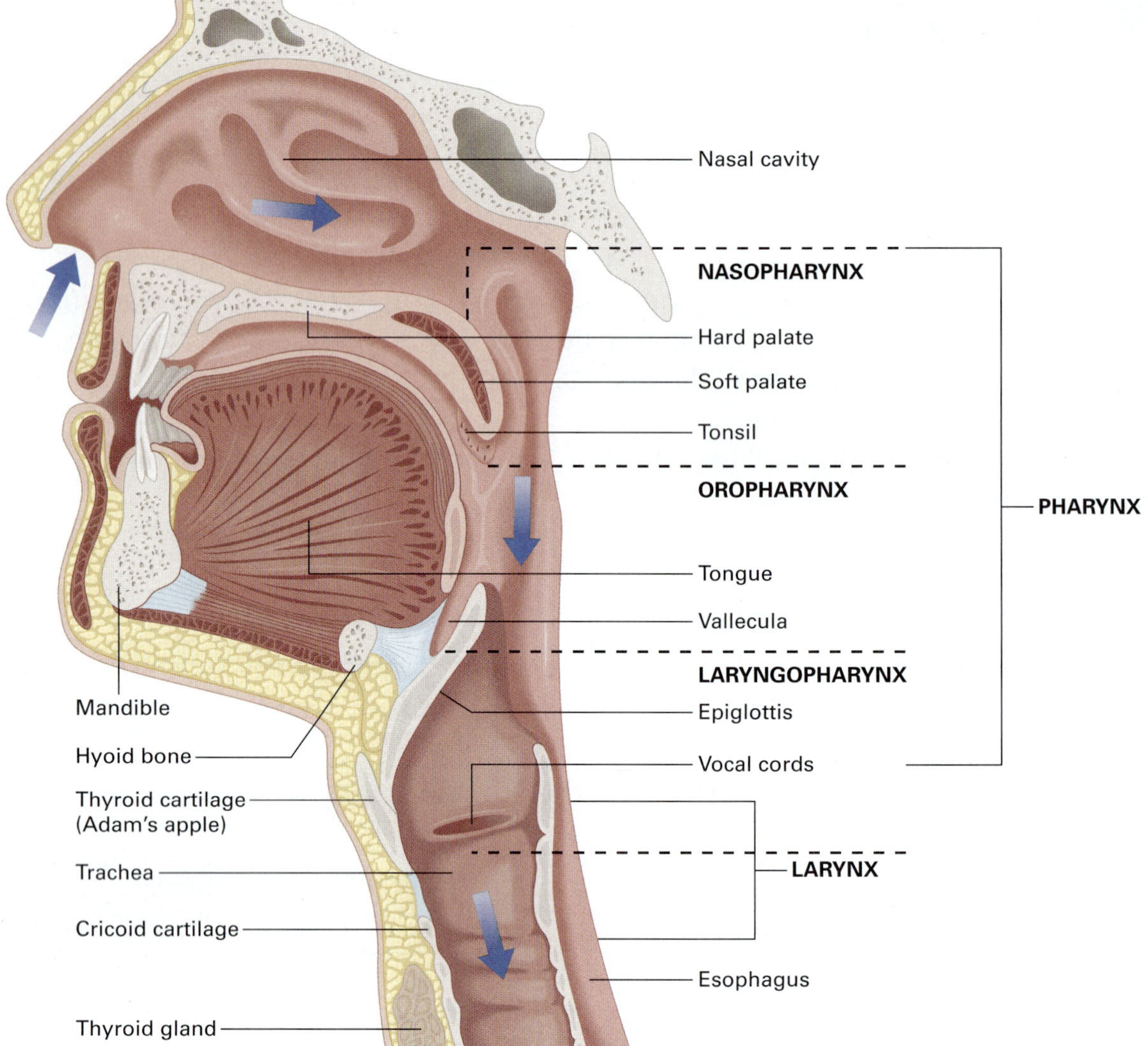

Figure 7–1 Anatomy of the upper airway.

it is up to 60 breaths per minute. Adequate breathing is regular in rhythm and free of unusual sounds, such as wheezing or whistling. The chest should expand adequately and equally with each breath. The depth of the breaths should also be adequate.

Breathing should be virtually effortless. It should be accomplished without the use of accessory muscles in the neck, shoulders, and abdomen.

Infants and Children

When treating infants and children, remember the anatomical differences between their respiratory system and that of an adult. The differences include the following (Figure 7–3):

- All structures, including the mouth and nose, are smaller than those of adults. They are more easily obstructed, even by small objects, blood, or swelling. Take extra care to keep the airways of infants and children open.
- The tongue of an infant or child takes up proportionally more space in the pharynx than that of an adult. It can therefore block the airway more easily.
- The trachea of an infant or child is narrower than an adult's. It is also softer and more flexible. Tipping the infant's or child's head too far back or allowing it to fall forward can close the trachea. Because the head of an infant or young child is quite large relative to the body, a folded towel or similar item under the shoulders of a supine patient may be needed to keep the airway aligned and open.
- Because their chest walls are softer, infants and children tend to rely on the diaphragm

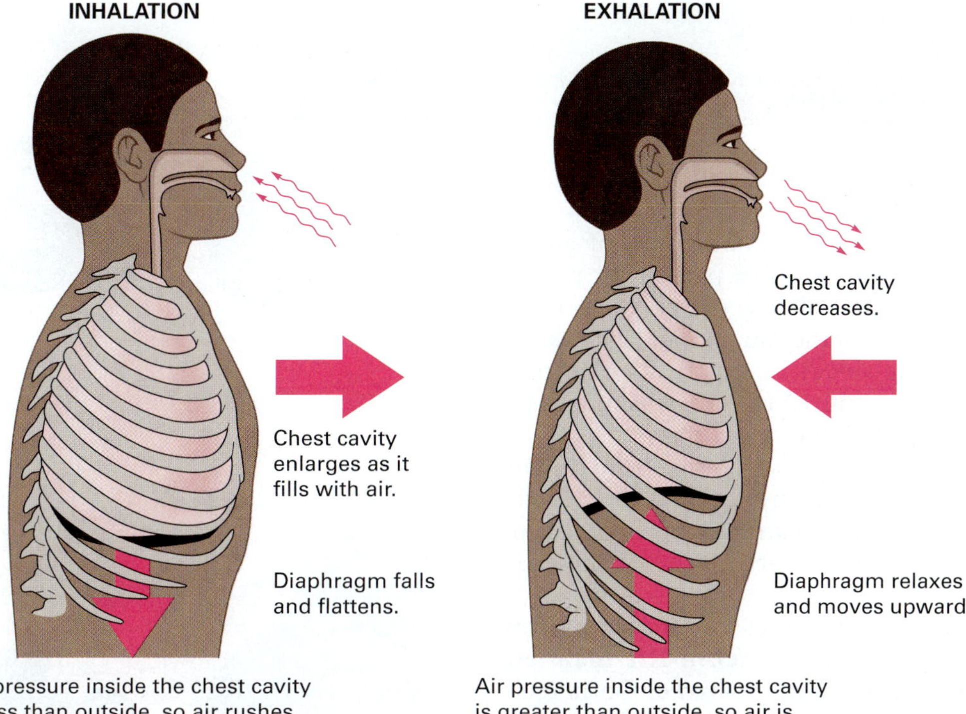

Figure 7–2 How respiration works.

for breathing. Watch for excessive movement there—it can alert you to respiratory distress. Remember, the primary cause of cardiac arrest in infants and children is an uncorrected respiratory problem.

Just a reminder: Whether your patient is an infant, child, or adult, remember that family members also need you. Be calm and caring, as well as professional. The patient's interests are paramount, but keep the family's feelings in mind as well.

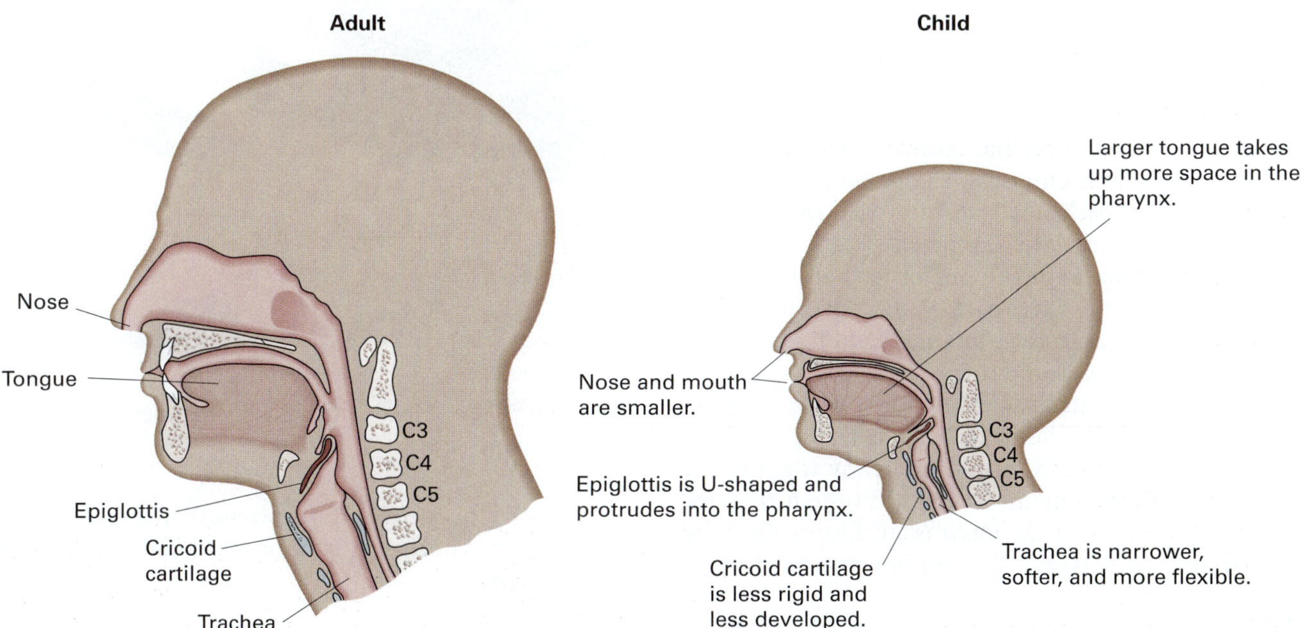

Figure 7–3 Comparison of the airways of an adult and an infant or child.

SECTION 2
PATIENT ASSESSMENT GUIDELINES

Opening the Airway

The tongue is the most common cause of airway obstruction in an unresponsive patient. A patient who loses consciousness will lose muscle tone. When that happens, the base of the tongue can fall back and **occlude** (block) the airway. The patient's efforts to breathe then create negative pressure, which pulls the tongue, epiglottis, or both into the throat.

In some cases, patients require **ventilation** (assistance with breathing by forcing air into the patient's lungs). Before a patient who is breathing inadequately can receive assistance, he or she must have an open airway.

There are two manoeuvres commonly used to open an airway: the **head-tilt/chin-lift manoeuvre** and the **jaw-thrust manoeuvre**. Both techniques move the tongue from the back of the throat and allow air to pass into the lungs. The tongue is attached to the lower jaw. Moving the lower jaw forward will relieve the obstruction.

Head-Tilt/Chin-Lift Manoeuvre

The head-tilt/chin-lift manoeuvre is the method of choice for opening the airway of an uninjured patient. The **Heart and Stroke Foundation of Canada (HSFC)** recommends it for opening the airway of patients who do not have injuries to the head, neck, or spine. Use it first on unresponsive patients who are not injured.

To perform the manoeuvre, do the following (Figure 7–4):

1. Place your hand on the patient's forehead. Use the hand that is closest to the patient's head.
2. Apply firm, backward pressure with the palm of your hand to tilt the head back.
3. Place the fingertips of your other hand near the chin under the bony part of the patient's lower jaw. If the patient is an infant or child, place only your index finger under the jaw.
4. Lift the chin upward. At the same time, support the jaw and tilt the head back as far as possible. The patient's teeth should be nearly together. If the patient is an infant or child, tilt the head back only slightly, as if the child is sniffing (called the **sniffing position**). Remember not to overextend the head.
5. Continue to press the other hand on the patient's forehead to keep the head tilted back.

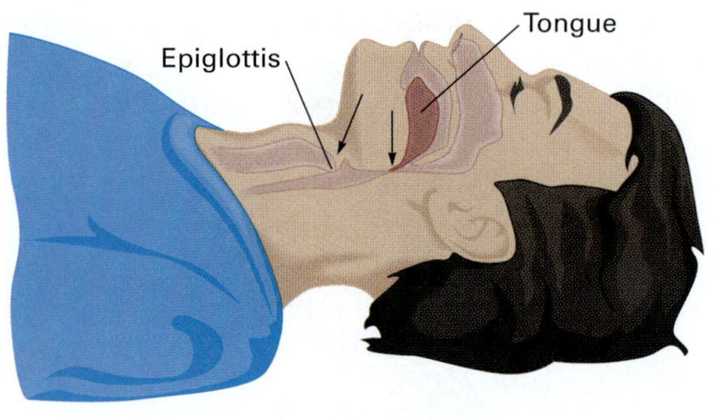

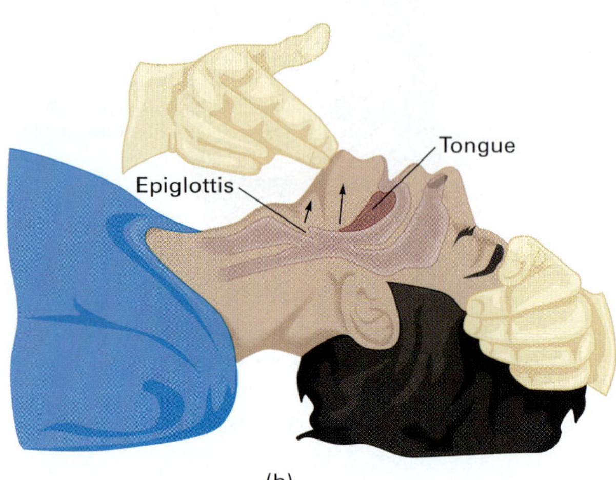

Figure 7–4a Head-tilt/chin-lift manoeuvre on an adult.

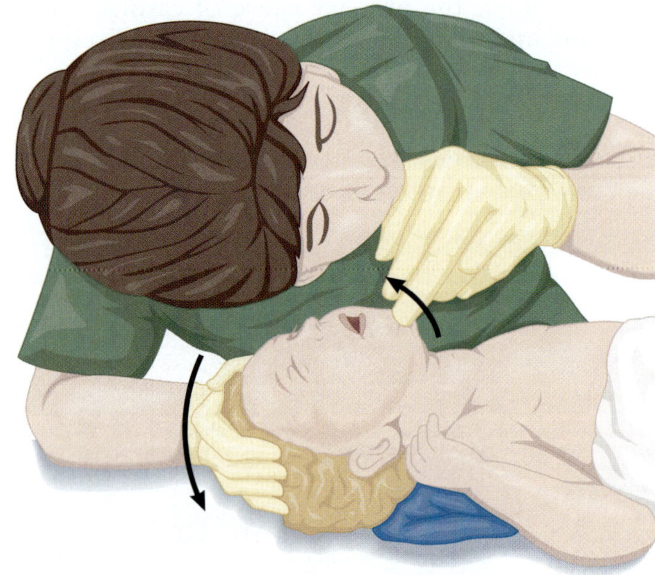

Figure 7–4b Head-tilt/chin-lift manoeuvre on an infant.

There are several important precautions to remember when performing the head-tilt/chin-lift manoeuvre:

• Never let your fingers press deeply into the soft tissues under the chin. You could block the patient's airway.

- If necessary, use your thumb to press on the patient's lower lip, keeping the patient's mouth slightly open. Never use your thumb to lift the patient's chin.
- Do not let the patient's mouth close unless you are giving mouth-to-nose ventilation.
- If the patient has dentures (false teeth), try to hold them in place. This will help prevent the patient's lips from interfering with breathing. If you are unable to manage the dentures, remove them.

Jaw-Thrust Manoeuvre

A jaw-thrust manoeuvre may be used instead of the head-tilt/chin-lift manoeuvre. Note, however, that it is tiring and technically difficult. It is, however, the safest approach to opening the airway in a patient with suspected spinal injury. The patient's head and neck are brought into a neutral position, so the head is not turned to the side, tilted forward, or tilted back.

Use the jaw-thrust manoeuvre on unresponsive patients who are injured or who have suspected spinal injury. To perform it, do the following (Figure 7–5):

1. Kneel above the patient's head. Place your elbows on the surface where the patient is lying. Place one hand on each side of the head with your thumbs on the patient's cheek bones.
2. Grasp the angles of the patient's lower jaw on both sides. If the patient is an infant or child, place two or three fingers of each hand at the angle of the jaw.
3. While keeping your thumbs on the cheeks, with both hands use a lifting motion to move the jaw

up and away from you. This pulls the tongue away from the back of the throat.

4. Keep the patient's mouth slightly open. If necessary, pull back the lower lip with the thumb of one gloved hand.

If the jaw-thrust manoeuvre does not open the patient's airway, try again. Reposition the jaw and determine whether or not the airway is open. If repositioning does not work, insert an airway adjunct (described later in this chapter) or use the head-tilt/chin-lift manoeuvre.

Inspecting the Airway

Assess the airway of every one of your patients. A clear and open airway, or **patent airway**, is absolutely necessary for adequate breathing.

You can determine that a patient's airway is patent if he or she is alert, conscious, and talking to you in a normal voice. If you see that his or her mental status is altered, however, you will have to look more closely. A patient who is drowsy, disoriented, confused, or unresponsive may have blood, vomit, or excess saliva in the airway.

To inspect the airway of an unresponsive patient, first open the patient's mouth with a gloved hand. If necessary, use the **cross-finger technique**. To do so, kneel next to the patient's head and cross the thumb and forefinger of one hand. Place the thumb on the patient's lower incisors and the forefinger on the upper incisors. Then use a scissors-like or finger-snapping motion to open the patient's mouth. When the mouth is open, look inside for fluids and solids, including broken teeth or dentures that may

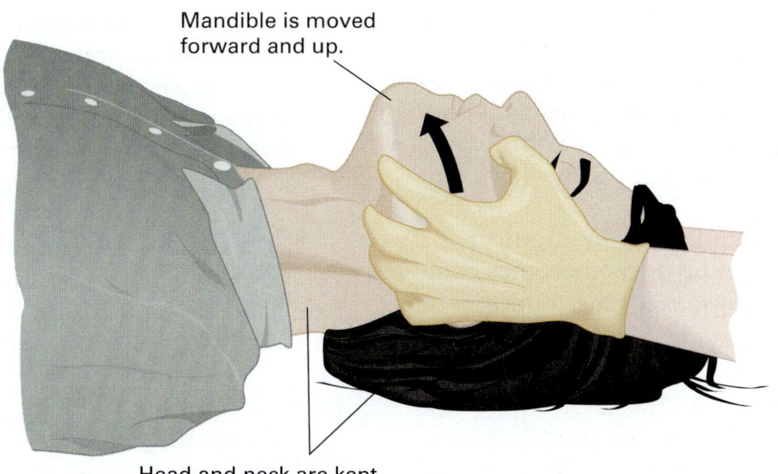

Figure 7–5 Jaw-thrust manoeuvre.

be blocking the airway. Finally, listen for unusual sounds.

Respiration sounds that may indicate an airway obstruction include the following:

- *Snoring.* This sound may indicate that the upper airway is blocked by the tongue or by relaxed tissues in the throat.
- *Crowing.* This sounds like the cawing of a crow and may mean that the muscles around the larynx are in spasm.
- *Gurgling.* Blood, vomit, mucus, or another liquid may be in the airway.
- *Stridor.* This harsh, high-pitched sound during inhalation may indicate that the larynx is swollen and blocking the upper airway.

Airway Adjuncts

Once the airway is open, it may be necessary to insert an **airway adjunct** (an artificial airway). There are two kinds: the **oropharyngeal airway** and the **nasopharyngeal airway**. Both extend down to, but do not pass through, the larynx. They are often used when patients are being artificially ventilated. (Artificial ventilation is covered in Section 3 of this chapter.)

When using airway adjuncts, remember the following:

- The airway adjunct must be clean and clear of any obstructions.
- The proper size must be used to be effective and to prevent complications.
- A patient with an airway adjunct can still aspirate secretions, blood, vomit, or other foreign substances into the lungs.
- The patient's mental status and gag reflex will tell you if an airway adjunct is appropriate. In general, if the patient is unresponsive with no gag reflex, use the oropharyngeal airway to help maintain or open the airway. If the patient is responsive or has a gag reflex, use the nasopharyngeal airway. Using an oropharyngeal airway may cause vomiting or spasm of the vocal cords, which will further compromise the airway.
- You must continually and carefully monitor the patient's mental status. If he or she becomes completely responsive or gags, you must remove the airway adjunct.

Oropharyngeal Airway

The oropharyngeal (oral) airway is a semicircular device made of hard plastic or rubber (Figure 7–6). It is designed to hold the tongue away from the back

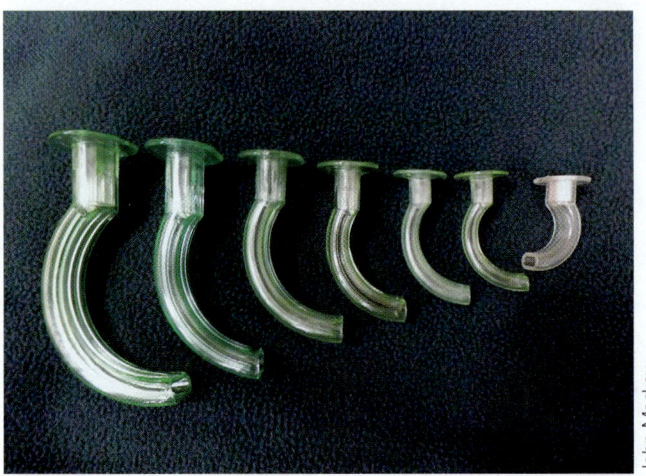

Figure 7–6 Oropharyngeal (oral) airways.

of the throat at the level of the pharynx. It also allows secretions to drain in a patient without a gag reflex.

There are two common types. One is tubular and the other has a channelled side. Both types are disposable and come in a variety of infant, child, and adult sizes.

To insert an oropharyngeal airway, follow these steps (Figure 7–7):

1. *Select the proper size.* The airway adjunct should extend from the corner of the lip to the angle of the jaw or to the tip of the earlobe. If the device is too long, it can push the epiglottis over the opening of the trachea, closing off the airway completely.
2. *Open the patient's mouth.* If necessary, use the cross-finger technique.
3. *Insert the airway upside down.* Be sure the tip is pointing toward the roof of the patient's mouth.
4. *Advance the airway gently.* Stop when you encounter resistance. This will happen when the device comes into contact with the soft back of the roof of the mouth.
5. *Turn the airway 180°.* Do so while continuing to advance it until the flat flange at the top rests on the patient's front teeth. The airway follows the natural curve of the tongue and the oropharynx.

If the patient gags at any time during insertion, *remove the oropharyngeal airway* by gently pulling it out and down. Do not rotate the device during removal. It may then be necessary to use a nasopharyngeal (nasal) airway or no airway adjunct at all. If the patient tries to dislodge the device, remove it. Be prepared for the patient to vomit.

If the patient is an infant or child, a preferred alternative is to use a tongue depressor (blade) to help insert the device. Proceed as follows (Figure 7–8):

INSERTING AN OROPHARYNGEAL AIRWAY

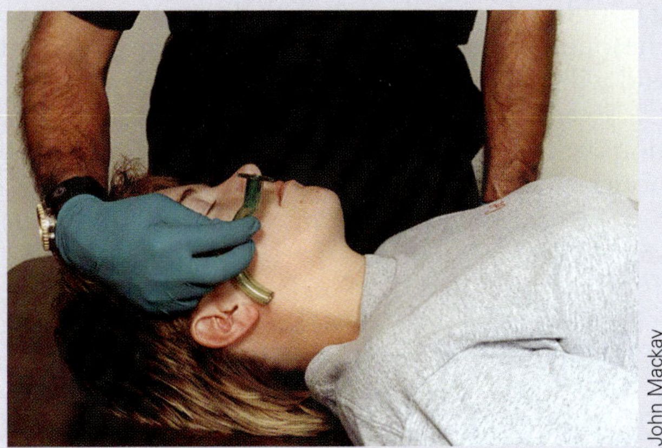

Figure 7–7a Measure the oropharyngeal airway to ensure the correct size.

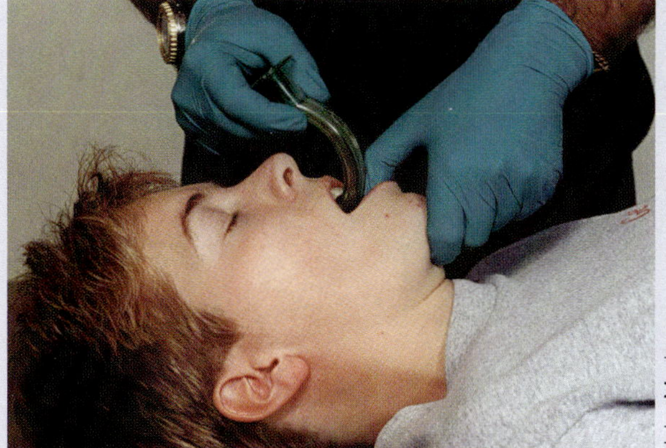

Figure 7–7b Insert it with the tip pointing toward the roof of the mouth.

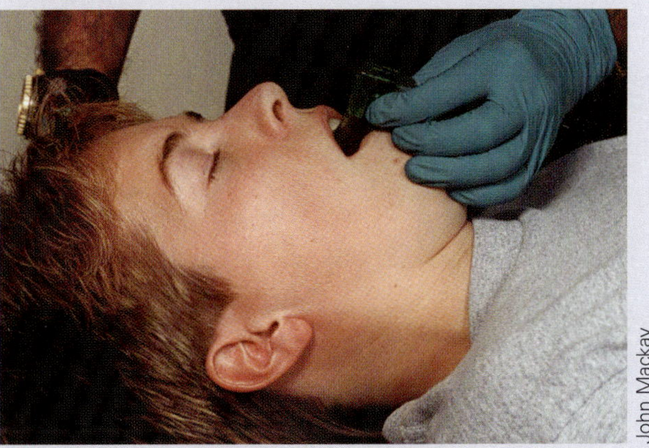

Figure 7–7c Gently rotate the airway until it reaches its proper position.

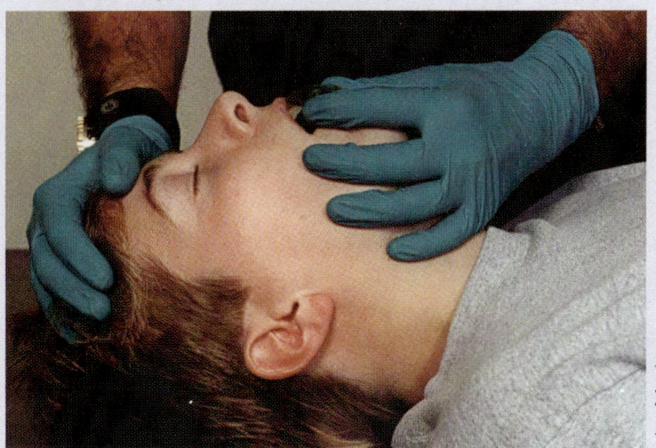

Figure 7–7d Continue inserting until the flange rests on the patient's teeth.

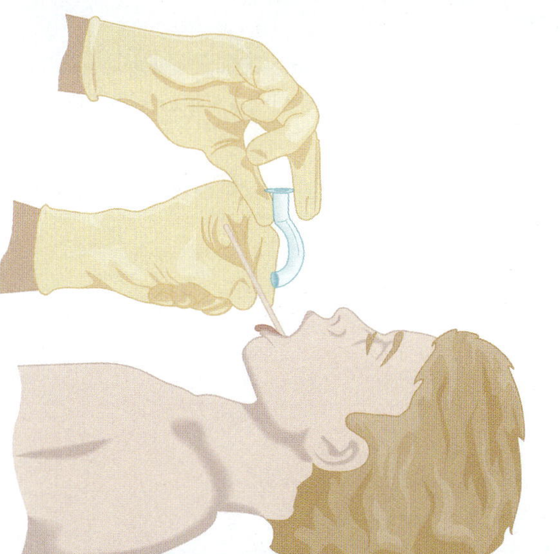

Figure 7–8 Inserting an oropharyngeal airway in an infant or child.

1. *Select the proper size.*
2. *Open the patient's mouth.*
3. *Insert the tongue depressor.* Stop when its tip is at the base of the tongue. Press the tongue depressor, and therefore the tongue, down toward the floor of the mouth and away from the opening of the throat.
4. *Insert the airway in its normal upright position.* Stop when the flange is seated on the patient's teeth. Do not insert it upside down as you would in an adult. If you do, it could cause bleeding in the airway.

Nasopharyngeal Airway

The nasopharyngeal (nasal) airway is a curved, hollow tube of soft plastic (Figure 7–9). It has a flange or flare at the top and a bevel at the bottom. It comes in a variety of sizes.

Nasal airways are less likely to cause vomiting than oral airways. This is because the soft tube

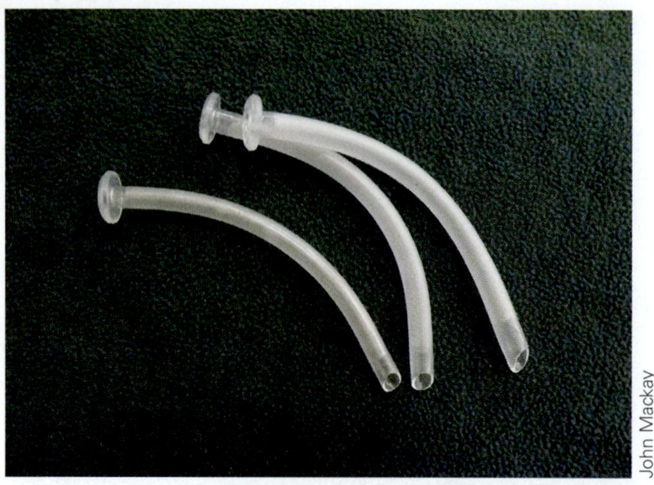

Figure 7–9 Nasopharyngeal (nasal) airways.

moves and yields when the patient swallows. Use it to keep the tongue from blocking the airway in patients who are not fully responsive or who have a gag reflex. Use it also when the patient cannot take the oral airway or if the teeth are clenched tightly and will not open.

Even though a nasal airway is lubricated, insertion can be painful and may cause the lining of the nose to bleed into the patient's airway.

To insert a nasopharyngeal airway, follow these steps (Figure 7–10):

1. *Select the proper size.* The airway adjunct should extend from the tip of the patient's nose to the tip of the earlobe. The diameter should fit

INSERTING A NASOPHARYNGEAL AIRWAY

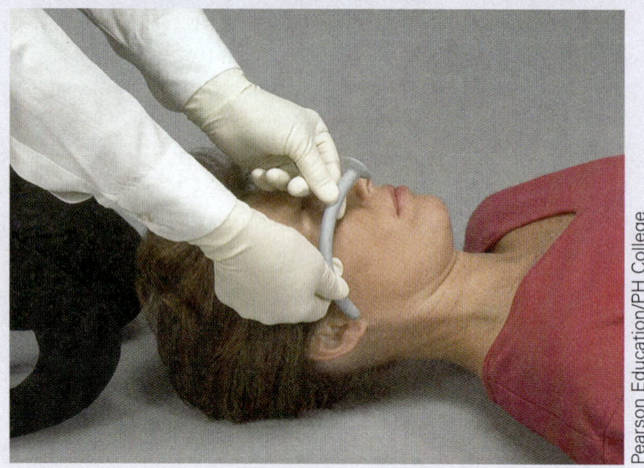

Figure 7–10a Measure the nasopharyngeal airway to ensure the correct size.

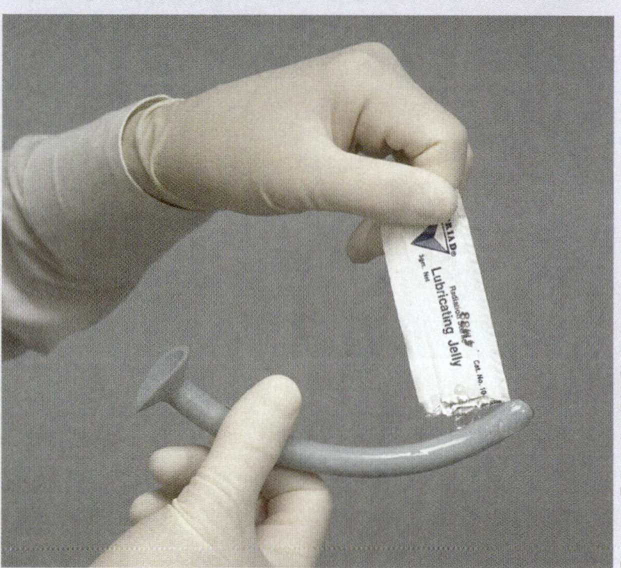

Figure 7–10b Lubricate it with a water-soluble lubricant.

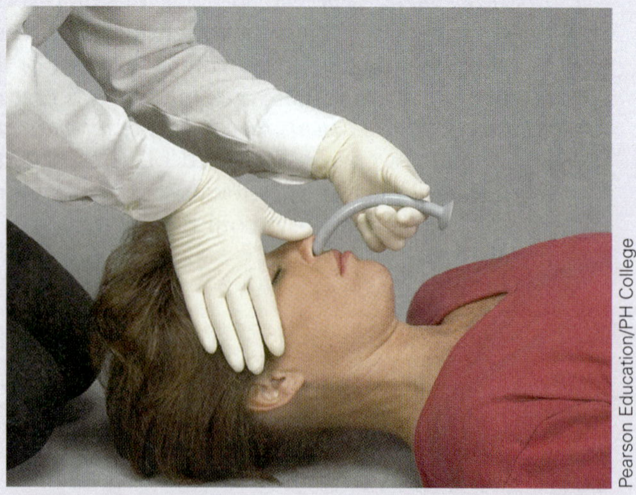

Figure 7–10c Insert the airway adjunct.

inside the nostril without **blanching** (causing loss of colour from) the skin of the nose. If it is too long, it could send air into the stomach instead of into the lungs, causing massive **gastric distention** (inflation of the stomach) and inadequate ventilation.

2. *Lubricate the device.* Use a sterile, water-soluble lubricant. This makes it easier to insert the airway. It also reduces the chances of injuring the nasal lining. Do not use petroleum jelly as it can damage the lining of the nose and throat.

3. *Insert the airway posteriorly.* The bevel, when it is inserted into the right-side nostril, should point toward the **septum**. (The septum is the wall dividing the two nostrils.) Insert the device close to the midline, along the floor of the nostril, and straight back into the nasopharynx. When the airway is properly inserted, the flange should lie against the flare of the nostril.

4. If the airway cannot be inserted into one nostril, try the other nostril. Do not force a nasal airway into place. If you meet resistance, gently rotate it. If you still feel resistance, remove the airway.

After insertion, check to see that air is flowing through the airway as the patient breathes. If the patient is breathing spontaneously, but no air movement is felt through the tube, remove it immediately and try inserting it into the other nostril.

Note that it is still necessary to maintain a head-tilt/chin-lift or jaw-thrust manoeuvre once the device is inserted.

Clearing the Airway

The recovery position, **finger sweeps**, and **suctioning** are three ways that an EMR can clear an airway of secretions. These techniques are not performed sequentially. The technique you choose depends on the patient's condition.

Recovery and Haines Positions

If the patient is breathing adequately and has a pulse, the HSFC recommends that you place him or her in the **recovery position** (Figure 7–11a). It is the first step in maintaining an open airway.

This position uses gravity to keep the airway clear. It allows fluids to drain from the mouth instead of into the airway. The patient's airway is likely to remain open and obstructions are less likely to occur. Note that even though the patient is in the recovery position, you should continue to monitor him or her until the paramedics arrive and take over care. In fact, the HSFC discourages the use of the recovery position with infants and children since the airway may become blocked if their head is not properly supported.

Do not move the patient into the recovery position if you suspect trauma or spinal injury. The position should only be used with an unresponsive, uninjured patient who is breathing adequately. He or she should stay in that position until the ambulance arrives. (If the patient is not breathing, or breathing inadequately, he or she must remain supine so that you can provide **artificial ventilation**, or artificial respiration.)

To move a patient into the recovery position, perform the following:

1. Lift the patient's left arm above his or her head. Then, cross the patient's right leg over the left leg.

2. Support the patient's face as you grasp the right shoulder.

3. Roll the patient toward you onto one side (the left side, preferably). Then, place his or her right hand under the side of the face. If possible, move the patient's head, shoulders, and torso simultaneously as a unit without twisting. The head should be as close to a midline position as possible.

4. Flex the patient's top leg at the knee.

If there is a suspected spinal injury or even a potential mechanism for injury, use the **HAINES recovery position** (High Arm IN Endangered Spine; Figure 7–11b) if you must turn an unconscious patient onto his or her side.

To move a patient into the HAINES position, perform the following:

1. Position the patient's left arm straight above his or her head with the palm facing up. Then, cross the patient's right arm over their chest and bend their right knee so that their right foot is positioned with the sole on the floor.

2. Support the patient's head with your left hand while your left forearm is positioned slightly below the patient's right shoulder.

3. Roll the patient away from you onto their left side by pushing their right knee over their left leg. Then, place his or her right hand toward the left armpit to help maintain a neutral position while the left arm remains under the head. Try to move the patient's head, shoulders, and torso simultaneously as a unit without twisting.

4. Flex the patient's top leg at the knee.

Alternatively, you may use your opposite arms in step 2 and roll the patient toward you if you are more comfortable. Turning the patient toward you increases the chance of your contact with **vomitus** but may offer you better control and support as you complete the move.

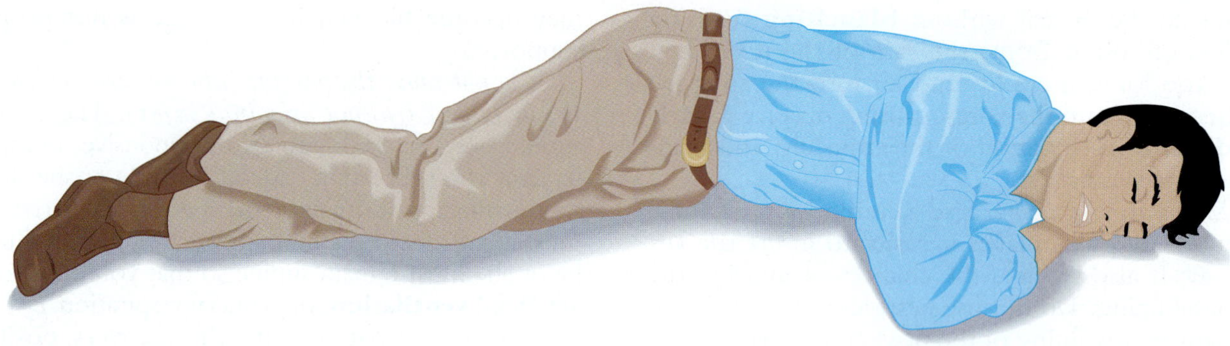

Figure 7–11a The recovery position.

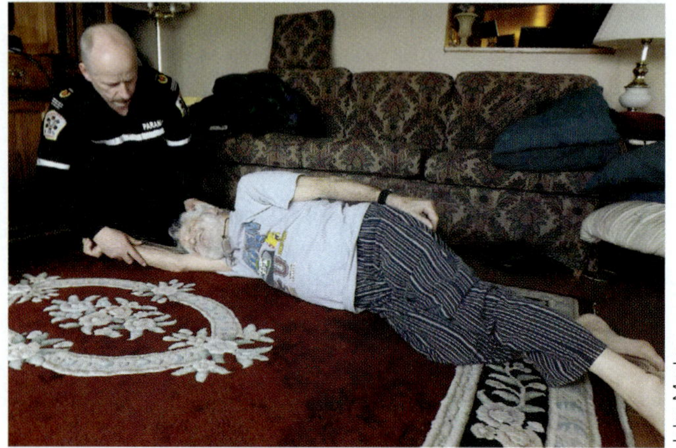

Figure 7–11b The HAINES recovery position.

Finger Sweeps

A finger sweep is performed only on unconscious patients. In a finger sweep, you use your finger to remove solid objects from the airway once you have seen them. Always wear latex gloves when performing a finger sweep. Foreign material or vomit in the mouth should be removed quickly. Never probe deeply with your fingers in an infant's or child's mouth. (This is called a blind finger sweep.) If you do not see an object in the infant's or child's mouth, do not perform a finger sweep.

To perform a finger sweep on an uninjured, unresponsive patient, do the following:

1. Roll the patient onto his or her left side. This position allows material to drain out of the mouth. It also helps keep the tongue away from the back of the throat.
2. Open the patient's mouth using the **tongue-jaw lift** technique and look inside. The tongue-jaw lift is performed by placing your fingers under the patient's chin and hooking your thumb over the lower teeth (Figure 7–12). If you see liquids or semi-liquids, cover your gloved index and middle fingers with a cloth.

3. Wipe the inside of the patient's mouth. Insert your index finger. Pass it along the inside of the cheek and into the throat at the base of the tongue. (Use your little finger for an infant or child.) Hook your finger around any foreign object to dislodge and remove it. Take extreme care that you do not force an object deeper into the patient's throat.

Suctioning

Suction devices use negative pressure to keep the airway clear. They remove blood, vomit, secretions, and other liquids from the mouth and airway. If you hear a gurgling sound during assessment or artificial ventilation, immediately suction the airway.

Most suction units cannot remove solid objects like teeth, particles of food, and other foreign bodies. Some cannot remove very thick vomit. In such situations, you may need to use an alternative piece of suction equipment or a finger sweep.

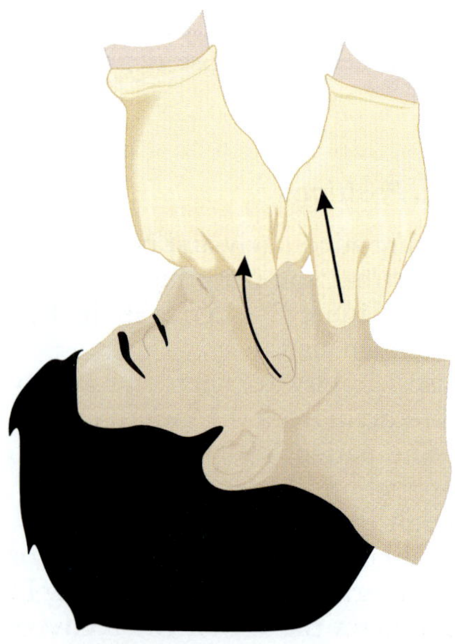

Figure 7–12 A finger sweep with tongue-jaw lift.

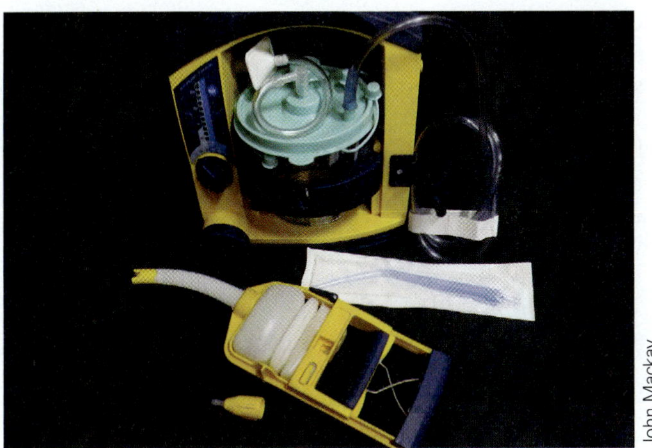

Figure 7–13 Portable suction units.

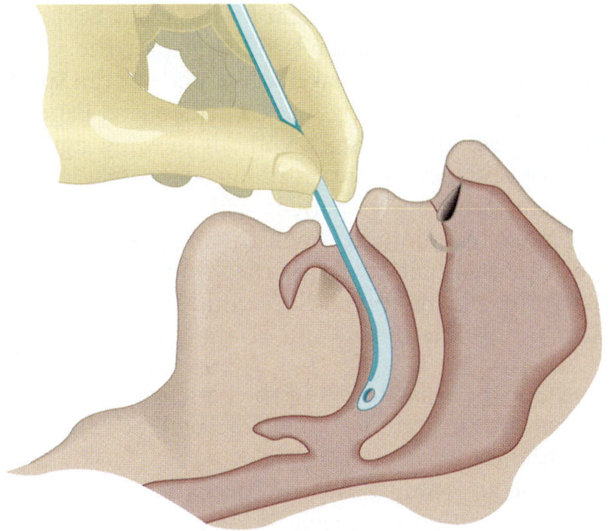

Figure 7–14 Suctioning technique.

Suctioning Equipment. Portable suction units (Figure 7–13) can be manually or electrically powered. Some are oxygen or air powered. All produce a vacuum that can suction substances from the throat. Each should be inspected before a shift or on a regular basis.

Manual units do not require an energy source other than the person operating them. As a result, they lack some of the typical problems associated with electric- or oxygen-powered devices. They can also more effectively suction heavy substances such as thick vomit.

Electric units must have fully charged batteries to function effectively. A low battery charge reduces the vacuum and the length of time the unit can be used. Some units allow for constant charging so that batteries remain full.

Any type of suction unit must have the following:

- Wide-bore, thick-walled, non-kinking tubing that fits a standard suction catheter
- Several sterile disposable suction catheters
- An unbreakable collection bottle or container
- A supply of water for rinsing and clearing tubes and catheters
- Enough vacuum pressure and flow to effectively suction substances from the throat

Principles of Suctioning. The procedure for suctioning varies depending on the type of unit and catheter used. However, the following general principles apply:

1. Be sure to take BSI precautions. Suctioning involves removal of body fluids. The potential for coughing and splatters is high. Wear protective eyewear, a mask, and gloves. If you suspect TB, wear appropriate protection the entire time you are in contact with the patient.
2. Use the type of catheter that is correct for your patient. Use a tonsil tip or tonsil sucker catheter to suction the mouth and throat of an unresponsive patient or an infant or child. Use a flexible, or French, catheter to suction the nose.
3. Insert the catheter, without suction, only to the base of the tongue. Place the convex (bulging) side of the catheter against the roof of the patient's mouth (Figure 7–14).
4. Apply suction by moving the catheter from side to side. Stop after 5 seconds in an infant, 10 seconds in a child, and 15 seconds in an adult.

Do not exceed the maximum times noted above. Air and oxygen are removed during suctioning. This can cause a quick drop in blood oxygen levels and changes in heart rate. In an adult, watch for rapid, slow, or irregular heart rates. In an infant, watch for a decreased heart rate. If a decrease is noted, stop suctioning and reapply oxygen or ventilate for at least 30 seconds prior to suctioning again.

Assessing Breathing

A pulseless patient will not be breathing. If your patient has a pulse but is unresponsive, you must establish an open airway and determine if the patient's breathing is adequate. The brain, heart, and liver are most sensitive to inadequate oxygen. Brain cells start to die within minutes without an oxygen supply.

Determining the Presence of Breathing

Breathing should be effortless. Watch to determine whether or not the chest rises and falls as the patient breathes. Check to see if the patient is using accessory muscles to breathe; look for excessive use of the neck muscles. Also look for excessive inward pulling of the muscles between the patient's ribs.

Observe a responsive patient for the ability to speak. This ability means that air is moving past the vocal cords. If the patient can make only sounds or can speak just a few words, breathing may be inadequate. Patients who can speak full sentences, without showing signs of distress or obstruction, are breathing adequately.

In an unresponsive patient with a pulse, use the cross-finger technique to open the mouth if needed. Then, open the airway with the head-tilt/chin-lift or jaw-thrust manoeuvre. Place your ear close to the patient's mouth and nose and do the following:

- *Look* for the rise and fall of the patient's chest.
- *Listen* for air coming out of the patient's nose or mouth.
- *Feel* for air coming out of the patient's nose or mouth against your cheek.

If the airway is obstructed, the patient's chest may still rise and fall. However, air will not be moving in and out of the patient's nose or mouth. Assessing breathing need only be done for five to ten seconds to determine if respirations are present.

Note that **agonal respirations** (reflex gasping with no regular pattern or depth) may occur with cardiac arrest. They may also be a late sign of impending respiratory arrest. These reflex gasps should not be confused with breathing.

Signs of Inadequate Breathing

It is very important for you to recognize the signs of inadequate breathing. Some are subtle and require careful evaluation. If you are not sure that a patient needs breathing assistance, it is better to err on the side of safety and provide ventilation.

Inadequate breathing is characterized by the following signs (Figure 7–15). Note, however, that not all the signs will be present at the same time. Any one of them may be reason enough to ventilate a patient without delay.

- *Too fast or too slow a breathing rate.* Rates of fewer than 20 respirations per minute in an infant, fewer than 10 in a child, and fewer than 8 in an adult are ominous signs of inadequate breathing.
- *Inadequate chest wall motion.* Adequate breathing is normally accompanied by the rise and fall of the chest. If the chest wall is not rising and falling as it should, or if the sides of the chest rise and fall unequally, breathing is inadequate.
- **Cyanosis.** This is a bluish discolouration of the skin and mucous membranes. It is a sign that body tissues are not receiving enough oxygen.
- *Mental status changes.* Remember that the mental status of a patient typically correlates with the status of his or her airway and breathing. A patient who becomes drowsy, disoriented, confused, or unconscious may not be breathing adequately.
- *Increased work of breathing* (WOB). Normal breathing is effortless. When you see a pronounced use of abdominal muscles to breathe, the patient is pushing on the diaphragm to force air out of the lungs. You may note retractions (inward pulling) between the ribs, above the collarbone, in the neck muscles, or below the rib cage as the patient inhales. An infant may develop a see-saw motion in which the abdomen and chest move in opposite directions. Flaring of the nostrils during inhalation is another sign more commonly seen in infants and children.
- *Gasping and grunting.* These sounds mean that the patient is having a difficult time moving air through the respiratory tract. Be alert for other abnormal sounds, such as snoring, crowing, gurgling, or stridor.
- *Slow heart rate accompanied by slow breathing rate.*

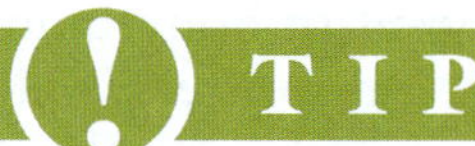

Figure 7–15 Signs of inadequate breathing.

T I P

These guidelines for assessing breathing and artificial ventilation are your priority only in patients with a pulse. As you will see in Chapter 8, cardiac compressions receive priority in a pulseless patient.

SECTION 3
GUIDELINES FOR EMERGENCY CARE

Artificial Ventilation

If a patient is breathing inadequately or is not breathing at all, that patient needs your immediate assistance. Artificial ventilation is a way of breathing for these patients.

The air we inhale contains about 21 percent oxygen. Only a small percentage of it is used by the body. The air we exhale contains about 17 percent oxygen and 4 percent carbon dioxide. Since the air you breathe into a patient contains more than enough oxygen to keep him or her alive, artificial ventilation is sufficient to support life until high-concentration oxygen is available.

When performing artificial ventilation, monitor the patient continuously to make sure your breaths are adequate. Indications of adequate ventilations include the following:

- The rate of respiration is adequate—once every three to five seconds for infants and children, once every five to six seconds for adults.
- The force of air is consistent and sufficient to cause the chest to rise during each ventilation.
- The patient's heart rate decreases or returns to normal. However, underlying medical conditions may prevent this from happening even when ventilations are adequate.
- The patient's colour improves.

Inadequate ventilation may occur because of problems with the patient's airway or because of improper use of a ventilation device. Indications of inadequate ventilations include the following:

- The chest does not rise and fall with each ventilation.
- The ventilation rate is too fast or too slow.
- The heart rate does not decrease or return to normal.

The risk of coming into contact with a patient's secretions, blood, or vomit while you are ventilating is high. Therefore, you must take BSI precautions. At a minimum, use gloves, eyewear, and a pocket face mask or other barrier device with a one-way filter. If large amounts of blood or secretions are present, use a face mask.

There are many techniques for artificial ventilation. An EMR must be competent in three, listed here in order of preference: **mouth-to-mask ventilation**, **mouth-to-barrier device ventilation**, and **mouth-to-mouth ventilation**.

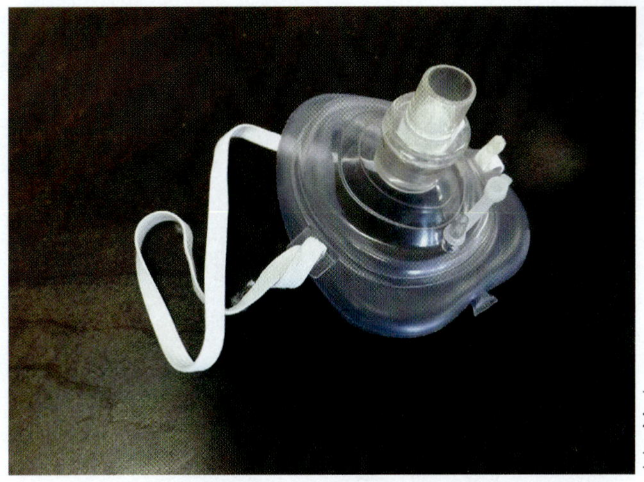

Figure 7–16 A pocket face mask with a one-way valve and oxygen port.

Mouth-to-Mask Ventilation

The most effective EMR technique for ventilation is mouth-to-mask. A pocket face mask with a one-way valve is used to form a seal around the patient's nose and mouth (Figure 7–16). You blow into a port at the top of the mask to deliver the ventilation. The one-way valve diverts the patient's exhaled breath.

Mouth-to-mask is the preferred technique because it eliminates direct contact with the patient's nose, mouth, and body fluids. It prevents exposure to the patient's exhaled air. It also allows you to deliver ventilations of adequate force. The mask you use should have the following characteristics:

- It should be transparent so that you can see vomit, blood, or other substances in the patient's mouth.
- It must fit snugly enough on the patient's face to form a good seal.
- It should be available in an average adult size and in additional sizes for infants and children.
- It must have a one-way valve, or it must be able to connect to a one-way valve at the ventilation port.
- If you have oxygen available, the mask must have an oxygen inlet port.

Mouth-to-mask ventilation is very effective because both your hands are used to create a seal around the mask. To perform the technique, position yourself at the top of the patient's head or at the side. Attach oxygen to the mask if it is available. Then follow these steps (Figure 7–17):

1. *Position the mask on the patient.* The narrower top portion of the mask should be seated on the bridge of the nose. The broader portion should fit in the cleft of the chin. The position of the

ARTIFICIAL VENTILATION

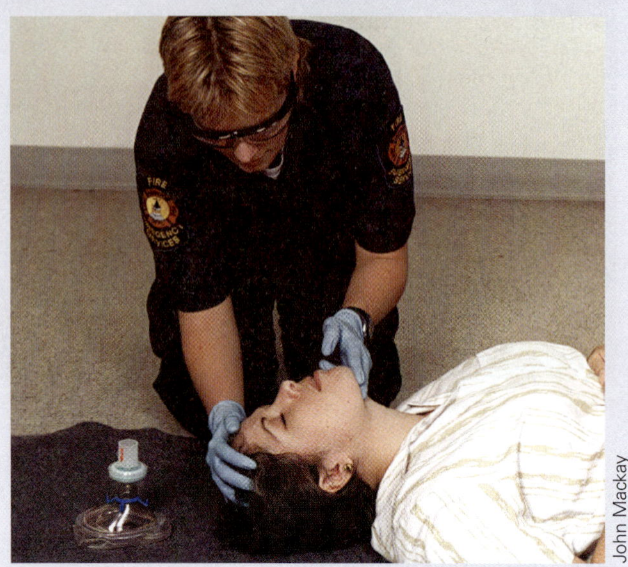

Figure 7–17a Open the airway with a head-tilt/chin-lift manoeuvre.

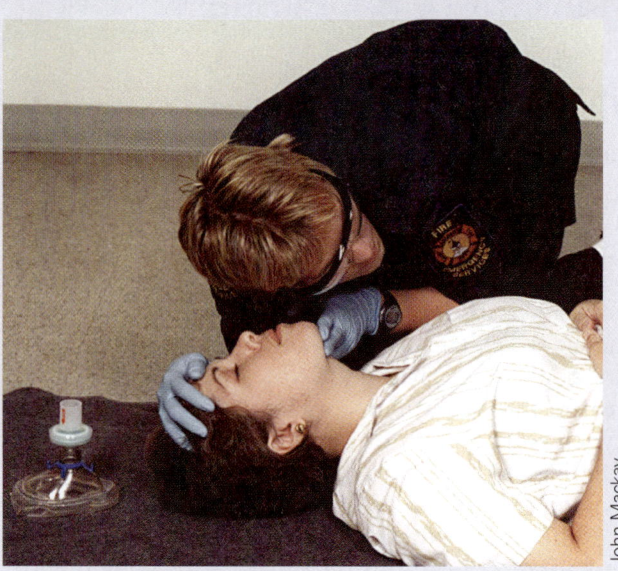

Figure 7–17b Look, listen, and feel to establish breathlessness.

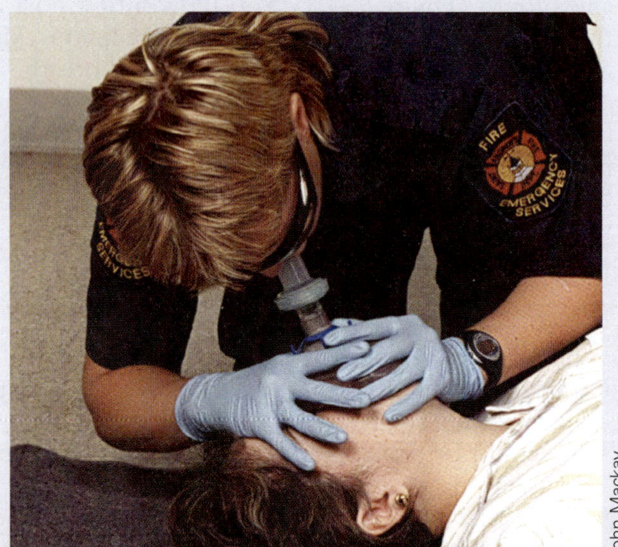

Figure 7–17c Deliver two slow full initial breaths, taking a deep breath before each.

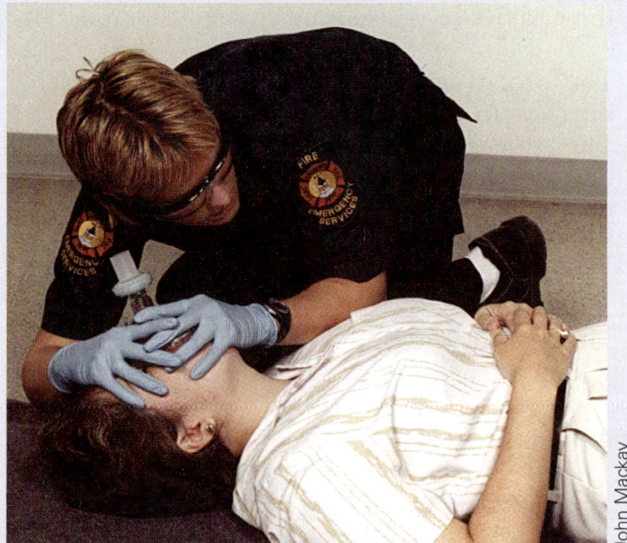

Figure 7–17d If ventilations are adequate, you will see the chest rise and fall and feel the exhaled air on your cheek.

mask is critical. If it is wrong, it will leak and prevent you from delivering adequate ventilations.

2. *Seal the mask.* If you are positioned at the top of the patient's head, place the roots of both thumbs on the top portion. Place the heels and palms of both hands along the sides. Compress the mask firmly around the edges to form a good seal.

3. *Open the patient's airway.* Place your index fingers on the part of the mask that covers the chin. Using the middle and ring fingers of both hands, grasp along the mandible (the bony part of the jaw). Pull upward to perform the manoeuvre. Use a jaw-thrust manoeuvre if trauma is suspected (Figure 7–18).

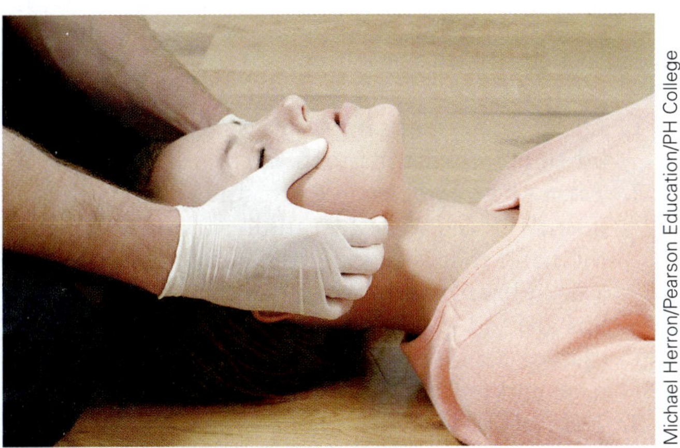

Figure 7–18a Artificial ventilation: Jaw-thrust manoeuvre; side view.

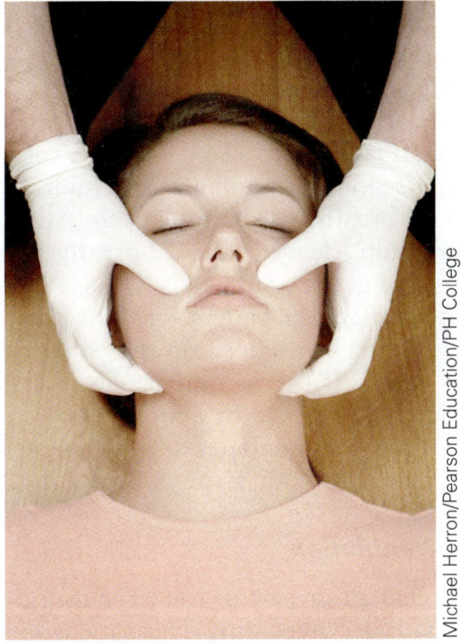

Figure 7–18b Artificial ventilation: Jaw-thrust manoeuvre; front view.

TABLE 7–2	
ARTIFICIAL VENTILATION RATES	
Patient	**Ventilation Rate**
Newborn	40–60 breaths per minute at 1 second each
Infant/child	12–20 breaths per minute at 1 second each (approximately 1 breath every 3–5 seconds)
Adult	10–12 breaths per minute at 1 second each (approximately 1 breath every 5–6 seconds)

infants and children, deliver 12 to 20 breaths per minute, with each breath lasting 1 second. For adults, deliver 10 to 12 breaths per minute, with each lasting 1 second.

7. If you cannot ventilate the patient, or if the chest does not rise adequately, reposition the patient's head and try again. (Improper head position is the most common cause of difficulty with ventilation.) If the second try also fails, assume that the airway is blocked by a foreign object. Then follow the guidelines (later in this chapter) for removing it.

Mouth-to-Barrier Device Ventilation

A barrier device, such as a face shield, can be used during ventilation (Figure 7–19). It provides some of the same protection to the EMR as a pocket face mask. A thin and flexible plastic face shield can also be folded and carried easily. Some are available in key-ring and belt-storage containers.

Barrier devices are thin enough to provide very low resistance to the ventilations you deliver to

4. *Deliver two effective initial breaths.* Place your mouth around the one-way valve and blow into the ventilation port. Each breath should be delivered over one second. It should also be steady and of sufficient volume to make the chest rise, usually 800 to 1200 mL (millilitres) in an average adult. Make sure that you do not deliver too much air too fast, or you will force air into the patient's stomach.

5. *Determine if ventilations are adequate.* Watch the chest to see if it rises and falls. Listen and feel for air escaping when the patient exhales.

6. *Continue ventilations at the proper rate* (Table 7–2). For newborns, deliver 40 to 60 breaths per minute, with each breath lasting 1 second. For

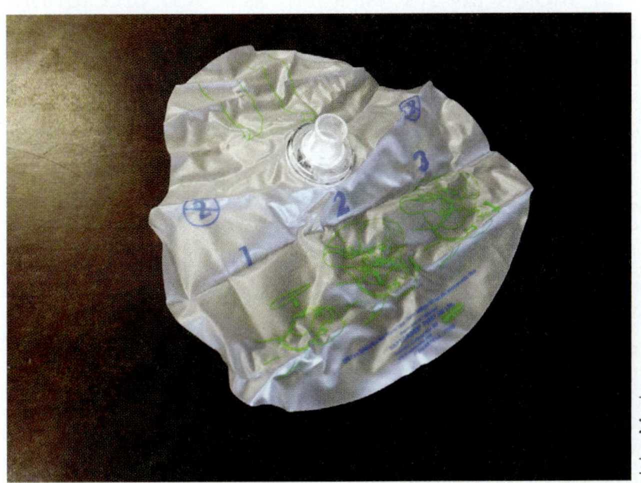

Figure 7–19 Example of a barrier device.

the patient. And they can provide some protection against contamination from body fluids. However, many do not have a one-way valve that diverts the patient's exhaled air.

To provide ventilations using a barrier device, kneel at the patient's head. Then, follow these steps:

1. *Position the device on the patient.*
2. *Open the patient's airway.* Use a head-tilt/chin-lift or jaw-thrust manoeuvre.
3. *Deliver two effective initial breaths.* Place your mouth over the barrier device and blow into it. Each breath should be slow (delivered over one second). It should also be steady and of sufficient volume to make the chest rise. Make sure that you do not deliver too much air too fast, or you will force air into the patient's stomach.
4. *Determine if ventilations are adequate.* Watch the chest rise and fall. Listen and feel for air escaping when the patient exhales.
5. *Continue ventilations at the proper rate.* For newborns, deliver 40 to 60 breaths per minute, each breath lasting 1 second. For infants and children, deliver 12 to 20 breaths per minute, each lasting 1 second. For adults, deliver 10 to 12 breaths per minute, each lasting 1 second.
6. If you cannot ventilate the patient, or if the chest does not rise adequately, reposition the patient's head and try again. If the second try also fails, assume that the airway is blocked by a foreign object. Then, follow the guidelines (later in this chapter) for removing a foreign body airway obstruction.

Mouth-to-Mouth Ventilation

The risk of contracting infectious diseases makes mouth-to-mouth ventilation too dangerous for regular use by EMRs. As described earlier, barrier devices and face masks with one-way valves are available. You should always use them as a BSI precaution. However, your decision is a personal one. Mouth-to-mask and mouth-to-barrier device techniques should not replace training in mouth-to-mouth ventilation.

Mouth-to-mouth ventilation is a quick, effective method for delivering oxygen to a non-breathing patient. It involves ventilating the patient with your exhaled breath while making mouth-to-mouth contact. Use the mouth-to-mouth technique only in emergency situations in which no protective devices are available. For example, you may find that you need to perform mouth-to-mouth ventilation on a family member at home, where a barrier device is not available.

In mouth-to-mouth ventilation, you form a seal with your mouth around the patient's mouth. The obvious risk to you is exposure to body fluids and, thus, to infectious diseases.

To perform the technique, kneel at the patient's head. Then, follow these steps:

1. *Open the patient's airway.* Use a head-tilt/chin-lift or jaw-thrust manoeuvre.
2. *Form an airtight seal.* Gently squeeze the patient's nostrils closed with the thumb and index finger of the hand that is holding the patient's head. Take a deep breath and form an airtight seal with your lips around the patient's mouth. If you are ventilating an infant or small child, cover both the nose and mouth with your lips.
3. *Deliver two effective initial breaths.* Each breath lasts one second. Each breath should be steady and of sufficient volume to make the chest rise. Make sure that you do not deliver too much air too fast, or you will force air into the patient's stomach.
4. *Determine if ventilations are adequate.* Watch the chest to see if it rises and falls. Listen and feel for air escaping when the patient exhales.
5. *Continue ventilations at the proper rate.* For newborns, deliver 40 to 60 breaths per minute, each breath lasting 1 second. For infants and children, deliver 12 to 20 breaths per minute, each lasting 1 second. For adults, deliver 10 to 12 breaths per minute, each lasting 1 second.
6. If you cannot ventilate the patient, or if the chest does not rise adequately, reposition the patient's head and try again. If the second try also fails, assume the airway is blocked by a foreign object. Then, follow the guidelines (later in this chapter) for removing a foreign body airway obstruction.

Mouth-to-Stoma Ventilation

A patient who has had all or part of the larynx surgically removed has had a laryngectomy. This patient will have a **stoma**, a permanent opening that connects the trachea directly to the front of the neck (Figure 7–20). These patients (neck breathers) breathe only through the stoma.

To perform artificial ventilation on a patient with a stoma, remove all coverings, such as scarves or ties, from the stoma area. Then follow these steps:

1. *Clear the stoma of any foreign matter.* Use a gauze pad or handkerchief. Do not use tissue, which can shred and cling.
2. *Form an airtight seal around the stoma.* Whenever possible, use a barrier device such as a pocket face mask or shield.
3. *Blow slowly through the stoma for one second.* Use just enough force to make the patient's chest rise.
4. *Determine if ventilations are adequate.* Allow time for exhalation. Watch for the patient's chest to fall. Feel to make sure air is escaping back through the stoma as the patient exhales.

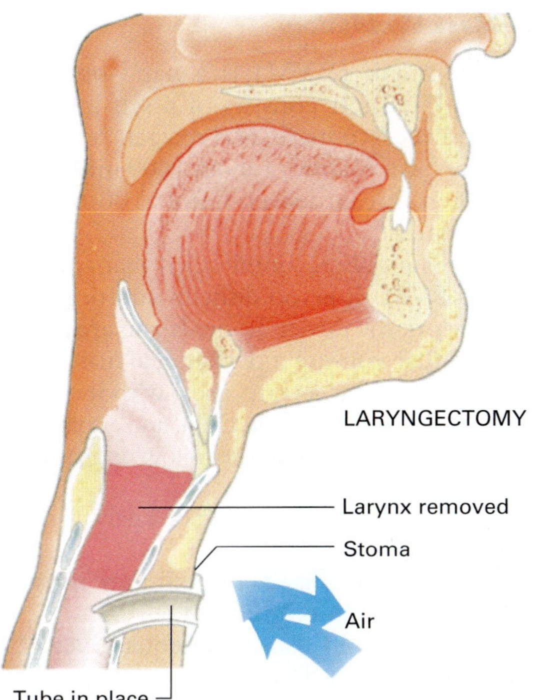

Figure 7–20 The neck breather's airway has been changed by surgery.

5. *Continue ventilations at the proper rate.* For newborns, deliver 40 to 60 breaths per minute, each breath lasting 1 second. For infants and children, deliver 12 to 20 breaths per minute, each lasting 1 second. For adults, deliver 10 to 12 breaths per minute, with each lasting 1 second.

If the chest does not rise, the patient may be a partial neck breather. This patient has had only part of the larynx removed. He or she can breathe through both the stoma and the nose or mouth. Seal the patient's nose and mouth with one hand. Pinch the nose between your third and fourth fingers (Figure 7–21). Seal the lips with the palm of the same gloved hand. Hook your thumb under the patient's chin and press up and back. Continue ventilations through the stoma.

Infants and Children

Many of the steps involved in managing the airway of an infant or child are the same as those for an adult. However, remember that there are important differences.

You must position the head carefully when preparing for artificial ventilation. Keep an infant's head in a neutral (sniffing) position. You can extend the head slightly beyond neutral if the patient is older than one year, but do not extend the infant's or child's head too far. The airway is more flexible than

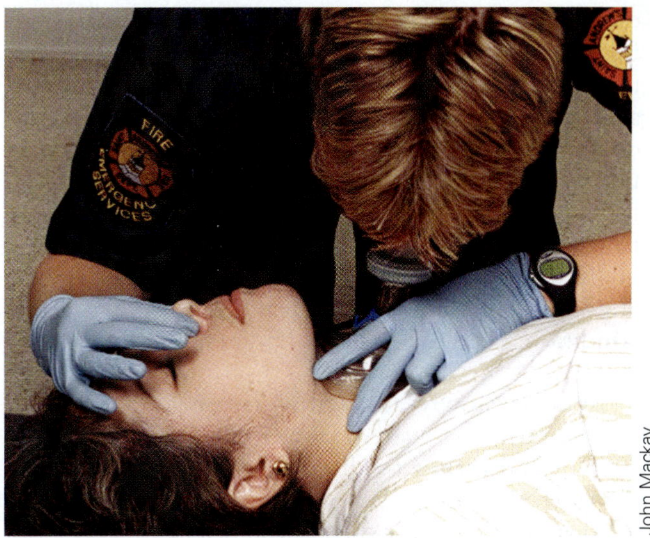

Figure 7–21 Mask-to-stoma ventilation.

an adult's and can be easily overextended, which in itself can block the airway.

Consider an oral airway adjunct for an infant or child. The primary cause of blocked airway in these patients is the tongue. Try positioning the head and pulling the jaw forward to move the tongue away from the back of the throat. If that is unsuccessful, use an oropharyngeal airway to keep the tongue away from the throat and the airway open.

Depending on the age and size of an infant, you may be able to form a seal with your mouth over the infant's mouth and nose. Use a proper-sized mask if possible. If an adult pocket face mask must be used, position the mask with the orientation of the narrow nose part and the broad chin part reversed (Figure 7–22).

Guard against gastric distention. This is common in infants and children who are being ventilated. During artificial ventilation, air may get into the

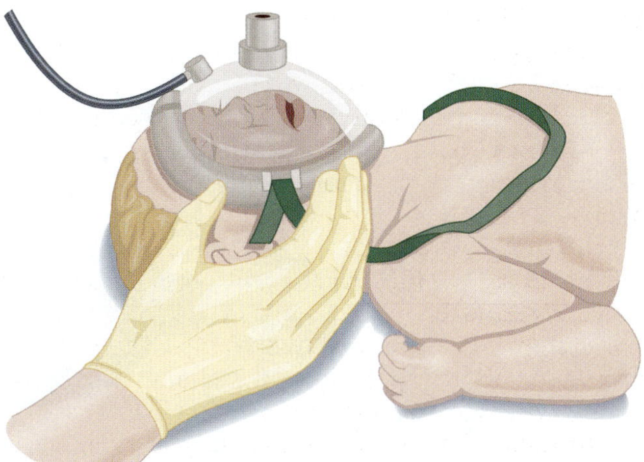

Figure 7–22 On an infant, the orientation of the adult pocket face mask is reversed.

esophagus and stomach if ventilations are too forceful. Because it puts pressure on the diaphragm, gastric distention may significantly impair your attempts at ventilation, limiting the amount of air that can enter the lungs. Monitor the infant or child carefully to make sure the chest is rising and falling with ventilations. Listen and feel for exhaled air. Watch carefully to make sure the abdomen does not start to extend.

The HSFC recommends against pressing on the abdomen to relieve gastric distention. To avoid this condition, keep the following points in mind:

- Breathe slowly and with just enough force to make the chest rise. If you notice that the abdomen is starting to distend, reduce the force of your ventilations.
- Keep the infant's or child's head in a neutral position.
- Allow the infant or child to exhale between ventilations.
- Monitor against vomiting. If it looks like the infant or child is about to vomit, immediately stop ventilating and roll him or her onto his or her side. This position allows the vomit to flow out from the mouth rather than into the lungs. If the infant or child vomits, suction or quickly wipe the mouth with gauze pads. Wipe the face, and return to ventilation.

Patients with Dental Appliances

If the patient has dentures that are secure in the mouth, leave them in place. It is much easier to create an airtight seal with them there. If the dentures are extremely loose, remove them so they do not block the airway. Partial dentures—plates and bridges—may also become dislodged. If they are loose, remove them.

In patients who have dental appliances, reassess the mouth frequently to make sure that they have not come loose.

Bag-Valve-Mask Ventilation

The **bag-valve-mask (BVM)** is a hand-operated device (Figure 7–23). It consists of a self-inflating bag, one-way valve, face mask, and oxygen reservoir. The BVM device has a volume of about 1600 mL. When used with oxygen, it can deliver almost 100 percent oxygen to the patient.

Note that it is highly recommended that two rescuers operate a BVM. It is too difficult and tiring for one rescuer to work the device alone. If you are alone, we recommend that you use a pocket face mask, as it is easier for one rescuer to create a seal with it.

The BVM is available in infant, child, and adult sizes. Whatever the size, it should have the following features:

- Self-refilling bag that is disposable or easily cleaned and sterilized
- Non-jam valve that allows a maximum oxygen inlet flow of 15 L/min or greater
- No pop-off valve (can cause inadequate ventilations if present but not disabled)
- Standardized 15/22 mm (millimetre) fittings
- Oxygen inlet and reservoir that allow for a high concentration of oxygen
- True non-rebreather valve
- Ability to perform in all environments and at extreme temperatures

To provide artificial ventilation by way of a BVM, follow these steps:

1. *Open the patient's airway.* Note that an oral or nasal airway adjunct may be necessary in conjunction with the BVM. If you suspect injury to the head or spine, stabilize the patient's head between your knees or have an assistant manually stabilize it.
2. *Select the correct size of mask*—infant, child, or adult.

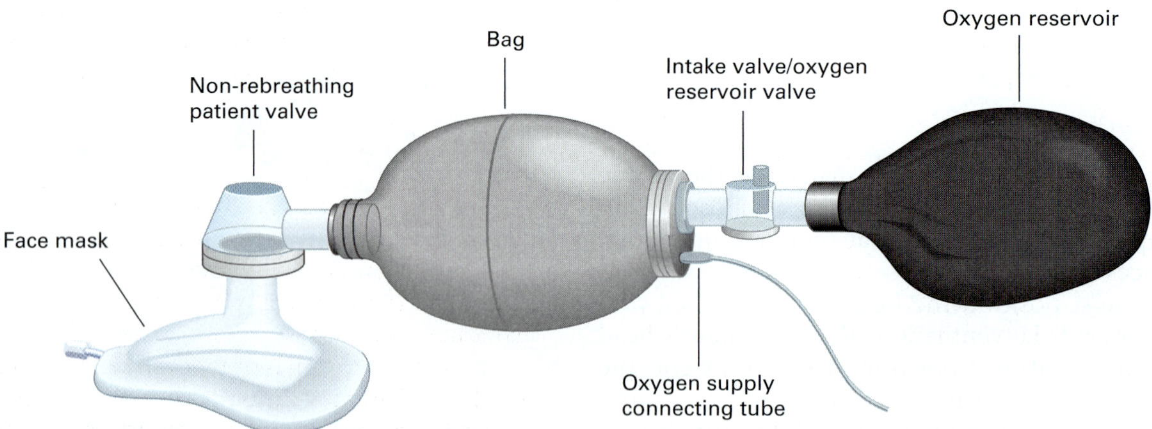

Figure 7–23 Bag-valve-mask (BVM) unit.

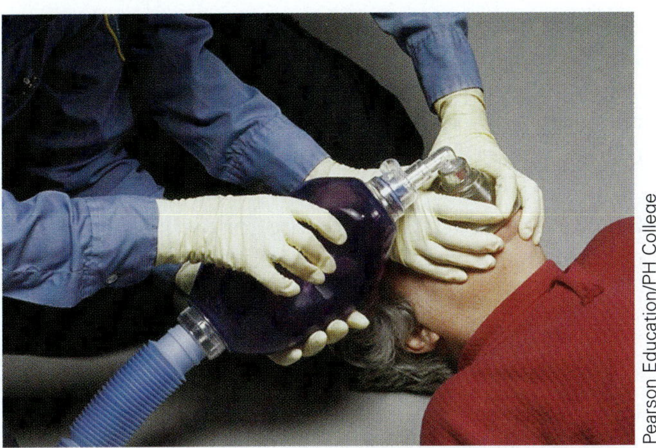

Figure 7–24 Two rescuers operating a bag-valve-mask unit.

3. *Position the mask.* Place your thumbs over the top half of the mask. Index and middle fingers should be over the bottom half. Then, put the narrow end (apex) of the mask over the bridge of the patient's nose. Lower the mask over the mouth and upper chin. If the mask has a large round cuff around a ventilation port, centre the port over the patient's mouth. Use your ring and little fingers to bring the jaw up to the mask. Use the jaw-thrust manoeuvre if you suspect head or spinal injury. Be sure to avoid tilting the head or neck.

4. *Connect the mask to the bag,* if it has not been done already.

5. *Operate the bag* (Figure 7–24). Your partner should squeeze the bag with two hands until the patient's chest rises. For infants and children, deliver 12 to 20 breaths per minute, with each lasting 1 second. For adults, deliver 10 to 12 breaths per minute, with each lasting 1 second.

If you are alone, form a "C" around the ventilation port with your thumb and index finger. Use your middle, ring, and little fingers under the jaw to maintain a chin lift and complete the seal. Squeeze the bag with your other hand while observing the chest to see if it rises and falls.

If the chest does not rise and fall with your ventilations, reposition the patient's head or jaw. Check again for an airway obstruction. If air is escaping from under the mask, reposition your fingers and check the position of the mask. If the patient's chest still does not rise, use an alternative method, such as mouth-to-mask ventilation.

Assisting Inadequate Breathing

If your patient is breathing inadequately, provide ventilations while the patient is inhaling.

Since inadequate breathing is often slower than usual, you will need to provide *additional* ventilations in between the patient's own attempts to inhale. If breathing is rapid or very shallow, provide assisted ventilations when the patient begins inhaling. You will find that providing a ventilation while the patient is exhaling can create resistance or an unusual noise.

Simply continue to time your assisted ventilations as best as you can with the patient's own respiratory effort. Recognizing inadequate breathing and assisting the patient with ventilations are among the best things you can do for your patient. Your intervention may prevent him or her from lapsing into complete respiratory and cardiac arrest.

Oxygen Therapy

Oxygen equipment can be an excellent tool for a well-trained EMR. It allows you to deliver oxygen to patients who desperately need it. However, if you are not allowed to administer oxygen in your EMS system, do not wait for it to arrive before providing emergency care.

Indications for Oxygen Therapy

Conditions that may require oxygen therapy include major injury, heart or breathing problems, shock, or any other condition that prevents the efficient flow of oxygen throughout the body. Signs and symptoms that indicate the need for oxygen are as follows:

- Poor skin colour (blue, grey, or pale)
- Unresponsiveness
- Cool, clammy skin
- Difficulty breathing
- Blood loss
- Chest pain
- Trauma (injury)

When you provide artificial ventilation, you can give a higher concentration of oxygen to the patient by connecting supplemental oxygen to the pocket face mask.

Oxygen Cylinders

All oxygen cylinders are manufactured according to strict government regulations. These regulations govern how often cylinders must be checked for safety. Labels on the cylinders warn of dangers and include handling precautions.

A number of different types of oxygen cylinders are available. They vary in size and volume (Figure 7–25). Even though the volume of oxygen may vary, all the cylinders, when full, are at the same pressure, about

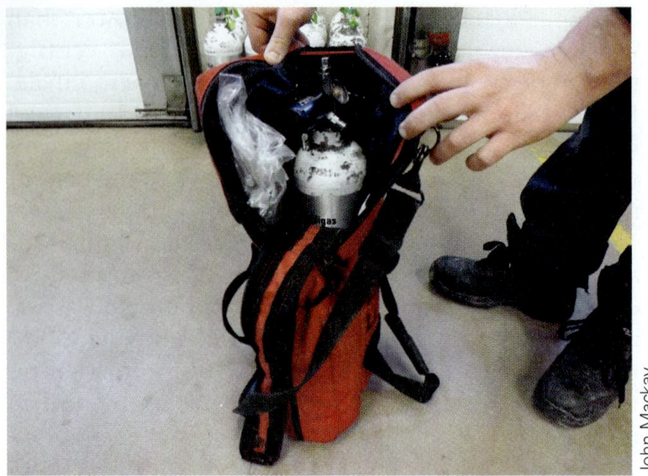

John Mackay

Figure 7–25 A portable oxygen cylinder and regulator.

2000 psi (pounds per square inch). Cylinder sizes are identified by letter. The following are sizes used in emergency medical care:

* D cylinder—350 L
* E cylinder—625 L
* M cylinder—3000 L
* G cylinder—5300 L
* H cylinder—6900 L

Gas flow from an oxygen cylinder is controlled by regulators. They reduce pressure in the cylinder to a safe range of about 50 psi and control the flow from 0.25 to 25 L/min. Regulators are attached to the cylinder by a yoke. Each yoke fits only the cylinders made for one type of gas. In addition, all gas cylinders are colour coded according to contents. Oxygen cylinders in Canada are generally aluminum grey.

Two types of regulators may be attached to oxygen cylinders. They are **high-pressure regulators** and **therapy regulators**.

The high-pressure regulator can provide 50 psi to power a demand-valve type resuscitator (flow-restricted, oxygen-powered ventilation device) or a suction device. It has a threaded outlet and one gauge, which registers the cylinder contents. It cannot be used interchangeably with the therapy regulator. It has no mechanism to adjust flow rate, and it is designed specifically for use with advanced oxygen delivery devices. To use a high-pressure regulator, attach the equipment supply line to the threaded outlet and open the cylinder valve fully. Then, close it one-half turn for safety.

The therapy regulator can administer oxygen at 0.25 to 25 L/min. It has two gauges. One shows cylinder contents and the other allows you to provide a metered flow of oxygen to the patient. The cylinder is full when the pressure is 2000 psi or greater. This

pressure drops in direct proportion to the contents. For example, if the pressure is 1000 psi, the cylinder is half full. Adjust the flow meter to provide oxygen appropriate to the device used and the condition of the patient. Follow local protocols.

Safety Precautions. Observe the following safety precautions when you handle oxygen cylinders:

* Never allow combustible materials, such as oil or grease, to touch the cylinder, regulator, fittings, valves, or hoses.
* Never smoke or allow others to smoke in any area where oxygen cylinders are in use or on standby.
* Store the cylinders below 50°C.
* Never use an oxygen cylinder without a safe, properly fitting regulator valve.
* Never use a valve made for another gas even if it has been modified.
* Keep all valves closed when the oxygen cylinder is not in use, even when a tank is empty.
* Keep oxygen cylinders secure to prevent them from toppling over. In transit, they should be in a carrier rack.
* Never place any part of your body over the cylinder valve. A loosely fitting regulator can be blown off with sufficient force to decapitate a person.
* Never stand an oxygen tank upright near the patient. If the tank is not in a commercial pack, lay it on its side by the patient.

Using the Cylinders. Prepare the tank, if it is not used every day, by following these steps (Figure 7–26):

1. Place the cylinder securely upright and confirm that it contains oxygen. Do not position yourself over any part of the cylinder as you remove the protective seal.
2. Using the supplied wrench, slowly open the cylinder valve for one second then rapidly close it to clear it of dust or debris.
3. Inspect the regulator valve to be certain that it is the right type for an oxygen cylinder. Be sure it has an intact washer. Place the yoke of the regulator over the cylinder valve and align the pins.
4. Hand-tighten the T-screw on the regulator.
5. Open the main cylinder valve to check the pressure. Make one half-turn beyond the point where the regulator valve becomes pressurized. Read the gauge to be sure that the tank has an adequate amount of oxygen. Most tanks will not function at less than 200 psi.
6. Attach the oxygen-delivery device to the regulator.
7. Adjust the flow meter to the appropriate litre flow.
8. Apply the oxygen-delivery device to the patient.

When you are ready to stop oxygen therapy, detach the mask from the patient. Then, shut off the control valve until the litre flow is at zero. Shut off the main cylinder valve. Then, bleed the other valves by leaving the control valve open until the needle or ball indicator returns to zero. Shut the control valve on all cylinders you carry.

It should be part of your daily routine to check the oxygen cylinder carried in your vehicle. You should open the main cylinder valve and check the pressure remaining in the cylinder. Many organizations have a policy of replacing or refilling oxygen cylinders that get below 500 psi. It is negligent, not to mention very frustrating, to arrive at the scene of a crash with lights, sirens, and other fanfare only to find that you have an empty oxygen cylinder.

Always replace a cylinder when the pressure is low. Have backup portable oxygen cylinders in your vehicle. Note that oxygen itself does not burn. It does, however, feed and support combustion, especially when the oxygen is pressurized. Make absolutely sure that there are no open flames in the area when you are using oxygen.

Oxygen-Delivery Equipment

A variety of devices are available to deliver oxygen to the patient. Proper training in their use is essential. Follow all local protocols.

Oxygen equipment delivers either low-flow or high-flow oxygen. Use low-flow oxygen through a **nasal cannula**. Use high-flow oxygen through a

OXYGEN ADMINISTRATION

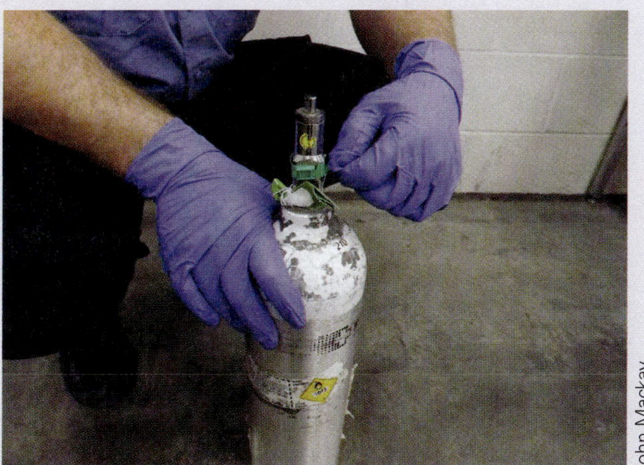

Figure 7–26a Confirm that the cylinder contains oxygen and remove the protective seal.

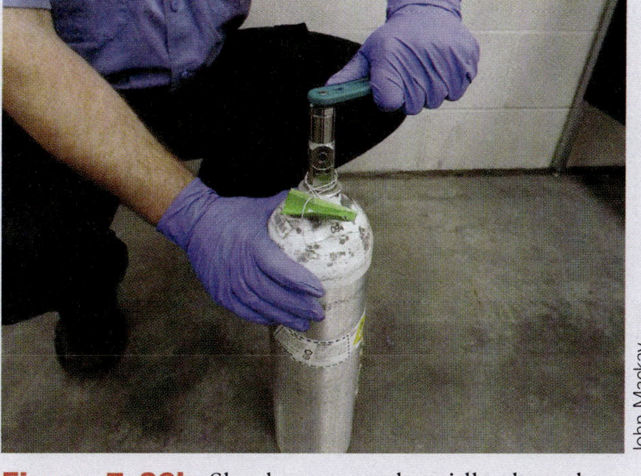

Figure 7–26b Slowly open and rapidly close the cylinder valve for one second to remove dust or debris.

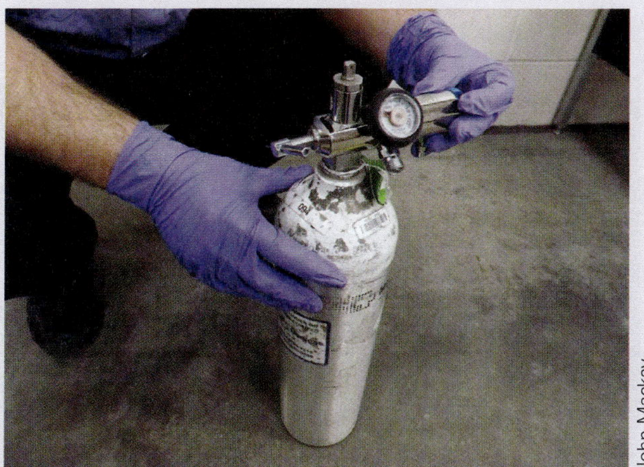

Figure 7–26c Place the yoke of the regulator over the cylinder valve and align the pins.

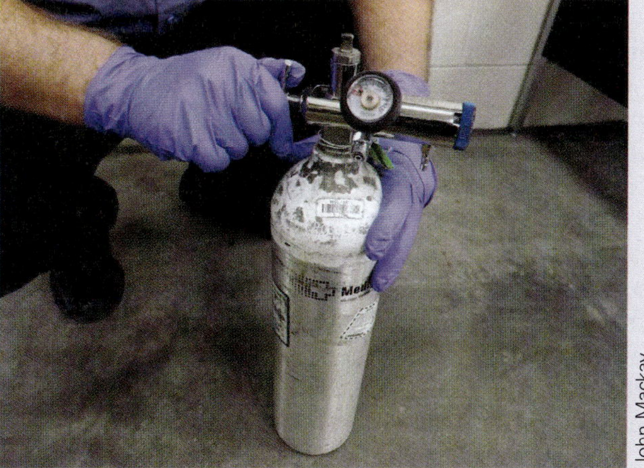

Figure 7–26d Hand-tighten the T-screw on the regulator.

(continued)

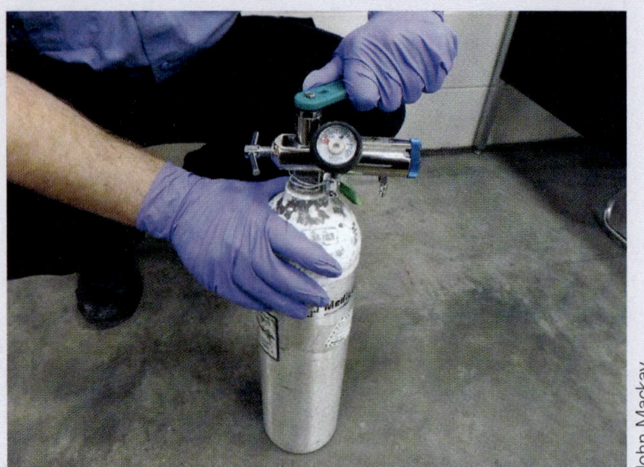

Figure 7–26e Open the main cylinder valve to check the pressure.

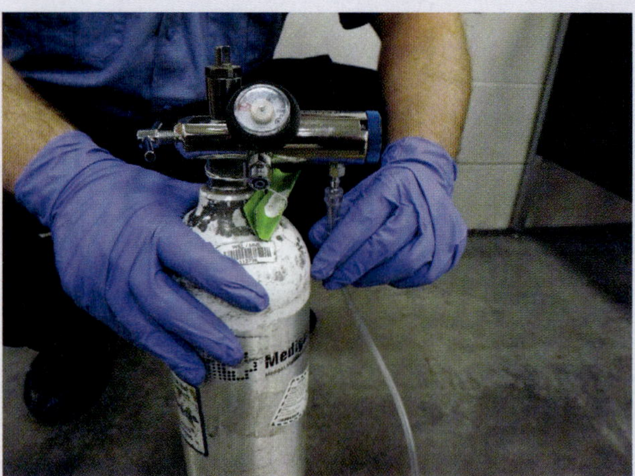

Figure 7–26f Attach the oxygen-delivery device to the regulator.

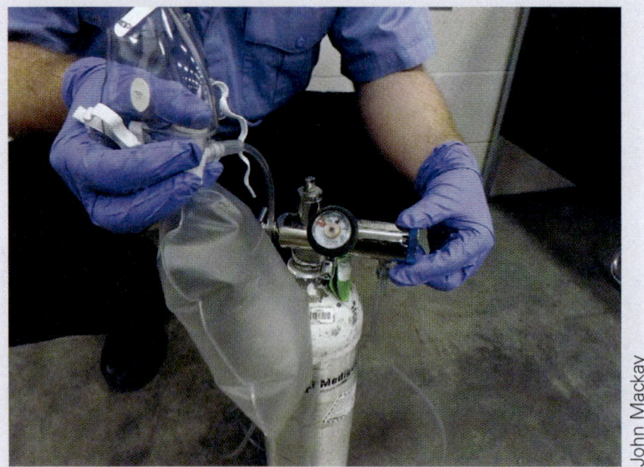

Figure 7–26g Adjust the flow meter to the appropriate litre flow.

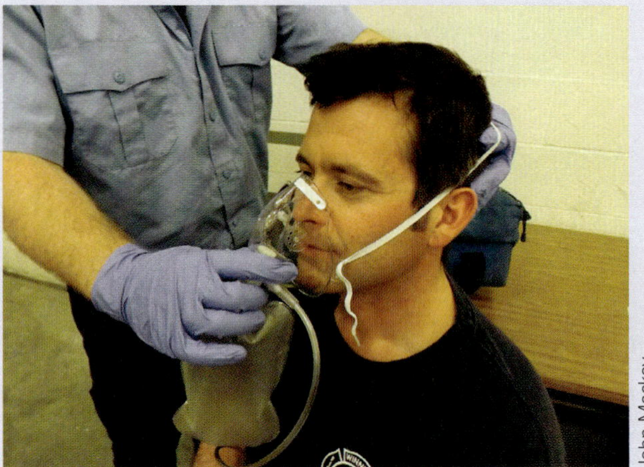

Figure 7–26h Apply the oxygen-delivery device to the patient.

non-rebreather mask. Note that the patient must be breathing in order for you to use either of these devices. If the patient is not breathing or is breathing inadequately, begin artificial ventilation with supplemental oxygen.

Nasal Cannula. One of the most common oxygen devices is the nasal cannula (Figure 7–27). Its two soft plastic tips are inserted a short distance into the nostrils. The tips are attached to the oxygen source with thin tubing. It is comfortable and convenient. Most patients are able to tolerate it with ease.

The nasal cannula provides safe, comfortable, low-flow oxygen in concentrations of 24 to 44 percent with a flow of 1 L to 6 L. It should be used at low rates of less than 6 L/min. Higher flows can cause headaches, drying of the nasal membranes, and nosebleeds.

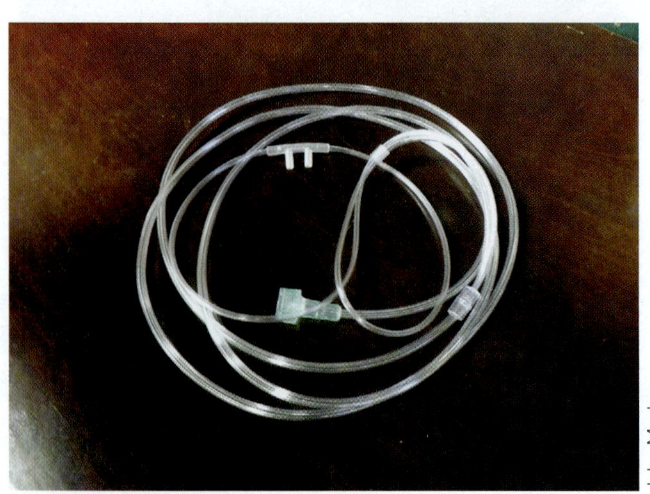

Figure 7–27 Nasal cannula.

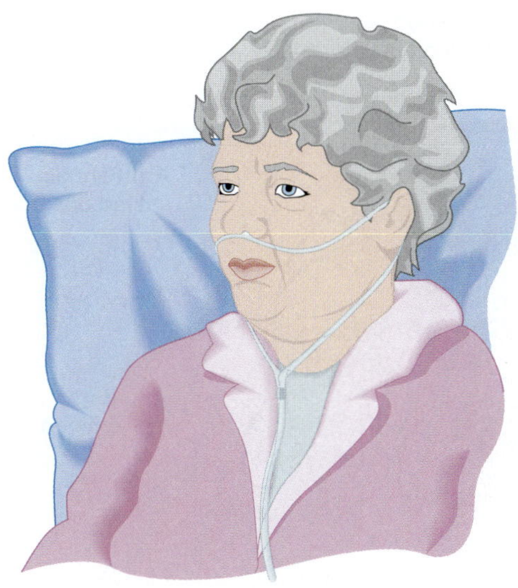

Figure 7–28 Nasal cannula applied to a patient.

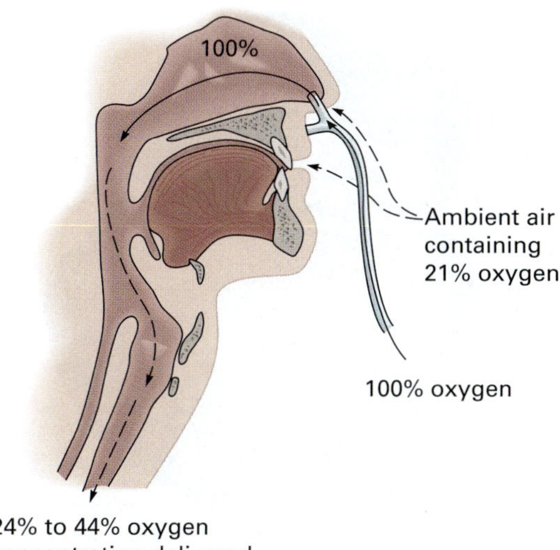

The nasal cannula is good for patients who are anxious about a mask, for patients who are nauseated or vomiting, and in situations in which you need to have the patient communicate with you.

To use a nasal cannula, follow these steps (Figure 7–28):

1. Set the litre flow to the desired rate. Make sure oxygen is flowing from the cannula tips.
2. Insert the two tips into the nostrils, with the tab facing out.
3. Position the tubing over and behind each ear.
4. Gently secure it by sliding the adjuster underneath the chin.

Do not adjust the tubing too tightly. If an elastic strap is used, adjust it so that it is secure but comfortable. If the tubing causes irritation, pad the patient's cheeks and behind the ears with 2″ × 2″ gauze pads. Be sure to check the placement often. The cannula can be dislodged easily.

Non-Rebreather Mask. A non-rebreather mask has an oxygen reservoir bag and a one-way valve (Figure 7–29). The one-way valve allows the patient to inhale from the bag and exhale through the valve. Adjust the oxygen flow to prevent the bag from collapsing during inhalation, using about 10 to 15 L/min.

A non-rebreather mask requires a tight seal. If fitted properly to the face, it can deliver oxygen concentrations of up to 90 percent. It is ideally suited for patients who have severe **hypoxemia**, such as those with chest pain or injuries. Remember that the flow rate must be adequate to keep the bag inflated as the patient inhales. If the bag collapses, the patient will not receive oxygen and may suffocate. Be ready to remove the mask if the patient vomits. Caution must be exercised when using this device on patients who have some chronic lung diseases. (See "Special Considerations" on the next page.)

To use the non-rebreather mask, follow these steps (Figure 7–30):

1. Select a mask with the oxygen supply tube pre-attached. The other end attaches to the oxygen source.
2. Turn on the oxygen at 10 to 15 L/min to fill the bag. Then, set the flow at the prescribed level. Make sure the bag is full before using it.
3. Gently place the mask over the patient's face. Slip the loosened elastic strap over the head so that it is positioned below or above the ears. Then, pull the ends of the elastic until the mask fits the patient's face.

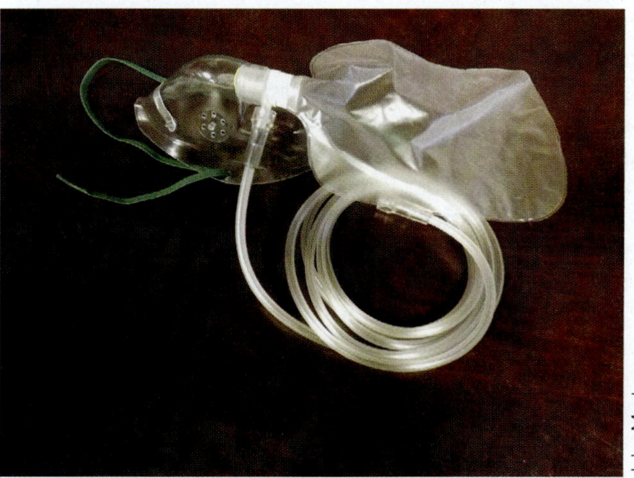

John Mackay

Figure 7–29 A non-rebreather mask.

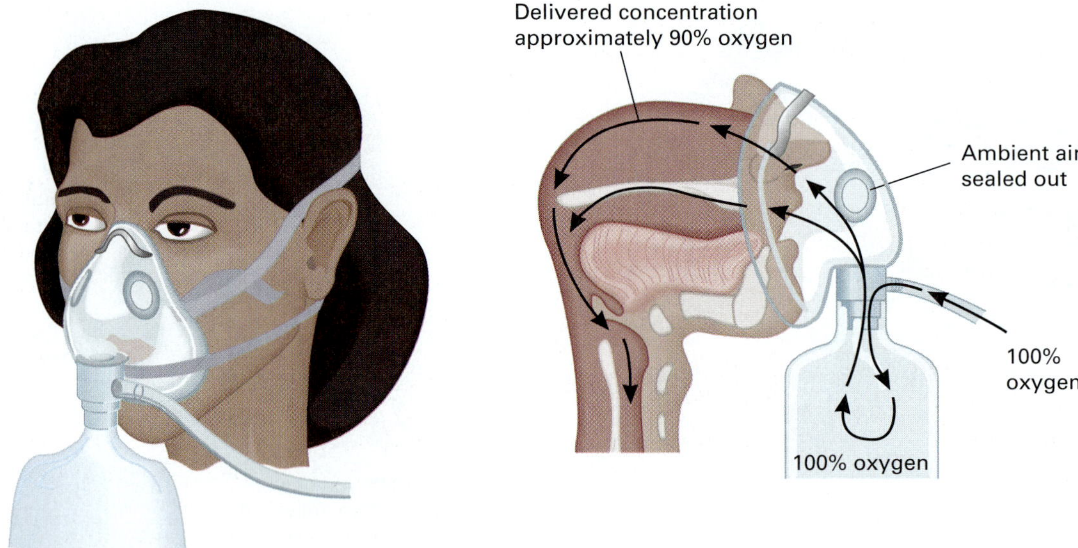

Figure 7–30 A non-rebreather mask applied to a patient.

You should not lift the head of a trauma patient. Such movement may worsen a spinal injury. Instead, gently tape the mask to the patient's cheeks. Then, monitor the airway.

Some masks have a thin metal strip where the mask covers the bridge of the patient's nose. To ensure a good seal, that strip should be pinched so that the mask conforms to the shape of the nose.

Patients who have trouble breathing or who are in shock may get anxious when you try to place a mask on their face. To these patients, it feels as if they are being suffocated. Try to persuade the patient to accept the mask. Explain to the patient what the mask is and why you are using it. You might tell him or her that the mask can feel confining but that it also provides the high concentration of oxygen he or she needs. As a last resort, use a nasal cannula to provide some oxygen.

Special Considerations

WARNING! The term *respiratory depression* refers to a slow breathing rate of fewer than eight breaths per minute. It sometimes results when oxygen is applied to patients who have **chronic obstructive pulmonary disease (COPD)**, such as emphysema or chronic bronchitis. Beware of this rare complication.

COPD patients cannot eliminate carbon dioxide properly. Their breathing centres have become used to high carbon dioxide and low oxygen levels. They are stimulated to breathe by oxygen receptors in the aorta and carotid arteries, so oxygen therapy may supply high enough oxygen levels to stop the body's messages to breathe.

Be sure to ask your patient if he or she has a history of respiratory disease before beginning oxygen therapy. If patients suffer from COPD, closely monitor their breathing as you give oxygen. If a COPD patient's breathing rate becomes very slow or shallow, or if the patient begins to get groggy or sleepy, assist ventilations with a pocket face mask or BVM unit.

> **T I P**
>
> Eliminating the **hypoxic drive** is, in reality, something that might be witnessed during long-term care in a hospital. Most EMRs and paramedics will never see this in the field. If the patient's respirations drop below eight per minute, then the individual needs assistance. As one paramedic so aptly put it, "If it really does happen, just bag 'em." Do not withhold oxygen from a patient displaying signs of shortness of breath.

Although caution must be exercised, oxygen should never be withheld from any patient who needs it. A COPD patient who has been injured in a motor vehicle accident (MVA), for example, will most likely need high concentrations of oxygen. A COPD patient who complains of minor respiratory distress may not need such aggressive care.

Foreign Body Airway Obstruction

An upper-airway obstruction is anything that blocks the nasal passages, the back of the mouth, or the throat. A lower-airway obstruction can be caused by aspirating a foreign body or by a severe spasm of the bronchial passages. *A* **foreign body airway obstruction (FBAO)** *is a true emergency.* It must be cleared from the airway before the patient can breathe and before you can give artificial ventilation.

The most common FBAO is food. If your patient was eating prior to collapsing, suspect that he or she may have choked on food. Elderly people are at risk of choking because they have a weaker gag reflex. They are frequently misdiagnosed as having heart disease when they collapse.

Other common causes of airway obstruction in a conscious patient are bleeding into the airway and aspirated vomit. Other causes include secretions, blood clots, cancerous conditions of the mouth or throat, enlarged tonsils, and acute epiglottitis.

Airway obstruction in a conscious patient can cause cardiac arrest. It can also be the result of cardiac arrest.

In an unresponsive patient, an FBAO may be caused by vomiting, loose or broken dentures or bridges, or injury to the face or jaw. The most common source of upper-airway obstruction in an unresponsive patient is the tongue.

Types of FBAO

There are two types of FBAO: partial and complete.

A **partial FBAO** means that an object is caught in the throat, but it does not totally occlude breathing. Even if a patient has good air exchange, you should *never leave a patient with a partial FBAO*. The obstruction can shift and become complete.

A patient with a partial FBAO but with good air exchange may do the following:

- Remain conscious
- Be able to speak
- Cough forcefully
- Wheeze between coughs

A patient with a partial FBAO and poor air exchange may have the following:

- Weak, ineffective cough
- High-pitched noise when inhaling
- Increased respiratory difficulty
- Cyanosis

In a **complete FBAO**, all air exchange has stopped because an object fully occludes the patient's airway. The patient may be either responsive or unresponsive, depending, in part, on how long the airway has been blocked.

A patient with a complete FBAO will be unable to breathe, cough, or speak. Such patients may clutch at the neck with the thumb and fingers (the universal signal for choking). The amount of oxygen in the blood will decrease rapidly when air cannot enter the lungs. This will result in unresponsiveness. Death will occur rapidly if the obstruction is not removed.

The way you manage an obstructed airway depends on whether the obstruction is partial or complete. Always approach a responsive FBAO patient with the question "Are you choking?" If the person can speak, breathe, or cough, do not interfere.

Partial FBAO with Good Air Exchange

A patient with a partial obstruction and good air exchange is responsive and able to cough forcefully. In this case, do the following:

- Do not interfere with the patient's own attempts to dislodge the obstruction by coughing.
- Encourage the patient to cough up the foreign body.
- Do not make any specific attempts to relieve the obstruction.
- Never leave the patient until you are certain the airway is clear and there are no other problems that threaten the airway.
- If the patient cannot dislodge the object on his or her own, even if good air exchange continues, activate the EMS system.
- Place the patient in a position of comfort in which it is easiest for him or her to breathe.

Partial FBAO with Poor Air Exchange or Complete FBAO in Adults and Children over One Year of Age

The HSFC recommends the **Heimlich manoeuvre** for conscious patients in cases of partial airway obstruction with poor air exchange and in cases of complete airway obstruction. Also called subdiaphragmatic abdominal thrusts, or simply abdominal thrusts, the Heimlich manoeuvre quickly pushes the diaphragm upward (Figure 7–31). This action can force enough air from the lungs to dislodge and expel the foreign object. *The HSFC recommends against the use of back blows on an adult.*

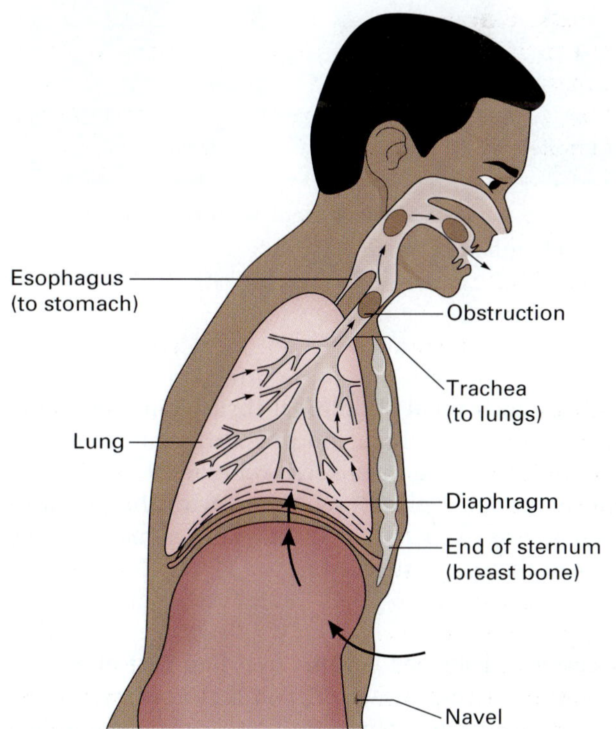

Figure 7–31 Abdominal thrusts push the diaphragm up, forcing air to expel the foreign object.

FOREIGN BODY AIRWAY OBSTRUCTION (FBAO)—RESPONSIVE ADULT

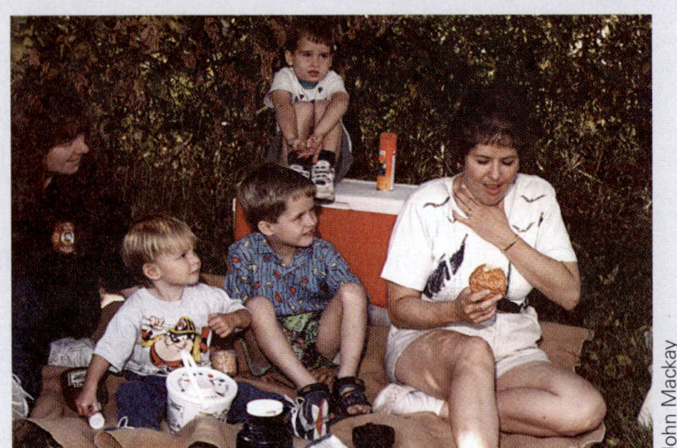

Figure 7–32a The universal sign for choking.

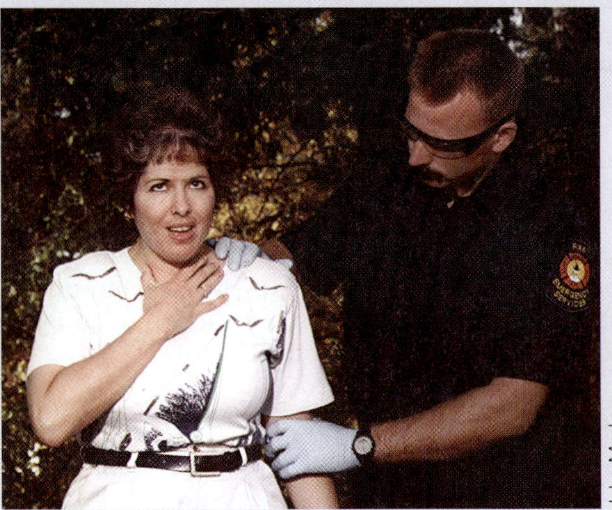

Figure 7–32b Determine whether the patient can speak or cough by asking, "Are you choking?"

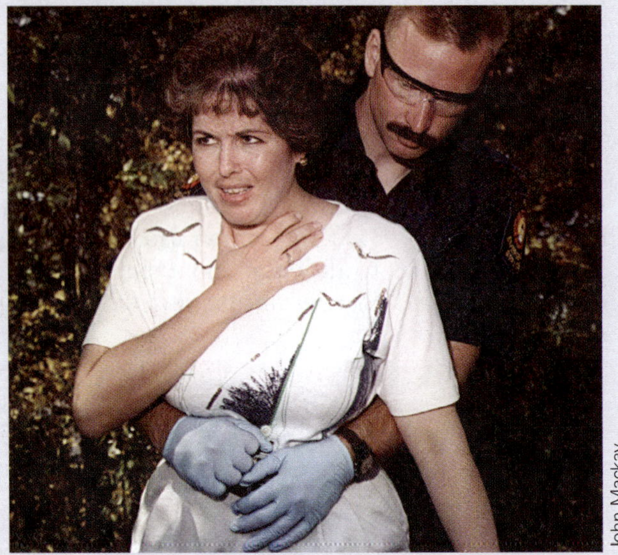

Figure 7–32c If the patient is choking, perform the Heimlich manoeuvre.

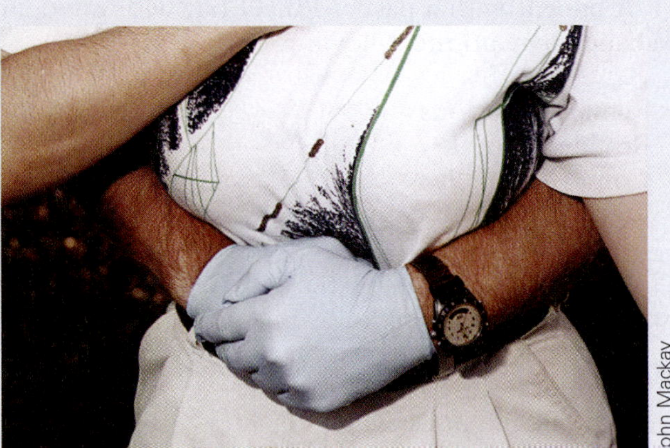

Figure 7–32d Hand position for the Heimlich manoeuvre.

Each individual abdominal thrust must be delivered with enough force and pressure to dislodge the foreign object. You must keep trying if the first thrust is unsuccessful. Deliver each thrust with the intent of relieving the obstruction. It may take as many as five or more thrusts to succeed.

Responsive Adults and Children over One Year of Age. If the patient is responsive, explain that you are trained and know how to help; then, perform the Heimlich manoeuvre as follows (Figure 7–32):

1. *Get in position.* Stand behind the patient. Wrap your arms around his or her waist. Keep your elbows out, away from the patient's ribs.
2. *Position your hands.* Make a fist with one hand. Place the thumb side of the fist on the middle of the abdomen slightly above the navel and well below the xiphoid process.
3. *Perform an abdominal thrust.* First, grasp your fist with your other hand, thumbs toward the patient. Then, press your fist into the patient's abdomen with a quick inward and upward thrust.

4. If the first thrust does not dislodge the foreign body, make each new thrust separate and distinct. Continue until the object is expelled or the patient becomes unresponsive.

Beware of certain dangers. First, if you are improperly positioned, or if you perform the thrusts too rapidly or too forcefully, you can lose your balance and fall against the patient. If your hands are positioned too high, you could cause internal injury. Finally, the Heimlich manoeuvre can cause vomiting. Correct hand placement and use of appropriate force minimize this risk.

Pregnant or Obese Responsive Adult. If the patient is in the advanced stages of pregnancy or is markedly obese, there may be no room between the rib cage and the abdomen to perform abdominal thrusts, or you may be unable to reach around the patient. If this is the case, perform chest thrusts as follows (Figure 7–33):

1. *Get in position.* Stand behind the patient. Place your arms directly under the patient's armpits. Wrap your arms around the patient's chest.
2. *Position your hands.* Make a fist with one hand. Place the thumb of your fist on the middle of the patient's sternum. If you are near the margins of the rib cage, your hand is too low.
3. *Perform a chest thrust.* First, seize your fist firmly with your other hand. Then, thrust sharply backward.
4. If the first thrust does not dislodge the foreign body, repeat thrusts until the object is expelled or the patient becomes unresponsive.

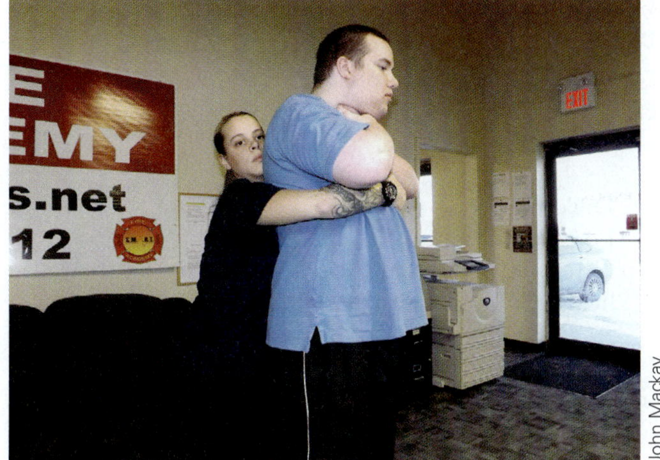

Figure 7–33 Chest thrusts on a standing obese patient with an FBAO.

Unresponsive Adult or Child over One Year of Age. If your patient is unresponsive when you find him or her or if the patient becomes unresponsive as you try to dislodge the obstruction, activate the EMS system. Then, place the patient in a supine position and proceed with the following:

1. *Get in position.* Kneel alongside the patient's chest (Figure 7-34a).
2. *Position your hands.* Use the same positioning as you would for CPR.
3. *Perform 30 chest thrusts* (Figure 7–34b). Do not check for a pulse. Current research has compelled the HSFC to direct that immediate cardiac compressions (see Chapter 8) are likely most beneficial for this patient.
4. *Look into the mouth* (Figure 7-35a). If you see an object in the back of the throat, remove it.
5. *Open the airway* using the head-tilt/chin-lift or jaw-thrust manoeuvre.
6. *Attempt to ventilate the patient* (Figure 7–35b). Try to ventilate using the mouth-to-mask device, mouth-to-barrier device, or the mouth-to-mouth technique. Use the jaw-thrust manoeuvre without the head tilt if a head, neck, or spinal injury is suspected.
7. If ventilation is unsuccessful, reposition the patient's head and try again. If ventilation is still unsuccessful, continue with chest compressions and attempted ventilations.
8. If the foreign body is not dislodged, repeat the sequence by alternating these manoeuvres in rapid sequence: repeated chest compressions, checking in the mouth, and attempted ventilation. Continue until the foreign body is expelled and ventilation is successful or until you are relieved by other EMS personnel.

Pregnant or Obese Unresponsive Adult. If you find an unresponsive patient who is in the late stages of pregnancy or is markedly obese, or if such a patient becomes unresponsive as you try to dislodge an obstruction, activate the EMS system. Then proceed with the same eight steps found in the previous section.

FBAO in Infants and Children up to One Year of Age

Manage a complete airway obstruction in children older than one year the same way you would in adults. Treatment for newborns, infants, and children up to one year of age is different.

Most childhood deaths from FBAO are in children younger than five years. Of those who die, the majority are infants. The most common causes of FBAO in infants and small children are toys, balloons,

FOREIGN BODY AIRWAY OBSTRUCTION (FBAO)—UNRESPONSIVE ADULTS AND CHILDREN OVER ONE YEAR OF AGE

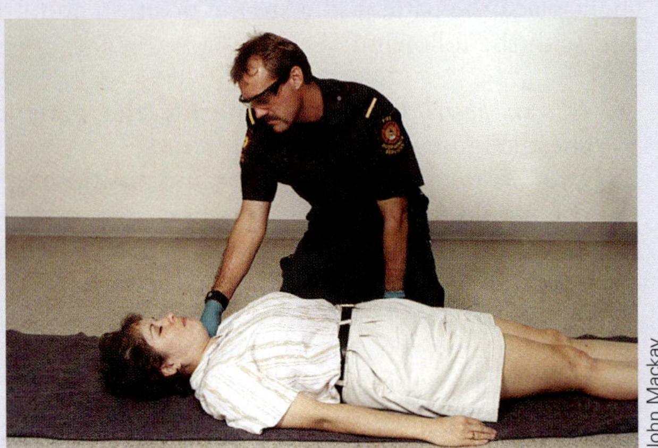

Figure 7–34a Position supine.

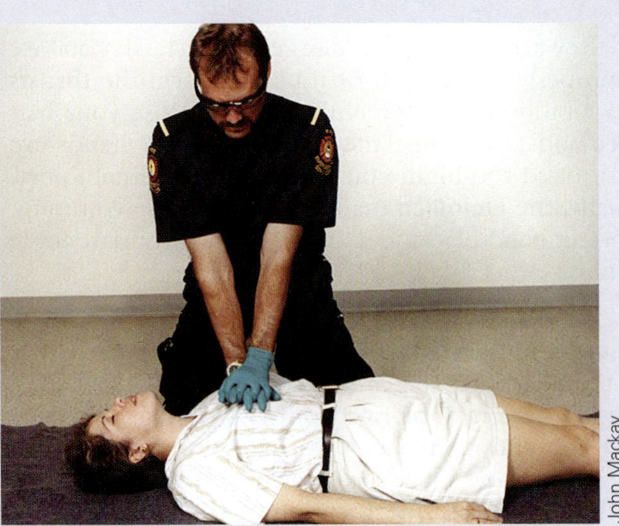

Figure 7–34b Deliver 30 chest thrusts without a pulse check.

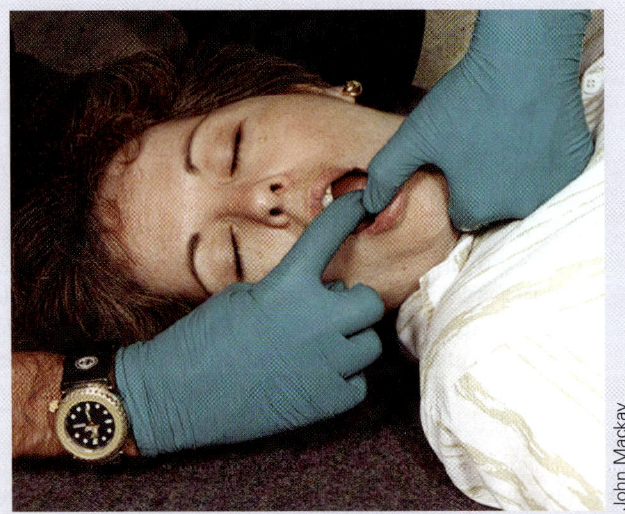

Figure 7–35a Look into the mouth and remove the object.

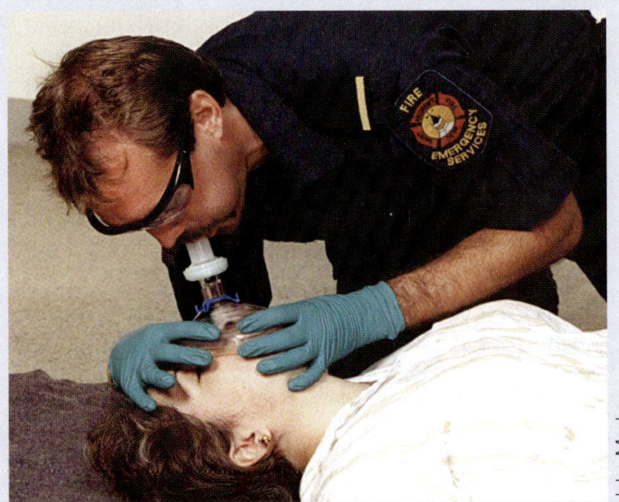

Figure 7–35b Attempt to ventilate the patient. Without performing a pulse check, continue chest compressions and attempted ventilations until effective or until advanced life support arrives.

small objects, and food such as hot dogs, round candies, nuts, and grapes.

Airway obstruction in an infant or small child can also be caused by swelling and infection. Both narrow the airway. Croup and epiglottitis can cause complete blockage of the airway.

Suspect that the obstruction is caused by infection, instead of by a foreign object, if you detect:

- Fever (especially if accompanied by congestion)
- Hoarseness
- Drooling
- Lethargy or limpness
- Unexplained unresponsiveness in a normally healthy infant or small child

If you suspect that the obstruction is caused by infection, arrange for immediate transport to a medical facility.

An FBAO should be suspected in an infant or child who has sudden onset of respiratory distress associated with coughing, gagging, stridor, or wheezing; a weak cry; and grey-blue colour of the lips and gums, especially when food or small items are found near the child. You should try to clear only a complete airway obstruction or a partial airway obstruction with poor air exchange.

Never perform a blind finger sweep on an infant or child. Perform a tongue-jaw lift, look into the airway, and use your finger to sweep the foreign body out *only* if you can actually see it.

Responsive Infant (or Child up to One Year of Age.) If the infant has a partial airway obstruction, but still has good air exchange, alert the incoming paramedic unit. Let the infant try to expel the object by coughing. Place the patient in a position of comfort (in the parent's arms, if possible) so that secretions and vomit will drain out of the mouth. The jaw will also fall forward, bringing the tongue and epiglottis away from the back of the throat.

If the infant has serious difficulty breathing, an ineffective cough, and no strong cry, he or she has a partial obstruction with poor air exchange.

According to the HSFC, you should perform the following procedure *only* if the infant has a complete FBAO or a partial obstruction with poor air exchange and *only* if the obstruction is due to a witnessed or strongly suspected foreign object. Do not perform the following procedure if you suspect that the obstruction is caused by infection. Instead, arrange for immediate transport to a medical facility.

If you are not able to clear the FBAO in an infant within *one minute* using the following procedure, then activate the EMS system.

To relieve an FBAO in a responsive infant (up to one year of age), do the following:

1. *Get in position.* Straddle the infant over one of your arms, face down with his or her head lower than the rest of the body. Rest your arm on your thigh for support. Support the infant's head by firmly holding the jaw with your hand.
2. *Deliver up to five back blows.* Use the heel of your hand between the shoulder blades (Figure 7–36).
3. *If the foreign body is not expelled, turn the infant face up.* Support him or her on your arm, with the head lower than the rest of the body.
4. *Position your hand.* Place your middle and ring finger over the middle of the infant's sternum. They should be just below an imaginary line drawn between the infant's nipples (Figure 7–37).
5. *Deliver up to five chest thrusts.* Use a quick downward motion.
6. *If the first set of thrusts does not dislodge the foreign body, do the following:* continue alternating sets of five back blows and five chest thrusts until the foreign body is expelled or the infant becomes unresponsive.

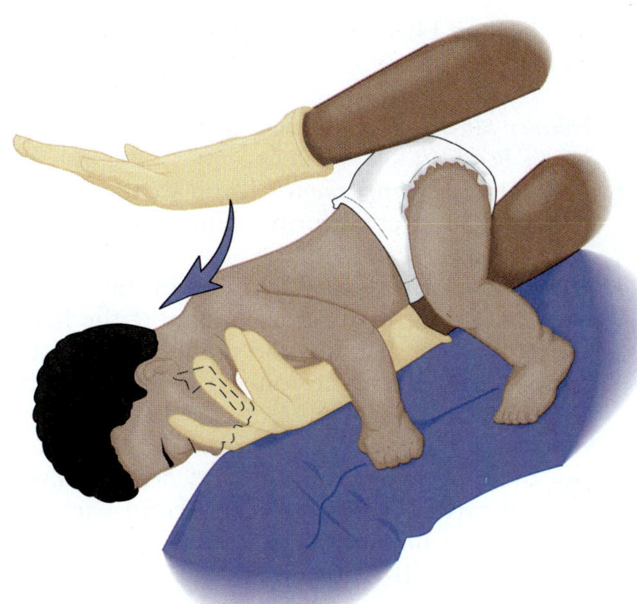

Figure 7–36 Back blows for an infant with an FBAO.

If a choking infant becomes unresponsive while you are attempting to clear an FBAO, have a second person activate the EMS. Perform a tongue-jaw lift and, if you can see the object, perform a finger sweep to remove it. If necessary, continue with airway care as described below for an unresponsive infant.

Unresponsive Infant. If you reach an infant who is unresponsive, have a second person activate the EMS system. If no one is available, make the call yourself. Remember to ensure scene safety, ensure your safety, and use barrier devices.

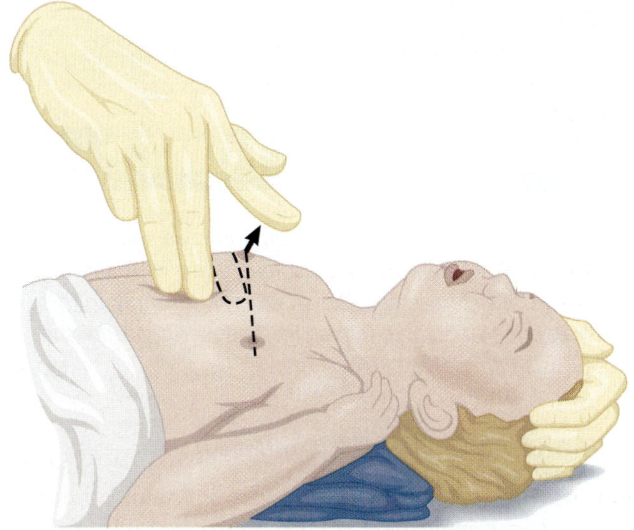

Figure 7–37 Locating the finger position for chest thrusts on an infant with an FBAO.

To relieve an FBAO in an unresponsive infant, do the following:

1. *Deliver 30 chest compressions while maintaining proper head tilt.*
2. *Look into the infant's mouth.* If you see the object, remove it. (Never perform a blind finger sweep on an infant.)
3. *Open the airway.* Place the infant on his or her back on a firm, hard surface. Support the head and neck. Note that the head should be in a neutral position. Overextension of the infant's neck can obstruct the airway.
4. *Attempt to ventilate the patient.* Create a good seal over the infant's mouth and nose. Deliver two effective breaths, at one second each. If ventilation is not successful, reposition the head and try again. If ventilation is still unsuccessful, repeat the procedure beginning with chest compressions. Continue with alternating sets of 30 chest compressions, looking for a foreign object in the back of the throat, and attempted ventilation until the foreign body is expelled or until you are relieved by another EMS worker.

When the foreign body is expelled, a responsive infant will usually start to cry or make a noise. An unresponsive infant may not make a noise or breathe spontaneously. You will need to determine if air is reaching the lungs and if there is a pulse. If there is no pulse, begin infant CPR as described in Chapter 8.

If the infant is breathing and has a pulse, place him or her in the recovery position. Monitor breathing and pulse while you maintain an open airway.

EMR FOCUS

The body requires oxygen to live. Without adequate respiration, we die. These statements alone provide your focus. As an EMR, you must evaluate respiration. Do everything possible to make sure that respirations continue adequately and without obstruction.

Consider this scenario. You come upon the scene of an MVC. You find a patient who has been ejected from the vehicle. He appears to have multiple injuries, and you immediately notice bleeding from the mouth and nose. The patient is unresponsive and is making gurgling sounds from his airway. He has a rapid, weak pulse.

After performing a scene assessment and taking BSI precautions, your next priority is the airway if the patient has a pulse. The patient needs suctioning. Depending on the amount of bleeding, he may need frequent suctioning. If you leave the airway, even briefly, to perform more of your assessment, the patient will lose his airway and die.

If all you do is take care of the airway, and you do it well, you have done everything possible to save a life. A nicely assessed and packaged patient who does not have an airway has not been properly cared for.

CASE STUDY FOLLOW-UP

At the beginning of this chapter, you read that EMRs were called to help an unconscious adult with snoring respirations. To see how the chapter skills apply to this emergency, read the following. It describes how the call was completed.

PRIMARY ASSESSMENT *(Continued)*

Since it was not possible to assess her while she was slumped in a chair, we quickly, but carefully, moved the patient to the floor. My partner, Pete, immediately checked her pulse and found that it was rapid and weak. He then performed a head-tilt/chin-lift manoeuvre. It eliminated the snoring sounds.

Pete suctioned the airway to remove the built-up secretions. Mrs. Constantino didn't have a gag reflex. She accepted the oropharyngeal airway well.

Our assessment of her breathing revealed that there was minimal chest movement and slow respirations. She was also beginning to show signs of blue colouration around her lips.

Realizing that Mrs. Constantino was breathing inadequately, we ventilated her using a BVM unit and supplemental oxygen.

PATIENT HISTORY

Mr. Constantino told us that his wife had had a heart attack several years before. She took medications for her heart condition and for high blood pressure. She had complained of a headache about an hour before she became unresponsive. She had eaten breakfast earlier. She had no allergies.

SECONDARY ASSESSMENT

We believed that Mrs. Constantino had a medical problem rather than a traumatic condition. I did a quick secondary assessment while my partner continued to assist ventilations. There were no signs of injury on Mrs. Constantino's head, neck, chest, abdomen, or extremities. Her pulse was 96 and bounding. The respiratory rate was 8 and shallow.

ONGOING ASSESSMENT

Our primary focus was making sure that Mrs. Constantino was ventilated properly. We made sure that we checked her pulse frequently. Her pulse on our second check was 104, bounding, and regular. Her respirations were about 6 and shallow, so we continued assisting her with a BVM unit.

TRANSFER OF CARE

We had the airway under control when the paramedics arrived. The patient's colour had improved. Her pulse had also slowed down a bit. Pete gave them the hand-off report:

"This is Mrs. Constantino. She is 74 years old. She had a headache about an hour ago. Her husband found her slumped over in a chair. We moved her to the floor and found that she had a rapid, weak pulse and inadequate ventilations. We began assisting with a BVM unit and oxygen. She groans with loud verbal stimulus. Her respiratory rate is about 6 and her pulse is 104 and bounding. She has a history of heart attack and high blood pressure. She ate breakfast. She has no allergies."

I saw Mr. Constantino in the grocery store recently. He told me that his wife had had a severe stroke. She remained in the hospital for some time and was eventually moved to a rehabilitation centre. He thanked me again and told me that he hoped his wife would be home soon.

NO AIRWAY = NO PATIENT

It has been said that the priorities in patient care are the airway, the airway, and the airway! By today's CPR standards, this is true only if a patient has a pulse or is already receiving cardiac compressions. However, without a clear and open airway, plus adequate ventilations, no patient can survive. So, even as you approach your patient's side, the first questions in your mind should be, "Is she breathing? Is she breathing adequately?" Check the pulse and begin cardiac compressions if necessary, but remember, without an airway, there is no chance of survival.

NOCPs

4.3 e Conduct respiratory system assessment and interpret findings **S**

4.4 b Assess respiration **S**

5.1 a Use manual manoeuvres and positioning to maintain airway patency **S**
 b Suction oropharynx **S**
 d Utilize oropharyngeal airway **S**
 e Utilize nasopharyngeal airway **X**
 i Remove airway foreign bodies (AFB) **S**

5.2 a Prepare oxygen delivery **A**
 b Utilize portable oxygen-delivery systems **S**

5.3 a Administer oxygen using nasal cannula **S**
 b Administer oxygen using low concentration mask **S**
 d Administer oxygen using high concentration mask **S**
 e Administer oxygen using pocket mask **S**

5.4 a Provide oxygenation and ventilation using manual positive pressure devices **S**

6.1 c Provide care to patient experiencing signs and symptoms involving respiratory system **S**

REVIEW QUESTIONS

Page references where answers may be found or supported are provided at the end of each question.

SECTION 1

1. What are the nine major components of the respiratory system? (p. 84)

SECTION 2

2. What are the two manoeuvres that you can use to open a patient's airway? Describe when you should use each one. (pp. 88–89)

3. What are the two types of airway adjunct? Describe when you should use each one. (pp. 90–93)

4. How can you find out if a patient is breathing? (pp. 95–96)

5. What is the HAINES position? Describe when you should use it. (p. 93)

6. What are the signs of inadequate breathing? (p. 96)

SECTION 3

7. What are the three techniques used by an EMR to artificially ventilate a patient? Name them in order of preference. (p. 97)

8. What are the signs that show your ventilations are adequate? (p. 97)

9. How do you perform artificial ventilation? Briefly describe each step, including rates for infants, children, and adults. (pp. 97–103)

10. How do you relieve an FBAO in a responsive adult? Briefly describe each step. (pp. 109–111)

11. How do you relieve an FBAO in an unresponsive five-year-old child? Briefly describe each step. (p. 111)

8

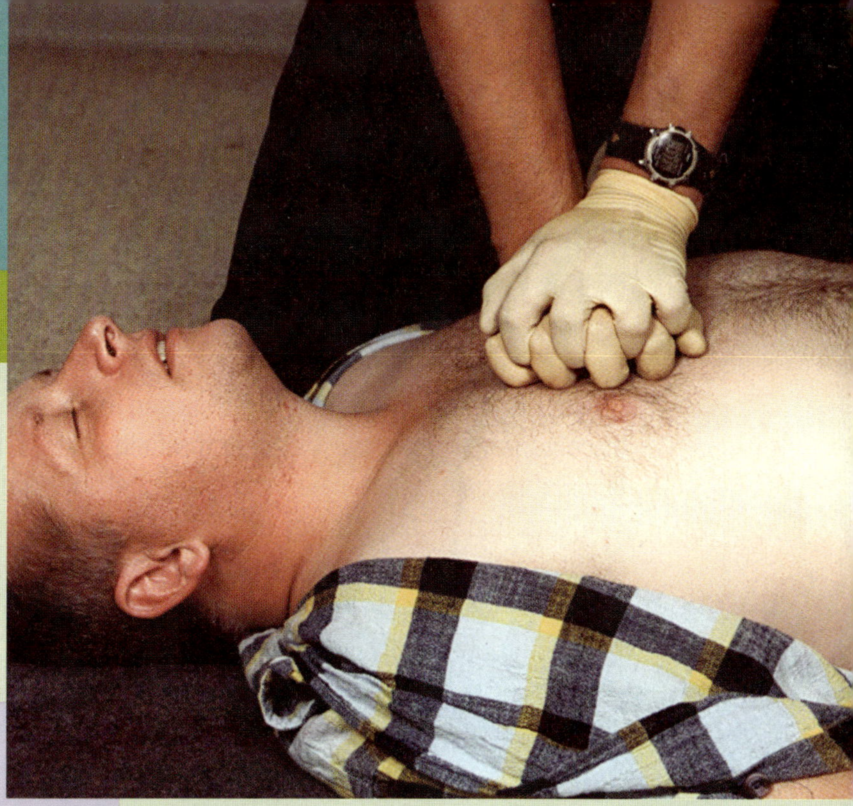
John Mackay

Circulation

OBJECTIVES

1. List eight reasons for the heart to stop beating.
2. Describe each of the five links in the Chain of Survival for adult and pediatric patients and how they relate to the EMS system.
3. Define the components of CPR.
4. Demonstrate the steps of infant, child, and adult one- and two-rescuer CPR.
5. Describe the technique for external chest compressions on infants, children, and adult patients.
6. Explain when the EMR is able to stop CPR.
7. Understand and be able to respond to the feelings of the family of a patient during a cardiac event.

INTRODUCTION

Heart attacks take the lives of about 23 000 Canadians each year, and 50 percent of these before they ever reach a hospital. The patients who can be saved need immediate CPR followed by advanced medical care, including **defibrillation**, within eight to ten minutes of collapse.

But even with CPR, many patients will not live. They may have been without a pulse or oxygen for too long, or the attack may have caused irreversible damage to the heart. Please do not let that discourage you. Emergency care in the field is still critical to saving many lives. And today's new hospital techniques often help to reverse the crippling effects of heart attack.

Note that several studies have shown that you can lose your CPR skills unless you have frequent practice and retraining. Retraining should occur often. Recertification should occur annually.

SECTION 1
THE CIRCULATORY SYSTEM

The circulatory system is responsible for delivering oxygen and nutrients to the body's tissues. It is also responsible for removing carbon dioxide and waste from the tissues. Its basic components are the heart, arteries, veins, capillaries, and blood (see Figure 4–11 on p. 48).

The heart is a hollow, muscular organ about the size of a fist. It lies in the lower left central region of the chest between the lungs. It is protected in the front by the ribs and sternum (breastbone). In the back, it is protected by the spinal column. The heart contains four chambers. The two upper ones are the left and right atria. The two lower ones are the left and right ventricles. The septum (a wall) divides the right side of the heart from the left side. The heart also contains several one-way valves that keep blood flowing in the right direction.

The circulatory system also contains blood vessels. These vessels transport blood throughout the body. You will recall from Chapter 4 that the arteries transport blood away from the heart. Veins carry blood back to the heart. The tiny capillaries allow for the exchange of gases and nutrients between the blood and the cells of the body.

How the Heart Works

The heart is like a two-sided pump (Figure 8–1). The left side receives oxygenated blood from the lungs and pumps it to all parts of the body. The right side receives blood from the body and then pumps it to the lungs to be re-oxygenated.

The blood is kept under pressure and in constant circulation by the heart's pumping action. In a healthy adult at rest, the heart contracts between 60 and 80 times per minute. The pulse is a sign of the pressure exerted during each contraction of the heart. Every time the heart pumps, a wave of blood is sent through the arteries. That wave is felt as a pulse. It can be palpated (felt) most easily where a large artery lies over a bone close to the skin. These sites include the carotid pulse in the neck, the brachial pulse in the upper arm, the radial pulse in the wrist, and the femoral pulse in the upper thigh.

The pulse is felt most easily over the carotid arteries on either side of the neck. A carotid artery should be palpated first if a patient is unconscious. The radial arteries on the thumb side of the inner surface of the wrists are also easy to feel. A radial artery should be palpated first if the patient is conscious.

The heart, lungs, and brain work closely together to sustain life. The smooth functioning of each is critical to the others. When one organ cannot perform properly, the other two are handicapped. If one fails, the other two will follow soon.

When the Heart Stops

Clinical death occurs when a patient is in **respiratory arrest** (not breathing) and **cardiac arrest** (the heart is not beating). Immediate CPR may reverse that state and restore the patient without damage. However, if a patient has been clinically dead for four to six minutes, brain cells begin to die. After eight to ten minutes without a pulse, irreversible damage occurs to the brain.

There are many reasons why a heart will stop, including heart disease, stroke, allergic reaction, diabetes, prolonged seizures, and other medical conditions. The heart may also stop because of a serious injury. In infants and children, respiratory problems are the most common cause of cardiac arrest. This is why airway care is so important in young patients.

CASE STUDY

Dispatch

Our engine company was dispatched for an EMS assist because the closest ambulance was unavailable. The call was for a cardiac patient. We knew that time would really count.

Scene Assessment

There were three of us on the pumper. I was the officer. I assessed the scene carefully from the cab before we got out. I reminded the others to remember their BSI equipment.

Primary Assessment

We observed a woman performing CPR on an older gentleman. The woman seemed to be doing pretty well, but she was getting tired. My crew approached and took over. We rechecked the patient's status, found no pulse or respirations, and continued CPR.

CPR is an important skill for the EMR. Though needed in only a small percentage of calls, when required, it is vitally important. In the scenario described above, the firefighters have begun CPR. How long do you think they should continue? Could CPR injure the patient? Will the patient live? Consider these questions as you read Chapter 8.

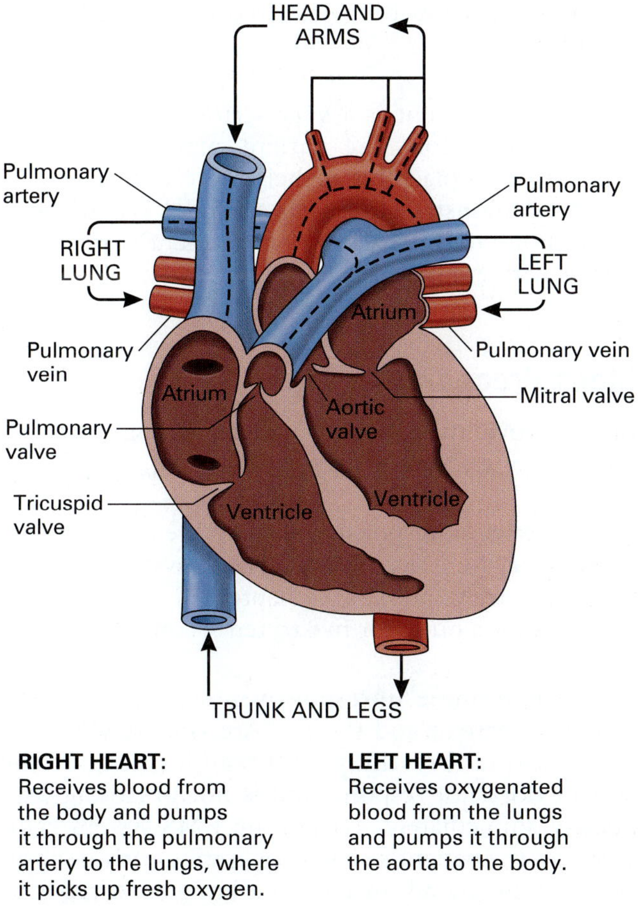
HEAD AND ARMS
Pulmonary artery
RIGHT LUNG
Pulmonary vein
Pulmonary valve
Tricuspid valve
Atrium
Ventricle
Pulmonary artery
LEFT LUNG
Atrium
Pulmonary vein
Aortic valve
Mitral valve
Ventricle
TRUNK AND LEGS
RIGHT HEART:
Receives blood from the body and pumps it through the pulmonary artery to the lungs, where it picks up fresh oxygen.
LEFT HEART:
Receives oxygenated blood from the lungs and pumps it through the aorta to the body.

Figure 8–1 The heart.

The adult patient in respiratory and cardiac arrest has the best chance of surviving if all the links in the **Adult Chain of Survival** come together (Figure 8–2). This chain, as identified by the Heart and Stroke Foundation of Canada (HSFC), contains five links:

1. *Immediate recognition of cardiac arrest* as well as prompt activation of the emergency response system.
2. *Early CPR,* with emphasis on high-quality chest compressions, must be started as quickly as possible after a patient's collapse to increase his or her chance of survival.
3. *Early defibrillation* is the most likely link for improving adult victim survival rates. Public access defibrillation (PAD) programs are attempting to increase survival rates by placing more trained rescuers in the community with access to an automated external defibrillator (AED).
4. *Effective advanced life support* is provided by trained personnel. Aspirin and clot-busting

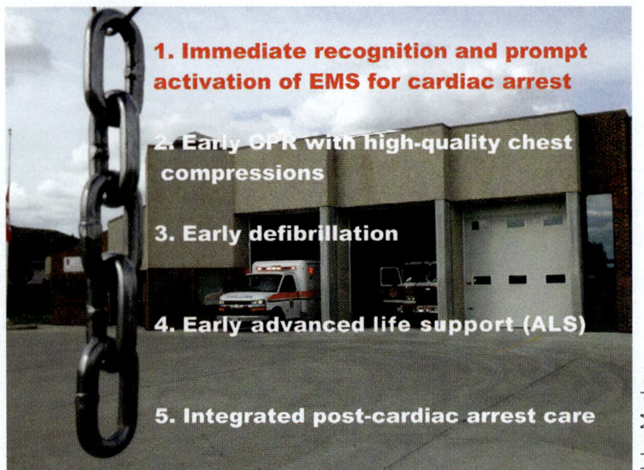

Figure 8–2 Adult Chain of Survival.

medications may be given by paramedics and hospital staff to help minimize the damage to the heart.

5. *Integrated post-cardiac arrest care* is provided by multi-disciplinary teams at cardiac centres. These hospitals provide advanced care such as ventilatory support, hemodynamic stabilization, neurological and glycemic monitoring, therapeutic hypothermia, percutaneous coronary intervention (PCI), and more.

As an EMR, you have an important role. You can provide early CPR and, if permitted in your area, defibrillation.

The principle of CPR is to circulate oxygenated blood for the patient until defibrillation and advanced care can be given. Any delay in starting CPR increases the chances of nervous system damage and death. The faster the response, the better the patient's chances are. Survival rates improve when the time between the arrest and the delivery of defibrillation and other advanced measures is short. (The Pediatric Chain of Survival is discussed on page 129.)

SECTION 2
CARDIOPULMONARY
RESUSCITATION (CPR)

According to the HSFC, proper assessment of the patient's circulation, airway, and breathing is critical to successful CPR. No patient should undergo the intrusive procedures of CPR until the need is clearly established.

You can establish the need for CPR by determining that the patient is unconscious, breathless, and pulseless. The HSFC 2010 guidelines recommend that you recognize abnormal breathing (gasping or the absence of breathing) and check for a pulse for at least five but no more than ten seconds.

To provide CPR, you must provide artificial circulation by means of chest compressions, maintain an open airway, and provide artificial ventilation. (For a detailed discussion of airway maintenance and artificial ventilation, see Chapter 7.)

It was once thought that chest compressions work because they squeeze the heart between the sternum and backbone to force blood out. Newer evidence indicates that they produce pressure changes inside the chest cavity. This pressure may be responsible for increased circulation to the body.

Therefore, be sure to pay as much attention to the duration as to the rate of chest compressions. Be sure to stay current on new CPR developments.

CPR must begin as soon as possible and continue until any of the following occurs:

- The EMR is exhausted and is unable to continue.
- The patient is handed over to another trained rescuer or to hospital staff.
- The patient is resuscitated.
- The patient has been declared dead by a proper authority.

A cardiac event is a very serious one. Without your intervention, the patient may not survive. Remember to place his or her interests first and be sure to demonstrate a caring attitude. When possible, respond to the feelings of the patient's family and friends with empathy.

Steps Preceding CPR

Before providing CPR to a patient, you must first do the following (Figure 8–3):

- Determine unresponsiveness and breathlessness.
- Activate the emergency response system and call for or retrieve an AED (Chapter 9).
- Assess for a pulse for five to ten seconds.

To determine unresponsiveness, tap or gently pinch the patient and shout, "Are you okay?" Look for abnormal breathing or breathlessness. If the patient does not respond and is not breathing adequately, immediately activate the EMS system. This increases the patient's chance of getting early defibrillation and early advanced care. Then continue with your assessment.

STEPS PRECEDING CPR

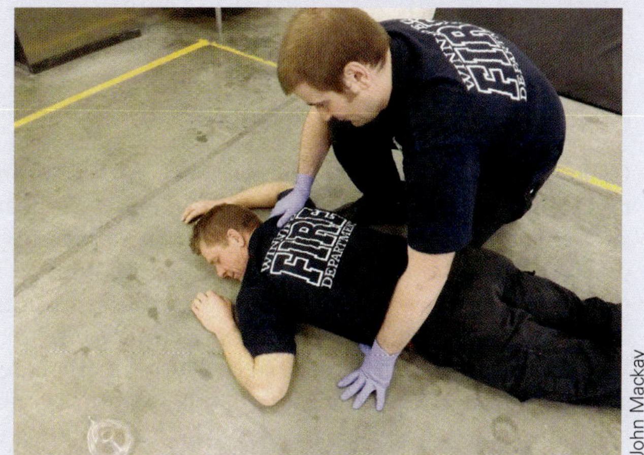

Figure 8–3a Determine unresponsiveness.

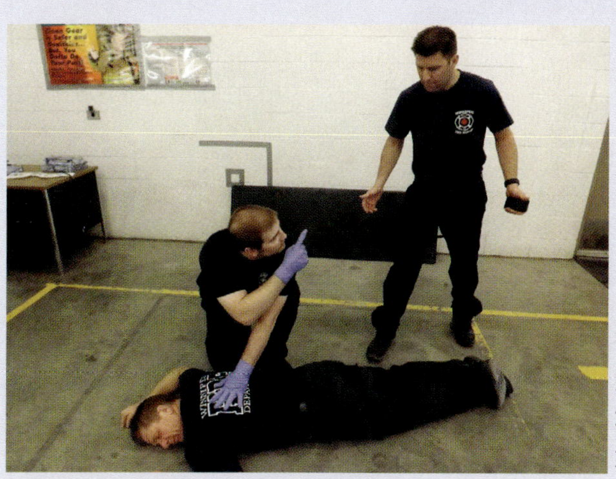

Figure 8–3b Activate the EMS system.

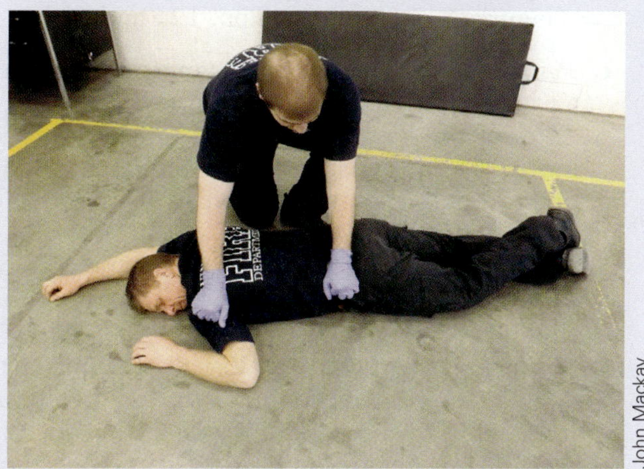

Figure 8–3c Position the patient on a firm, flat surface.

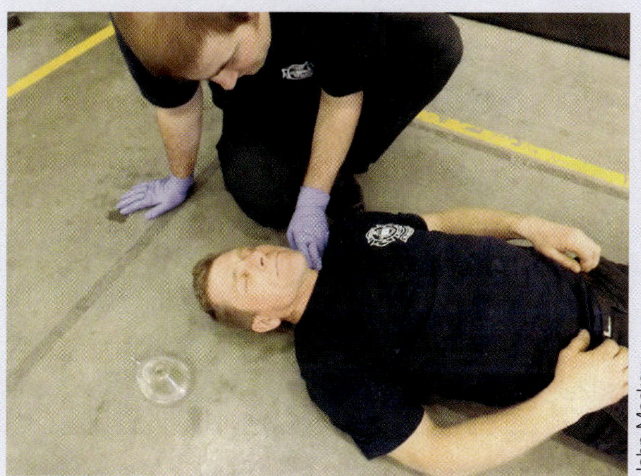

Figure 8–3d Look for signs of breathing and check pulse.

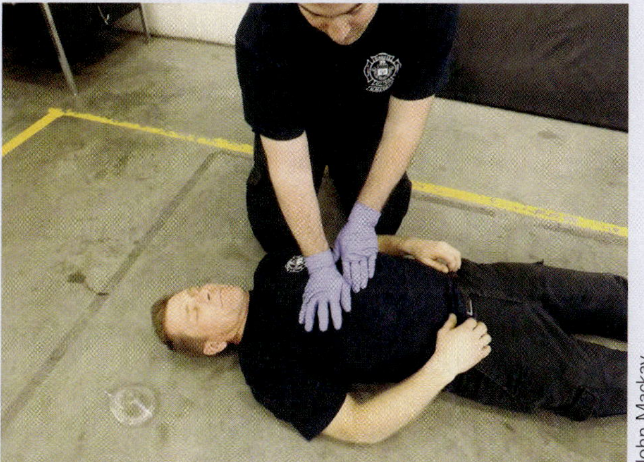

Figure 8–3e If no pulse, begin chest compressions.

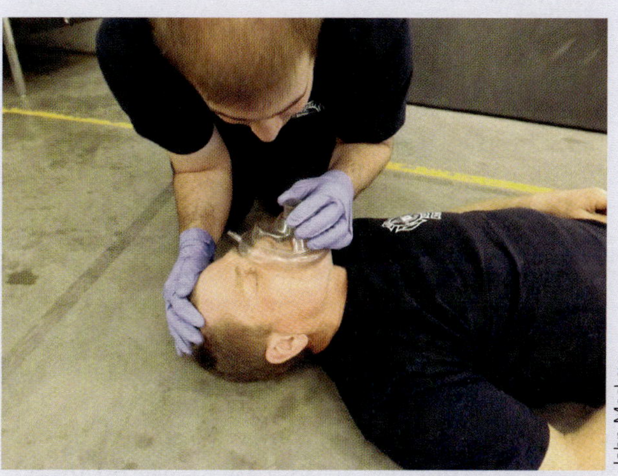

Figure 8–3f Perform artificial ventilation.

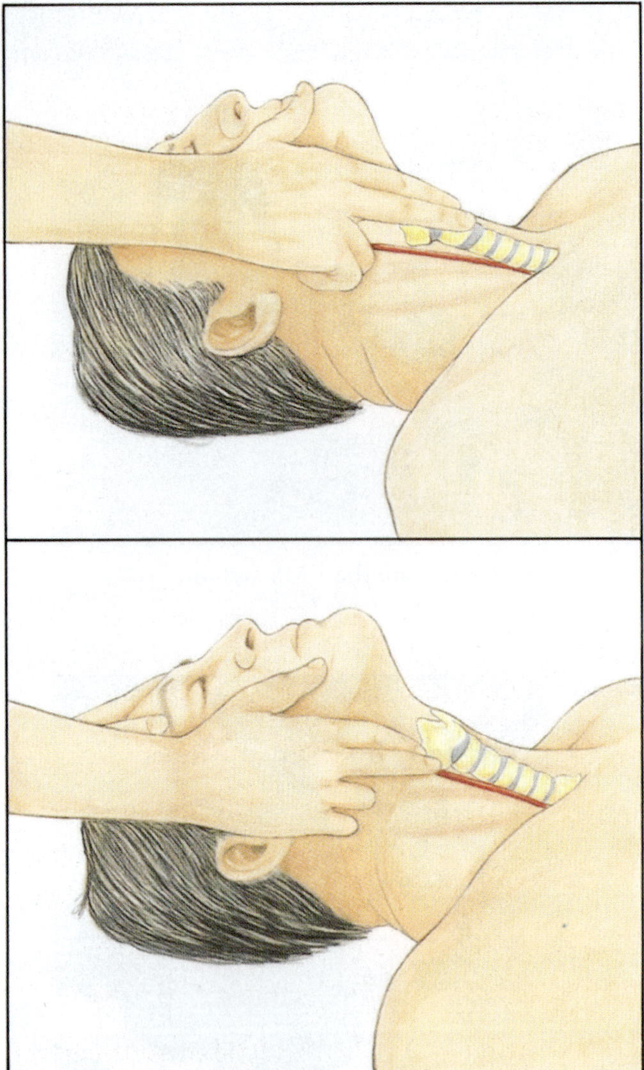

Figure 8–4 Locating the carotid artery.

To assess circulation, check for a pulse. To determine pulselessness, find a carotid artery pulse point (Figure 8–4):

1. Place two fingers on the larynx ("Adam's apple").
2. Slide your fingers to the side. Stop in the groove between the larynx and the large neck muscle.
3. Feel for the pulse. Press for at least five but no more than ten seconds. Do not use your thumb. Do not rest your hand across the patient's throat, but rather check the carotid pulse on the same side of the patient on which you are positioned.

If the patient has a pulse—even a weak or irregular one—do not begin chest compressions. You could cause serious problems. If the patient has no pulse, assume that he or she is in cardiac arrest. Begin CPR immediately.

Note that for you to perform CPR correctly, your patient must be in a supine position on a firm, flat surface such as the floor.

You may wish to refer to the CPR summary, Table 8–1, as you read the rest of this chapter.

CPR for Adults

CPR involves a combination of skills. Most important is cardiac compressions. When a patient's heart suddenly stops, their blood volume may still be well oxygenated. The patient's best chance of survival is provided by prompt, high-quality cardiac compressions followed by effective artificial ventilations.

Chest compressions consist of rhythmic, repeated pressure over the lower half of the sternum. They cause blood to circulate as a result of the buildup of pressure in the chest cavity. When combined with artificial ventilation, they provide enough blood circulation to maintain life.

To perform chest compressions, follow these steps (Figures 8–5 and 8–6 on pp. 124 and 125):

1. *Position the patient.* He or she must be supine on a firm, flat surface such as the floor.
2. *Uncover the chest.* Remove the patient's shirt or blouse. Do not waste time unbuttoning it. Rip it open or pull it up. Cut a woman's bra in two or slip it up to her neck.
3. *Get in position.* Kneel close to the patient's side. Have your knees about as wide apart as your shoulders.
4. *Locate the compression site.* Visualize an imaginary line running down the middle of the breastbone intersected by a second line connecting the nipples. These lines should cross at mid-sternum. Improper placement of your hands can fracture the sternum or ribs and lacerate the heart, lungs, or liver.
5. *Position your hands.* Place the heel of one hand where the two lines meet and place the heel of your other hand on top of the first hand. An alternative position for large hands, and hands or wrists with arthritis, is to grasp the wrist of the hand on the patient's sternum.
6. *Position your shoulders.* Put them directly over your hands with straight arms.
7. *Perform chest compressions.* Keeping your arms straight and your elbows locked, thrust from your shoulders. Push hard and fast. Depress the sternum at least 5 cm (2 inches) in an adult. Be sure the thrust is straight down into the sternum. If it is not, the torso will roll and part of the force of the thrust will be lost.

Bend at the hips, using the weight of your body as you deliver the compressions. If necessary, add force to the thrusts with your shoulders. Never

TABLE 8–1
CPR SUMMARY

	Adult (puberty and older)	Child (1 year to puberty)	Infant (under 1 year)
Hand Position	Heel of one hand on centre of breastbone between nipples, other hand on top	Heel of one hand (two hands for larger patients) on centre of breastbone between nipples	Two fingers just below nipple line on breastbone (two thumbs encircling hands for two-rescuer CPR)
Compressions	At least 5 cm (2 inches) in depth	At least one-third the depth of the chest (2 inches)	At least one-third the depth of the chest (1½ inches)
Breaths	Two breaths, each 1 second in duration	Two breaths, each 1 second in duration	Two breaths, each 1 second in duration
Cycle	30 compressions, two breaths (one- or two-rescuer CPR)	30 compressions, two breaths for one-rescuer CPR (15:2 for two-rescuer CPR)	30 compressions, two breaths for one-rescuer CPR (15:2 for two-rescuer CPR)
Rate	At least 100 per minute	At least 100 per minute	At least 100 per minute

add force with your arms—the force is too great and could fracture the sternum. Compressions should be 50 percent of the cycle. This means that the compression and release time should be about equal.

8. *Completely release pressure after each compression.* Let the sternum return to its normal position and allow blood to flow back into the chest and heart. If you do not allow full chest recoil after each compression, blood will not circulate properly. Do not lift or move your hands in any way. You could lose proper positioning. Avoid sudden, jerky movements. Effective compressions provide only one-fourth to one-third of normal blood circulation. Anything less is ineffective.

9. *Count as you administer compressions.* You should be able to say (and do) the following in slightly less than two seconds:

- One—push down
- and—let up
- Two—push down
- and—let up

Your goal is to administer at least 100 compressions per minute. Practise until you can perform 30 complete compressions in just under 20 seconds. Beware of becoming hyperventilated. If you find you are, continue breathing at a regular tempo, but not at the same rhythm you used before.

One-Rescuer CPR

To perform CPR alone, you must take the following steps. Determine unresponsiveness and breathlessness. Activate the EMS system. Absence of a patent airway and breathing are addressed after the first 30 cardiac compressions. If the patient is breathing and has a pulse, place him or her in the recovery position. Do not begin CPR.

If the pulse is absent, begin CPR as follows (Figure 8–7 on p. 126):

1. *Get in position.* Locate the proper hand position (described earlier).
2. *Perform 30 chest compressions.* Perform 30 chest compressions at a rate of at least 100 per minute. Either count out loud or use some other way to

LOCATION OF XIPHOID PROCESS

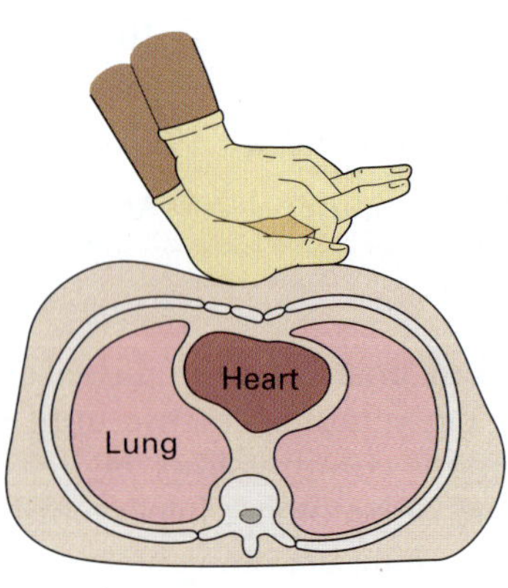

Posterior movement of xiphoid process may lacerate the liver. Lowest point of pressure on the sternum must be above, not on, the xiphoid process.

LOCATING XIPHOID PROCESS

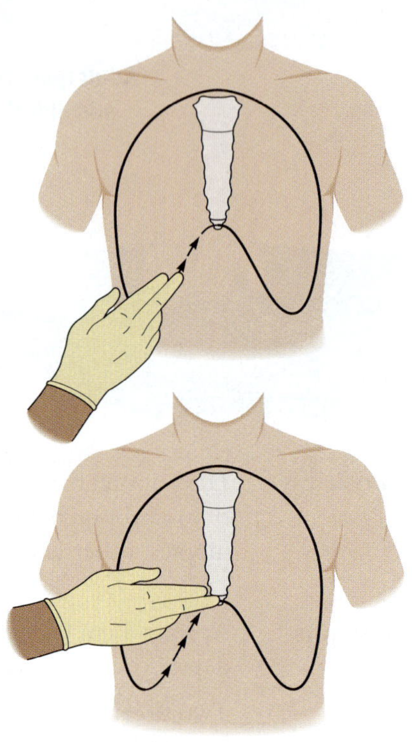

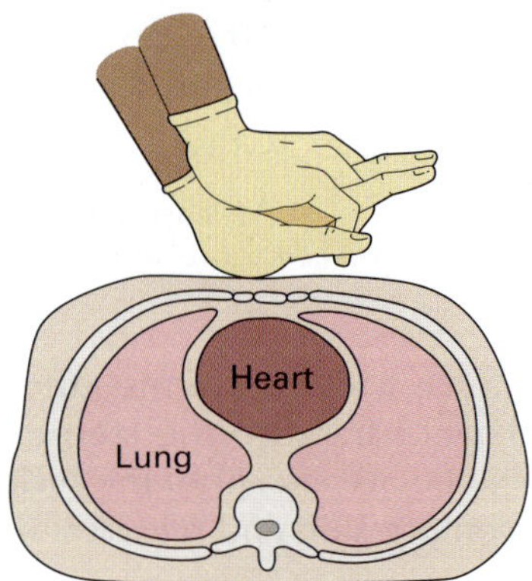

COMPRESSION   **RELEASE**

Figure 8–5 Locating proper hand placement for CPR.

keep track of the number of compressions you deliver.

3. *Deliver two breaths.* After completing 30 compressions, open the airway. Then deliver two breaths, each lasting one second. Be sure you inhale sufficiently between breaths, and make sure that the patient's chest is rising.

4. *Continue until you have completed five cycles of 30 compressions and two ventilations.* (About two minutes.)

5. *Check the patient's pulse.* Check for at least five but no more than ten seconds at the carotid artery. If the pulse has returned, place the patient in the recovery position. Monitor the patient's pulse and breathing closely until the paramedics arrive. If the pulse has returned, but the patient is not breathing, provide artificial ventilation at one breath every five to six seconds, or ten to twelve breaths per minute. If there is still no pulse, resume CPR. Check again for pulse and breathing every five cycles.

If another EMR trained in CPR arrives on the scene, he or she should do two things. First, the new rescuer should verify that the paramedics have been alerted to the patient's condition and are responding. Have him or her activate the EMS system if necessary. Second, the new rescuer should take over cardiac compression when the first rescuer has completed a cycle of 30 compressions.

CORRECT POSITIONING FOR CPR

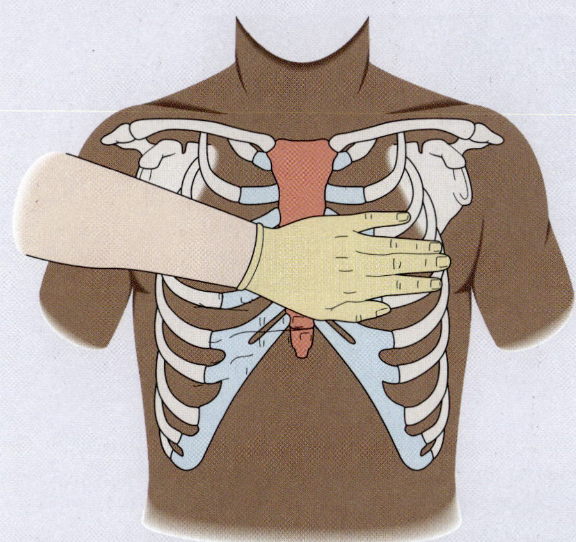

Figure 8–6a Place the heel of your hand on the patient's sternum between the nipples.

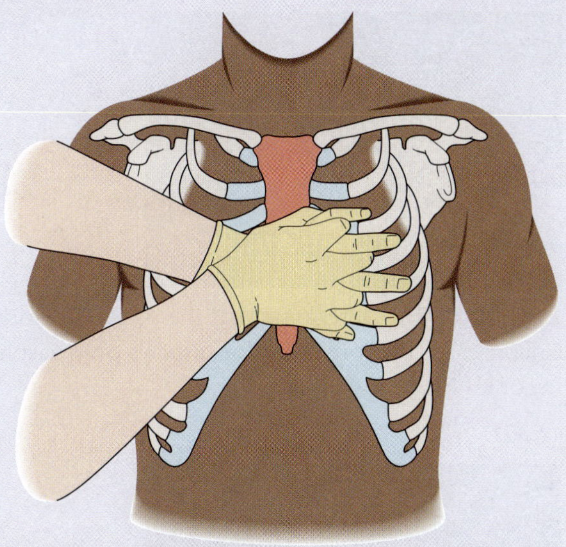

Figure 8–6b Interlace your fingers.

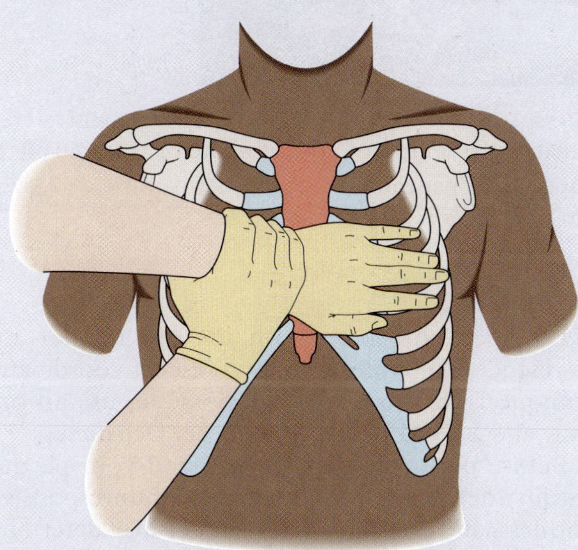

Figure 8–6c Alternative hand placement for CPR.

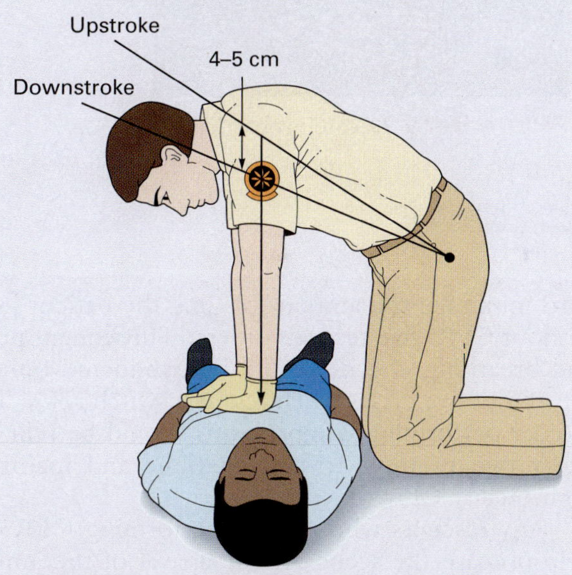

Figure 8–6d Position your shoulders and then perform chest compressions.

To relieve the first rescuer with as little interruption as possible, follow these steps:

- If the first rescuer is performing chest compressions when the second rescuer arrives, the second rescuer should take a position at the patient's head. The second rescuer should then check the pulse while the first rescuer continues compressing the chest. Adequate CPR will usually create a carotid pulse. When the first rescuer completes the 30 compressions, the second rescuer should provide two ventilations. The second rescuer can then resume CPR.
- If the first rescuer is performing ventilations when the second rescuer arrives, the second rescuer should prepare to perform compressions. After the first rescuer completes two ventilations, the second rescuer should begin compressions.

There is no exact sequence to cover all situations. The examples above are efficient ways to change rescuers when CPR is performed. The main objective

ONE-RESCUER ADULT CPR

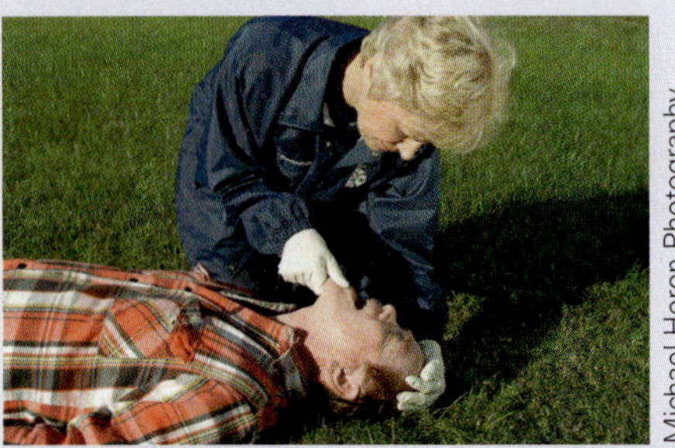

Figure 8–7a Determine that the patient is both unconscious and breathless or displays only gasping (agonal) breathing attempts.

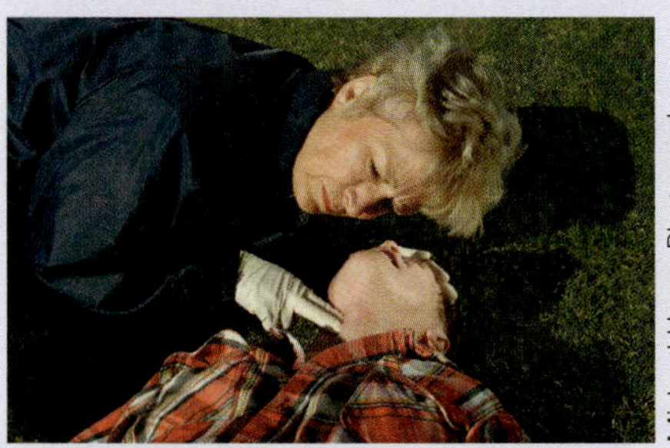

Figure 8–7b Determine pulselessness.

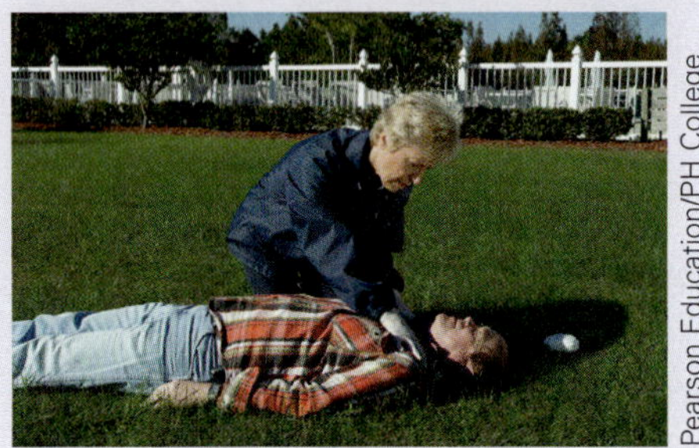

Figure 8–7c Locate proper hand position.

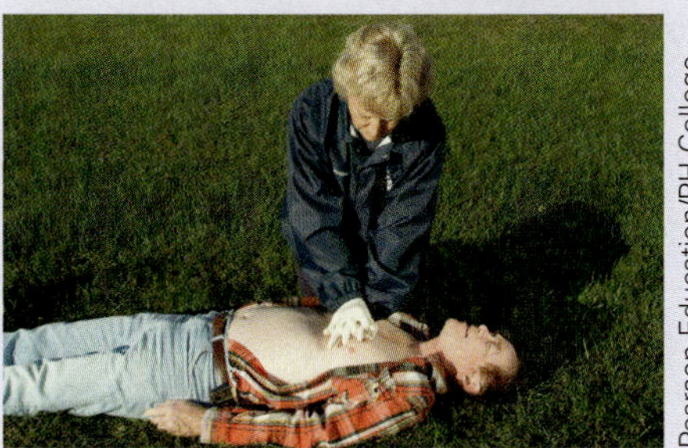

Figure 8–7d Perform chest compressions and ventilations at a ratio of 30:2 at a rate of at least 100 compressions per minute.

is to minimize the amount of time the patient goes without CPR (five seconds or less). Subsequent pulse and breathing checks should be conducted only at the end of five cycles when rescuers switch roles. The rescuer performing compressions should be relieved every two minutes to avoid fatigue and maintain high-quality CPR.

Any rescuers who are not performing CPR can help prepare the scene for the arrival of the ambulance. Paramedics require space for stretchers, equipment, and additional personnel. Moving furniture away from the patient may help create extra space. Directing the ambulance crew to the patient is also valuable. If time permits, find out from family or bystanders the exact sequence of events leading to the time the patient's heart stopped.

> ### (!) T I P
>
> If more than two rescuers are available, the compressor role should switch every two minutes. A third rescuer can assist by helping with the BVM if it is being used.

Two-Rescuer CPR

All EMRs should learn both the one-rescuer and two-rescuer techniques. The two-rescuer coordinated technique is less tiring. When possible, use an oral airway and a BVM device or a pocket face mask.

Before performing CPR, you and your partner must first determine that the patient is unresponsive, breathless, and pulseless. One rescuer may determine unresponsiveness and absence of effective breathing and check the pulse. At the same time, the second rescuer can activate the EMS system and prepare to do compressions.

If the patient is unresponsive, breathless, and pulseless upon your initial assessment, proceed with CPR as follows (Figure 8–8):

1. *Get in position.* The rescuers, if possible, should take positions on opposite sides of the patient. One rescuer kneels by the patient's side for compressions. The other kneels at the patient's head to provide ventilations.
2. *Perform 30 chest compressions.* Perform 30 chest compressions in under 20 seconds so that they can be achieved at a rate of at least 100 per minute. The

TWO-RESCUER ADULT CPR

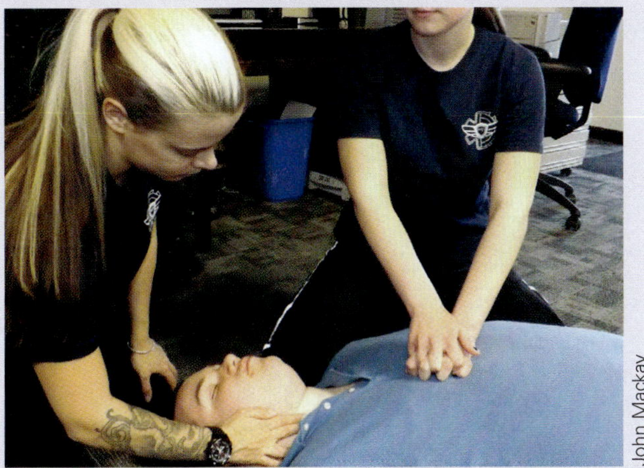

Figure 8–8a The first rescuer delivers 30 chest compressions to a depth of at least 5 cm (2 inches) at a rate of at least 100 per minute while allowing for full chest recoil between compressions.

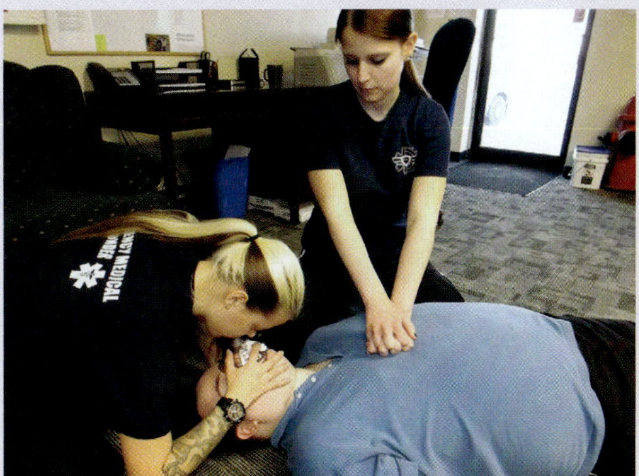

Figure 8–8b The second rescuer then gives two breaths, while maintaining the airway and watching for chest rise and fall.

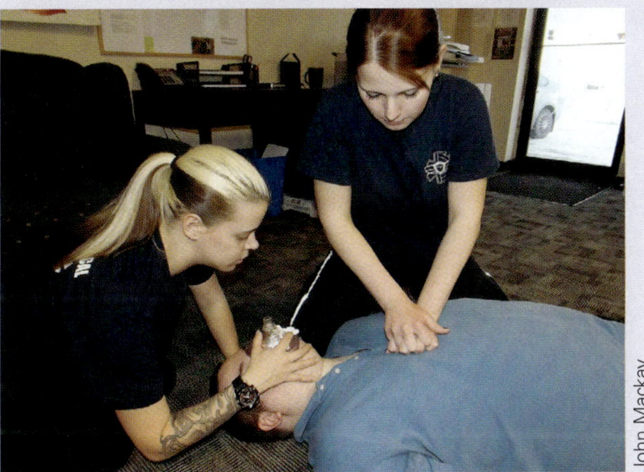

Figure 8–8c Continue compressions and ventilations at a ratio of 30:2 at a rate of at least 100 per minute. Pause CPR to assess the carotid pulse after five cycles and every two minutes thereafter.

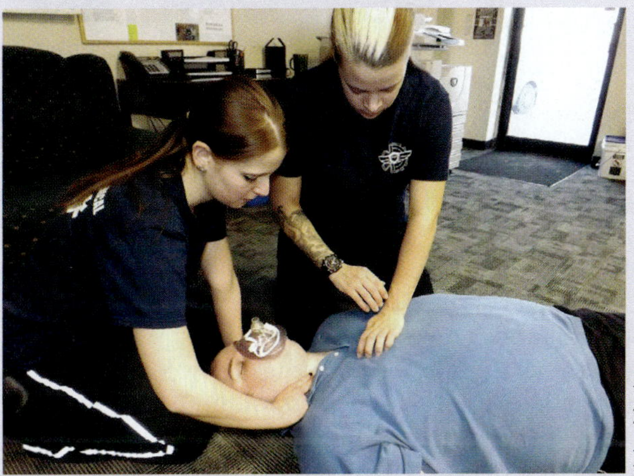

Figure 8–8d Switch roles every five cycles in order to minimize fatigue and maximize high-quality chest compressions.

compression rescuer should count the sequence out loud. Use an audible count of "one and two and three and four and five and six and . . ."

3. *Deliver two breaths.* The ventilation rescuer should take a deep breath on "28," get into position to ventilate on "29," and begin breathing into the patient after "30." The compression rescuer pauses for three to four seconds so that the patient receives two full, one-second breaths. If you have the proper equipment and training, ventilate with 100 percent oxygen.

4. *Continue until you have completed five cycles of 30 compressions and two ventilations.*

5. *Check the patient's pulse.* Check for at least five but no more than ten seconds at the carotid artery. If the pulse has returned, monitor the patient's pulse and breathing closely until the paramedics arrive. If the pulse has returned but the patient is not breathing, provide artificial ventilation at ten to twelve breaths per minute every five to six seconds. If there is still no pulse, resume CPR. Check again for pulse and breathing every two minutes or five cycles.

Note that in two-rescuer CPR, the ratio of compressions to ventilations remains 30:2 (30 compressions

CHANGING POSITIONS

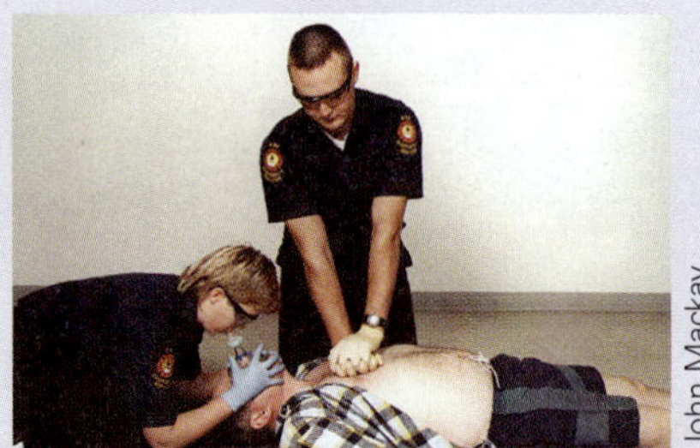

Figure 8–9a Two-rescuer CPR.

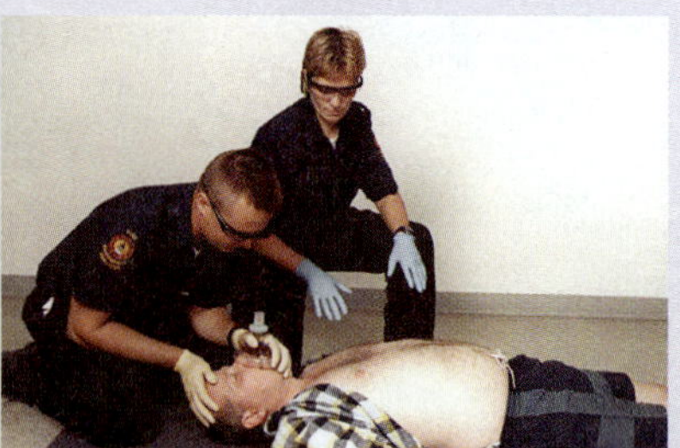

Figure 8–9b Rescuers change positions with little interruption.

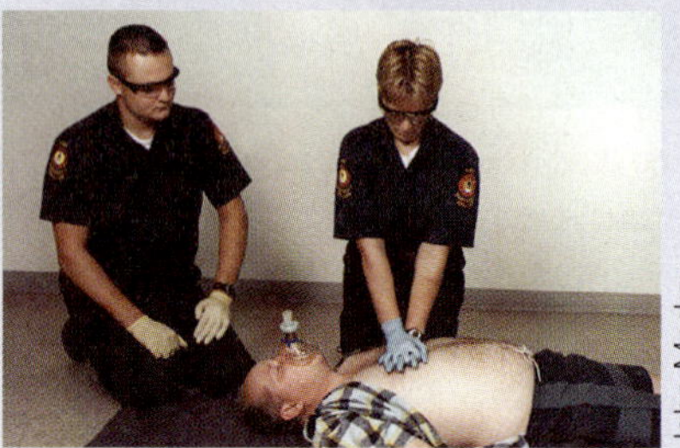

Figure 8–9c One-rescuer CPR.

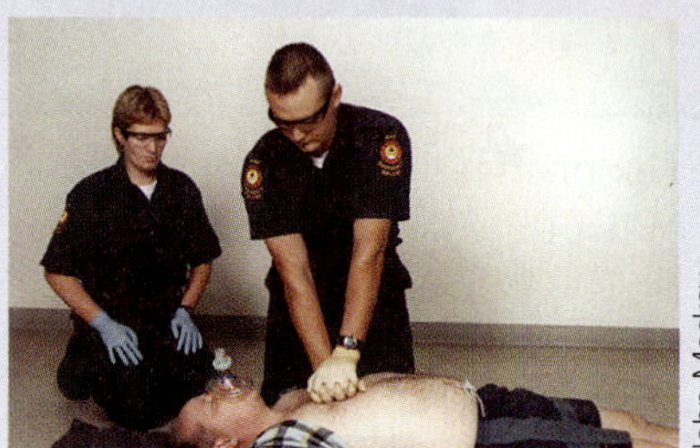

Figure 8–9d Second rescuer takes over one-rescuer CPR.

and then two ventilations). The ventilations should be delivered during a three- to four-second pause after every thirtieth chest compression.

Rescuers should change positions after every five cycles or about two minutes of CPR. Whether rescuers are changing positions during two-person CPR (Figures 8–9a and 8–9b) or switching rescuers and resuming one-person CPR (Figures 8–9c and 8–9d), the rescuers should take less than five seconds to switch. When changing positions during two-person CPR, resume the sequence with a pulse check, followed by 30 compressions and two rescue breaths.

Monitoring the Patient

The patient's condition needs to be monitored throughout CPR. This will ensure that rescue efforts are effective. It also lets you know when spontaneous breathing and the pulse return.

In two-rescuer CPR, there is a ventilation rescuer and a compression rescuer. To monitor the effectiveness of the chest compressions, the ventilation rescuer should feel for a pulse at the carotid artery during compressions. To determine if a spontaneous pulse has returned, the ventilation rescuer should check the carotid artery for five to ten seconds at the end of five cycles of CPR and every two minutes thereafter. Note that the pulse must also be checked when CPR is not in progress.

In general, CPR should not be interrupted for more than five seconds. One of the few exceptions to this rule applies to moving a patient. It may not be possible to perform CPR in a cramped bedroom or other small areas. In this case, it is acceptable to move the patient so that proper CPR can be performed. These actions must be kept as close to five seconds as possible.

Signs of Successful CPR

Signs of successful CPR include the following:

- Each time the sternum is compressed, you feel a pulse in the carotid artery. It will feel like a flutter.
- The chest rises and falls with each ventilation.
- The pupils react or appear to be normal. (Pupils should constrict when exposed to light.)
- A heartbeat returns.
- A spontaneous gasp occurs.
- The patient's skin colour improves or returns to normal.
- The patient moves his or her arms or legs.
- The patient tries to swallow.

Remember that successful CPR does not mean that the patient will live. It means only that you performed CPR correctly.

Very few patients will survive if they do not receive advanced cardiac life support (ACLS). The goal of CPR is to prevent the death of cells and organs for a few crucial moments. Hopefully, ACLS providers will arrive in time.

Mistakes in Performing CPR

The most common ventilation mistakes are as follows:

- Failing to maintain an adequate head tilt
- Failing to maintain an adequate seal around the patient's mouth, nose, or both with a pocket face mask or face shield
- Failing to release the seal when the patient exhales
- Completing two breaths in longer than four seconds
- Failing to watch and listen for exhalation
- Not giving one-second breaths
- Providing breaths too rapidly

Common chest compression mistakes include the following:

- long pauses in compressions
- Bending the elbows instead of keeping them straight
- Not aligning the shoulders directly above the patient's sternum
- Placing the heel of the bottom hand too low or not in line with the sternum (Figure 8–10)
- Not depressing the sternum to a proper depth
- Allowing the fingers to apply force to the chest away from the sternum
- Pivoting at the knees, instead of at the hips
- Compressing at an incorrect rate
- Moving the hands from the compression site between compressions

Complications Caused by CPR

Even properly performed, CPR may cause rib fractures in some patients. Other complications that can occur even with proper CPR include the following:

- Fracture of the sternum
- Pneumothorax (collapse of the lungs caused by air in the chest)
- Hemothorax (collapse of the lungs caused by bleeding in the chest)
- Cuts and bruises to the lungs
- Lacerations (cuts) to the liver

These complications are rare. However, you can help minimize the risk by giving careful attention to your performance. Remember that effective CPR is necessary, even if it results in complications. After all, the alternative is death.

Note that the rib cartilage in elderly patients separates easily. You will hear it crunch as you compress, but do not stop. Be sure that your hand is positioned correctly with these patients and that you are compressing to the correct depth.

CPR for Infants and Children

Infants (up to one year old) and children (one year old to puberty) need slightly different care.

Cardiac arrest in these patients is rarely caused by heart problems. The heart nearly always stops beating because of too little oxygen due to injuries, suffocation, smoke inhalation, sudden infant death syndrome (SIDS), or infection.

The Pediatric Chain of Survival differs from that of adults in that it emphasizes the importance of prevention of arrest in infants and children (Figure 8–11). The HSFC recognizes four links in this chain:

1. Prevention of arrest
2. Early and high-quality CPR performed by bystanders
3. Rapid activation of the EMS system
4. Early and effective advanced life support (ALS) intervention and transport
5. Integrated post-cardiac arrest care

See Chapter 7 for ways to determine if an infant or child patient is unresponsive and breathless. Follow the directions there, too, for caring for an infant or child who is not breathing. Unlike the HSFC guidelines for adult CPR, once pulselessness is established you should complete five cycles of CPR before summoning help. Then proceed with activating the EMS system. If you are in the capacity of an EMS professional called to the scene, you should then update the paramedics as to the patient's condition if they are not already on scene.

Determining that an infant or child patient is pulseless is important. Check for visible signs of circulation and pulse. For an infant, check the brachial pulse on the inside of the upper arm between the elbow and shoulder. Press the artery gently with your index and middle fingers. Never use your thumb. In a child, check the pulse at the carotid or femoral artery. A femoral pulse is palpated with two fingers on the inner thigh between the hip and pubic bones.

It can be difficult to find a pulse in an infant or child. You should not spend more than 10 seconds trying to locate one. In addition to the pulse, the signs of circulation include normal breathing, coughing, or movement in response to rescue breathing.

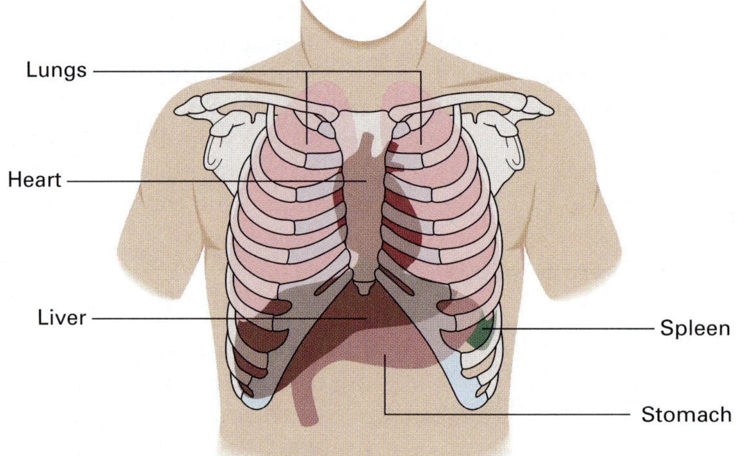

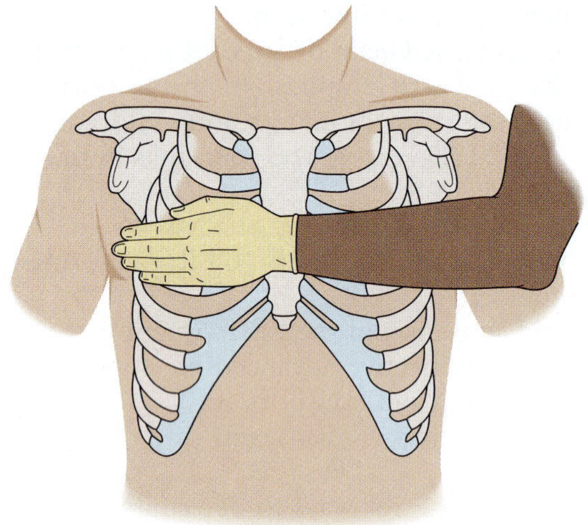

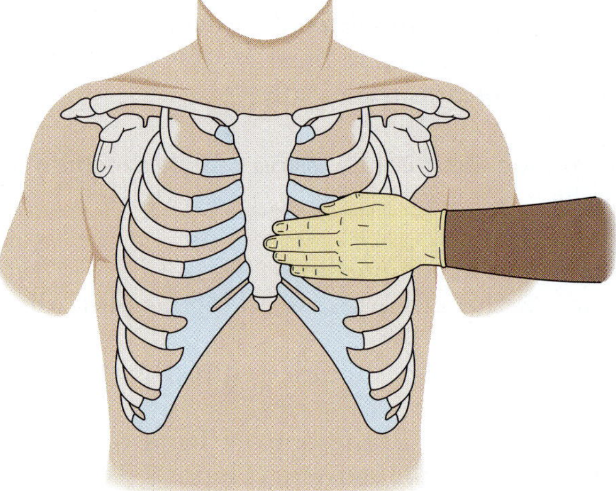

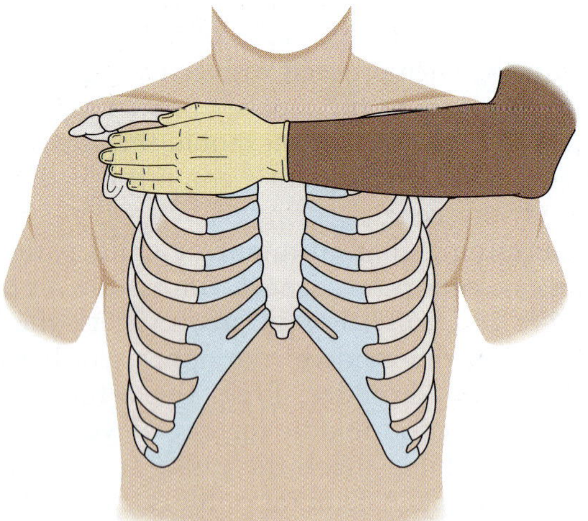

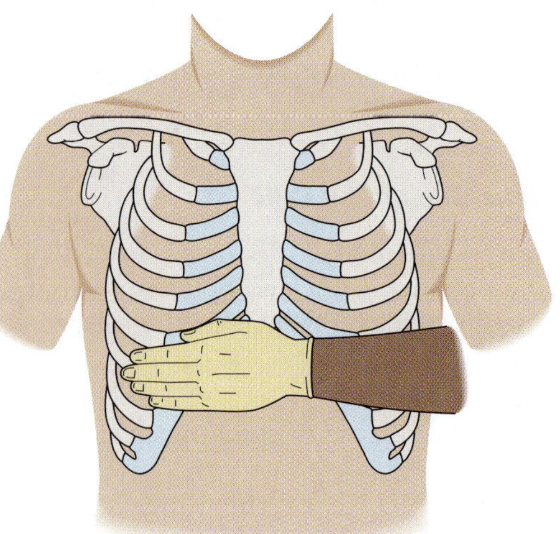

Figure 8–10 Consequences of improper hand placement.

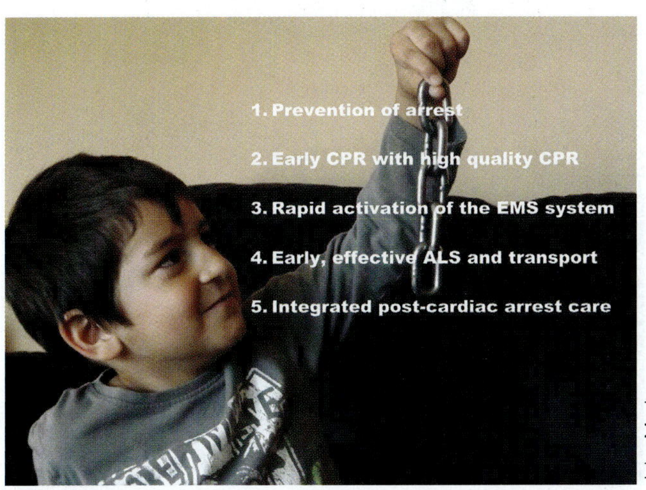

Figure 8–11 Pediatric Chain of Survival.

Performing CPR

If the infant or child is breathless and pulseless, or if the pulse is slower than 60 beats per minute with signs of poor perfusion, then begin CPR. Follow these guidelines to perform chest compressions (Figures 8–12 and 8–13):

1. *Position the patient.* Make sure the patient is lying on a firm, flat surface. If the patient is an infant, put him or her in your lap with the head supported in a neutral (sniffing) position. Use your palm to support the infant's back. Make sure his or her head is not higher than the rest of the body.
2. *Locate the compression site.* For an infant, it is just below an imaginary line between the nipples.

INFANT AND CHILD CPR

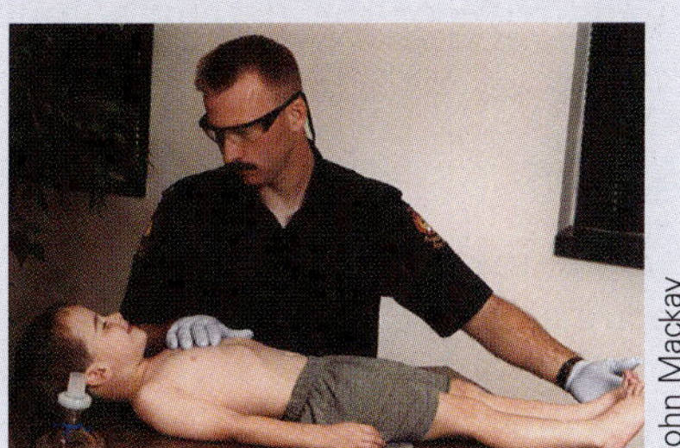

Figure 8–12a After determining unresponsiveness and breathlessness or insufficient breathing, activate EMS.

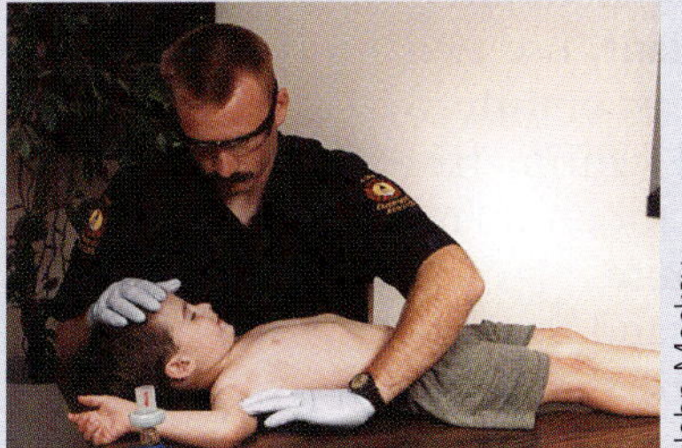

Figure 8–12b Determine pulselessness at the infant's brachial artery or the child's carotid or femoral artery.

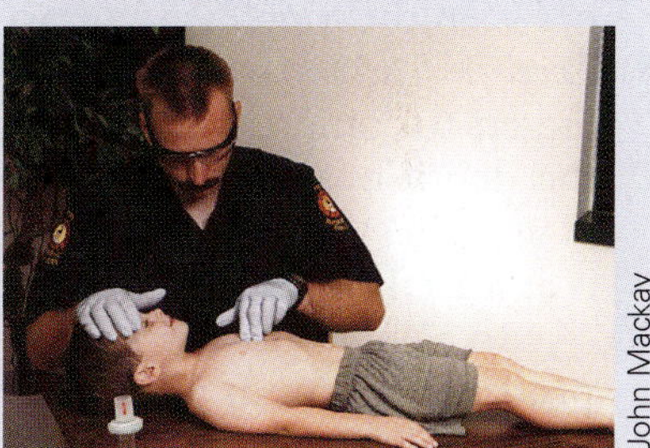

Figure 8–12c Locate the correct hand position.

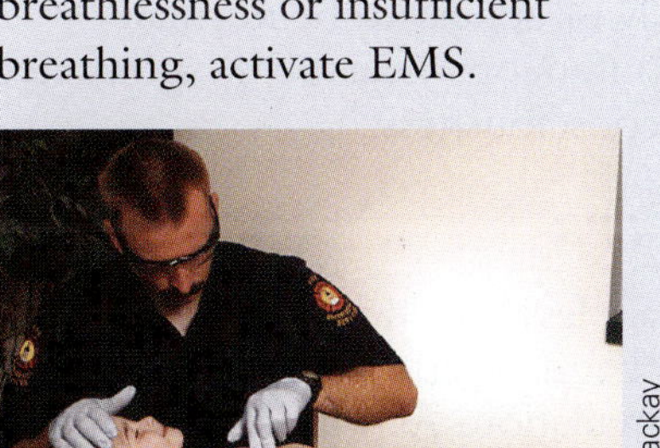

Figure 8–12d Compress the sternum at a rate of at least 100 per minute.

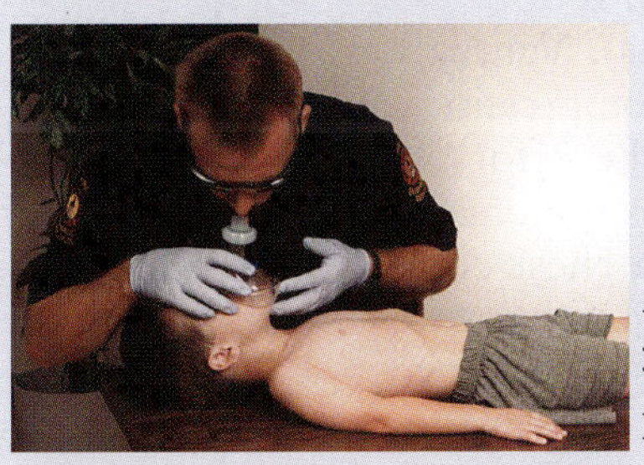

Figure 8–12e Cover the infant's mouth and nose with a pocket mask. Then ventilate.

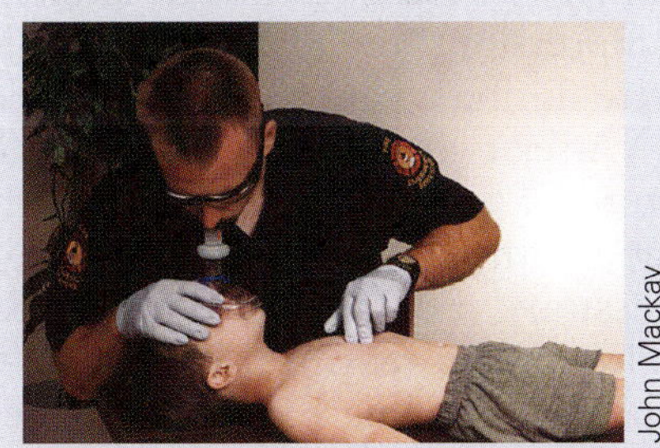

Figure 8–12f Give two one-second breaths after every thirtieth compression.

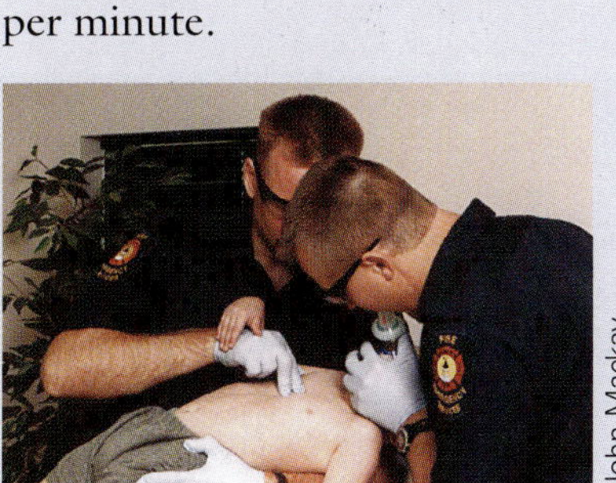

Figure 8–12g Perform CPR while carrying the patient.

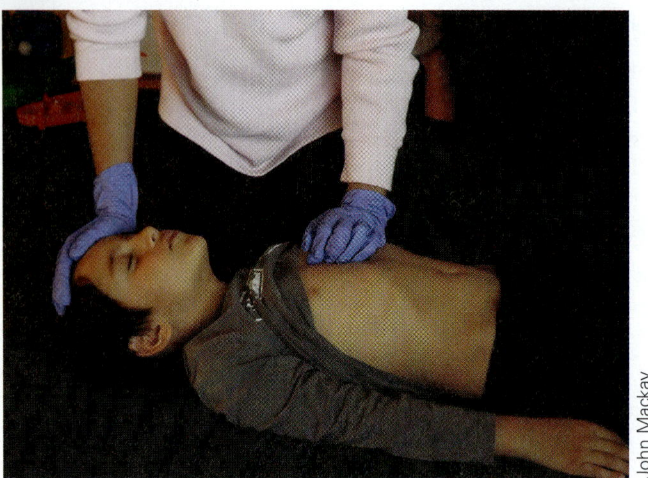

Figure 8–13 Chest compressions on a bigger child.

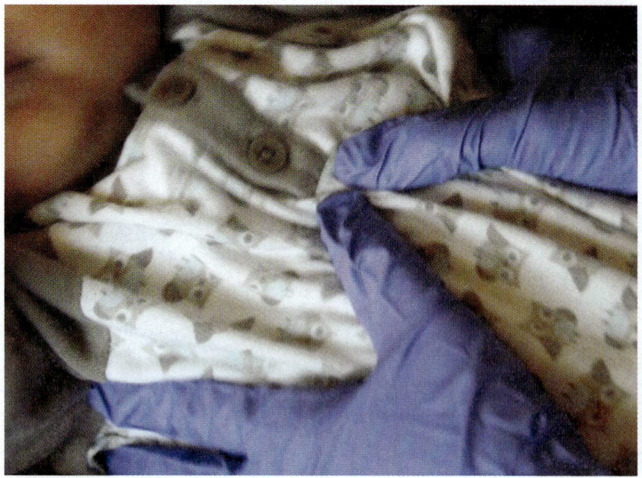

Figure 8–14 Two thumbs encircling hands technique on an infant.

For a child, locate the centre of the breastbone between the nipples as you would for an adult.

3. *Perform chest compressions.* In an infant, use two fingers to compress the sternum at least one-third the depth of the chest or at least 4 centimetres (1½ inches). The compression rate for an infant is at least 100 compressions per minute.

   In a child, use the heel of one hand to compress the sternum at least one-third the depth of the chest or approximately 5 centimetres (2 inches). The compression rate for a child is at least 100 compressions per minute.

The ratio of compressions to ventilations in one-rescuer CPR in both infants and children is 30:2 (30 compressions and then two ventilations). Ventilate twice during a pause after the thirtieth compression.

After two minutes, or five cycles, check for the return of a spontaneous pulse. If there is none, continue with sets of 30:2, beginning with chest compressions. For two-rescuer CPR on infants and children, the ratio is 15:2. Consider using the two thumbs-encircling hands technique for compressions (Figure 8–14) where the rescuer's hands encircle the infant's thorax with the thumbs over the lower half of the sternum. The second rescuer provides ventilations.

Reassess and switch compressors every two minutes until ACLS personnel arrive or the patient's condition changes.

Signs of Successful CPR

The methods for checking for successful CPR in infants and children are almost the same as for adults:

- Check the patient's pulse every five cycles or two minutes. In the infant, check the brachial pulse. In the child, check the carotid or femoral pulse.
- Check the pupils. CPR is successful if they are reacting normally or appear to be normal.
- Watch for a spontaneous heartbeat, spontaneous breathing, and consciousness.

Complications of CPR

While rib fractures are less likely with the softer skeleton of a child, correct hand positioning is imperative for effective artificial circulation. As with adults, improper positioning can cause gastric distention and vomiting, which can interfere with efficient CPR. One of the most common complications with injury and sudden illness in children is hypothermia (below-normal body temperature). Therefore, keep the infant or child warm.

EMR FOCUS

Circulation, like respiration, is essential to life. If a patient's heart fails to beat, he or she will surely die unless actions are taken to restore the heartbeat. As an EMR, you will help take these actions.

CPR is the first step in saving the life of a patient whose heart has stopped beating. The sooner CPR is started, the better. Permanent brain damage may occur after as few as four minutes without oxygen.

Over the years, scientists have discovered that CPR has limitations. It is not nearly as effective as the patient's own heartbeat. This is why the CPR procedure calls for you to activate EMS before beginning CPR. This allows other members of the EMS system to respond while you perform CPR.

The next chapter covers automated external defibrillation using an **automated external**

defibrillator (AED). The AED is a device that applies an electric shock to the patient's chest to restore a heartbeat. You will recall that the Adult Chain of Survival requires early recognition, early CPR, and early defibrillation, together with early advanced care and integrated post-cardiac arrest care, for an optimal chance of survival.

Perform CPR in accordance with HSFC standards when you are called to do so. Be sure you have a barrier device with you at all times.

CASE STUDY FOLLOW-UP

At the beginning of this chapter, you read that EMRs took over CPR from a bystander. To see how the chapter skills apply to this emergency, read the following. It describes how the call was completed.

PATIENT HISTORY

I talked to a bystander, who told me that the patient had been mowing the lawn when he collapsed. He wasn't sure how long his neighbour had been down, but he thought it was less than five minutes.

The patient's wife told me that her husband was 71 and had had bypass surgery two years before, after a heart attack. He was on medication for his heart and high blood pressure. She went to get the medicine as I radioed the incoming EMS units with an update.

SECONDARY ASSESSMENT

Our first concern was providing good CPR. Two men in my crew were doing that. A thorough physical exam would have to wait. The patient was on the grass and didn't appear to have any injuries from falling to the ground.

ONGOING ASSESSMENT

All we could do at this point was monitor the success of the CPR. We checked the carotid pulse during chest compressions and the chest rise and fall during ventilations.

TRANSFER OF CARE

When the paramedics arrived, I told them that the patient was a 71-year-old male. He was found in cardiac arrest by his wife, who had begun CPR. The patient was unresponsive, with no pulse or respirations, when CPR was continued by our crew. I told them I didn't believe that the patient had any injuries. He had a history of bypass surgery and high blood pressure and took medication. I gave them the patient's medication vials.

The paramedics continued emergency care as we watched. It took three shocks from the semi-automated external defibrillator to get the patient's heart started again. But he still had no respirations. One of them continued to ventilate the patient, while the others put the patient on a backboard. The backboard would give them a hard surface to compress against, in case they had to start CPR again.

Later, the paramedics told me that the patient had improved slightly in the ambulance and had been transferred to the cardiac unit at the hospital. Not all patients survive. I was happy we helped one who did.

> Cardiovascular disease is still the major cause of death and disability in Canada in people over 45 years of age. Be prepared to provide CPR to any patient who needs it. Remember to take refresher courses frequently and to get recertified according to local protocols every one or two years.

NOCPs

4.3 c Conduct cardiovascular system assessment and interpret findings **S**

4.4 a Assess pulse **S**

5.5 a Conduct cardiopulmonary resuscitation **S**

6.1 a Provide care to patient experiencing signs and symptoms involving the cardiovascular system **S**

6.2 a Provide care for the neonatal patient **S**

b Provide care for the pediatric patient **A**

c Provide care for the geriatric patient **A**

6.3.1 a Conduct ongoing assessments based on patient presentation and interpret findings **S**

b Re-direct priorities based on assessment findings **S**

REVIEW QUESTIONS

Page references where answers may be found or supported are provided at the end of each question.

SECTION 1

1. What is the name and location of each of the four chambers of the heart? (p. 118)
2. What is a pulse? Where can you best palpate it? (p. 118)
3. What are the links in the Adult Chain of Survival? (pp. 119–120)
4. What is PAD and why is it important? (p. 119)
5. What are the links in the Pediatric Chain of Survival? (p. 129)

SECTION 2

6. Before performing CPR on your patient, what must your assessment of his or her condition reveal? (pp. 120–122)
7. When should you activate EMS if your patient is an unconscious adult? An unconscious infant? (p. 120)
8. How can you find the correct CPR compression site on an infant, child, and adult? (pp. 122, 131, 132)
9. What are the appropriate compression depths for an infant, child, and adult? (pp. 122, 132)
10. Why is it essential to perform CPR in spite of the problems it may cause? (p. 132)

9

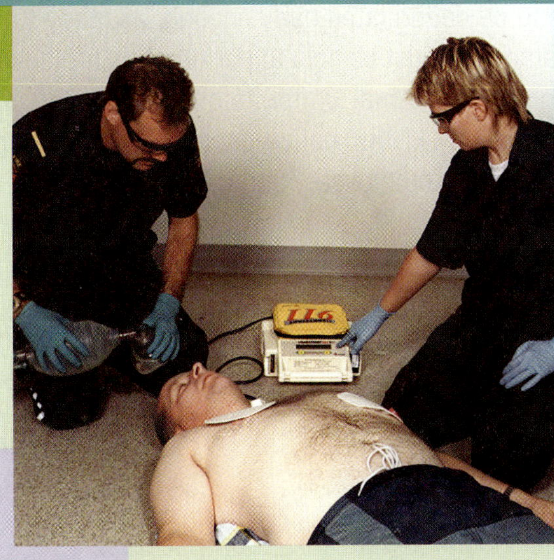

John Mackay

Automated External Defibrillation

OBJECTIVES

1. Define defibrillation and describe the indications for and purpose of automated external defibrillation.

2. Identify the two types of automated external defibrillator (AED).

3. List the contraindications for the use of automated external defibrillation.

4. Explain how to operate an automated external defibrillator.

5. Demonstrate how to integrate CPR procedures and automated external defibrillation procedures.

6. Explain how to adapt the AED procedure to unconscious patients.

7. List the eight components of an AED that should be checked every shift.

INTRODUCTION

As you will recall from Chapter 8, early defibrillation is part of the Chain of Survival. In order for patients to be defibrillated early enough, as many trained people as possible, not just physicians and paramedics, must be able to perform this life-saving skill.

Automated external defibrillators have made **public access defibrillation (PAD)** possible. Now many EMRs, police personnel, security guards, airline staff, sports and recreation personnel, office employees, and other members of the public are able to defibrillate a patient when it is needed.

SECTION 1
ABOUT DEFIBRILLATORS

Defibrillation is the application of an electric shock to the chest of a patient who is in cardiac arrest—a non-breathing and pulseless patient. It has been used for many years by physicians and paramedics. Most of them use *manual* defibrillation. This means that they interpret the information provided by the defibrillator, decide if shocks are indicated, and then deliver the shocks themselves by applying paddles or hands-free defibrillation pads to the patient's chest.

The automated external defibrillator (AED) can perform all those tasks. The AED has a microprocessor that actually interprets the heart rhythm, just as a physician would. When necessary, shocks are delivered by the device directly to the patient.

The shocks are delivered to the chest through adhesive pads. These pads are connected to the AED through cables, which can transmit a shock to the chest that is powerful enough to correct a lethal heart rhythm. The pads make defibrillation safer since no one needs to touch the patient at all during analysis or shocks.

EMS systems that allow EMRs to use AEDs should have all of the following in place:

- All the EMS links of the *Chain of Survival.* Without immediate recognition of cardiac arrest and prompt activation of EMS, early CPR, early defibrillation, early advanced life support, and integrated post-cardiac arrest care, the patient will not have the best chance of survival.
- *Medical direction.* A physician must issue standing orders for EMRs to use an AED.
- *Quality improvement programs* to monitor the use of AEDs in the field.
- Mandatory *continuing education* for AED users.

Types of AED

There are two types of automated defibrillators— one that is fully automated and one that is semi-automated (Figure 9–1). The operator attaches a fully automated defibrillator to the patient, turns it on, and the device does the rest. The **semi-automated external defibrillator (SAED)** is the most common defibrillator used by EMRs and PAD programs. Often referred to under the generic term AED, it performs the same tasks as a fully automated defibrillator, but it is a safer machine because the operator must push a button to analyze the patient's heart rhythm and to deliver the shock.

Components of AEDs

There are many brands of AEDs. They include some or all of the following components:

- *On/off button.* This button controls power to the AED.
- *Analyze button.* Press this button to instruct the AED to analyze the patient's heart rhythm.
- *Shock button.* Press this button to deliver an electric shock to the patient.
- *Voice synthesizer.* Some units have an electronic voice that prompts you to perform specific actions. The voice may direct you to analyze rhythm or to shock at the appropriate time.
- *Tape recorder.* Some units have a built-in microphone and a tape recorder that tapes the events of a cardiac arrest. The recording can then be used at a later date for training or quality improvement.
- *Electrocardiogram (ECG) screen or light.* Even though EMRs do not analyze heart rhythms, some AEDs have a built-in screen or light that shows the electrical activity of the heart.

CASE STUDY

Dispatch

Our engine company was sent on a call to an unconscious woman at 326 Riverview Lane.

Scene Assessment

We approached the scene carefully and saw a man frantically waving to us. We were alert to the possibility of danger as we pulled closer.

When we got to the house, the man said his neighbour, a nurse, was performing CPR. We saw her working on an elderly woman who was lying on the lawn. "My wife collapsed while she was carrying in the groceries," the man said. "Please help her. Please!"

There was only one patient. We called for the medics right away. After putting on our gloves and grabbing pocket face masks, we joined the nurse in doing CPR. She was doing a good job.

Primary Assessment

We checked the patient's pulse and respirations. There weren't any.

> Cardiac arrest is literally a life or death situation. Some patients may be saved through the use of an AED. Consider this patient as you read Chapter 9. See if you can decide if she needs defibrillation. If she does, how and when would you apply it? When should you stop?

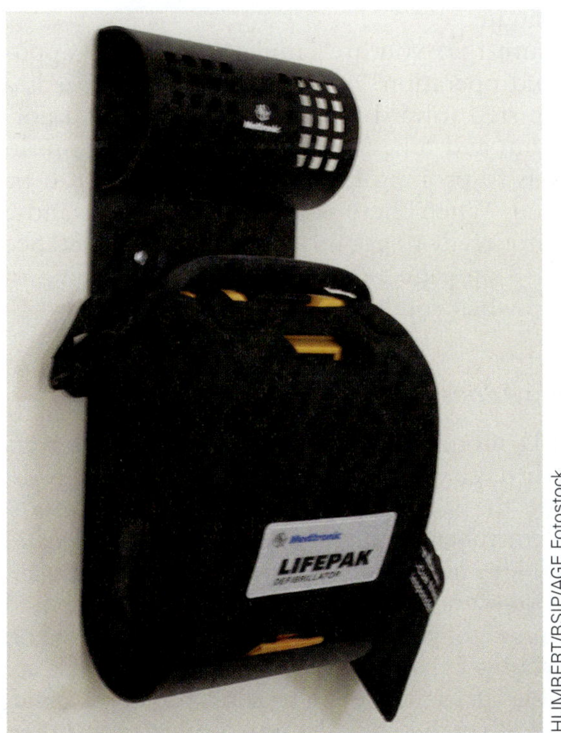

Figure 9–1a Example of a fully automated external defibrillator.

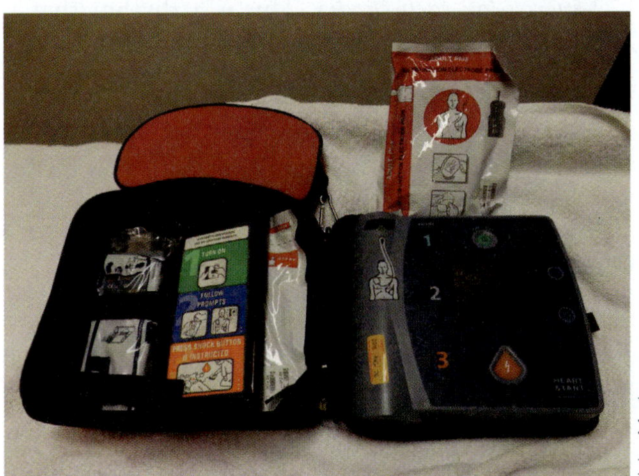

Figure 9–1b Example of a semi-automated external defibrillator.

SECTION 2
OPERATING A DEFIBRILLATOR

AEDs are very safe and accurate. Even so, you must carefully follow operation guidelines. This will ensure safe and proper use of the defibrillator:

- Become familiar with the AED you are using.
- Make sure the AED batteries are fully charged. Carry extra fully charged batteries.
- Carefully follow your local protocols regarding AED use in your area.
- Make sure no one touches the patient while the AED is analyzing the heart rhythm or while a shock is being delivered. If someone is in contact, the shock may be transferred to that person. Touching the patient or cables may also cause interference with the accuracy of the AED.
- Do not apply the AED to a patient with a pulse. The shock could cause the heart to stop.

Local protocols may limit the use of an AED on patients who are in cardiac arrest due to injury or hypothermia.

Heart Rhythms

The normal electrical impulses of the heart occur in an orderly, rhythmic fashion. When you place an AED on a patient, it evaluates the patient's heart rhythm (Figure 9–2).

There are two specific rhythms that do require an AED shock. They are as follows:

- *Ventricular fibrillation*. This is a chaotic, unorganized heart rhythm. It cannot create a pulse or circulate blood to sustain life.
- *Ventricular tachycardia*. This is a rhythm that is more organized, but very rapid and inefficient. It is capable of producing a pulse. (Note that AED shocks must be delivered only to patients without a pulse, so administer an AED shock for ventricular tachycardia only if a pulse is not being produced.)

Heart rhythms that do *not* require an AED shock are as follows:

- *Pulseless electrical activity (PEA), otherwise known as electro-mechanical disassociation (EMD)*. If you were to look at an ECG displaying this rhythm, you might think nothing was wrong. You would find electrical activity on the display, but you would not find a pulse. PEA indicates that the trouble with the heart is not lack of electrical activity, so administering an AED shock will not help.

- *Asystole*. Also known as flatline, this is a condition in which there are no electrical impulses present and, therefore, no pulse. The ECG shows a flat line. Contrary to what movies show, an AED will not help in this case.

Common advice to paramedics and doctors also applies to EMRs who use AEDs: "Treat the patient, not the machine." For example, if the AED reads a flatline, it may only mean that one of the electrodes or cables has become detached from the patient. Also, mechanical or electrical interference with the tracing on the screen, called **artifact**, can mimic ventricular fibrillation, suggesting the need for defibrillation. At other times, an AED might read normal electrical activity when there isn't any. If you were to pay attention only to the machine's monitor screen, you would not realize that a PEA patient needed CPR immediately. Remember, the AED only analyzes heart rhythms. It does not check the pulse.

Always follow your local protocols when determining if a patient is a candidate for defibrillation. If you have questions, contact the medical director. Also, be sure to practise AED procedures frequently and attend continuing education sessions.

Operation Guidelines

Automated defibrillation is easy to learn. An AED may be applied and the patient defibrillated in less than a minute.

Be sure that you are familiar with AED application and operation. Always remember that it is a definitive step toward returning the heart to a normal rhythm and function. CPR is vital, but its main purpose is to prolong life until defibrillation can be performed. When there is a pulseless patient and a defibrillator ready to go, use the defibrillator first! See Figure 9–3 on page 140 for the ideal positioning of personnel when conducting defibrillation.

Applying Adhesive Pads

The AED monitors the heart rhythm and delivers shocks through the electrodes in the adhesive pads. Therefore, the pads must be placed in very specific locations. Remember, all directions refer to the *patient's* right and left, not yours. Defibrillation pads are available in two sizes: adult and child. Adult pads are used on patients eight years and older. They may be used on a child younger than eight years only if child pads are unavailable. If using the larger adult pads on a child, make sure that the pads do not contact each other. Child pads may not be used on an adult. The lower electrical dosage used for children may not be effective

HEART RHYTHMS

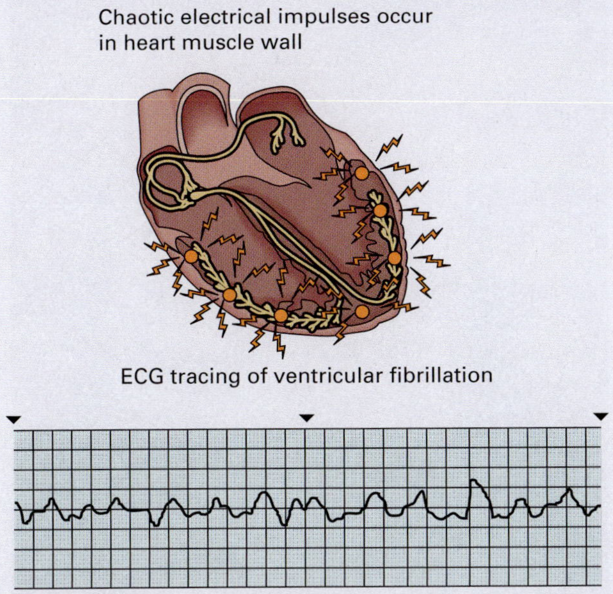

Chaotic electrical impulses occur in heart muscle wall

ECG tracing of ventricular fibrillation

Figure 9–2a Ventricular fibrillation.

Electrical impulses start in a ventricle

ECG tracing of ventricular tachycardia

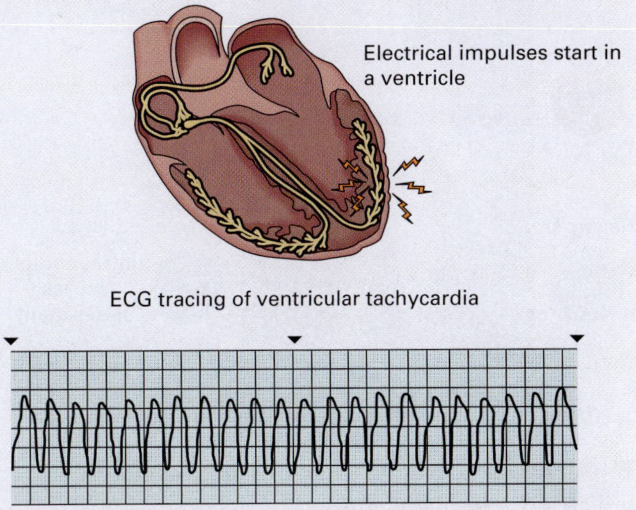

Figure 9–2b Ventricular tachycardia.

No electrical impulses

ECG tracing of asystole

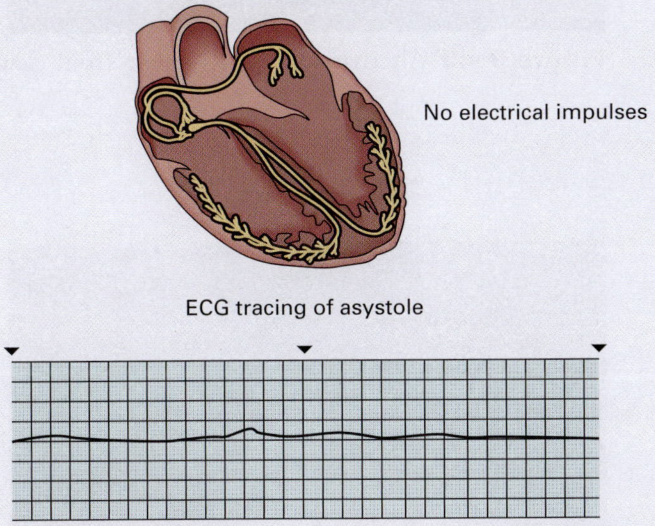

Figure 9–2c Asystole.

on adults. When using the AED on a child, be sure to use the child key switch. Child pads are designed for patients one to eight years of age. The HSFC has no recommendations for or against the use of an AED in children younger than one year of age.

Adhesive pads should be securely applied to the chest. This may not be possible if the patient is extremely hairy. Be sure to carry a razor in your AED kit. Use it to quickly but safely shave the areas where the pads are to adhere. Remove the protective liner from the self-adhering pads and apply them to the torso as follows. Place one pad just below the patient's right clavicle and to the right of the sternum. Place the other pad over the patient's left lower ribs (Figure 9–4a). For colour-coded pads, the mnemonic "white to right, red to ribs" may help you remember where the pads and cables are to be placed. Familiarize yourself with the pads you will be using as they will display specific instructions for placement. Insert the connector for the pads into the AED or into the therapy cable as appropriate for your hardware.

Occasionally, you will find patients who have nitroglycerin patches on their chests. Do not place pads on or near these patches because they can cause arcing or burning of the patient's skin. Instead,

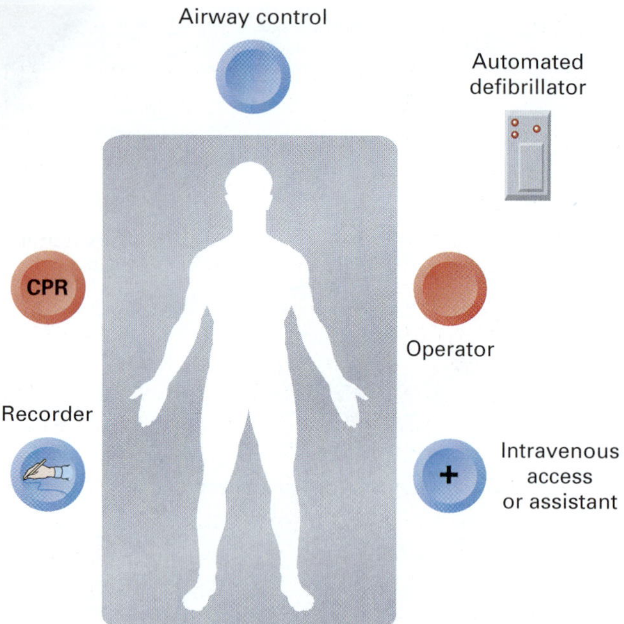

Figure 9–3 Ideal positioning of personnel for defibrillation. (Alternatives may be needed.)

remove the patches and use a towel to wipe away any paste that remains.

Be sure the adhesive pads are not positioned over a pacemaker. It is possible to observe or feel a pacemaker once you bare the patient's chest. You may also be told by a family member that the patient has one. Place the adhesive pads so that they are not touching the pacemaker.

An alternative pad placement (Figures 9–4b and 9–4c) is the anterior/posterior (A/P) positioning. A/P placement of the defibrillator pads can avoid an implanted pacemaker, and actually offers a superior pathway for the electrical current to pass through the heart.

It is also critical to make sure that the patient's chest is dry. Wipe the patient so that water cannot conduct energy away from where it is needed. Always remove a victim from any water.

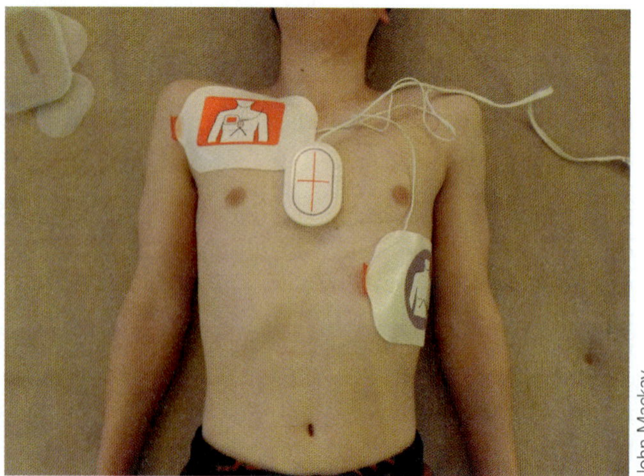

Figure 9–4a Defibrillator pad placement.

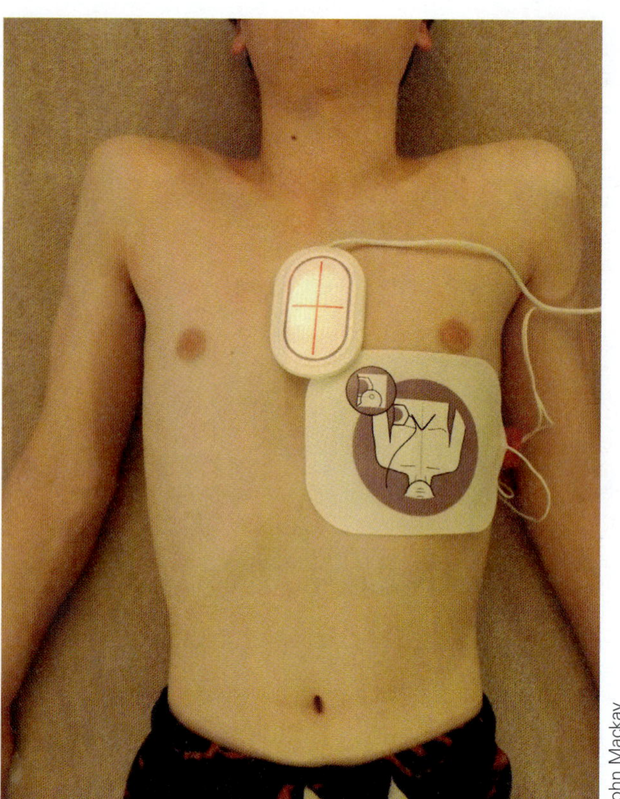

John Mackay

Figure 9–4b Alternative pad placement, front view.

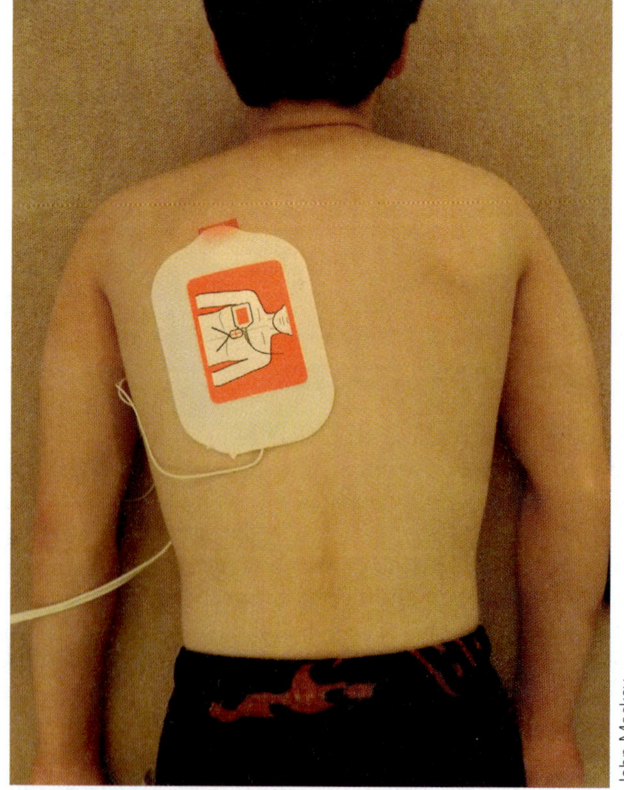

John Mackay

Figure 9–4c Alternative pad placement, back view.

Procedure for Patients with CPR in Progress

After assessing the scene and taking BSI precautions, perform a primary assessment. If CPR is in progress, stop it to check the patient's pulse and respirations (Figure 9–5). If there is no pulse, do the following:

1. Turn on the AED power.
2. Apply the appropriate-sized adhesive pads. Then attach the end of the cable to the AED if it is not already connected. If there will be a delay in administering a shock, resume CPR.
3. Stop CPR and instruct everyone to stay clear of the patient.
4. Press the analyze button.

If the AED advises to administer a shock, make sure everyone is still clear:

5. Deliver the shock.
6. Resume chest compressions immediately. The AED will prompt you to repeat steps 3 and 4 after two minutes or five cycles of CPR. The AED will then re-analyze the heart rhythm.

If the AED advises NOT to administer a shock, follow these steps:

1. Recheck the patient's pulse.
2. If a pulse is present, check respirations. If breathing is inadequate, assist with ventilations. If the pulse is not present, perform CPR for two minutes and then analyze the heart rhythm once again.

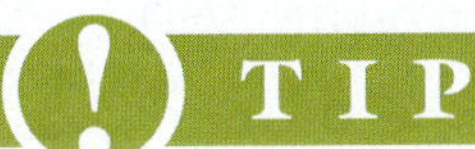

TIME = MUSCLE. The longer a heart has to endure a non-life-sustaining rhythm, the more the heart muscle will weaken. Work quickly!

Procedure for Unconscious Patients

If you are alone and find an unconscious patient, do the following:

1. Assess the patient's breathing and pulse. If these are absent *and* the elapsed time from the call to your arrival is more than four to five minutes, provide about two minutes of CPR before using the AED.
2. If you witnessed the collapse or the patient has been down for less than four minutes, apply the AED and analyze the heart rhythm immediately. Do not begin CPR first. Defibrillation is more important at this point and may be more beneficial to the patient.
3. Follow the instructions outlined above for "If the AED advises to administer a shock."

Post-Resuscitation Care

In some cases, your patient will regain a pulse. This is exciting, but there is much more to be done. Your patient is still in serious condition. Remember the following points when caring for a patient whose pulse has returned:

- Monitor the pulse carefully; it may disappear.
- Many patients will not breathe even though a pulse has returned. This is common. Ventilate the patient or assist ventilations as necessary.
- If your patient has regained a pulse and has adequate respirations—and has not been injured—place him or her in a recovery position.
- Apply high-concentration oxygen if you are trained and allowed to do so by local protocol.
- Keep the AED attached to the patient. EMS personnel who take over care will want it attached during transport.
- Your assessment of the patient should be ongoing until you hand over care.

It will help the patient if advanced care is also available. Arrange for the paramedics to rush to the scene if you have not done so already. Whether the advanced care is performed by them or by physicians, advanced care includes medication and other interventions that will help stabilize the patient and prevent another cardiac arrest. If the advanced care paramedics cannot respond in a reasonable amount of time, an ambulance should promptly transport the patient to the nearest hospital emergency department.

Call Review

After using an AED, the call should be reviewed by a quality improvement committee. (Your medical director will be involved.) The committee reviews all AED calls to determine if protocols were followed. This review uses the run report and, if your AED was equipped with a recorder, the tape recording of the call.

While the call review looks for problem areas, it is not designed to get people into trouble. If needed, the committee may recommend further training for some or all rescuers who use AEDs. The goal of the review is to have trained EMRs providing quality care to patients.

AED Maintenance

The AED is a vital piece of equipment. It would be devastating to arrive at the side of a patient in cardiac arrest with a machine that is not working. Such an occurrence may also be a cause of liability against you and your agency. Consequently, complete the AED

USING A SEMI-AUTOMATED DEFIBRILLATOR

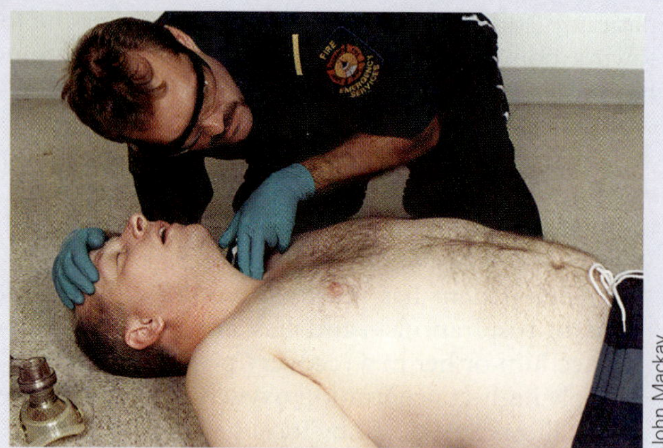

Figure 9–5a Determine that the patient is breathless and pulseless.

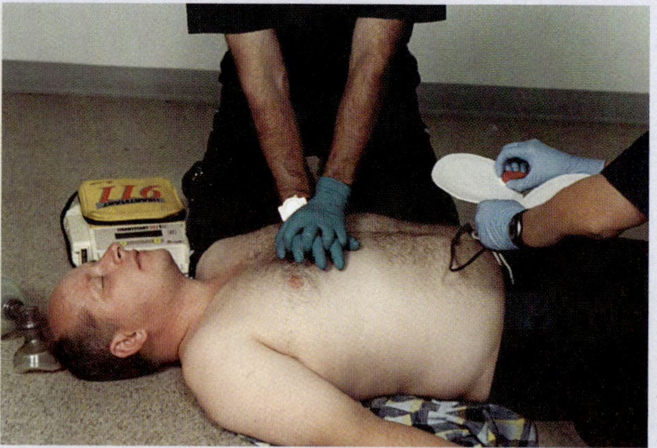

Figure 9–5b One rescuer initiates CPR, while the other prepares the AED.

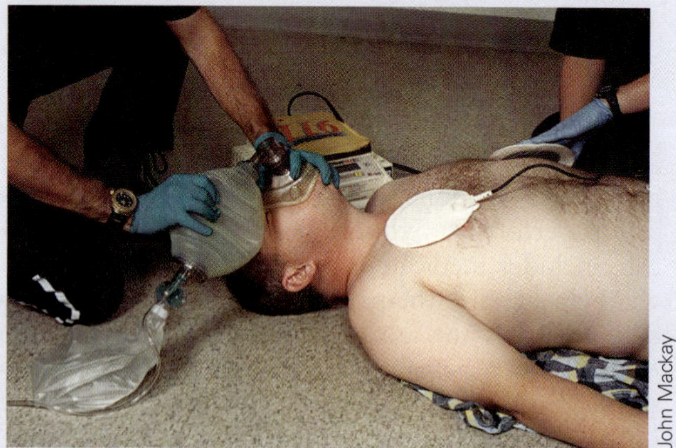

Figure 9–5c Place adhesive pads on the patient's chest.

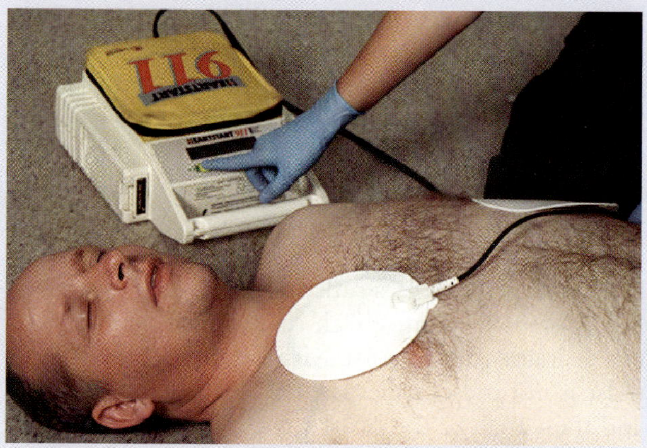

Figure 9–5d Turn on the AED.

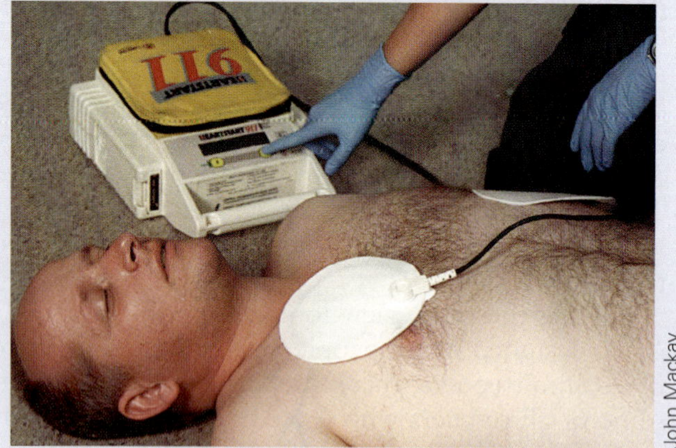

Figure 9–5e Stop CPR and get clear of the AED as it analyzes the heart rhythm.

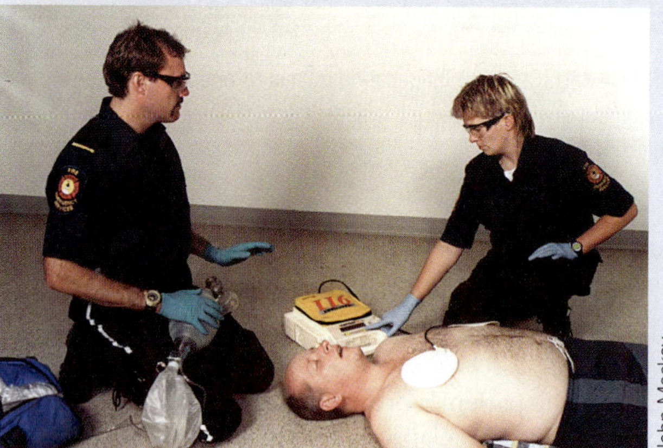

Figure 9–5f If a shock is advised, clear all others from the patient and deliver the shock.

operator's shift checklist at the beginning of every shift (Figure 9–6). Make sure that the AED battery and a spare are fully charged and ready. Make sure the leads are with the unit and there are several sets of adhesive pads available. Always handle the AED carefully. Do not expose it to unnecessary jarring or other rough moves. Finally, follow the manufacturer's guidelines for maintenance.

AUTOMATED DEFIBRILLATORS: OPERATOR'S SHIFT CHECKLIST

Date: _____________   Shift: _________________________   Location: _______________________

Mfr/Model No.: _____________________   Serial No. or Facility ID No.: _______________________

At the beginning of each shift, inspect the unit. Indicate whether all requirements have been met. Note any corrective actions taken. Sign the form.

	Okay as found	Corrective Action/Remarks
1. Defibrillator Unit		
Clean, no spills, clear of objects on top, casing intact		
2. Cables/Connectors		
a. Inspect for cracks, broken wire, or damage b. Connectors engage securely		
3. Supplies		
a. Two sets of pads in sealed packages, within expiration date b. Hand towel c. Scissors d. Razor * e. Alcohol wipes * f. Monitoring electrodes *g. Spare charged battery *h. Adequate ECG paper *i. Manual override module, key or card *j. Cassette tape, memory module, and/or event card plus spares		
4. Power Supply		
a. Battery-powered units (1) Verify fully charged battery in place (2) Spare charged battery available (3) Follow appropriate battery rotation schedule per manufacturer's recommendations b. AC/Battery backup units (1) Plugged into live outlet to maintain battery charge (2) Test on battery power and reconnect to line power		
5. Indicators/*ECG Display		
* a. Remove cassette tape, memory module, and/or event card b. Power on display c. Self-test okay * d. Monitor display functional *e. "Service" message display off *f. Battery charging; low battery light off g. Correct time displayed — set with dispatch centre		
6. ECG Recorder		
a. Adequate ECG paper b. Recorder prints		
7. Charge/Display Cycle		
* a. Disconnect AC plug — battery backup units b. Attach to simulator c. Detects, charges and delivers shock for "VF" d. Responds correctly to non-shockable rhythms *e. Manual override functional f. Detach from simulator *g. Replace cassette tape, module, and/or memory card		
8. *Pacemaker		
a. Pacer output cable intact b. Pacer pads present (set of two) c. Inspect per manufacturer's operational guidelines		
☐ **Major problem(s) identified** **(OUT OF SERVICE)**		

Applicable only if the unit has this supply or capability

Signature: _________________________________

Figure 9–6 Operator's shift checklist for an AED.

EMR FOCUS

Automated external defibrillation saves lives. It is a skill that the HSFC believes should be taught to every EMR.

Remember that CPR will sustain life for a period of time until more advanced care can be provided. An automated defibrillator can actually shock certain abnormal heart rhythms back to normal. Never delay defibrillation. If you have a choice between CPR and defibrillation, choose defibrillation. The earlier the shock is applied, the better chance you have of restoring a normal heart rhythm in your patient.

Finally, when you are called to the scene of a patient in cardiac arrest, there will be considerable stress, especially if you have not been on many such calls. The old adage "Practice makes perfect" applies here. If you practise with your AED frequently, and if you are familiar with protocols, you will perform better, even under the stress of the situation.

CASE STUDY FOLLOW-UP

At the beginning of this chapter, you read that EMRs were at the scene of a patient in respiratory and cardiac arrest. To see how the chapter skills apply to this emergency, read the following. It describes how the call was completed.

PRIMARY ASSESSMENT *(Continued)*

I had the AED. It took only a few seconds to hook up the electrodes and cables while CPR continued. I turned on the AED and instructed everyone to clear the patient while it analyzed the heart rhythm. The machine advised me to press the shock button.

After making sure everyone was clear, I shocked the patient. We resumed CPR for two minutes while the AED went back to the analyze mode. It instructed me to shock again. Everyone was clear and I shocked the patient again. After two more minutes of CPR, the AED analyzed again. It then told me to check the pulse. I couldn't believe it. There was a pulse.

We immediately checked the patient's respirations. There weren't any. We hooked oxygen into the pocket face mask and ventilated her.

PATIENT HISTORY

Among the facts the patient's husband, Mr. Jones, told us was that his wife was in good health. She hadn't been to a doctor in years. She took no medication. She had no complaints before she collapsed. They had had sandwiches for dinner two hours before. She had no allergies. "She was always so healthy. I just don't understand," he said.

SECONDARY ASSESSMENT

We checked quickly for any obvious signs of injury and found none.

ONGOING ASSESSMENT

We never got to the ongoing assessment. The medics were already on the scene.

TRANSFER OF CARE

The hand-off report to the medics was as follows:

"This is Georgia Jones. She is 66 and was carrying groceries into the house when she collapsed on the grass. A nurse who lives next door started CPR. She was doing a good job. We hooked up the AED and gave two shocks. This caused the pulse to return, but no respirations. We ventilated the patient and monitored her pulse until you arrived. Georgia hasn't been to the doctor recently, has no meds, and no allergies. Her husband says she is in good health, and there were no problems before she collapsed. There appear to be no injuries from the fall. She had a sandwich two hours ago for dinner."

The medics initiated **advanced life support (ALS)**. They started IVs, put in airway adjuncts, and gave medication. The patient went back into cardiac arrest once while they were caring for her. They used their manual defibrillator and got her pulse back with one shock. Georgia made it to the hospital with a pulse, but the doctors said her heart and brain had suffered too much damage to survive.

After a day in the cardiac unit, Georgia died. We were sad and disappointed to hear it. We realized that we had done the best we could. Many patients don't survive a heart attack. I know that. The next time maybe we'll get to shake the hand of the person we help when she or he walks out of the hospital.

> SPECIAL NOTE: The AED is a device that has tremendous potential to save lives. But there are some patients who will not be saved. Some may have been down too long or suffered heart damage so great that they could not be saved even if they were in a hospital. Do your best for all patients. If a patient does not survive, even with your best efforts, it is not your fault.
>
> Watching a patient die is a difficult experience. Remember that you have done everything that could be done to help by offering your best efforts. Focus on the good you have done for prior patients and the good you will do for future ones. Also seek out experienced members of your agency. They have undoubtedly felt the same at some point in their career. If necessary, speak to your medical director about the call.

NOCPs

5.5 i Conduct automated external defibrillation **S**

6.1 a Provide care to patient experiencing signs and symptoms involving cardiovascular system **S**

6.3 a Conduct ongoing assessments based on patient presentation and interpret findings **S**

   b Re-direct priorities based on assessment findings **S**

REVIEW QUESTIONS

Page references where answers may be found or supported are provided at the end of each question.

SECTION 1

1. What is the difference between automated and semi-automated external defibrillators? (p. 136)

SECTION 2

2. What role does medical direction play in the use of an AED? (pp. 136, 138, 141)

3. Why is it so important to make sure that no one is touching the patient while the AED analyzes or shocks the patient? (p. 138)

4. If given a choice between performing CPR and using an AED, which should be performed first? Explain your answer. (p. 138)

5. For what age of patient should child defibrillator pads be used? (p. 138)

6. Where on the patient are the AED adhesive pads placed? (pp. 139–140)

7. Identify four special situations that may require extra consideration before attaching an AED. (pp. 139–140)

8. When should the patient's pulse be checked—before or after the first shock? What might you do for the cardiac arrest victim between subsequent shocks? (pp. 141–142)

CHAPTER 10

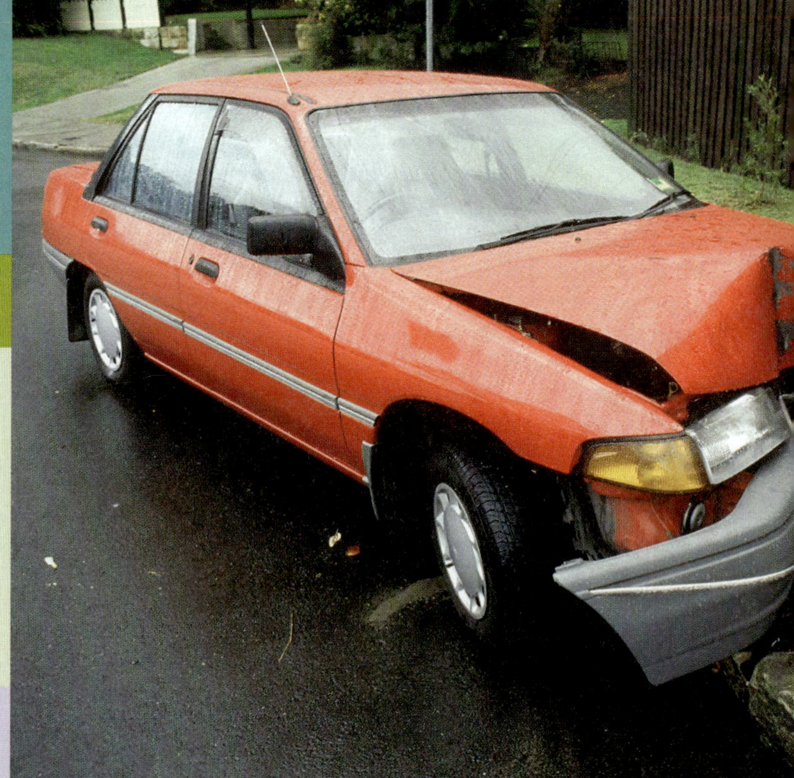

Phillip Hayson/Photolibrary/Getty Images, Inc.

Scene Assessment

OBJECTIVES

1. List the three components of scene assessment.
2. Describe common hazards found at medical or trauma scenes.
3. Explain how a patient's presentation affects your evaluation of the mechanism of injury or the nature of the illness.
4. Discuss the four common mechanisms of injury.
5. Discuss the reason for identifying the total number of patients at the scene.

INTRODUCTION

The purpose of **scene assessment** is to ensure the safety of the people at the scene, to identify the mechanism of injury or nature of the illness, and to determine the necessary additional resources. Most likely, you will not have contact with your patient during scene assessment. Even so, your observations, decisions, and actions provide the foundation for the success of the entire call.

SECTION 1
ENSURING PERSONAL SAFETY

Personal Protective Equipment

Body substance isolation (BSI) precautions must be taken on every call. See Chapter 2 for a full discussion. What follows is a brief review.

Personal protective equipment (PPE) includes the following:

- *Gloves.* Wear them when there is any chance of coming into contact with a patient's blood or other body fluids.
- *Eye protection.* Wear it when there is any chance of blood or other body fluids spraying or splashing into your eyes.
- *Mask.* Wear one when there is any chance of blood or other body fluids spraying or splashing into your nose or mouth.
- *Gown.* Wear one when there is any chance of clothing becoming soiled with blood or other body fluids.

Remember that you should always have PPE available. When you approach the scene, anticipate which items may be needed and put them on. Waiting too long may cause you to become so involved in patient care that you forget to protect yourself.

Nothing is more important at the emergency scene than your safety. Hazards may include obvious situations such as violence, downed power lines, or hazardous materials. Do not overlook the dangers at other scenes, such as potential crashes, unstable vehicles, unstable surfaces (slopes, ice, and so on), and dangerous pets. Place your safety first. If you do not, you may become a patient yourself and quite possibly prevent others from caring for the patient you were sent to help.

The vast majority of calls go by uneventfully. When there is danger, three words sum up the actions required to respond appropriately: *plan, observe,* and *react* (Figure 10–1).

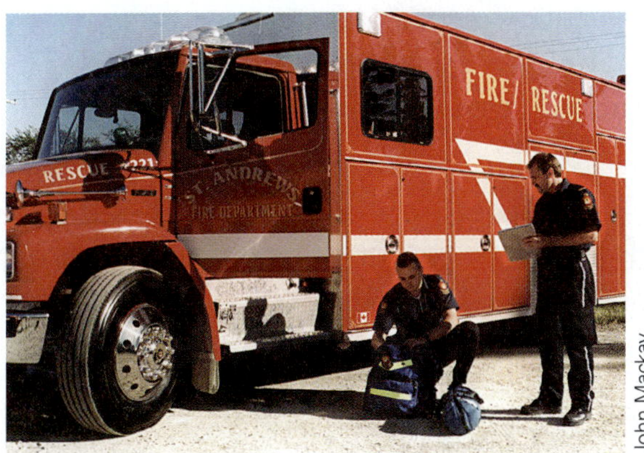

Figure 10–1a Plan for the possibility of a dangerous scene.

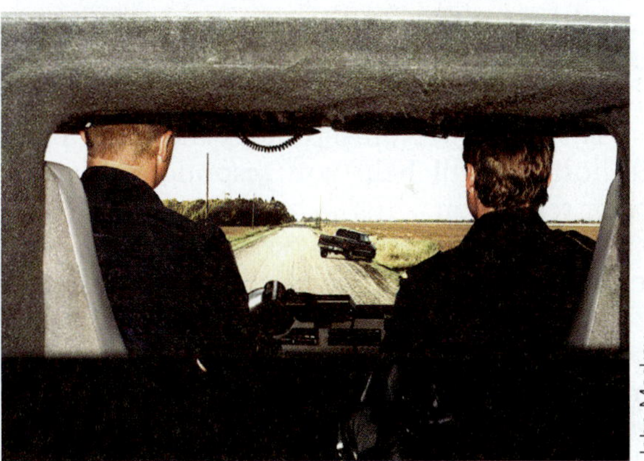

Figure 10–1b Observe the scene for signs of potential danger.

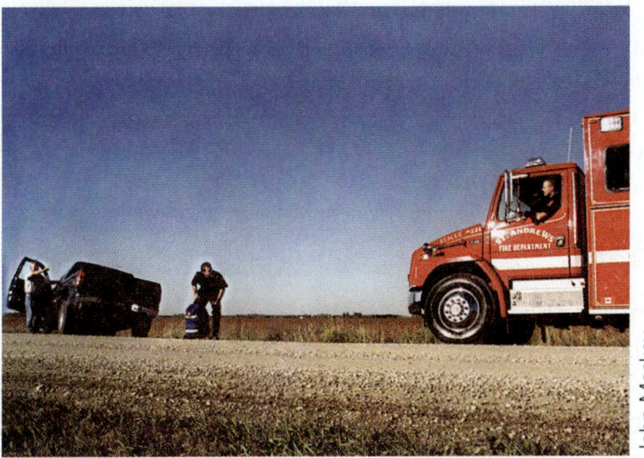

Figure 10–1c React to danger appropriately—retreat, radio, and re-evaluate.

CASE STUDY

Dispatch

I am an EMR for the fire department. My partner and I were dispatched to an MVA at the corner of Central and Devine. The caller indicated that the crash seemed pretty bad.

Scene Assessment

When we approached the scene, we saw that the caller was correct. It was a head-on into a telephone pole.

> The scene assessment on this call will be very important. As you read Chapter 10, consider what the EMRs should do to assess the scene in addition to handling other parts of the call.

Plan

Many EMRs work together to prevent danger and know what to do when danger strikes. However, scene safety begins long before the actual emergency. For example, you should do the following:

- *Wear safe clothing.* Non-slip shoes and other practical clothing will help you respond to danger without restriction.
- *Prepare your equipment properly.* Make sure your first response kit is not cumbersome. Remember that you will be carrying it into emergencies. If it is too heavy or large, it will distract your attention from where it should be—on the scene.
- *Carry a portable radio.* A radio allows you to call for help if you are separated from your vehicle.
- *Plan safety roles.* If there will be more than one rescuer on any call, tasks can be split. For example, one rescuer can care for the patient while the other observes for safety. The observer could look for nearby weapons or other threats, for example, and for clues to the patient's condition, such as prescription medicines.

Observe

Remember that it is always better to prevent danger than to deal with it. Observation and awareness are the best ways to accomplish this goal.

Observation begins early in the call. As you approach the scene, turn off your lights and sirens to avoid broadcasting your arrival and attracting a crowd. Observe the neighbourhood as you look for house numbers. If possible, do not park directly in front of the call address. This provides two benefits. First, you may be able to approach the scene unnoticed, which allows you to assess it without distraction. Second, since many EMR units do not transport, the area directly in front of the call address is left open for the ambulance.

As you approach an emergency scene, look for the following signs of potential danger:

- *Violence.* Any indication that violence has taken place or may take place is significant. These signs include arguing, threats, or other violent behaviour. Also note any broken glass, overturned furniture, and the like.
- *Weapons of any kind.* If a weapon is on the scene, it is a serious potential danger.
- *Signs of intoxication or drug use.* When people are under the influence of alcohol or drugs, their behaviour is unpredictable. In addition, even though you see yourself as being there to help, other people may not. You may be mistaken for the police because you are in uniform and you drove up in a vehicle with lights and sirens.
- *Anything unusual.* Even an awkward silence should cause you to be wary. Emergencies are usually very active events. In situations where you observe an unusual silence, a certain amount of caution is advisable.

Note that nothing in this book is meant to create fear or unwarranted suspicion. Remember that the vast majority of EMS calls will go by uneventfully. Some calls, however, do pose a threat. Those calls usually provide subtle clues that may be picked up *before* the danger strikes. Use your observation skills on every call to determine important safety information.

Remember, the general rule is this: If you are trained to do so, make an unsafe scene safe. If not, **do not enter** and call for the appropriate teams to handle the situation.

React

If you find danger at the scene, there are three "Rs" of reacting: *retreat, radio,* and *re-evaluate.*

Retreat

With the exception of police who train with this book, it is not an EMR's responsibility to subdue violent persons or wrestle weapons away. A clear and justified course is to retreat from danger.

There are some ways to retreat that are safer than others. When leaving the scene of danger, remember the following points:

- *Flee far enough away that danger will not threaten you again.* Retreating only a short distance keeps you in danger. In addition, when fleeing a scene of danger, place two major obstacles between you and it. If a dangerous person moves in your direction and gets through one obstacle, the second obstacle acts as a buffer.
- *Take cover.* Cover and concealment are important considerations. Take cover by finding a position that hides your body and protects it from projectiles (for example, getting behind a brick wall). This is preferred over concealment, which only hides your body but offers no protection (for example, getting behind a shrub).

When fleeing danger, moving a considerable distance from the scene and taking cover are usually the best options.

- *Discard your equipment.* Do not get weighed down. The equipment you carry can be thrown at the threatening person's feet to give you additional time to retreat.

Radio

The portable radio is an important piece of safety equipment. Its main function is to call for police assistance and to warn other rescuers of impending danger. When using the radio, speak clearly and slowly. Advise the dispatcher of the exact nature and location of the problem. Specify how many people are involved and whether or not weapons were observed.

Remember that the information you have must be shared as soon as possible to prevent others from coming up against the same danger.

Re-evaluate

Do not re-enter the scene until it has been secured by the police. Even then, keep in mind that violence may begin again. Emergencies are situations packed with stress for families, victims, rescuers, and bystanders, so maintain a high level of observation throughout the call.

After the call, document the situation on your patient care report. Occasionally, the danger may cause delays in reaching the patient. Courts have held this as acceptable, provided that there has been a real and documented danger.

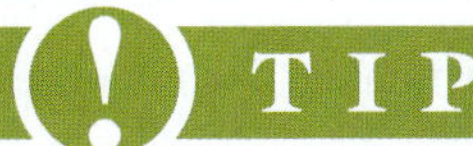

When taking cover behind a vehicle, use the vehicle's engine and front tires. These are more likely to stop a bullet, which can penetrate doors, windows, and vehicle compartments.

SECTION 2
MECHANISM OF INJURY AND NATURE OF ILLNESS

During scene assessment, you must determine the source and nature of the patient's problem. You may already have some idea from dispatch whether your patient is a **medical patient** (ill) or a **trauma patient** (injured). So, when you scan the scene for safety factors, also try to determine if the patient is ill or injured.

A medical patient's condition is caused by some internal factor, such as a heart or breathing problem. There is nothing at the scene that suggests injury. In this case, speak to the patient, family, or bystanders to determine why EMS was called and what the **nature of the illness** might be.

When you scan a trauma scene, note the **mechanism of injury** (how the injury occurred, including the forces that caused it). For example, if your patient fell from a ladder, it would be important to note how far the patient fell. The greater the distance, the more serious and extensive the injuries may be.

Occasionally, a patient may have a combination of illness and injury. Consider the patient who fell from a ladder, for instance. What if she or he passed out due to a medical problem and then fell to the

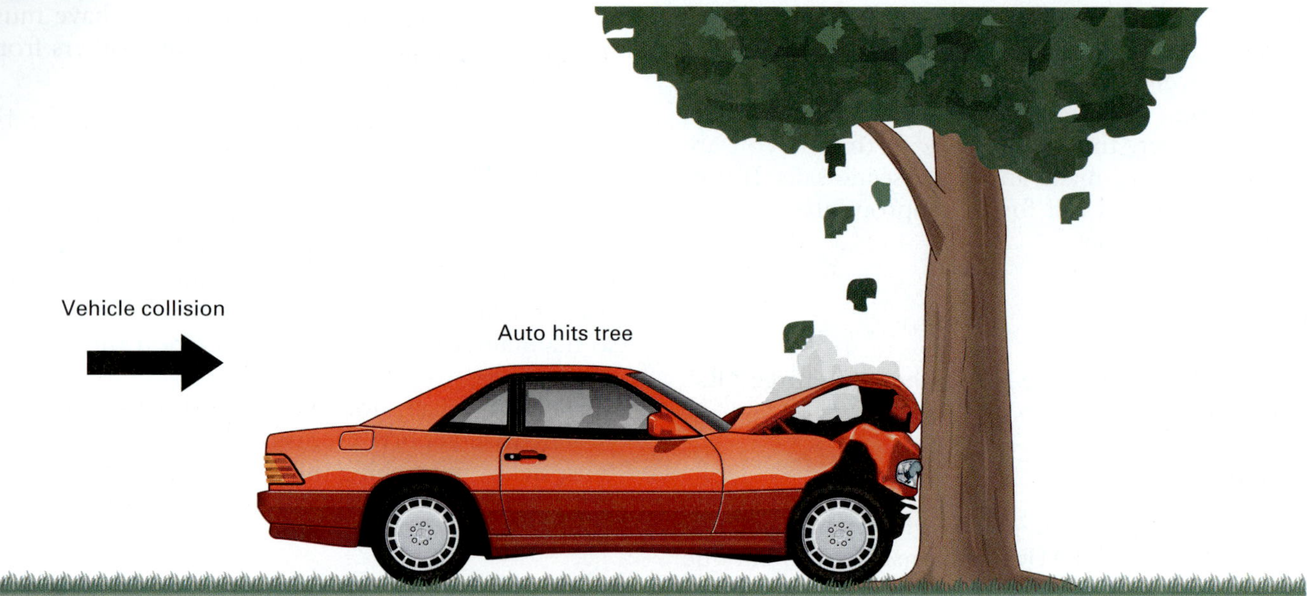

Figure 10–2a Impact 1—the vehicle strikes an object.

ground? As you approach the scene, the mechanism of injury may be obvious. The illness may not be. It will be your examination of the scene, as well as the eventual patient history, that will make a difference. (See Chapter 11 for instructions on how to gather a patient history.)

Kinematics of Trauma

Trauma is the leading cause of death among people between the ages of 14 and 40. It is also the third leading cause of death overall—behind only heart disease and cancer.

Emergency medical treatment of trauma depends on the extent of the injuries. However, it is not quite so simple. Too often, hidden injuries prove to be fatal. In order to understand how seriously a patient may be injured, you must determine the mechanism of injury. It will tell you what injuries or patterns of injury the patient may be suffering from.

The science of analyzing the mechanism of injury is called the **kinematics of trauma**. The process is based on physical laws; for example, that an object (mass) in motion contains energy, and that energy is influenced by the interaction of **velocity** (speed) and mass.

Kinetic energy is the total amount of energy contained by an object in motion. When the weight of that object is doubled, its energy is also doubled. In other words, a 2 kg rock causes twice as much damage as a 1 kg rock.

Velocity is the speed at which an object moves. According to physical laws, velocity is more important than weight in producing kinetic energy. The higher the speed of an object, the more energy it has. The rate at which an object changes speed (its acceleration and deceleration) is also significant. As you know, the faster a car travels, the longer it takes to stop.

The process of gaining and losing velocity occurs with each impact in a crash. The number of impacts varies, but there are three basic ones (Figure 10–2). First, the car impacts the object. Then, the occupant impacts the interior of the car. Finally, the occupant's organs impact the surfaces inside the body.

Each impact in a crash has the potential to cause harm. The amount of kinetic energy that is absorbed on impact, however, depends on how much energy

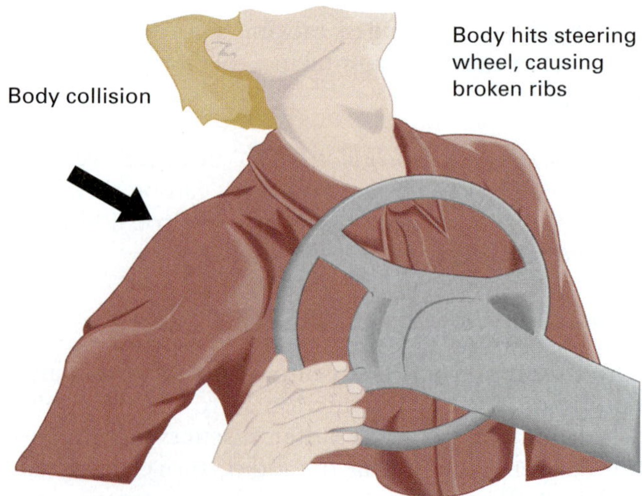

Figure 10–2b Impact 2—the occupant continues to move forward and collides with the steering wheel.

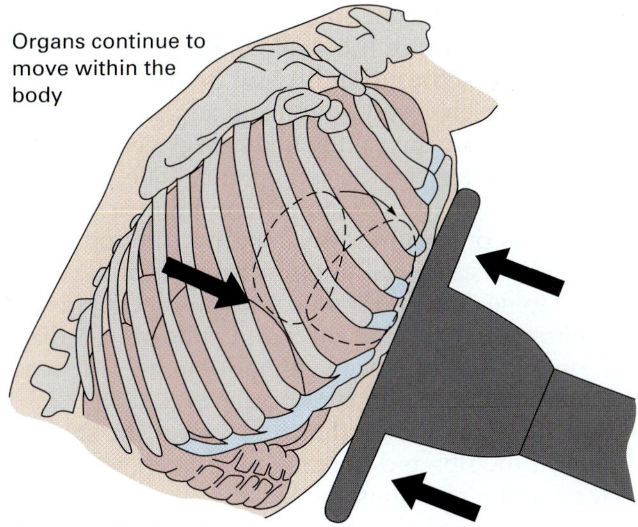

Figure 10–2c Impact 3—the internal organs continue to move forward and collide with other organs and the inside surface of the chest.

is absorbed by the surface that the body lands on or against. For example, a person who falls on freshly plowed soil will not be injured as severely as the person who falls the same distance onto cement pavement.

Remember that the mechanism of injury is an important part of your assessment of a trauma patient. It can suggest which body parts are injured and how severe the injuries might be. Whenever you care for a trauma patient, maintain a high **index of suspicion** and take note of the following:

- The body position at the time of impact
- The part of the body that first impacted a surface
- The surface the body landed on
- The object that penetrated the body
- The distance involved, if any

The common mechanisms of injury are vehicular crashes, falls, penetrating objects such as bullets and knives, and explosions.

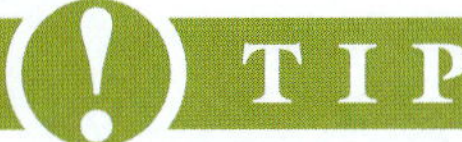

As you roll up to a motor vehicle accident (MVA) and before you even get out of your vehicle, there are some important observations you can make that can help you piece together and preserve the scene. Observe the posted speed limit and road conditions. Look for skid patterns or marks from the application of brakes.

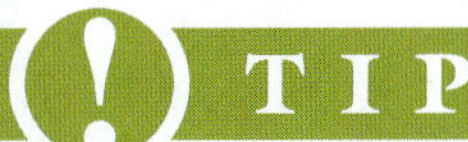

Try to avoid disturbing the skid marks, as police traffic analysts may need such evidence to recreate the scene. Picking up objects or debris can destroy evidence, since their distances from the point of impact can be used to determine prior velocity.

Motor Vehicle Accidents

There are five basic types of MVA: head-on impact, rear impact, side impact, rotational impact, and rollover. Each one has its own predictable pattern of injury.

Head-On Impact

A head-on impact occurs when a car hits an immovable object such as a tree (Figure 10–3). The greater the car's speed, the greater the energy and the greater

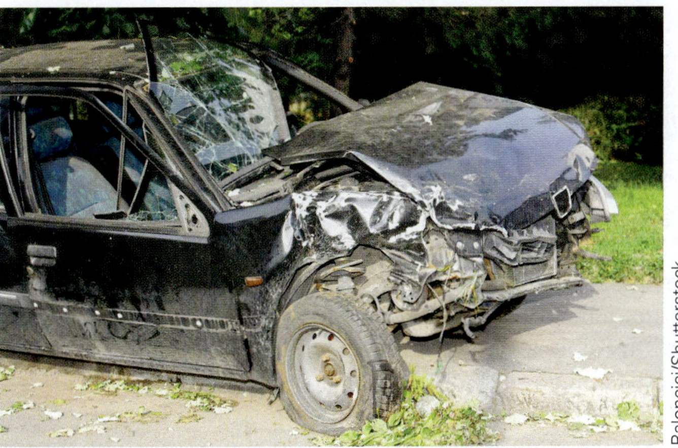

Baloncici/Shutterstock

Figure 10–3 Head-on impact.

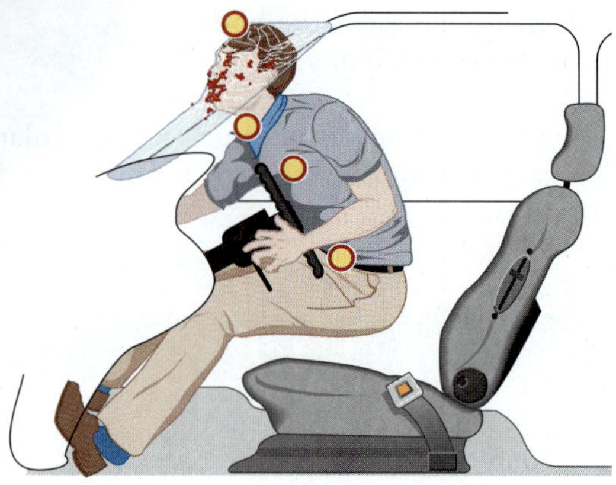

a.

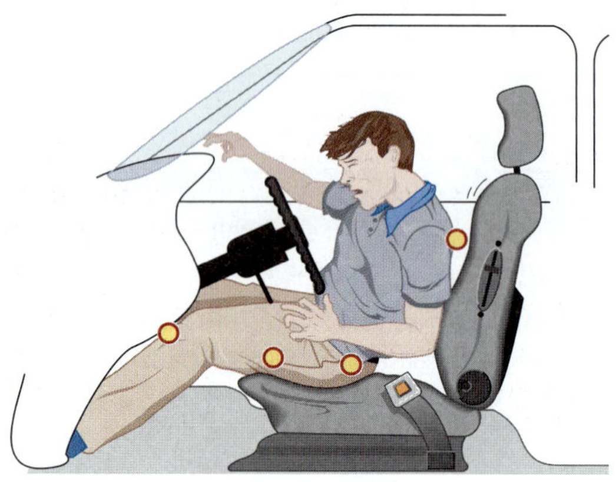

b.

Figure 10–4 In a head-on impact, the patient is forced either (a) up and over or (b) down and under.

the damage. When the car stops, its occupants continue to travel forward. They take one of two possible pathways of motion—up and over or down and under (Figure 10–4). Each pathway has a distinctive pattern of injury, which can be affected by the use of a seat belt.

In the up-and-over pathway of motion, the torso may be thrown over the steering wheel. The face, head, and neck then strike the windshield. The chest and abdomen may then strike the steering wheel. Note the following patterns of injury:

- *Face, head, and neck injuries.* Look for obvious clues, such as hair, tissue, or blood on the windshield or rear view mirror. The windshield also may bulge out in a classic bull's eye or spider web pattern.
  - The face can sustain extensive soft tissue damage. However, bleeding from its rich supply of blood vessels may not be as serious as it looks. Watch for airway problems if there is bleeding from the mouth, nose, or face.
  - Skull fracture may occur. Almost all head injuries have the potential to cause damage to the brain.

Brain tissue can compress, rebound against opposite sides of the skull, and bruise. Brain tissue can also be cut or bruised on the floor of the skull, which is very rough and jagged.
  - Energy can travel down the neck, causing the potential for cervical spine injury. The neck may be flexed or extended too far, resulting in whiplash injuries or fractures. An impact at the top of the head can cause compression fractures of the cervical spine. The anterior neck can also be injured by hitting the steering wheel or dashboard. Cartilage rings in the trachea (windpipe) can become separated and, thus, impair breathing.
- *Chest injuries.* When the chest strikes the steering wheel, the ribs and sternum may break, which can then injure the lungs and heart.
  - The heart may be compressed and bruised, making it unable to pump blood effectively. The aorta may be torn, resulting in life-threatening bleeding.
  - As the lungs are compressed, they can be bruised or ruptured.
- *Abdominal injuries.* When the abdomen strikes the steering wheel, the liver, spleen, and other organs are compressed. Sometimes they are cut.
  - The liver may be cut in half as it is forced against the ligament that holds it in place.
  - The spleen may be torn from its attachment, resulting in severe internal bleeding.

In the down-and-under pathway of motion, the body slides under the steering wheel. The knees strike the dashboard. Energy travels up the legs. The abdomen and then the chest strike the steering wheel. Classic injuries include dislocated hip and broken patella (kneecap), femur (thigh bone), and pelvis.

Rear Impact

Rear impact occurs when a car is struck from behind by another vehicle travelling at greater speed (Figure 10–5). The car that is hit accelerates suddenly, and the occupant's body is slammed backward and then forward (Figure 10–6). Suspect the same kinds of injuries as discussed for head-on collisions. If positioned properly, a headrest will prevent the head from whipping back. If the headrest is not in place, suspect soft tissue injury to the neck, compression of the cervical spine, and cervical spine fractures.

Side Impact

The side impact is often called a broadside or T-bone collision. The person closest to the impact absorbs more energy than the person on the opposite side. As the energy of the impact is absorbed, the body is

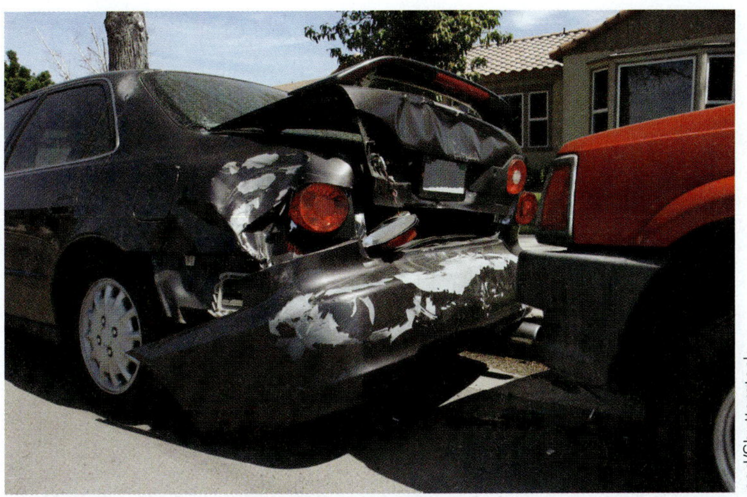

Figure 10–5 Rear impact.

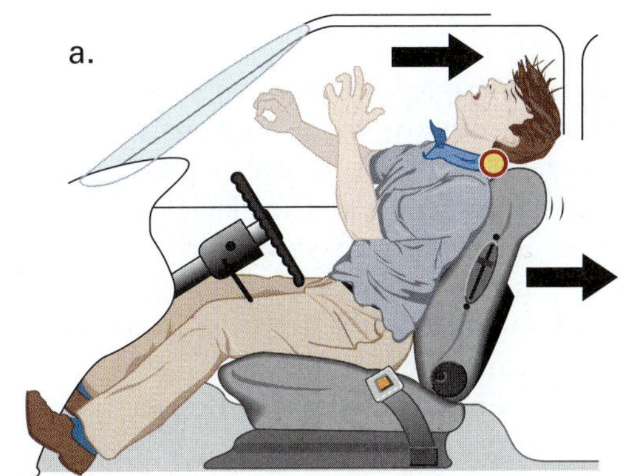

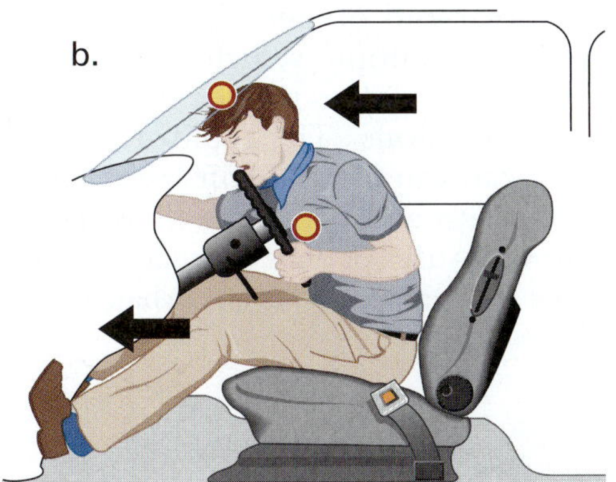

Figure 10–6 A rear impact forces the patient (a) backward and then (b) forward.

pushed sideways and the head moves in the opposite direction. The following injuries commonly occur:

- *Head and neck injuries.* The head often impacts the door post. This can result in skull injury, brain injury, and tears in neck muscles and ligaments. Cervical spine fractures are common, since the vertebrae are not designed for extreme lateral movement.

- *Chest injuries.* If the door slams against the shoulder, the clavicle will probably break. If the arm is caught between the door and the chest, or if the door impacts the chest directly, broken ribs and possible breathing problems may occur. Fractures low in the rib cage can injure the liver and spleen.
- *Pelvic injuries.* Lateral impact to the pelvis often causes fractures of the pelvis and femur.

The person on the opposite side of the car is subject to similar kinds of head and neck injuries.

In addition, if there is more than one person sitting on a seat, their heads often collide.

Rotational Impact

In a rotational impact, the car strikes an object and rotates around it until the car either loses speed or strikes another object. The sturdiest structures in the car (such as the steering wheel, dashboard, door posts, and windows) are the ones that cause the most serious injuries. A variety of injury patterns may occur due to the initial strike and subsequent striking of stationary objects. Look for the same kinds of injuries that occur with head-on and side impacts.

Rollover

During a rollover (Figure 10–7), occupants change direction every time the car does (Figure 10–8). Every fixture inside the car becomes potentially lethal. A specific pattern of injury is impossible to predict, but rollovers almost always cause injuries to more than one body system.

If the occupants are not wearing seat belts, they have a much greater chance of being ejected from the car, either partially or fully. Common injuries include severe soft tissue injuries, multiple broken bones, and

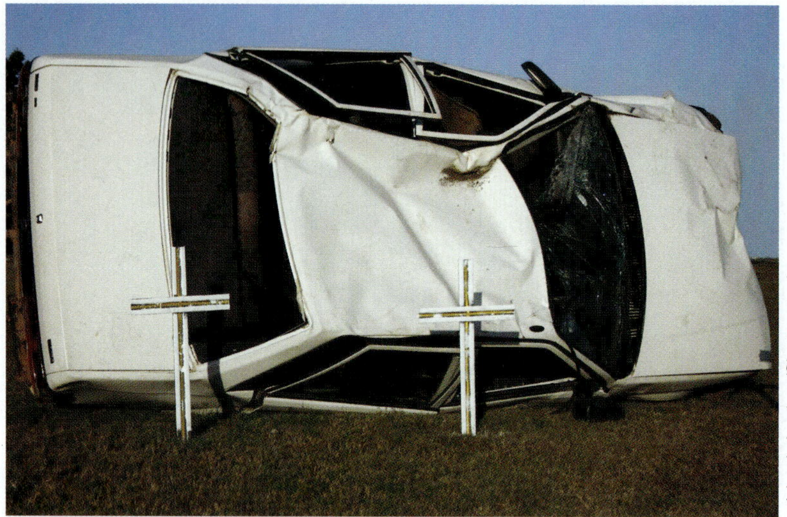

Figure 10–7 Rollover impact.

crushing injuries resulting from the car rolling over the occupant.

Restraints

Restraints help reduce the severity of injuries. However, the occupants of a car can still be injured, especially if restraints are not used properly.

- *Lap belt.* When worn properly, a lap belt can prevent the occupant from being thrown out of the car, but it does not prevent the head, neck, and chest from striking the steering wheel or dashboard. When the torso is thrown forward, compression fractures of the lower back can occur. If the belt is worn across the upper abdomen instead of over the pelvis, the spleen, liver, intestines, or pancreas can be injured. There may also be enough pressure in the abdomen to injure the diaphragm and force the abdominal contents into the chest cavity.

- *Lap and shoulder belt.* This type of restraint can prevent the occupant from striking the steering wheel or dashboard. A severe impact can cause the shoulder belt to break the clavicle. Even when properly used, a lap and shoulder belt does not prevent the head and neck from moving sideways or forward and back. If a headrest is not in place, suspect cervical spine injury.

- *Air bag.* An air bag cushions the occupant and absorbs energy in a head-on crash (some vehicles also contain side-impact air bags). Without a seat belt, however, an air bag is not effective in rollovers, rear-end or side collisions, or collisions involving multiple vehicles and repeated impacts. Air bags are often triggered during even lower speed collisions. The rapid deployment of an airbag can cause facial soft-tissue injuries around the mouth and nose, as well as the eyes, particularly when the patient is wearing glasses. The powder used in packing an airbag can also

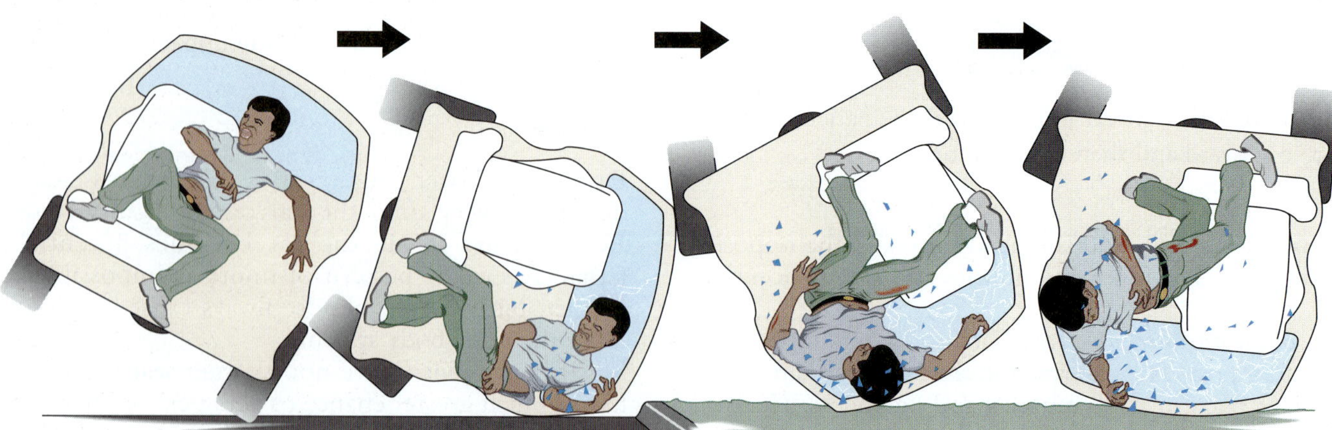

Figure 10–8 In a rollover, the occupant changes direction every time the car does.

be a skin irritant. Serious, even fatal, injuries have occurred in children in the front passenger seat when air bags deploy.

- *Car seat.* An infant car seat that faces backward in an upright position minimizes risk in a head-on collision. In a crash, all unrestrained parts of an infant's body continue to move forward. The greatest danger is to the neck. An infant's head is large for the body, and it tends to snap forward with great force. Suspect injury to the neck any time the mechanism of injury indicates it may be possible, even if the patient appears to be uninjured.

Motorcycle Crashes

Motorcycle crash injuries are greatly reduced when the rider wears a helmet. With no helmet, chances of severe head injury and death increase dramatically. There are three types of impact in motorcycle accidents: head-on, angular, and ejection. Laying the bike down, often an evasive action, can prevent serious injuries but can cause extensive scrapes, bruises, and burns.

Head-On Impact

In a head-on impact, the rider generally impacts the handlebars at the same speed the bike was travelling. A variety of injuries can be expected. For example, if the rider's feet get caught, the thighs or pelvis will strike the handlebars, resulting in fractures.

Angular Impact

In this type of impact, the rider strikes an object at an angle. The object then usually collapses on the rider. Common objects are signs, outside mirrors of cars, and fence posts. Severe amputations can result.

Ejection

If the rider clears the handlebars, ejection occurs. The body is thrown until it hits a stationary object or the ground. The body may hit several objects or strike the ground many times before stopping. Expect severe head and facial injuries if the rider is not wearing a helmet. Fractures and internal injuries are likely. If the rider is not wearing boots and leather clothing, expect severe soft tissue damage.

Laying the Bike Down

A rider who anticipates a crash may try to lay the bike down. This means that the rider may turn the motorcycle sideways and drag a leg on the ground to lose enough speed to get off. If successful, the rider slides along the ground, clearing the bike and the object it hits. Expect severe abrasions (scrapes) from contact with the ground. Many victims are also burned by contact with the motorcycle's hot exhaust pipe.

Recreational Vehicle Crashes

Injuries caused by recreational vehicle crashes are similar to those caused by motorcycles. However, since all-terrain vehicles (ATVs) are often used on fields and hilly terrain, patients can be harder to reach. One of the most dangerous ATV crashes occurs when a rider runs into an unseen wire fence. Cut neck vessels, severed windpipes, and even decapitations have resulted.

ATVs are prone to collision with other vehicles. Expect head, neck, and extremity injuries. The three-wheel ATV is especially unstable. A simple turn can cause a rollover, resulting in head and crush injuries. Unfortunately, many of those who ride ATVs are children. Their lesser body weight makes ATVs even more unstable.

Another type of recreational vehicle is the snowmobile. It is often driven at high speeds. When there is a crash, riders sustain severe head and neck injuries. Rollovers are also common.

Falls

The most common mechanism of injury is a fall. Falls account for more than half of all trauma-related accidents. The severity of injury depends on the following:

- The distance of the fall
- Anything that interrupts the fall
- The body part that first impacts a surface
- The surface on which the victim lands

Some experts say that the surface on which a victim lands is more important than the height of the fall. For example, diving into deep water from a high diving board is a recreational activity. Diving the same distance onto a concrete sidewalk is not.

Generally, a fall of two times a patient's height onto an unyielding surface is considered severe. You should have a high degree of suspicion about internal injuries, no matter how the patient looks.

Feet-First Falls

A feet-first landing causes energy to travel up the skeleton (Figure 10–9). If the knees are flexed when the person lands, injury to the bones will be less severe. Common injuries include fractures of the spine, hip

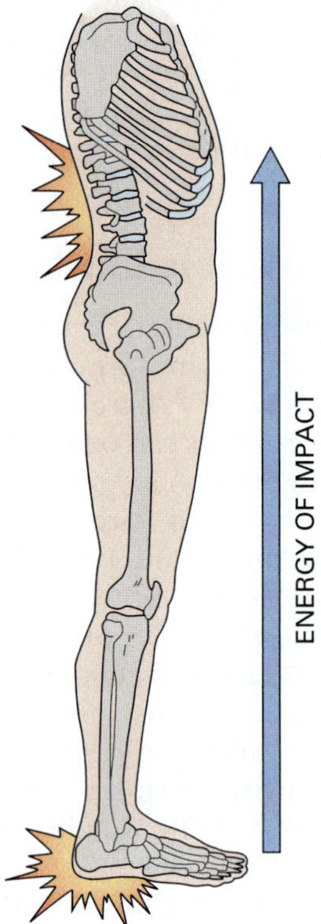

Figure 10–9 In feet-first falls, the energy of impact is transmitted up the skeleton.

socket, femur, heel, and ankle. Head, back, and pelvic injuries are common if the victim falls backward. If the victim extends his or her arms to break a forward fall, expect broken wrists. A broken shoulder and clavicle are also common.

In falls of 5 m or more, internal organs are likely to be severely injured from sudden deceleration. The liver may be sliced in two. The spleen or kidneys may be torn from their attachments. The heart may be torn from the aorta.

Head-First Falls

In head-first falls, the pattern of injury begins with the arms and extends up to the shoulders. Head and spinal injuries are very common. There is usually extensive damage to the neck. When the body is falling, the torso and legs are thrown either forward or backward, commonly causing chest, lower spine, and pelvic injuries.

Penetrating Trauma

This kind of injury occurs when an object penetrates the surface of the body. Hand-powered weapons, such as knives or arrows, generally cause low-velocity injuries. These are limited to the immediate site of impact. Projectiles powered by another source, such as bullets from a handgun, cause medium-velocity or high-velocity injuries. These affect tissues far from the site of impact.

When you encounter a scene of violence, it is absolutely essential that you make sure the scene is safe before you try to reach a patient. Follow local protocols.

Low-Velocity Injuries

Among the factors that help determine the severity of a low-velocity injury are the gender of the offender, the position of the victim when attacked, and the length of the object used to penetrate the body.

The gender of the offender can give you important clues. Women generally have less upper-body strength. They usually stab overhand or downward. Men have more upper-body strength, so they usually stab up and out. For example, if a standing victim was stabbed on the right side by a man, the most likely injuries would be to the liver, kidney, and intestines. If the victim was stabbed by a woman, the most likely injury would be to the lungs.

The length of the weapon also gives valuable clues. For example, a person stabbed in the chest with a 6 cm paring knife would probably suffer a pneumothorax (collapse of the lungs due to air in the chest). The same stab wound inflicted by a 20 cm knife could cut the pulmonary veins, the aorta, and the heart muscle itself.

Medium-Velocity and High-Velocity Injuries

In general, medium-velocity weapons include shotguns and handguns. High-velocity weapons include high-powered rifles. Knowing a weapon's velocity helps to determine how severe an injury might be. Other factors include the following:

- Trajectory—the path the bullet travels after it enters the body
- Drag—the factors that slow a bullet down
- Impact point—the bullet's point of entry into the body
- Whether or not the bullet fragments, or breaks apart
- The kind of pressure wave caused by the energy of the bullet as it travels through body tissue

The injury can also be complicated by clothing, gunpowder, bacteria, and any other foreign matter that is pulled into the wound. A soft-nose, high-velocity bullet is especially destructive. It can cause a wave of energy through the body 30 times the diameter of the bullet (Figure 10–10).

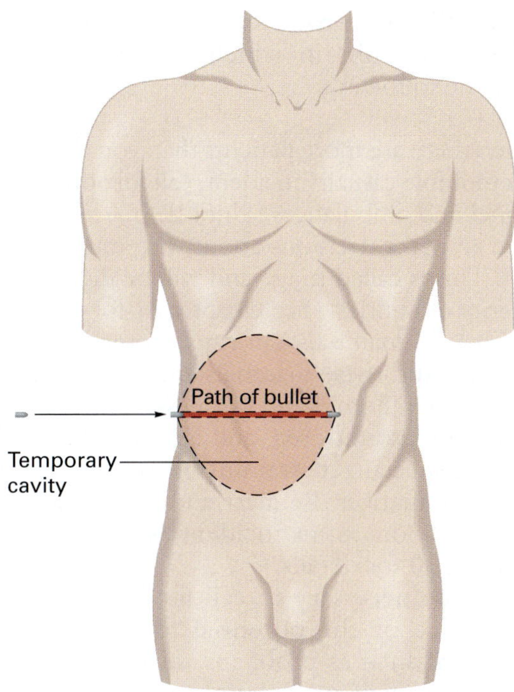

Figure 10–10 A gunshot wound can cause devastating damage, much more than a surface wound might indicate.

As you care for a gunshot victim, remember that tissue damage can be much more widespread than the surface wound indicates. A bullet wound that bleeds very little can be accompanied by a devastating internal injury.

If all the energy of a bullet is absorbed by the body, the bullet will remain there. If all the energy is not absorbed, the bullet will exit the body. You need to assess the victim carefully. Look for both entry and exit wounds. Note that an exit wound can be much larger than the entry wound.

Blast Injuries

The most common explosions involve natural gas, gasoline, fireworks, and grain elevators. Explosion injuries occur in three phases, and each type of injury has a typical pattern (Figure 10–11):

- *Primary.* The pressure wave of an explosion can injure gas-containing organs, such as the lungs, stomach, intestines, inner ears, and sinuses. The blood vessels and membranes of the organs can be ruptured. Death can occur without any obvious external injury. Common primary blast injuries

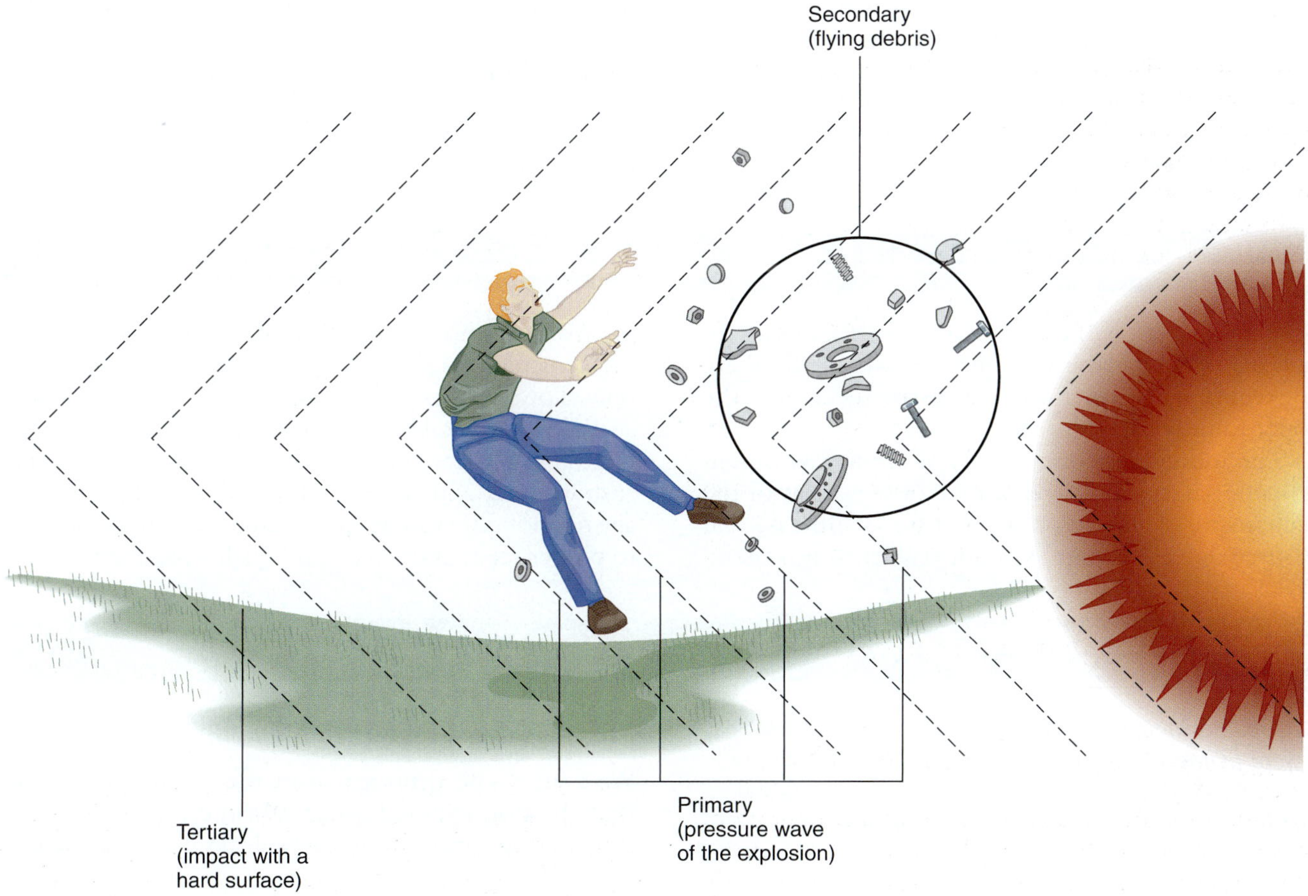

Figure 10–11 Phases of a blast injury.

include pneumothorax, pulmonary contusion (bruising of the lungs), and perforation of the stomach and intestines.

- *Secondary.* Injuries result from flying debris created by the force of the blast. Unlike primary blast injuries, these are obvious. They most commonly include open wounds, impaled objects, and broken bones.
- *Tertiary.* Injuries in this phase occur when the victim is thrown from the source of the explosion and impacts a surface. They are basically the same as those of a victim who is ejected from a car during a collision.

SECTION 3
RESOURCE DETERMINATION

Once you have ensured scene safety and determined the mechanism of injury or nature of the illness, you must make sure you have the appropriate resources. For example, if the scene involves hazardous materials, you need to call for a specialized HazMat team. If you have two or more patients, you may need to call for extra EMS personnel and ambulances.

If special teams or extra units will be required, call dispatch to request them. Do this before you begin patient care. Experience has shown that getting immersed in patient care can cause an EMR to forget to call for additional help. Call first. It will help prevent inefficiency and confusion later.

Never be too proud to ask for help when you need it! Situations in which you may need help include the following:

- When there are more patients than you can deal with in a multiple casualty incident, call for additional personnel and ambulances. Until help arrives, you will need to make decisions about who must be treated first. This is called triage and will be dictated by the severity of injuries. (See Chapter 31 for details.)
- Hazardous materials can cause complicated emergencies. And these materials are everywhere. They are stored in homes and businesses. They are transported by ground, sea, and air. HazMat incidents require specialized training in management and decontamination. Be alert and call for a HazMat team as soon as an incident is suspected. (See Chapter 30 for details.)
- It may be necessary to call for law enforcement if violence or the potential for violence exists. Situations such as problems with traffic, bystanders, and crowds or violations of the law will also require the police. Occasionally, weapons or illegal drugs may be found while you are assessing your patient. Notify the police immediately.

Other situations may require the fire service for firefighting or rescue, or the power company for dealing with downed wires. Confined space rescue, high- and low-angle rescues, and helicopter rescue or evacuation may also be needed. Call immediately for the resources you need. If later you find they are not needed, they may be cancelled. Time is of the essence.

EMR FOCUS

Scene assessment is the first step of every call you go on. This is one of the few rules for which there are no exceptions. Proper scene assessment creates the proper foundation for a call.

The individual components of scene assessment are scene safety, BSI precautions, observation of the mechanism of injury or the nature of illness, and resource determination. Do not rush through them.

You may notice experienced EMRs responding to each emergency calmly. A calm, observant approach not only allows you to perform optimal scene assessment, it also allows you to keep your wits about you. Some experienced EMS personnel who feel that they are starting to rush will stop and count to three. This brief pause, usually not noticed even by crew members, returns the focus to proper scene assessment and quality patient care.

CASE STUDY FOLLOW-UP

At the beginning of this chapter, you read that EMRs were at the scene of an auto crash. To see how the chapter skills apply to this emergency, read the following. It describes how the call was completed.

SCENE ASSESSMENT (*Continued*)

We kept a safe distance from the car. We could see that the pole seemed intact and there were no wires down. There were no gasoline leaks either. I saw that there was one patient in the car. He was conscious, so I told him not to move.

The patient had blood on his face. Looking at the mechanism of injury, I felt that he could be seriously injured. There was a lot of damage to the front of the car, including a large star in the windshield where the patient's head had hit. So I called the dispatcher to make sure the paramedics were on the way. We also called for an extrication truck.

We put on turnout gear and eye protection. Over our latex gloves, we put on heavy-duty gloves to protect ourselves from all the broken glass.

PRIMARY ASSESSMENT

The car was stable and safe, so I climbed into the back seat and held the patient's head and neck in a neutral in-line position. I asked him some quick questions and saw that he was alert.

The blood on the patient's face wasn't causing any airway problems. He was breathing deeply and at a good rate. This was a 30-year-old man who could be seriously injured due to the mechanism of injury.

My partner went to the window nearest the patient. She talked to him to calm him down. We saw no severe bleeding and his pulse was good. My partner placed him on oxygen and then updated the incoming units.

SECONDARY ASSESSMENT

The man had cuts and bruises to his forehead, which were oozing blood. He admitted that he had not been wearing a seat belt at the time of the crash. He complained of pain in his neck and chest. His neck was tender upon palpation. The left side of his chest was also tender, but there were no signs of broken ribs or open wounds. My partner listened to the patient's lungs. She said that air was moving in and out of both lungs. The man had no problems in his abdomen or hips. We could not get to his legs.

PATIENT HISTORY

We had not gotten far into the SAMPLE history (see Chapter 11) when extrication started. It was more important to get the patient out of the car. We could not hear or do much while the tools were in operation anyway.

ONGOING ASSESSMENT

We continued to monitor the patient's breathing and pulse during extrication. We also protected him from flying debris.

TRANSFER OF CARE

When the patient was extricated, the paramedics took over care. We told them what we had found so far: respiratory rate and pulse, the patient's complaints, our physical findings. We also told them that we had him on oxygen.

We stuck around and helped with the backboarding. Later we found out that the man got worse in the ambulance. He had a hemothorax, with blood accumulating around his left lung. Fortunately, the ambulance went to a trauma centre, where he was rushed into surgery. He was in the hospital for a while and recovered fully.

> As you can see, scene assessment is an important part of any call. It begins as you approach the scene, even before you see the patient. Scan for dangers, additional patients, and the mechanism of injury. Do not rush in. Determine right away whether or not you will need help and what kind. Then call for it.

NOCPs

1.6 b Practise effective problem solving **S**

2.3 d Recognize and react appropriately to non-verbal behaviours **A**

3.3 a Assess scene for safety **S**

    b Address potential occupational hazards **S**

4.2 f Obtain information regarding incident through accurate and complete scene assessment **S**

6.3 b Re-direct priorities based on assessment findings **S**

REVIEW QUESTIONS

Page references where answers may be found or supported are provided at the end of each question.

SECTION 1

1. What are the components of scene assessment? (pp. 148–149)

2. What are some signs of potential danger at an emergency scene? (pp. 148–149)

3. What is a general rule you can follow if you find a scene to be unsafe? (p. 149)

4. Which part of a vehicle provides the best cover from projectiles? (p. 149)

SECTION 2

5. What is the effect of mass (weight) and velocity (speed) on the severity of injuries? (p. 150)

6. What are the three impacts that may occur in a crash? (p. 150)

7. What trauma can be expected from the down-and-under and up-and-over pathways of injury in an MVA? (pp. 151–152)

8. What factors affect the seriousness of the injuries caused by a fall? (p. 155)

SECTION 3

9. What are some of the resources you should consider calling to a scene? (p. 158)

10. At what point should you call for extra resources at a scene? (p. 158)

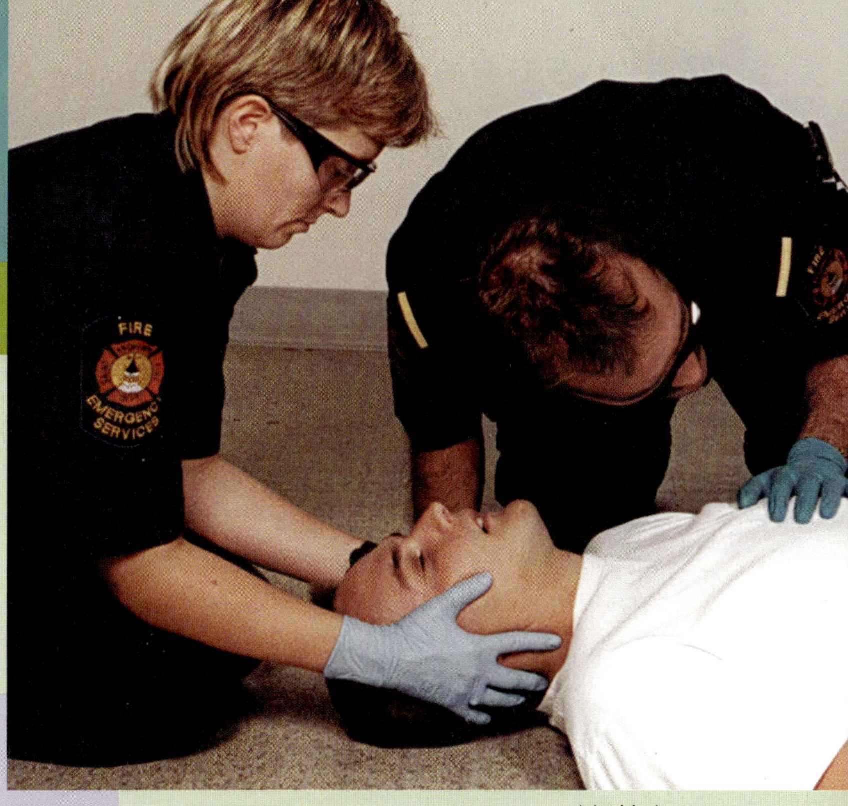

John Mackay

Patient Assessment

OBJECTIVES

1. Summarize the reasons for forming a general impression of the patient.
2. Describe methods and demonstrate techniques for the primary assessment, including level of consciousness, airway, breathing, and circulation.
3. Explain the reason for prioritizing a patient for care and transport.
4. Discuss the DOTS mnemonic involved in the secondary assessment.
5. Explain and demonstrate the assessment of the five vital signs.
6. Differentiate between a sign and a symptom.
7. Discuss the components of the SAMPLE history.
8. Discuss the four components of the ongoing assessment.
9. Explain the rationale for the feelings that the patient may be experiencing.
10. Describe the information included in the EMR hand-off report.
11. Demonstrate a caring attitude toward the patient and family during patient assessment while giving priority to the interests of the patient.

INTRODUCTION

EMRs must be able to assess a patient's condition quickly and accurately. This chapter will help you learn how. It presents a step-by-step routine used by many experienced emergency care providers. The routine includes scene assessment, primary assessment, secondary assessment, patient history, ongoing assessment, and patient hand-off (Figure 11–1).

As you already know from Chapter 10, scene assessment is always the first step. When the scene is safe to enter, the next step is to identify immediate threats to the patient's life. This is called primary assessment. You will perform a more thorough secondary assessment and get a patient history afterwards. The ongoing assessment follows. It is an organized way of monitoring the patient's condition while you wait for help. Finally, there's the patient hand-off. It is a summary of the patient's condition, which you report to the paramedics when they take over patient care.

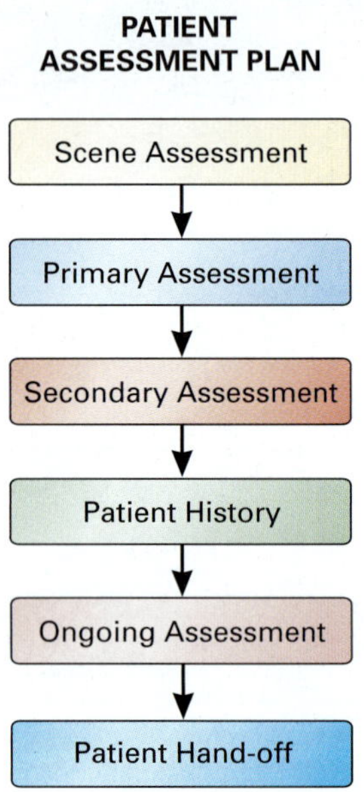

Figure 11–1 Patient assessment plan.

SECTION 1
PRIMARY ASSESSMENT

The **primary assessment** may be the most important part of the patient assessment process. During it you must identify and treat conditions that cause an immediate threat to the patient's life. Such threats usually involve breathing problems or severe bleeding.

The primary assessment includes getting a general impression of the patient, assessing consciousness, assessing the ABCs (including identification and control of external hemorrhage), and updating incoming EMS units about the patient's condition (Figure 11–2).

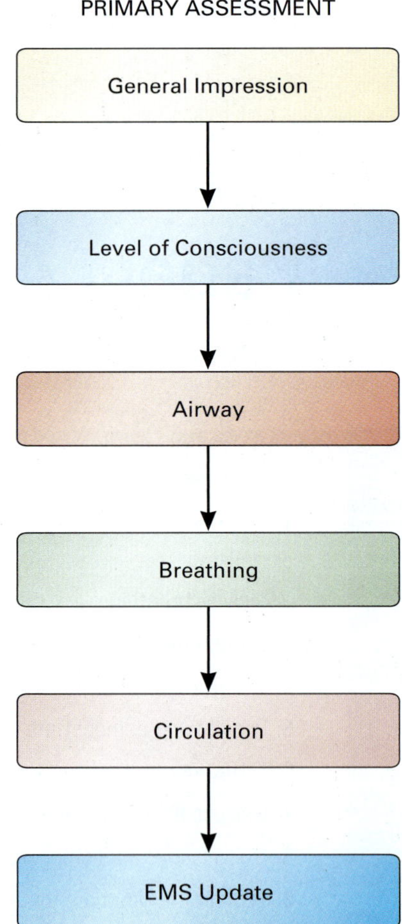

Figure 11–2 The primary assessment takes about a minute.

General Impression

Form a general impression as you approach the patient (Figure 11–3). It should include the patient's

CASE STUDY

Dispatch

My partner and I were dispatched to a call for an unconscious man at 46 Wilson Avenue. The dispatcher told us that the caller said she was unable to wake her husband up after a nap.

Scene Assessment

We approached the scene carefully, as we always do. This call was in a quiet section of town, but you never can tell. We realized that an unconscious person could mean anything from a drunk to a cardiac arrest, so we had all our protective equipment ready.

A woman, who was quite upset, met us at the door. She was about 60. We heard a dog in the yard, but the woman assured us that it couldn't get into the house. There was only one patient. The woman was sure her husband didn't fall or anything. We felt sure we had a medical problem on our hands.

Primary Assessment

We identified ourselves to the man but received no response. As my partner assessed the patient's level of consciousness, I took the pillows out from under his head and assessed his airway. I heard some gurgling, so I suctioned him out. This helped. His respirations were slow and shallow. My partner found a pulse, which was rapid. There was no external bleeding visible. Our general impression was of a male who was unconscious due to unknown causes and required ventilation assistance.

> Patient assessment is an important process for all levels of EMS practitioners. Here, the EMRs performed a scene assessment and a primary assessment. Consider this patient as you read Chapter 11. What else may be done to assess and care for the patient's condition?

chief complaint and a brief immediate assessment of the environment in which the emergency has taken place.

The chief complaint is the reason that EMS was called. It is generally the response to the question, "Can you tell me why you called EMS today?" Record the response on your forms in the patient's own words. "I fell down the stairs" or "My chest hurts" are examples of chief complaints. If the patient is unconscious, get information from the person who called EMS.

The general impression is not designed to be the final word on the patient's condition. Rather, it lets you get started on the right track with patient care. During this phase of the primary assessment, you determine if the situation is a trauma (injury) complaint or a medical (illness) complaint. Do so by listening to what the patient or bystanders tell you. Also, look around the scene to gain a quick impression of the forces involved in an injury.

If your general impression is that you are facing a patient with a potentially serious injury or illness, you may wish to ask EMS dispatch for advanced life support or additional units to assist. (You may have already done this during the scene assessment.)

To complete your general impression, you must also determine the patient's age and gender.

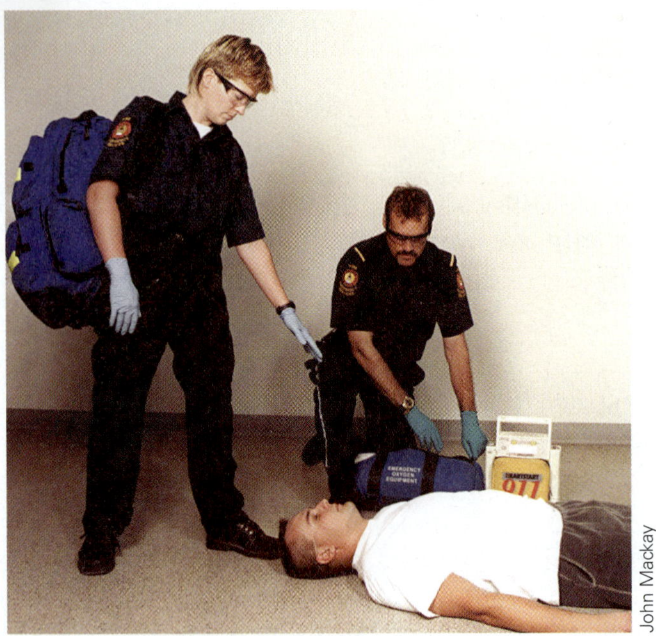

Figure 11–3 Form a general impression as you approach the patient.

Consider the following general impressions:

- A 12-year-old male patient, who was riding his bicycle, was struck by a dump truck. Your observation of the scene reveals that the boy's bicycle has been mangled by the truck. The boy appears to be unconscious.
- A 58-year-old woman is complaining of abdominal pain. She seems to be speaking normally, without any sign of strain. However, she is protecting her abdomen with one hand.
- A 26-year-old man is found unconscious on the floor of his bathroom. No one is quite sure what happened.

In the first case, the general impression leads you to believe the boy could be seriously injured. The second case appears to be a medical patient who is not in severe distress. The third case gives you little additional information on how to proceed. However, the mere fact that the man is unconscious can tell you that certain precautions must be taken.

Level of Consciousness

The next part of the primary assessment is determining the patient's **level of consciousness** (Figure 11–4). This is important for many reasons. One of the most important cases is the patient who has an **altered mental status** (a change in his or her normal mental state). That patient may need airway care as well as other lifesaving aids.

If the patient is confused, be sure to let him or her know who you are. Always make your identity clear as you approach a patient. State your name. Then explain that you are an EMR and you are there to help.

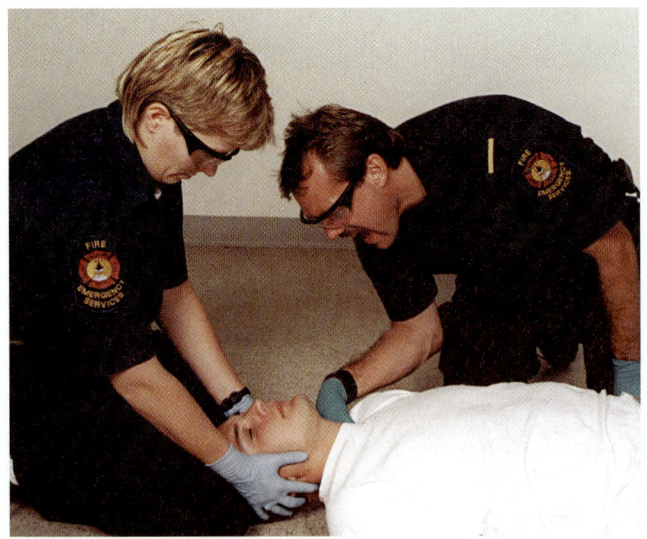

Figure 11–4 Assess the patient's level of consciousness.

If the mechanism of injury suggests a possible spinal or head injury, take **spinal precautions** at this time. This means holding the patient's head and neck stable, in a neutral position (Figure 11–5). If the spinal injury patient moves, further injury could occur.

To stabilize the patient's head and neck, place your hands on either side of the head. Then, spread your fingers apart. The objective is to prevent movement. If the patient is conscious, explain what you are doing so that she or he is not alarmed. Your hand position may reduce the patient's hearing. Be aware of the anxiety this may cause. (Spinal injuries are covered in depth in Chapter 25.)

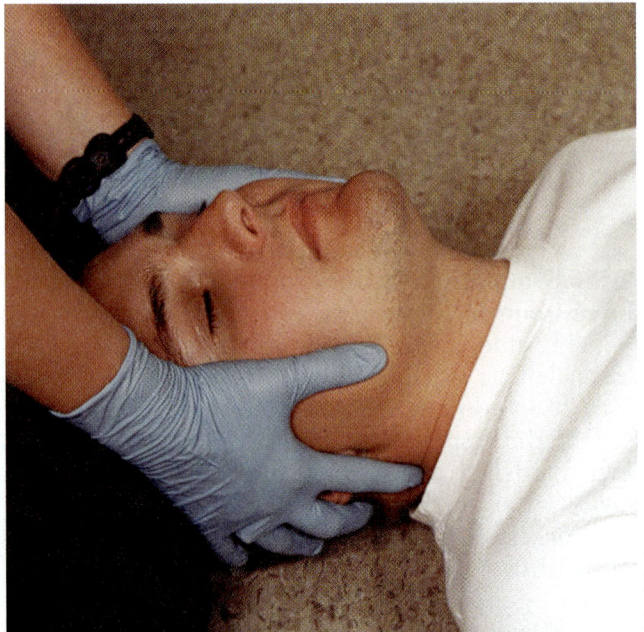

Figure 11–5 If there is a possibility of spinal or head injury, immediately stabilize the patient's head and neck.

Four levels of consciousness are commonly used to classify patients. The levels are *alert, verbal, painful,* and *unconscious.* Use the mnemonic **AVPU** to remember these terms. The classifications, when applied to patients, are as follows:

A — *Alert.* An alert patient is conscious and oriented. This means that the patient is aware of his or her surroundings, the approximate time and date, and his or her name. This is commonly referred to as being conscious to person, place, and date, or oriented 3. Each distinction is important. Some patients may appear wide awake but, in fact, are not aware of their surroundings. It is important to determine a patient's mental status because it can indicate injury or illness.

V — *Verbal.* This patient is disoriented but responds when spoken to. We say that the patient responds to verbal stimulus. A patient who answers questions about place and date incorrectly is another example. He or she may be suffering from a medical condition such as seizures or diabetes or from a traumatic condition such as shock.

P — *Painful.* The patient responds only to a painful stimulus and does not answer questions or open his or her eyes in response to verbal commands. He or she only stirs or flinches. The stimulus may be a pinch or a firm but careful rub on the sternum in the absence of chest injuries. (Remember to first check consciousness by observation. If the patient is alert or verbal, there is no need to apply a painful stimulus.)

U — *Unconscious.* This patient does not respond to any stimulus. He or she does not open his or her eyes, respond verbally, or even flinch when pain is applied. This patient is deeply unconscious, most likely in a critical condition and in definite need of airway and other supportive care.

> REMEMBER: If a patient is unconscious you should quickly observe if he or she is not breathing or has only agonal (gasping) respirations. If this is the case, you should skip a detailed airway and breathing assessment and go straight to a pulse check and begin CPR if necessary. If a pulse is present, continue with the following primary assessment.

Determining the level of consciousness in infants, children, and older adult patients is different from determining it in adults. In infants and young children, assess their response to the environment. They should recognize their parents, and they usually wish to go to them. Expect your assessment to cause crying. Children who do not recognize their parents or who are indifferent to your assessment and treatment may be very sick.

In older adults, there are common diseases and conditions, such as Alzheimer disease, that cause changes in consciousness. In cases such as these, try to find out from the family if there has been a change. In other words, if the patient is normally somewhat confused, has it become worse with this episode?

Some elderly patients live alone and have neither the means nor any reason to keep track of the date and current events. If an older patient does not know the date or another piece of information, try other questions to determine orientation. You might ask about the immediate surroundings, for example, or about what you are doing there.

Airway

The patient's airway status is the foundation of patient care. No patient can survive without an adequate airway. Therefore, make sure the patient's airway is open and clear (Figure 11–6). How you assess the patient's airway depends on whether or not the patient is conscious.

- *The conscious patient.* When a patient can respond to your questions, note if he or she can speak clearly. Gurgling or other sounds may indicate that something, such as teeth, blood, or other matter, is in the airway. Also, make sure that the patient can speak in full sentences.
- *The unconscious patient.* A patient who is unconscious needs aggressive airway maintenance. Immediately make sure the airway is open. If the

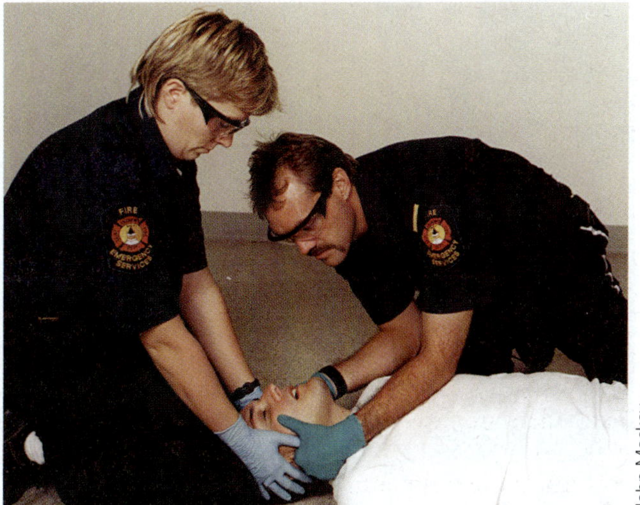

Figure 11–6 Open the patient's airway and make sure it is clear.

patient is ill, but with no sign of trauma, use the head-tilt/chin-lift manoeuvre to open the airway. If trauma is suspected, use the jaw-thrust manoeuvre, with great care to avoid tilting the head.

Inspect the airway for blood, vomit, or secretions. Also, look for loose teeth or other foreign matter that could cause an obstruction. Clear the airway using suction or a gloved finger.

Remember that the airway check is not a one-time event. Some patients with serious trauma or unconscious medical patients who are vomiting will need almost constant suctioning and airway maintenance.

Breathing

After securing an open airway, look, listen, and feel for breathing and signs of respiration (Figure 11–7). If there is breathing, determine if respirations are adequate. As you will recall from Chapter 7, breathing is not necessarily all or nothing. There will be times when a patient is breathing, but not at a sufficient depth or rate to sustain life.

Adequate breathing is characterized by three factors: adequate rise and fall of the chest, ease of breathing (breathing should appear effortless), and adequate respiratory rate.

Inadequate breathing may be identified by the following signs (Figure 11–8):

- Inadequate rise and fall of the chest
- Increased breathing effort
- Cyanosis (blue or grey colour to the skin, lips, or nail beds)

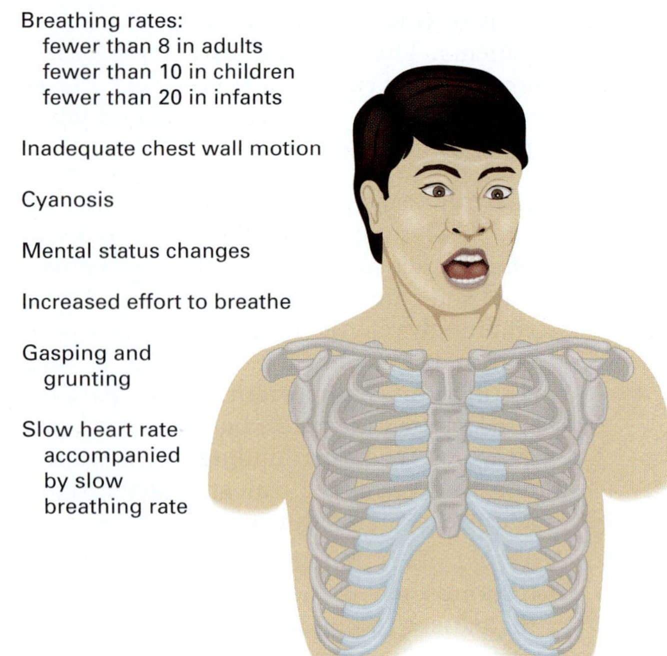

Figure 11–8 Signs of inadequate breathing.

- Mental status changes
- Inadequate respiratory rate (fewer than 20 breaths per minute in infants, fewer than 10 in children, and fewer than 8 in adults)

If the patient is breathing adequately, there may be no need to assist respiration in any way. However, during your assessment, you may determine that your patient would benefit from oxygen therapy. If you are

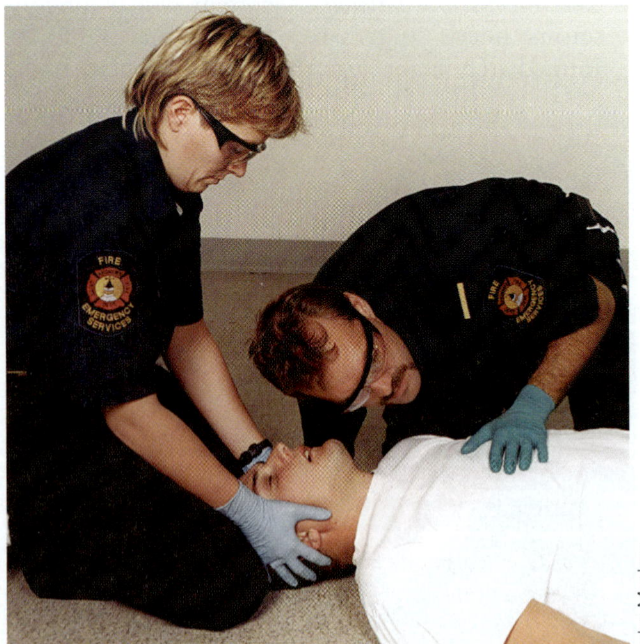

Figure 11–7 Look, listen, and feel for breathing and signs of respiration.

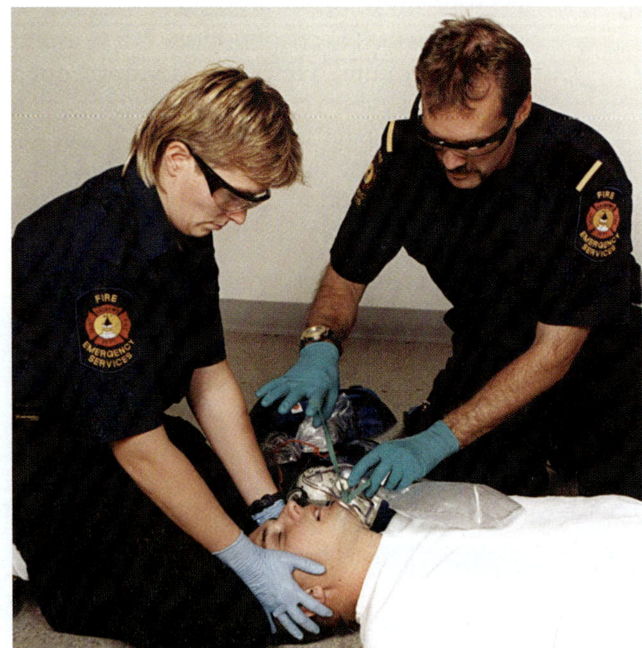

Figure 11–9 Apply oxygen if the patient needs it, and if you are permitted to do so.

trained and allowed to do so, administer oxygen to such patients (Figure 11–9).

If you determine that the patient's respirations are absent or inadequate, you must begin ventilating immediately. Do not stop until you are relieved by another trained rescuer or until the patient regains adequate respirations. In most cases, you will continue ventilating until the paramedics arrive.

Circulation

When you assess circulation, you are checking to ensure that the heart is pumping blood to all parts of the body. You must also make sure that the heart is pumping adequately and that there is no life-threatening external bleeding. To assess circulation, do the following (Figures 11–10 and 11–11):

- *The conscious patient.* If the patient is a verbally conscious adult, use the radial pulse to assess circulation.

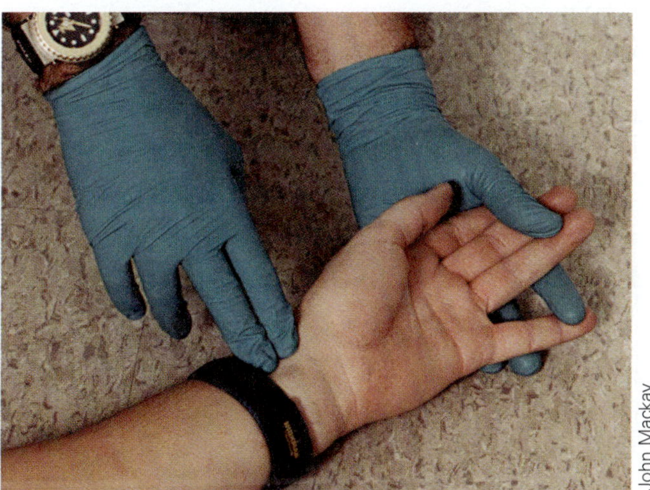

Figure 11–10a If the patient is conscious, assess the radial pulse.

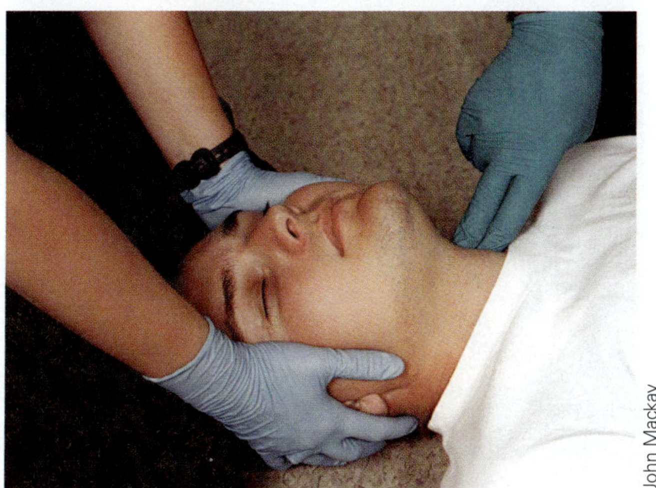

Figure 11–10b If the patient is unconscious or if there is no radial pulse, assess the carotid pulse.

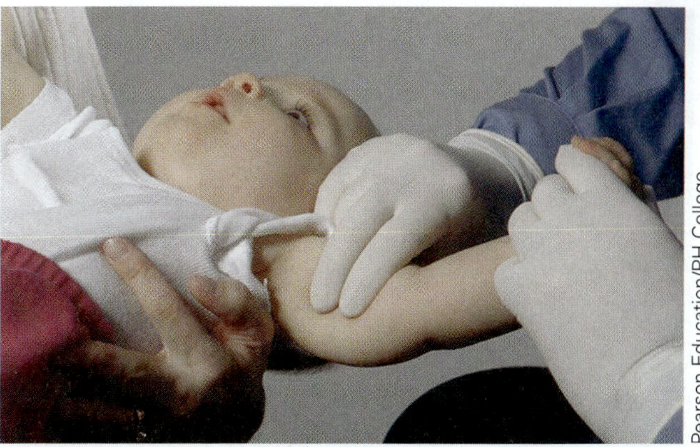

Figure 11-11a Assessing an infant's brachial pulse.

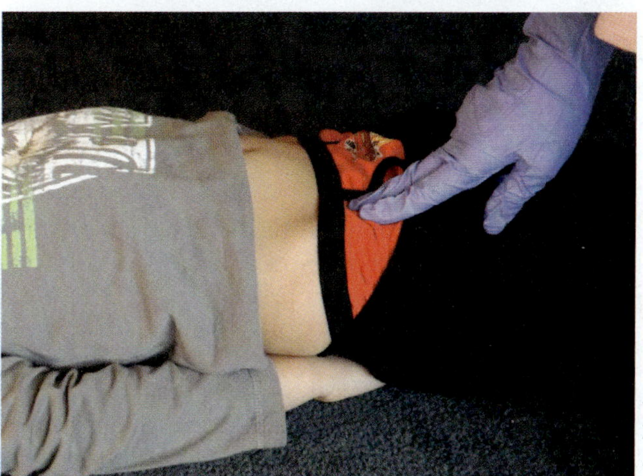

Figure 11–11b Assessing an unconscious child's femoral pulse.

Checking the carotid pulse may cause this patient undue anxiety. Always use the brachial pulse point in an infant. Use either the radial or brachial pulse point in the conscious child.

When checking the pulse, note the approximate rate and rhythm. If the pulse is very irregular or feels extremely slow or fast, be on the lookout for serious conditions.

Also, note the patient's skin at this time. Check the colour and temperature (Figure 11–12). Skin that is pale, cool, and moist may indicate shock.

- *The unconscious patient.* Check the pulse of an unconscious adult at the carotid artery. Check the pulse of unconscious children at the carotid or femoral artery. Remember, the pulse check for all infants is done at the brachial artery. If the pulse is absent, begin CPR.

After checking the patient's pulse, check for serious external bleeding (Figure 11–13). Remember that the primary assessment is designed to identify

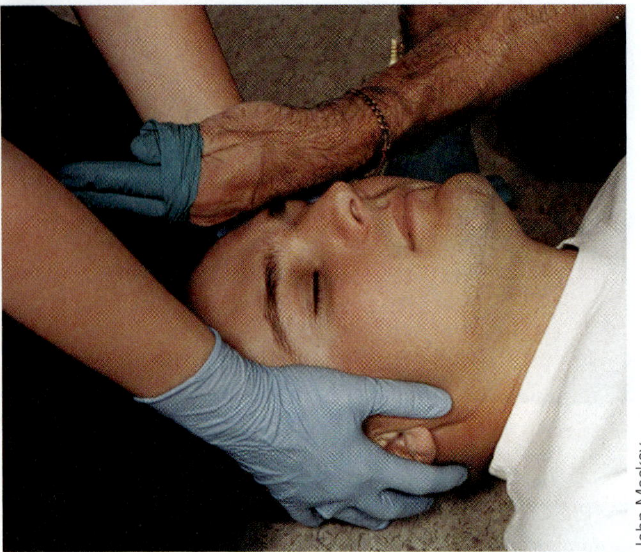

Figure 11–12 Assessing the patient's skin temperature.

and treat life-threatening problems. Be alert. Do not let minor wounds sidetrack you or keep you from caring for more serious injuries first.

Scan the patient for serious bleeding. Use your gloved hands to check areas that are hard to see, such as the small of the back and the buttocks. Remember that heavy clothes can absorb large quantities of blood. If serious bleeding is found, use the methods discussed in Chapter 19 to control the blood flow.

EMS Update

At this point, you will know if your patient is barely breathing and requires ventilation (a high priority) or if your patient is stable with a minor complaint. In either case, the EMS units currently en route to the scene will be interested in an update. The information you provide will allow them to prepare for the patient and provide more efficient care.

If you have a phone or radio available, report the following (Figure 11–14):

- Age and gender
- Chief complaint
- Level of consciousness
- Airway and breathing status
- Circulation status

Also, ask the incoming EMS units to give you their **estimated time of arrival (ETA)** so that you can continue patient care and prepare for their arrival.

The following is an example of a radio report. It might have been given by the EMRs in the Case Study that opened this chapter:

"Dispatcher, we have an approximately 60-year-old male who was found responsive only to painful stimulus. His airway required suctioning and we are assisting ventilations. The patient's pulse is rapid and weak."

After your report, the dispatcher will acknowledge your transmission and advise you of the ambulance's ETA.

> ## (!) TIP
>
> If patient transport is part of your job, life-threatening emergencies discovered in the primary assessment give you cause to load and go, unless ALS is present.

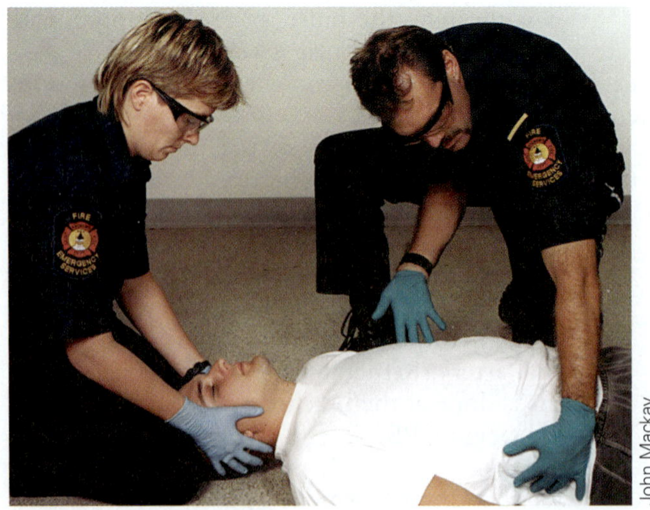

Figure 11–13 Assess for major bleeding.

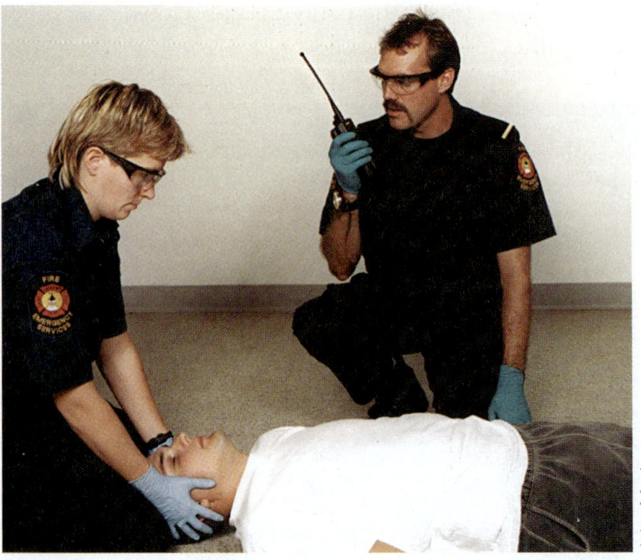

Figure 11–14 After the initial assessment, update incoming EMS units.

SECTION 2
SECONDARY ASSESSMENT

The primary assessment is designed to help you identify and treat life threats. However, not all problems will be life threatening. The EMR secondary assessment is a survey of the patient's entire body (Figure 11–15). It is meant to reveal any signs of illness or injury.

The secondary assessment is designed to be thorough. In some cases, you will have time to perform it. In others, you will have time for only a primary assessment before the paramedics arrive. When you have time and the patient does not need continued life-saving care, begin the secondary assessment.

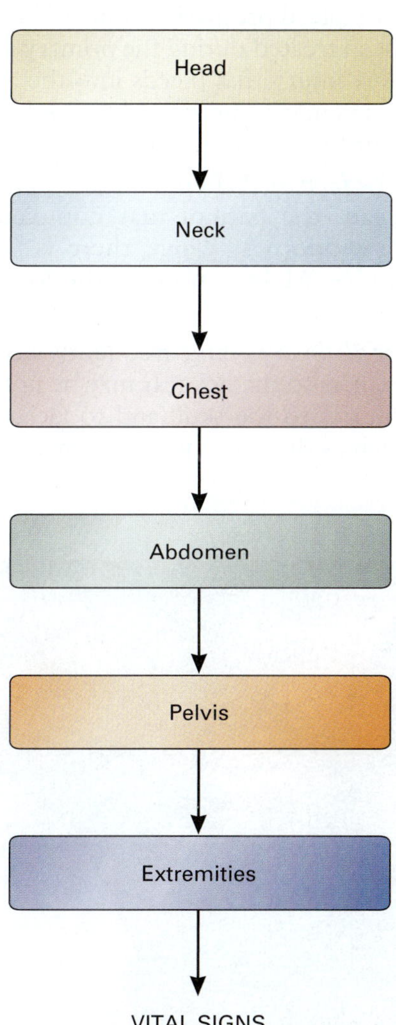

Figure 11–15 Components of the secondary assessment.

The secondary assessment proceeds in a logical order, usually from head to toe. It will be slightly different for each patient. If a patient falls a considerable height from a ladder, for instance, he or she could have injuries anywhere on the body. This patient would require a full assessment. In the case of an isolated cut to a finger, a complete hands-on examination would not be necessary.

Principles of Assessment

Patient assessment is a skill. Like other skills, the more you practise it, the better you will be. If you do not practise regularly, the result could be poor performance and missed injuries.

Methods of Examination

The patient assessment process involves the use of your senses. There are three methods you will use during your patient assessment: **inspection** (looking), **auscultation** (listening), and **palpation** (feeling).

- *Inspection.* The first method is the easiest. Simply make an overall observation of the patient. Then, observe the various parts of the body. What you see is very important throughout a call. As you approach a patient, even before you talk to him or her, you may observe that the patient is clutching a fist against his or her chest and appears to be uncomfortable. This could be your first indication of a heart problem.
- *Auscultation.* The most important listening you will do is for the sound of air entering and leaving the lungs. This sound will help you determine the status of the patient's breathing. If you are required by your EMS system to perform auscultation with a stethoscope, practise on your classmates. Become familiar with the sound of normal breathing.
- *Palpation.* Palpating, or feeling, with your fingertips is usually done last in the exam because it can cause pain. The actual pressure you apply depends on the area you are palpating and the type of problem you suspect. For example, if you observe a swollen lower leg, where the bone is normally near the surface, you would only need to palpate the area gently to determine if tenderness is present. Assessing the abdomen of an obese patient would require more pressure. Palpation will also identify areas where bones are rubbing together, abnormally rigid areas, skin temperature, and sweating.

Inspect, auscultate, and palpate each part of the body as applicable before you move on to the next area.

For example, observe whether the chest rises and falls with breathing. Then auscultate for adequacy of breathing and palpate for tenderness or other sensations. After examining the chest, you would move to the abdomen, where you would inspect, auscultate, and palpate as appropriate.

When conducting the exam, you will be looking for the following signs of injury:

- Deformities
- Open injuries
- Tenderness
- Swelling

Look at the first letters of each word listed above. The letters form the mnemonic **DOTS**. Use it to help you remember the signs you are looking for. Some signs will be obvious, such as a cut in the skin (open injury). Others, such as abdominal tenderness caused by internal injuries, will not be as obvious but are certainly serious.

As you proceed through the secondary assessment, be sure to listen to what your patient tells you. This may seem too obvious to even mention, but you could be distracted by other activities at a busy emergency scene. Listening shows that you care. It gives you important information necessary for the proper treatment of the patient. If you have to ask a patient to repeat something three or four times, the patient will stop answering your questions and believe that you do not care.

Finally, remember that your patient will be anxious or scared. It is important to reassure him or her throughout the call. When the paramedics arrive, be sure to introduce your patient to them and relay the special concerns or fears the patient may have discussed with you.

Medical vs. Trauma Patients

An examination of a trauma patient is different from an examination of a medical patient. It has been said that a trauma exam is 80 percent hands-on and 20 percent questioning, while a medical exam is 80 percent questioning and 20 percent hands-on. For example, once you have observed and examined an isolated injury, you do not need much more information. The physical signs of injury can be observed and palpated.

Compare that with the case of a patient who is having a heart problem. Chest pain is something you cannot observe or palpate. It can be felt only by the patient. In order to provide the appropriate emergency care, you must use questions to encourage the patient to describe the symptoms to you.

The Secondary Assessment

This section details the examination of specific areas of the body. Expose areas requiring detailed inspection and use the DOTS mnemonic to guide your assessment.

Examination of the Head

Assess all areas of the head, including the skull, face, and jaw (Figure 11–16). Also check the pupils for size. Note that injuries to the head may be serious. Bleeding can be severe. Many areas are covered by hair and can hide injuries. Use DOTS to guide you:

D — *Deformities.* Examine the skull, face bones, and jaw for signs of deformity (for example, depressions or indentations). Also look for deformities such as loose teeth, which can create airway problems.

O — *Open injuries.* Open injuries to the head may bleed profusely. As such, they may have been treated during the primary assessment. Any injury that bleeds into the airway is of particular concern. Also, look under the hair for injuries that may be hidden.

T — *Tenderness.* When you are palpating the head, the patient may complain of pain or tenderness where there is no obvious injury. Make a note of the locations that are tender.

S — *Swelling.* Swelling frequently accompanies injuries to the head. It may be noted around injuries to the skull and to facial structures such as the eyes, nose, and mouth.

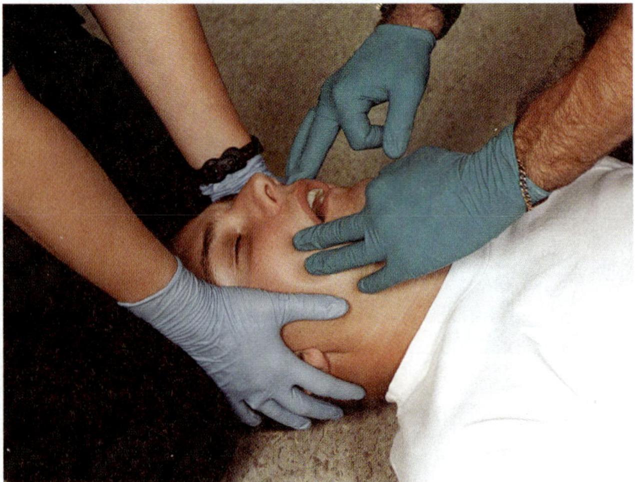

Figure 11–16 Assess all areas of the head.

Examination of the Neck

There are large blood vessels and major airway structures in the neck. Injuries can be quite serious. To examine the neck, also use DOTS as a guide (Figure 11–17):

D — *Deformities.* Look to see that the trachea is not deformed or shifted. Either condition can indicate a critical development, such as excessive pressure in the chest cavity. Palpate the vertebrae in the back of the neck.

O — *Open injuries.* Open injuries to the neck may result in serious blood loss. Bandage them immediately. Use an occlusive (airtight) dressing, which prevents air from entering the neck.

T — *Tenderness.* Palpate the soft tissues, trachea, and vertebrae for tenderness.

S — *Swelling.* Examine for swelling. The neck may accumulate blood. Also, air may escape from the trachea or other airway structure and cause a popping or crackling sound under the skin.

Whenever there is a possibility of spinal injury, maintain manual stabilization of the head and neck until the patient can be completely immobilized. If you are equipped, trained, and allowed to do so, apply a rigid cervical collar at this time (Figure 11–18). See Chapter 25 for a detailed discussion.

Examination of the Chest

Any injury to the chest may involve injury to the vital organs or to major blood vessels. Be sure to include the shoulders in this exam.

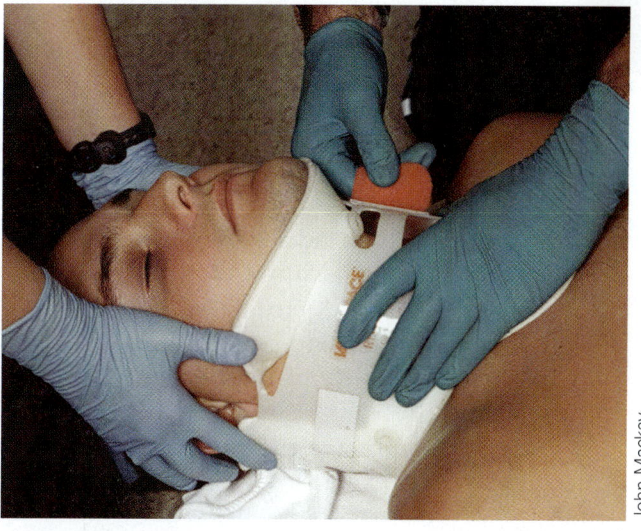

Figure 11–18 Apply a rigid cervical collar if the patient needs it and if you are permitted to do so.

If you are trained to do so, listen to the chest with a stethoscope. Determine if an adequate amount of air is entering the lungs. Compare both sides. The sounds you hear should be equal. Consider DOTS as you examine the chest:

D — *Deformities.* Feel the rib cage for signs of deformity (Figure 11–19). Remember that the ribs extend all the way back to the spine. Injuries to the back pose the same grave dangers as those to the front of the chest. Do not move the patient in order to examine the back until appropriate spinal precautions have been taken. Palpate the sternum. If the patient is conscious, ask him or her to take a deep breath. Determine if it causes pain.

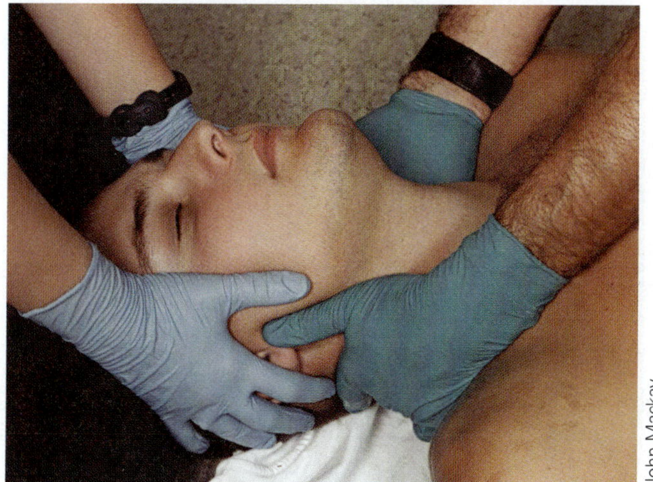

Figure 11–17 Examine both the front and back of the neck.

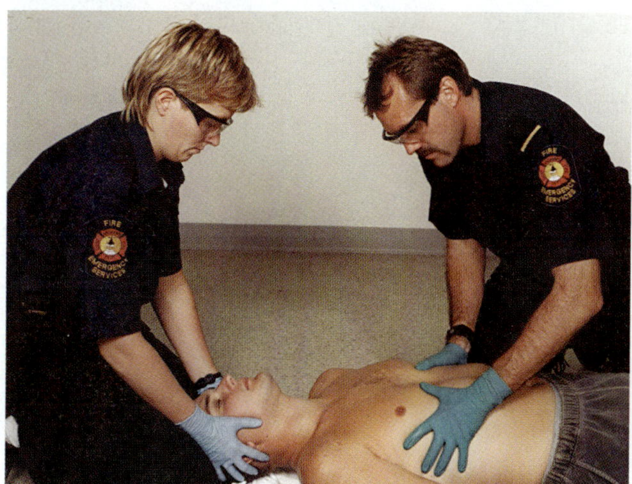

Figure 11–19 Examining the chest.

O — *Open injuries.* Open injuries are of particular concern when they occur in the chest. If a wound extends into the chest cavity, air may enter the area around the lungs and cause a serious condition called a sucking chest wound (which sometimes makes a sucking sound during respiration). Immediately bandage open wounds to the chest. Use an occlusive dressing.

T — *Tenderness.* While palpating the chest, ask the patient if there is any pain. Even when there is no obvious injury, internal injuries may be present.

S — *Swelling.* Observe the chest for swelling. If there is swelling or any other sign of possible injury, assess for underlying breathing problems.

Examination of the Abdomen

As you will recall from Chapter 4, there are many organs within the abdominal cavity that can be injured. (Though the spine lies to the rear of the abdomen, it is not palpated in this examination.) To examine the abdomen (Figure 11–20), again use the DOTS mnemonic:

D — *Deformities.* Deformity of the abdomen usually refers to rigidity (hardness) or distention.

O — *Open injuries.* Open injuries to the abdomen include cuts and scrapes (lacerations and abrasions), penetrating wounds (from a knife or gunshot), or protruding organs (eviscerations). These wounds are severe because of the potential for bleeding and infection.

T — *Tenderness.* Tenderness is an important symptom because it may indicate underlying injury. Recall the abdominal quadrants from Chapter 4. The quadrant where the patient complains of pain should be palpated last. If you examine this area first, you could cause severe pain, making the examination of the other quadrants impossible or inaccurate.

S — *Swelling.* Swelling or discoloration of the skin is another indication of abdominal injury. Check the flanks (the lateral sides of the hips and buttocks) for pooling of blood.

Examination of the Back

While it is important to check the patient's back, you must also realize that moving a patient could result in making a neck or spinal injury worse. If there are enough rescuers present who are trained in moving or rolling the patient, you may wish to check the back.

If you suspect a spinal injury and a long backboard is available, you may wish to move it under the patient while the patient is being rolled. But do so only if you are trained in its use and have enough help to do so safely.

Check the patient's back according to DOTS (Figure 11–21):

D — *Deformities.* Check for chest wall deformity, which may indicate broken ribs. Look for obvious deformity along the length of the spine.

O — *Open injuries.* Injuries to the posterior chest can cause the same serious conditions that occur on the anterior chest. Observe for scrapes, cuts, and other open injuries. Look for both entry and exit gunshot wounds.

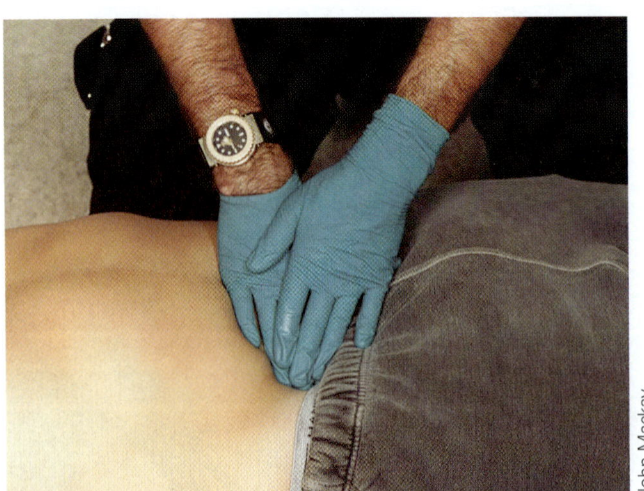

Figure 11–20 Palpate each quadrant of the abdomen.

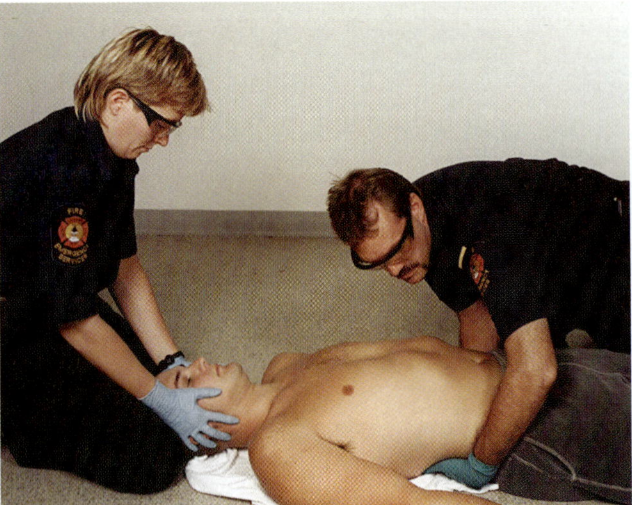

Figure 11–21 Examine the patient's back, keeping the head and neck in alignment at all times.

T — *Tenderness.* Tenderness may indicate a broken rib or an abdominal injury. Tenderness along the spine may indicate serious injury to the spinal cord.

S — *Swelling.* Look for blood accumulation in the flanks, which could indicate bleeding in the abdomen. Swelling anywhere indicates some type of injury.

Examination of the Pelvis

The pelvis is a large, bony structure. As you may recall, it is composed of left and right ileum, ischium, and the pubic bone. Palpate each of these areas for injury. The pelvis may be fractured, which could result in blood loss of 2 L or more. This amount of blood loss is life-threatening. Be sure to identify any possibility of pelvic injury during the assessment process:

D — *Deformities.* Unlike the bones of the arms and legs, deformities of the pelvis are not always obvious. Palpate the bones to feel for deformity (Figure 11–22).

O — *Open injuries.* There may be open injuries to the pelvis, although this is not as common as in other areas of the body.

T — *Tenderness.* Assess for tenderness. Palpate with less force if the bones of the pelvis are close to the skin. Palpate with more force if the patient is obese, with bones under a considerable amount of tissue. Though

you may feel awkward assessing the pubic (groin) bone, be sure to check it.

S — *Swelling.* Look for swelling and discoloration around the hips.

Examination of the Extremities

The extremities are common sites of injury. Do not rush your examination. Be sure to inspect and palpate each one (Figure 11–23):

D — *Deformities.* Because the bones are close to the surface, deformities may be seen easily in the extremities. Check the entire length of each bone and all joints for deformity.

O — *Open injuries.* Look for open injuries, which are quite common in the extremities.

T — *Tenderness.* Just as in other areas of the body, there may be underlying injury without obvious deformity. So, palpate each extremity for tenderness.

S — *Swelling.* Since injuries to the extremities are often close to the skin, swelling and discoloration may be evident. Any extremity that is painful, swollen, or deformed may be broken and should be manually stabilized until it can be splinted.

The extremities may also be checked by feeling for a pulse (Figure 11–24). The radial pulse in each wrist will tell you if circulation in the entire arm is adequate. There are two pulses in the feet, either of which may be palpated to see if circulation is adequate in the lower extremities. They are the **dorsalis pedis pulse** and the **posterior tibial pulse**.

The ability to move an extremity, such as wiggling fingers or toes, is also an important sign

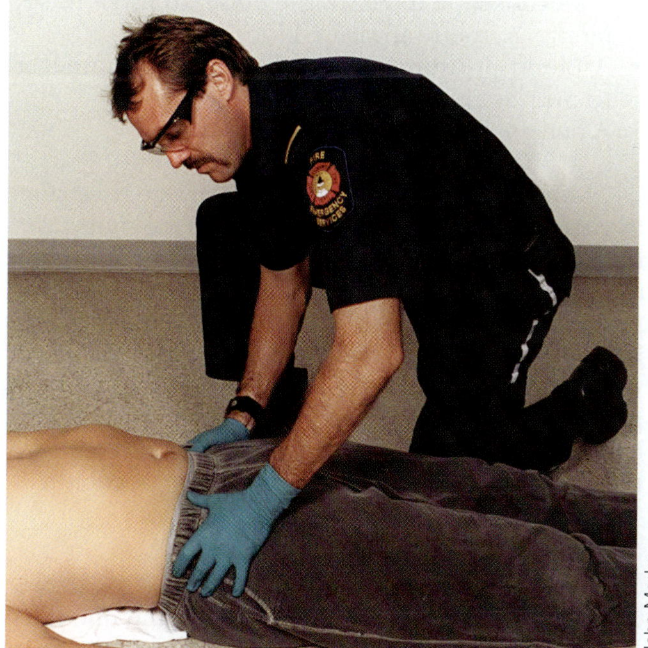

Figure 11–22 Examine the pelvis by applying gentle pressure.

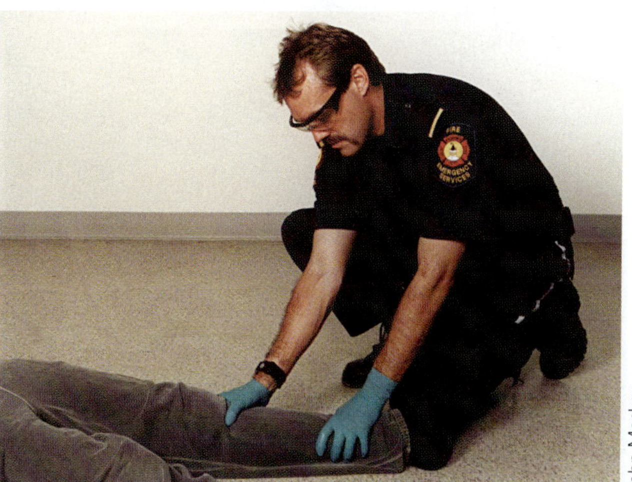

Figure 11–23 Visually inspect and palpate each extremity.

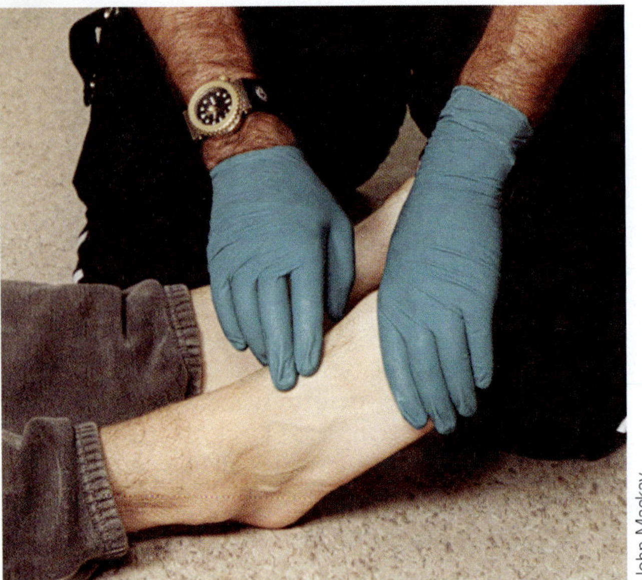

Figure 11–24 Check the pulse in each extremity.

(Figure 11–25). Movement means that impulses from the nervous system can reach these points. If there is no movement, there may be a problem with a nerve. No ability to move one side of the body, or below a certain point, could indicate problems in the central nervous system.

For the same reason, check to see that the patient has sensation in the limbs. Gently squeeze one extremity and then the other. As you do so, ask questions such as "Can you feel me touching your fingers?" or "Where am I touching you now?"

Vital Signs

Vital signs include the patient's respiration, pulse, skin, pupils, and blood pressure (Figure 11–26). You

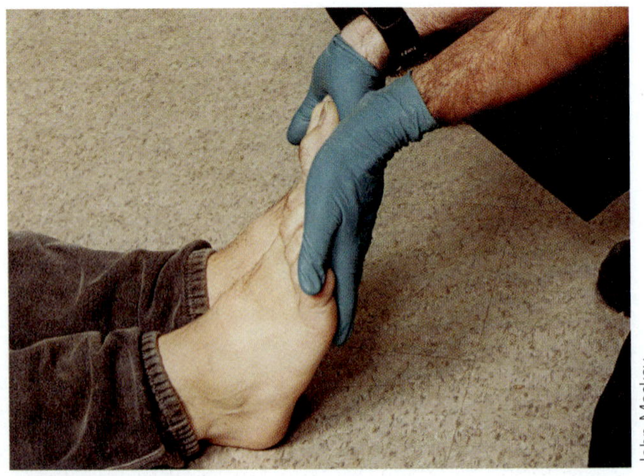

Figure 11–25 Check for sensation and the ability to move fingers and toes.

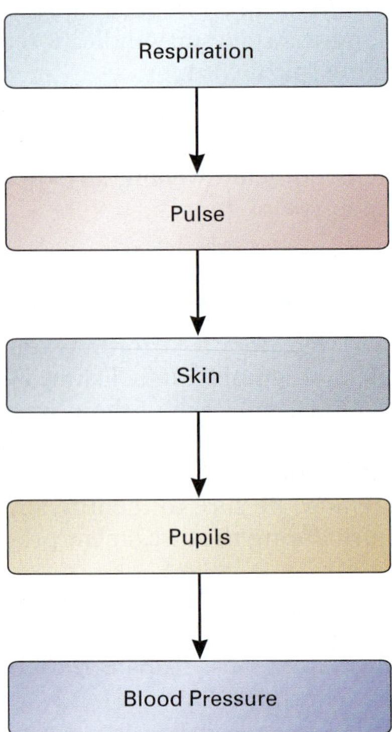

Figure 11–26 Vital signs.

can assess and monitor most vital signs by inspection, auscultation, and palpation. However, it is best if you have proper equipment, such as the following:

- A wristwatch to count seconds
- A penlight to examine the pupils
- A **stethoscope** to check the pulse, to listen to respirations, and to measure blood pressure
- A blood pressure cuff, or **sphygmomanometer**, to measure blood pressure
- A pen and notebook to take notes

More important than any one vital sign is a change in vital signs over time. The baseline vital signs taken by an EMR are particularly important because they are taken early in the call. Paramedics and hospital personnel will refer to them to see if the patient has improved or deteriorated over time. For example, if you check the pulse and obtain a reading of 90 beats per minute, and later the pulse rises to 120, a serious condition may be developing. Without your early readings, this observation would not be possible.

Respiration

A respiration consists of one inhalation and one exhalation. The normal number of respirations per minute varies with gender and age. In an adult, that number is between 12 and 20 per minute (Table 11–1).

TABLE 11–1
NORMAL RESPIRATORY RATES

Patient	Respiratory Rate*
Infant	Up to 60
Child	20–40
Adult	12–20

*Approximate rate per minute at rest.

Count your patient's respirations by doing the following (Figure 11–27):

1. Place your hand on the patient's chest or abdomen.
2. Count the number of times the chest (or abdomen) rises during a 30-second period. Then multiply that number by two.

The depth of respiration gives a clue to the amount of air that is inhaled. You can gauge depth by placing your hand on the patient's chest and feeling for chest movement. Feel the abdomen to see if it is moving instead of the chest.

Normally, the work required to breathe is minimal. Some effort is required to inhale, but almost none is required to exhale. For this reason, normal inspiration takes slightly longer than normal exhalation. When exhaling is prolonged, the patient may have a chronic obstructive pulmonary disorder such as emphysema.

Common signs and symptoms of respiratory distress include the following:

- Gasping for air
- Breathing that is unusually fast, slow, deep, or shallow
- Wheezing, gurgling, high-pitched shrill sounds, or other unusual noises

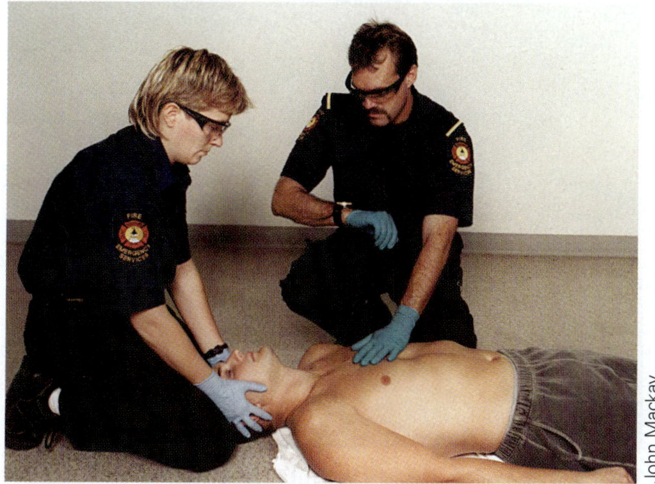

Figure 11–27 Assessing respirations.

- Unusually moist, flushed skin that may appear pale or turn bluish as the oxygen level in the blood falls
- Difficulty speaking (able to say only a few words without catching his or her breath)
- Dizziness, anxiety
- Chest pain and tingling in the hands and feet

Abnormal breathing conditions you should know about include the following:

- Shortness of breath or breathing difficulty
- Abnormally slow breathing
- Abnormally deep, rapid breathing

If the patient is aware that you are assessing his or her respirations, he or she may not breathe naturally. This can give a false reading. To get around this, check the pulse with the patient's arm draped over his or her chest or abdomen. Count the pulse for 15 seconds. Then, without moving the patient's arm, count respirations for the next 30 seconds. Readings are easily obtained by observing and feeling the chest rise and fall with your hand that is already on the patient's torso.

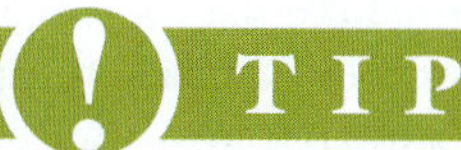

There is no "about" in vitals signs measurement. All vital signs must be accurate, and they should be taken at regular intervals. If you are uncertain of a reading, take it again. In most cases, you will observe pulse and respirations for 30 seconds and multiply by two. You will never get an odd number when multiplying by two. Practise both the technique and the math of vital signs assessment.

Pulse

Each time the heart beats, the arteries expand and contract with the blood flow. The pulse is the pressure wave generated by the heartbeat. It directly reflects the rate, relative strength, and rhythm of the contractions of the heart. Normal pulse rates are listed in Table 11–2.

When you check the pulse, note the following:

- Is the pulse rate slow or fast?
- What is the strength of the pulse? A normal pulse is full and strong. A thready pulse is weak and rapid. A bounding pulse is unusually strong.
- What is the rhythm of the pulse? A normal pulse has regular spaces between beats. An irregular one is spaced irregularly. You can describe the pulse of a patient, for instance, as "72, strong, and regular." The rate, strength, and regularity of a pulse tell what the heart is doing at any given time.

TABLE 11–2
NORMAL PULSE RATES

Patient	Pulse Rate*
Infant	120–150
Child	80–150
Adult	60–80

*Approximate rate per minute at rest.

The pulse can be felt at any point where an artery crosses over a bone or lies near the skin. EMRs often check the pulse at the wrist. This is where the radial artery crosses over the end of the forearm bone, or the radius.

To assess the radial pulse (Figure 11–28), carry out the following steps:

1. Have the patient lie or sit down.
2. Gently touch the pulse point with the tips of two or three fingers. (Avoid using your thumb. It has a prominent pulse of its own, which can be counted by mistake.)
3. Count the number of beats you feel in 15 seconds. Then, multiply that number by four. This will give you the number of beats per minute. If a pulse is irregular, slow, or difficult to obtain, count the beats for 30 seconds and multiply by two for a more accurate reading.
4. Write down the pulse and any other vital signs immediately. Never rely on your memory.

Other points where a pulse may be taken include the brachial artery in the upper arm, the carotid artery in the neck, the femoral artery in the groin, the dorsalis pedis on the top of the foot, the posterior tibial artery on the medial surface of the ankle, and the **apical pulse** under the patient's left breast (requires a stethoscope).

Checking pulses in several areas will help to determine how well the patient's entire circulatory system is working. The absence of a pulse in a single extremity may indicate a blocked artery. If this condition is left untreated, numbness, weakness, and tingling follow pain. The skin also gradually turns mottled, blue, and cold.

The Skin

Assessment of the skin temperature, colour, and condition can tell you more about the patient's circulatory system.

Skin Temperature. The normal body temperature is 37°C. Although **tympanic thermometers**, which take a temperature reading in the ear canal (Figure 11–29), have become popular, the most common way EMRs take temperature is by touching a patient's skin with the back of the hand. This is called **relative skin temperature**. It does not measure exact temperature, but you can tell if it is very high or very low.

Changes in skin temperature can alert you to certain injuries and illnesses. A patient whose skin temperature is cool, for example, may be suffering from shock, heat exhaustion, or exposure to cold. A high temperature may be the result of fever or heat stroke. Body temperature can also change over a period of time, and it can be different in various parts of the body. For example, circulatory problems may be indicated by a cold arm or leg. An isolated hot area could indicate a localized infection. Be alert to changes and record them.

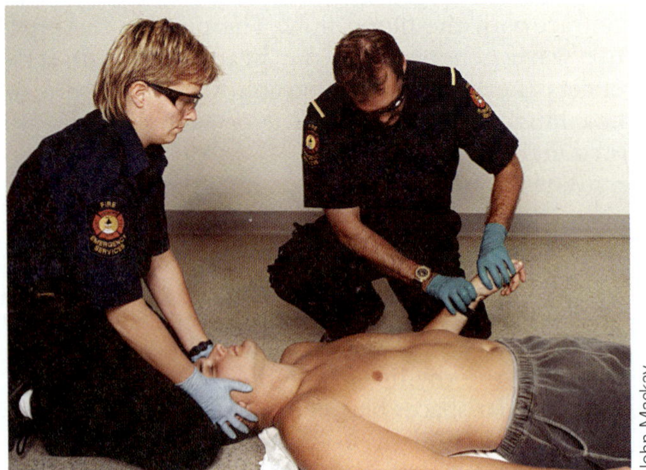

Figure 11–28 Assessing the pulse.

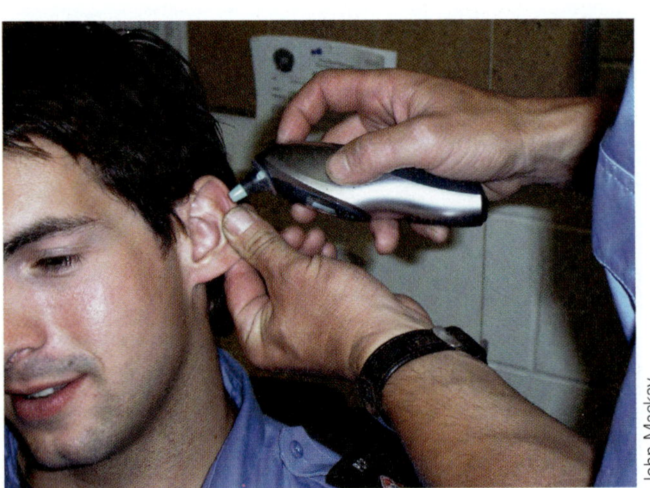

Figure 11–29 Taking temperature with a tympanic thermometer.

Skin Colour. Skin colour can tell you a lot about problems in a patient's heart and lungs, as well as other problems. In patients with medium to light skin colour, the following colour changes may be observed:

- Paleness may be caused by shock or heart attack. It may also be caused by fright, faintness, or emotional distress, as well as impaired blood flow.
- Redness (flushing) may be caused by high blood pressure, alcohol abuse, sunburn, heat stroke, fever, or an infectious disease.
- Blueness (cyanosis) is always a serious problem. It appears first in the fingertips and around the mouth. Generally, it is caused by reduced levels of oxygen, as in shock, heart attack, or poisoning.
- Yellowish colour may be caused by a liver disease.
- Black-and-blue mottling is the result of blood seeping under the skin. It is usually caused by a blow or severe infection.

In patients with dark skin colour, the above colour changes may be observed in the following areas of the body:

- Lips
- Nail beds and palms
- Earlobes
- Whites of the eyes and inner surface of the lower eyelid
- Gums and tongue

Checking the patient's nail beds is called assessing **capillary refill**. It is one way of checking for shock. Checking capillary refill is recommended only in children under six years of age. Research has proven that it is not always accurate in adults.

This procedure is performed by squeezing a fingernail or toenail (Figure 11–30). When squeezed, the tissue under the nail turns white. When you let go, the colour returns. To assess capillary refill, you have to measure the time it takes for the colour to return. Two seconds or less is normal. If refill time is greater than two seconds, suspect shock or decreased blood flow to that extremity.

Measure capillary refill time by counting "one 1000, two 1000," and so on. Capillary refill may be checked in infants by squeezing the palm of the hand or the sole of the foot and watching for the colour to return.

Note that when you recheck capillary refill in the ongoing assessment, you must be sure to do it in the same place. Different parts of the body may have different refill times.

Skin Condition. Normally, a person's skin is dry to the touch. When a patient's skin condition is wet or moist,

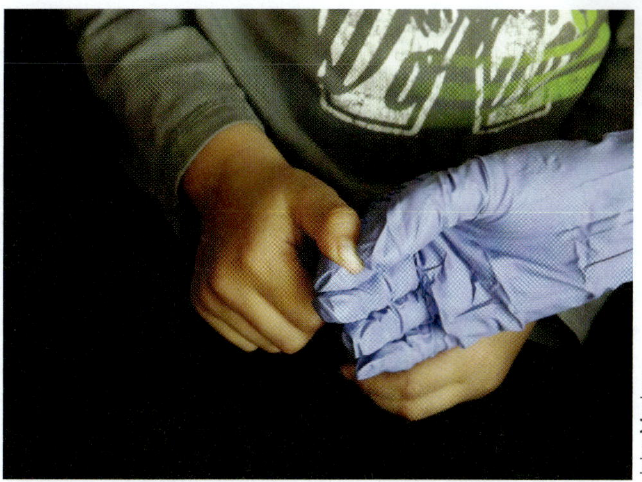

Figure 11–30 Assess capillary refill in children under six years of age.

it may indicate shock, a heat-related emergency, or a diabetic emergency. Skin that is abnormally dry may be a sign of spinal injury or severe dehydration.

Pupils

Normally, pupils **constrict** (get smaller) when exposed to light and **dilate** (enlarge) when the level of light is reduced. Both pupils should be the same size, unless a prior injury or condition changes this (Figure 11–31).

With these normal responses in mind, assess the patient's pupils. Shine your penlight into one of the patient's eyes and watch for the pupil to constrict in response to the light. If you are outdoors in bright light, cover the patient's eyes and observe for dilation of the pupils. Do not expose the patient's eyes to light for more than a few seconds, as this can be very uncomfortable for the patient.

Abnormal findings for pupils include the following:

- Pupils that do not react to light
- Pupils that remain constricted, or dilated (possibly caused by a drug overdose)
- Pupils that are unequal (possibly an indication of a serious head injury or stroke)

Blood Pressure

Some EMRs are taught to assess blood pressure. Others are not. Be sure to follow all local protocols.

Blood pressure is the amount of pressure the surging blood exerts against the arterial walls. It is an important index of the efficiency of the whole circulatory system. In part, it tells how well the organs and tissues are getting the oxygen they need. The blood pressure cuff is the instrument used to measure blood pressure.

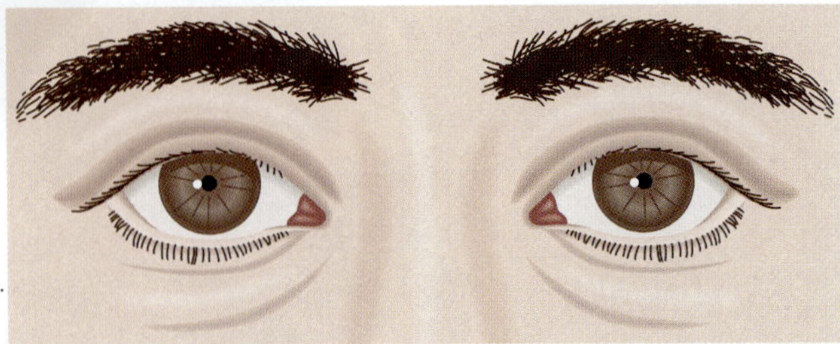

Constricted pupils

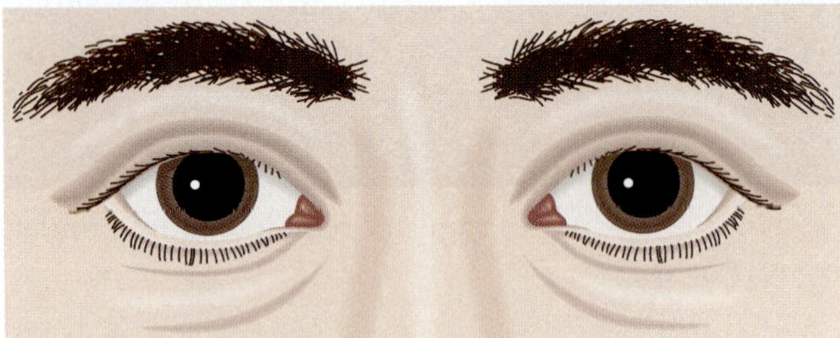

Dilated pupils

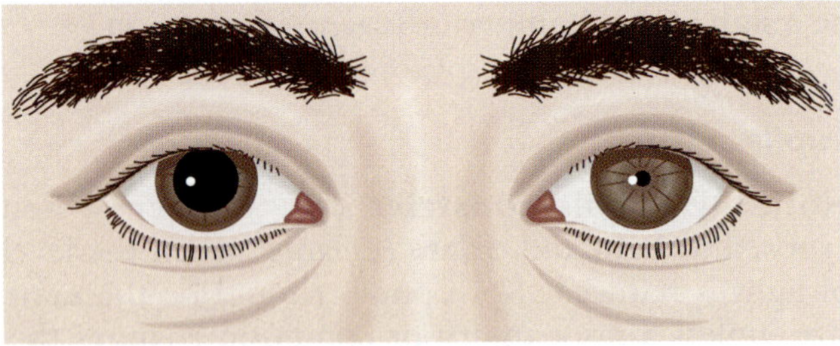

Unequal pupils

Figure 11–31 Check pupils for size, reactivity, and equality.

The pressure resulting from a contraction of the heart, which forces blood through the arteries, is called **systolic pressure**. The pressure resulting from the relaxation of the heart between contractions is called **diastolic pressure**. With most diseases or injuries, these two pressures rise or fall together.

Blood pressure normally varies with the age, gender, and medical history of the patient. The usual guide for systolic pressure is 100 plus the individual's age, up to 150 mmHg in the adult male or 140 mmHg in the female. Normal diastolic pressure in the male is 65 to 90 mmHg; in the female it is about 55 to 80 mmHg (Table 11–3). Blood pressure is reported as systolic over diastolic (for example, 120/80).

Measuring Blood Pressure. There are two methods of obtaining blood pressure with a blood pressure cuff. One is by *auscultation*, or by listening for the systolic and diastolic sounds through a stethoscope. The second method is by *palpation*, or by feeling for the return of the pulse as the cuff is deflated.

TABLE 11–3 NORMAL BLOOD PRESSURE RANGES		
Patient	**Systolic**	**Diastolic**
Child	2 × patient's age + 80	50–80 mmHg
Adult	Males: patient's age + 100 (up to 150 mmHg)	65–90 mmHg
	Females: patient's age + 100 (up to 140 mmHg)	55–80 mmHg

To assess blood pressure by auscultation (Figure 11–32), follow the steps described below:

1. Choose the proper size blood pressure cuff. It must be able to encircle the arm so that the Velcro strips on opposite ends meet and fasten securely. The cuff's bladder should cover half the circumference of the arm. If it covers less, it will not compress the blood vessels properly. If it covers more, it will suppress the pulse too quickly. The cuff should fit snugly, with the lower edge at least 2 to 3 cm above the **antecubital space** (the hollow, or front, of the elbow). The bladder should be centred over the brachial artery. It should not be too tight. You should be able to place one finger easily under its bottom edge. Some cuffs have markers for overlap placement, but they are not always in the correct location.

2. Now inflate the cuff rapidly with the rubber bulb. At the same time, palpate the radial pulse until it can no longer be felt. When that happens, make a mental note of the reading. Without stopping, continue to inflate the cuff to 30 mmHg above the level where the pulse disappeared.

3. Apply the stethoscope. Place the diaphragm of the stethoscope over the brachial artery just

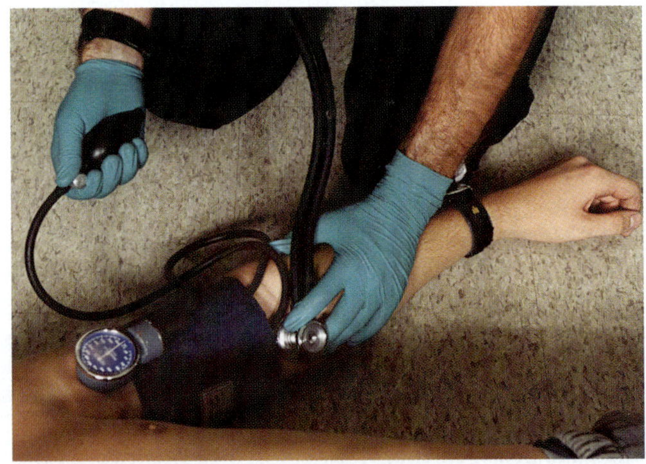

Figure 11–32 Taking blood pressure by auscultation.

John Mackay

above the hollow of the elbow. The diaphragm may be held with the thumb.

4. Deflate the cuff at approximately 2 mmHg per second (faster if skill permits). Watch the mercury column or needle indicator drop.

5. As soon as you hear two or more consecutive beats (clear tapping sounds of increasing intensity), record the pressure. This is the systolic pressure.

6. Continue releasing air from the bulb. At the point where you hear the last sound, record the diastolic pressure. Continue to deflate slowly for at least 10 mmHg. Remember that slow pulses require slower than normal rates of deflation. With children and some adults, you may hear sounds all the way to zero. In such cases, record the pressure when the sound changes from clear tapping to soft, muffled tapping.

7. Record on which limb the blood pressure was taken. Record the position of the person when the blood pressure was taken if other than supine. Record the size of the cuff if other than standard.

When it is too noisy for you to hear well enough to measure blood pressure by auscultation, palpate the blood pressure (Figure 11–33). Follow these steps:

1. Inflate the cuff rapidly. As you do so, palpate the patient's radial pulse.

2. Make a mental note of the level at which you can no longer feel the pulse.

3. Without stopping, continue to inflate the cuff another 30 mmHg. Then slowly deflate it.

4. Note the pressure at which the radial pulse returns. This is the systolic pressure.

5. Record it as a **palpated systolic pressure** (for example, 120/P).

Take several blood pressure readings during the time the patient is in your care. Watch for changes, as this may indicate changes in the patient's condition. Carefully record the blood pressure when you measure it, as well as the time it was taken.

It is not unusual for a patient's blood pressure to vary between the first reading on the scene and the reading at the hospital emergency department. Record the pressure accurately so that the receiving physician can tell how much it has changed.

Blood pressure may be normal even if the patient is seriously injured. You will learn in Chapter 19 that by the time the blood pressure drops, the patient is already in serious condition. It is almost always necessary to treat for shock when injuries are present.

> ## (!) T I P
>
> Blood pressures may be estimated by the location at which a pulse is found. Systolic pressure must be at least 60–70 mmHg to produce a carotid pulse, 70–80 mmHg for a brachial pulse, and at least 80–90 mmHg to produce a radial pulse. A patient with a blood pressure of 75/40 should have a carotid or brachial pulse but not likely a radial pulse. This minimum can be estimated when a BP cuff is not available.

Standards for Adults. Blood pressures vary greatly from person to person. Systolic blood pressures above 180 and below 90 usually indicate problems. Diastolic blood pressures above 90 and below 60 also indicate problems. The most common blood pressure problem observed in the field is low blood pressure. However, if blood pressure increases dramatically, the patient may suffer a stroke.

In general, blood pressure changes occur late in an emergency. A person who has a blood pressure of 132/82 could actually be developing severe shock. On the other hand, an uninjured person may normally have a blood pressure of 92/62 and be perfectly healthy. Ask the patient if they know their normal blood pressure range and make certain you consider all of their vital signs during the assessment.

Standards for Children. It is often difficult to take a child's blood pressure. Carrying a variety of cuff sizes is not always possible. But you must have a correctly fitting cuff if you are to get an accurate reading. Always try to get a complete set of vital signs. If a blood pressure reading is not readily attainable, the other vital signs may suggest the criticality of the child. Note that a blood pressure reading is not recommended in children under three years of age.

Average systolic blood pressure in children may be determined by the following formula: 80 plus two times the age in years. This formula works until the child is about 12 years of age. Average diastolic pressure is 50

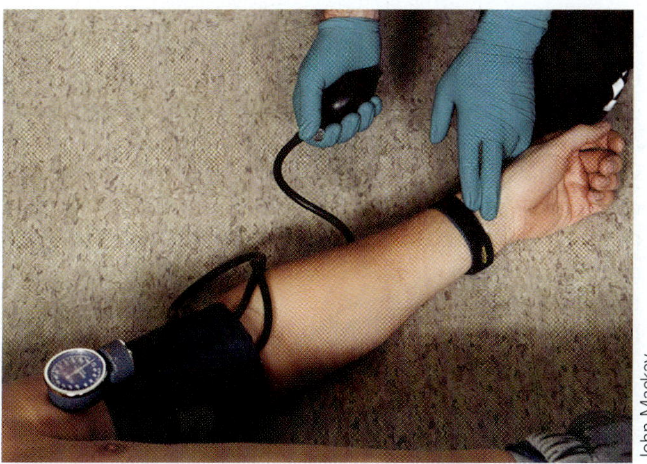

Figure 11–33 Taking blood pressure by palpation.

John Mackay

to 80 mmHg (see Table 11–3). From 12 years on, adult blood pressure values apply.

In children, adequate airway management is vital. Do *not* place blood pressure determination over assessment and treatment of life threats. A child's blood pressure may not begin to drop until well over 40 percent of blood volume is lost. If the mechanism of injury suggests it, treat for shock, regardless of vital signs.

Variable Factors. Factors that may increase blood pressure include conditions and substances that constrict blood vessels. They include the following:

- Cold environment
- High altitude
- Physical and emotional stress
- Pain
- Full urinary bladder
- Upper arm lower than heart level
- Cigarette smoke
- Caffeine (coffee, tea, cola, and some analgesic drugs)
- Decongestants

Heart failure, trauma, medications, and most types of shock can decrease blood pressure.

With the many possible variables that affect blood pressure, it is essential that you recognize the mistakes that can occur in taking a reading. The most critical of these possible errors are as follows:

- The rescuer does not hear accurately due to noise, head cold, or distractions.
- The stethoscope ear pieces are improperly placed.
- Improper conditions exist, such as a cuff not at heart level or a patient not sitting or lying down.
- The systolic pressure is not palpated at the highest level.
- The cuff is either too wide or too narrow.
- The bladder is too wide.
- The cuff is deflated too fast.

Pulse Oximetry

The oxygen in the blood is carried by **hemoglobin.** A **pulse oximeter** is a device that measures the percentage of the hemoglobin bound with a gas such as oxygen (Figure 11–34). This finding provides one representation of how much oxygen the patient has in his or her blood. For example, if the pulse oximeter reads 99 percent, it is indicating that 99 percent of the patient's hemoglobin is saturated with oxygen.

Any numerical score displayed on the pulse oximeter displays a percentage of oxygen-saturated hemoglobin. Normal readings are 95 percent to 100 percent in non-smokers. A reading of 90 percent to 94 percent indicates hypoxia (an insufficiency of oxygen in the

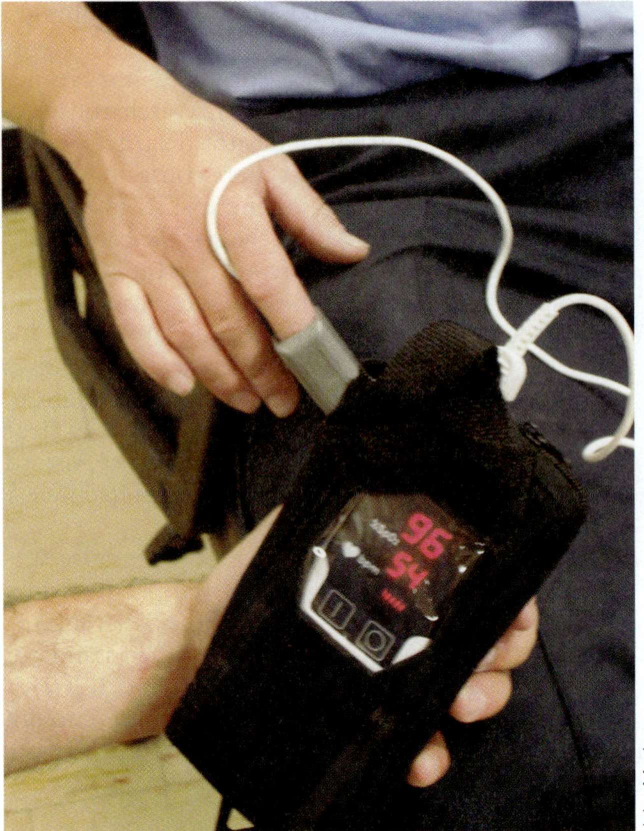

John Mackay

Figure 11–34 Using a pulse oximeter.

patient's tissues). Readings below 90 percent indicate severe hypoxia.

A significant limitation of the pulse oximeter is that it measures only oxygen in the blood, not in any other body tissue. Therefore, a patient in severe respiratory distress could have a reading of 97 percent, while a patient who has minimum distress could have a reading of 91 percent. This is why you will frequently hear, "Never withhold oxygen from a patient based on a 'normal' pulse oximetry reading." All patients with trauma, breathing difficulty, chest pain, or other serious pain should receive oxygen regardless of the pulse oximetry reading.

So, why use a pulse oximeter? The best reason is to identify changes (improvement or deterioration) in the patient's condition. Keep your pulse oximeter readily available in your kit, and place it on the patient before you administer oxygen. (NEVER delay administration of oxygen when pulse oximetry is not immediately available.) Observe an initial reading and then another after the patient has been receiving oxygen for a few minutes. If the patient reports feeling better or worse, this may correlate with changes on the pulse oximeter.

To use a pulse oximeter, follow these guidelines:

1. Turn on the device.
2. Check the patient. Make sure he or she is not wearing nail polish. Remove the nail polish, if necessary.

(Commercially prepared polish-removing wipes are available. Keep some with your oximeter.)

3. Place the oximeter on the patient's finger.

4. Observe for a light or a numerical reading, indicating capture of a pulse. If it matches the patient's pulse, which you take manually, this is a sign of proper functioning.

5. Observe and record the oxygen saturation reading. Remember: NEVER withhold supplementary oxygen from a patient based on normal pulse oximeter readings.

6. Be alert to changes in subsequent readings. Be sure to verify each reading. Never take subsequent readings without verifying each one with a radial or carotid pulse check.

Note that some circumstances make pulse oximetry not valuable or inaccurate:

- *Carbon monoxide poisoning.* Falsely high readings will occur because the hemoglobin is saturated, but not with oxygen. Carbon monoxide more readily binds with the hemoglobin molecule than oxygen does. (Note that some newer oximeters can differentiate between oxygen and carbon monoxide.)
- *Hypothermia.* Cold extremities and chronically reduced circulation will cause inaccurate readings.
- *Shock.* Shock is inadequate perfusion (blood supply to the body's tissues), so readings will be inaccurate in the extremities where perfusion is reduced. In some cases of shock, blood volume may be low due to internal or external bleeding. A pulse oximeter reading is irrelevant when there is not enough blood supply to the body.
- *Cardiac arrest.* In cardiac arrest, perfusion to the fingers is essentially absent, making readings unreliable. Realistically, there is usually no time to consider pulse oximetry during these emergencies. CPR and defibrillation are more important considerations.

SECTION 3
PATIENT HISTORY

The patient history is an important part of a thorough patient assessment. It involves gathering facts that you would not be able to gather otherwise. For example, the answer to a simple question such as "What happened?" can provide a good amount of information on the patient's condition and the events leading up to it.

Generally, you would ask the patient questions. If the patient is unconscious, however, you would

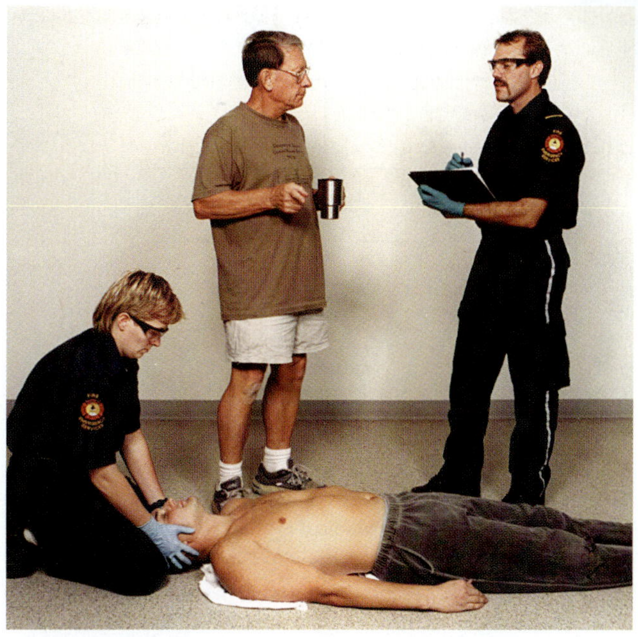

Figure 11–35 Gather facts from the patient or from family or bystanders.

gather facts by observing the scene, looking for medical identification tags and medications, and questioning family members and bystanders (Figure 11–35).

Remember the differences between a trauma patient and a medical patient. In trauma patients, you will most likely perform a secondary assessment before a patient history. In a medical patient, you may take the history before the secondary assessment.

The SAMPLE History

One way to remember the questions you need to ask is by using the mnemonic **SAMPLE**. Each letter identifies an important area of questioning (Figure 11–36):

S — Signs and symptoms
A — Allergies
M — Medications
P — Past medical history
L — Last oral intake
E — Events

Signs and Symptoms

Note a patient's signs and symptoms (Figure 11–37). A **sign** is something you can observe directly. You can see, feel, or hear signs. Examples include deformities (see), skin temperature (feel), and wheezing (hear).

A **symptom** cannot be observed by anyone but the patient. In order for you to be aware of symptoms, they must be described by the patient.

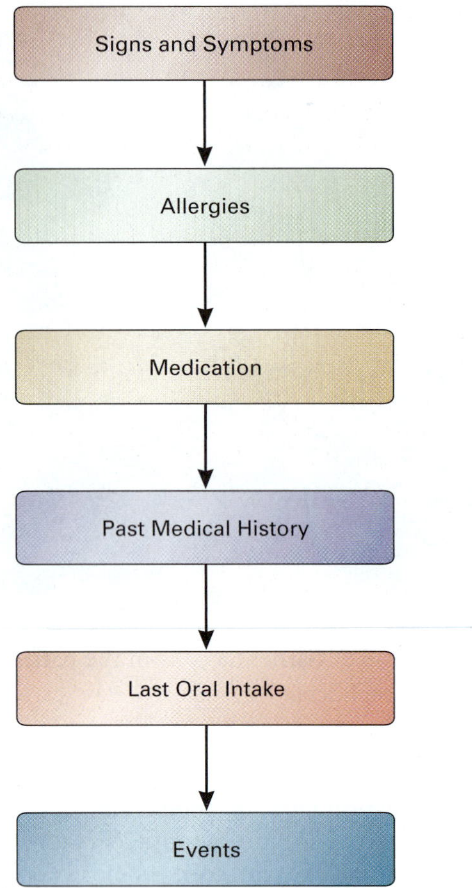

Figure 11–36 Components of the SAMPLE history.

Examples of symptoms include pain, tenderness, or difficulty breathing.

A good starting point to determine signs and symptoms is to ask the patient an open-ended question, such as "Why did you call today?" or "Can you describe how you feel?" This technique allows patients to answer without any restriction. They may even give you important information that you may not have thought to ask about.

Responses to such questions as "Do you have chest pain?" are restricted to a "yes" or "no" answer. They can cause you to miss important information. Such questions might be better rephrased as "What do you feel in your chest?" or "Tell me what the pain feels like."

You will find the signs and symptoms—as well as emergency care—for specific conditions described in later chapters. Remember that you are not required to diagnose any medical condition. An EMR's emergency care of a patient is based on assessment findings only.

Allergies

Determine if your patient is allergic to anything. This includes allergies to medications, foods, or substances

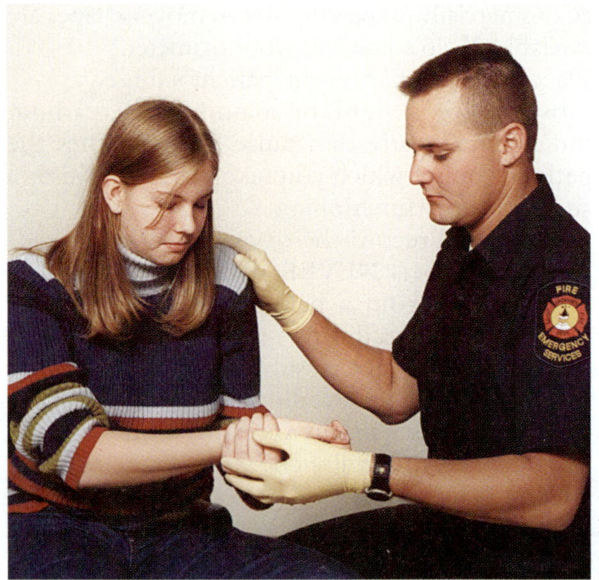

Figure 11–37a A *sign* is something EMRs can perceive, such as a deformed wrist.

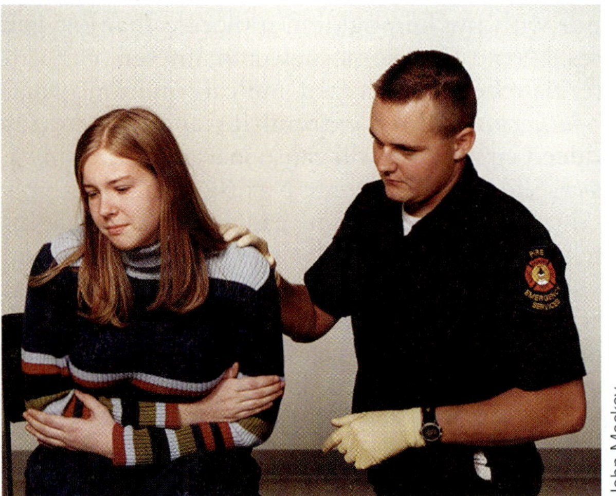

Figure 11–37b A *symptom* is something that the patient feels and describes, such as stomach pain.

in the environment. Being aware of an allergy can help determine the possible causes of the patient's condition. An allergic reaction can be very serious; in fact, it can be life threatening. Determining if a patient is allergic to a drug will help prevent other medical personnel in the field and in the hospital from administering it.

Medications

Identify all medications the patient is currently on or has recently taken. This information may help identify a medical condition. For example, a patient who takes insulin has diabetes. Other specific medicines are used for seizures, cardiac conditions, and respiratory problems. Many EMS rescuers carry a pocket guide that lists common prescription drugs and what they are used for.

Past Medical History

Most patients have had some type of medical condition in their lifetime. Some of these may be pertinent to the emergency care you provide to the patient. What is pertinent depends on the type of emergency.

For example, if a patient has shortness of breath, the fact that he has a history of heart problems is pertinent. The fact that he had foot surgery many years ago is not. However, if the patient's present emergency involves dropping a bowling ball on a foot that was once operated on, then the surgery is pertinent.

Patients and family members who are in the middle of a medical crisis may not know what to tell you. Some people say very little. Others are willing to tell you everything there is to know. It is your job to guide them.

Sometimes you need to ask more than one question to guide a patient to an answer. For example, you may begin by asking a patient to tell you about any medical problems she may have.

Your patient may answer "None," even though she has diabetes. This is because she may have understood her physician to say that she has "a little sugar problem," which is controlled with diet or pills.

So your next question might be, "Do you see a doctor for anything?" or "Have you ever been admitted to the hospital?" It may cause the patient to disclose the information you need.

Most patients do not withhold answers or answer incorrectly on purpose. Remember, they may be scared, confused, or both.

Last Oral Intake

You must find out the time of your patient's last oral intake. It may be pertinent in the patient who is unconscious or confused. It will also be important if the patient needs immediate surgery.

Do not ask "When was your last meal?" People may not consider a snack or several drinks a meal. Instead, ask "When was the last time you had anything to eat or drink?" This may include anything from a glass of water to a large meal.

Events

Such questions as "What were you doing when this happened?" help determine the events leading up to the incident. This information might not be as clear cut as it seems.

Say a patient falls from a ladder. You arrive to find her complaining of a possible broken arm. It is reasonable to assume that this is a trauma patient if she slipped on a rung of the ladder. However, if she fell as a result of getting dizzy or losing consciousness, then she may also be a medical patient.

If a person is driving, has a heart attack, and passes out behind the wheel, he will surely crash. Upon your arrival at the scene, you could assume that the patient has suffered serious trauma and is unconscious due to that trauma. It will be your assessment of the events that will help you determine what really happened. Keep an open mind and consider all factors. A passenger might tell you that he saw the driver clutch at his chest before the crash, or a medical information tag may alert you to a heart condition.

As you can see, the SAMPLE history is an important part of the patient assessment process in which information vital to patient care is obtained.

SECTION 4
ONGOING ASSESSMENT

Some patients are stabilized; others are not. However, your patient assessment process must go on. Continually reassess your patient until he or she is turned over to the paramedics (Figure 11–38).

Complete the following every 5 minutes in an unstable patient and every 15 minutes in a stable one:

- Reassess level of consciousness (AVPU).
- Reassess and correct any airway problems.

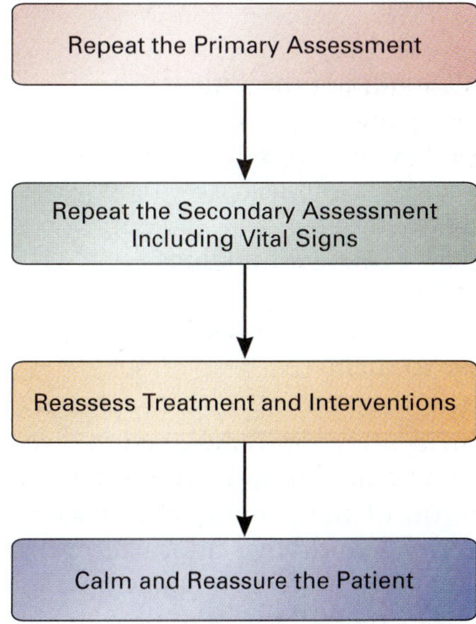

Figure 11–38 Components of the ongoing assessment.

- Reassess breathing for rate and quality. Ventilate if necessary.
- Reassess pulse for rate and quality.
- Reassess skin temperature, colour, and condition.
- Repeat any portions of the secondary assessment that might be necessary.
- Reassess your interventions (treatment) to see if they are effective.
- Continue to calm and reassure the patient.

Remember that the patients you come across are in crisis. They may be uncomfortable, confused, and possibly afraid that they will die. It is important for you to have a professional, calm, and caring attitude. Try to address the patient's concerns. For example, if you can protect the patient's modesty, do so. Do not leave the patient alone. If the patient feels cold—even if you do not—turn up the heating or provide another blanket.

The kindness and compassion you show will help calm the patient. It will also be remembered for a long time to come.

SECTION 5
HAND-OFF REPORT

When the paramedics arrive, you must be prepared to give them appropriate information about your patient and the care you have given. This is called your **hand-off report**.

The hand-off report contains the following (Figure 11–39):

- Age and gender of the patient
- Chief complaint
- Level of consciousness (AVPU)
- Airway and breathing status
- Circulation status
- Secondary assessment findings
- SAMPLE history
- Treatment, interventions, and the patient's response to them

The hand-off report is designed to give the transporting paramedics an up-to-the-minute account of the condition of the patient, what treatments have been performed, and other information that you feel is important. If you must complete a written report, many agencies require that you provide one copy to the paramedics at the scene.

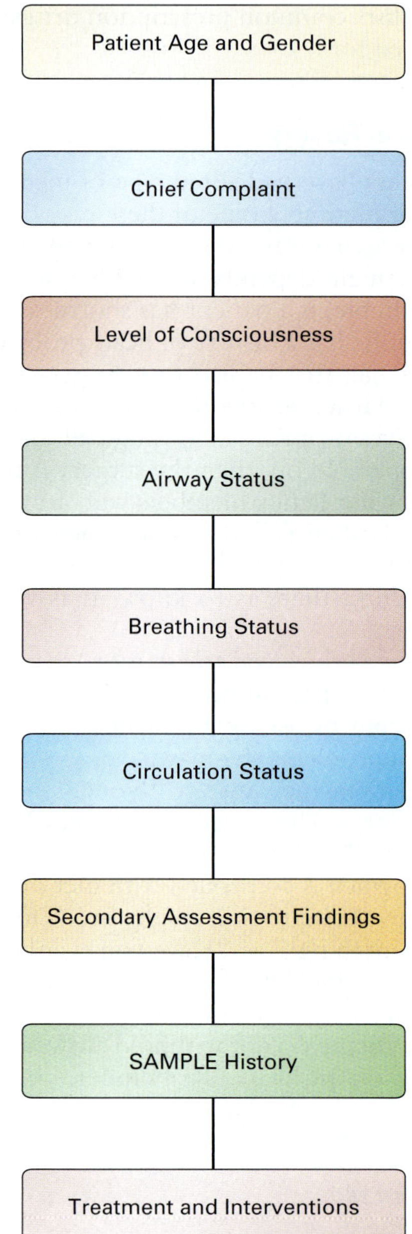

Figure 11–39 Information included in the hand-off report.

SECTION 6
CARING FOR UNIQUE PATIENT GROUPS

Other factors that may be relevant during patient assessment can be found in patients with physical or intellectual disabilities, those who are morbidly obese, and in older adult patients. Taking a history and being aware of these patients' conditions and limitations will assist you in your assessment and care.

The patient with a physical disability may normally present with a limited range of motion. Remember this during the secondary assessment. Physical impairments may also affect how you lift and handle the patient.

A patient with an intellectual disability may require extra patience and understanding from the EMR. Two-way communication may be ineffective, and this may limit your history gathering from the patient and your assessment of the patient's normal level of consciousness. Family or bystanders may be instrumental in helping you determine the normal mental status of the patient.

The morbidly obese, or bariatric, patient may present with both limited physical ability and a compounded list of medical issues. They may have skin deterioration and hygiene problems. Many of these patients have sheltered themselves from society as they feel ridiculed. Medical conditions may not yet be diagnosed as they have not been out of their home to attend a doctor's office.

It is important to speak directly to the patient in a friendly and confident manner. They may be able to help you determine how best to assist them in seeking definitive medical care. If the bariatric patient feels they are being stared at because of their size, you will have a difficult time getting the information you require to get them the assistance they need.

The older adult patient can present with any number of the physical or mental degenerative conditions that are most common in older people. While dementia and Alzheimer disease are two examples of mental conditions, the EMR should be aware that there are also many physical conditions that can afflict senior citizens. Maintain a high index of suspicion for fractures and head injuries from falls. Speak calmly and clearly and allow time for the patient to respond.

Explain what you will be doing to the patient, and always protect the patient's dignity during treatment and transport.

EMR FOCUS

Even after you have memorized the steps of the assessment process, you may still be amazed at the ease with which experienced EMRs and paramedics perform these complicated tasks. If you were to ask, many of them would tell you that patient assessment is an art.

You will see throughout the remaining chapters of this book that there are countless injuries and illnesses that patients can suffer. In every condition, the patient assessment finds injuries, signs, symptoms, and histories of past illnesses. All these are important to patient care.

One experienced EMR put it like this: "Patient assessment is like a puzzle. It's important to find all the pieces—the examination, the history—and put them together so that they make sense."

Proper patient assessment and history help you make sense of the patient's condition and provide quality patient care.

CASE STUDY FOLLOW-UP

At the beginning of this chapter, you read that EMRs were on the scene with an unconscious male patient. To see how the chapter skills apply to this emergency, read the following. It describes how the call was completed.

PATIENT HISTORY

Since the patient was unconscious, we asked his wife if he had any problems before he went to sleep. She didn't know of any. In response to further questioning, she told us that he had no allergies and that he was taking insulin for his diabetes. He had taken his insulin in the morning but had been working in the yard all morning after eating a small breakfast. His wife added that he had a similar episode last year.

SECONDARY ASSESSMENT

Although it seemed as if we had a medical problem, you can never be too sure, especially with a patient who cannot talk. I continued to assist ventilations and monitor the airway while my partner did a quick head-to-toe exam to check for injuries that may have been hidden. There were none. My partner then took a set of vital signs.

ONGOING ASSESSMENT

The patient required ventilation the entire time we were at the scene. I suctioned him one more time when I determined his secretions were building up. We continued to monitor the patient's mental status and spoke to him by name just in case he could hear. His wife was quite upset, so we tried to reassure her and keep her calm.

TRANSFER OF CARE

When the paramedics arrived, one of them performed an initial assessment. "Good job," he said after assessing the patient's airway. My partner gave them the hand-off report:

"This is Stan Wong. He is 62. His wife could not wake him up from a nap. He responds only to painful stimulus. We had to suction him and assist ventilations. The secondary assessment did not turn up anything, but his wife says he has diabetes. He took his insulin, had a small meal, then worked all morning in the yard. His wife says this has happened before. His vitals were pulse 110 and weak, respirations 10 and shallow, blood pressure 110/68. Pupils were equal and reactive, skin cool and moist."

The paramedics thanked us and took over care. We were then dispatched pretty quickly to another run. A few days later, I met one of the paramedics. He told me that they gave Mr. Wong glucose through an IV en route to the hospital. By the time they arrived at the hospital, he was sitting up and talking.

Patient assessment is performed on all patients that you come into contact with. The procedure may vary depending on whether your patient is suffering from a medical problem or trauma and whether the patient has minor injuries or serious ones. It is important to be thorough and work in a logical order. Practise your patient assessment skills frequently and become proficient.

NOCPs

4.2
a Obtain list of patient's allergies **S**
b Obtain patient's medication profile **S**
c Obtain chief complaint and/or incident history from patient, family members, and/or bystanders **S**
d Obtain information regarding patient's past medical history **S**
e Obtain information about patient's last oral intake **S**
f Obtain information regarding incident through accurate and complete scene assessment **S**

4.3
a Conduct primary patient assessment and interpret findings **S**
b Conduct secondary patient assessment and interpret findings **S**
c Conduct a cardiovascular system assessment and interpret findings **S**
d Conduct a neurological system assessment and interpret findings **S**
e Conduct a respiratory system assessment and interpret findings **S**
g Conduct a gastrointestinal system assessment and interpret findings **S**
i Conduct an integumentary system assessment and interpret findings **S**
j Conduct a musculoskeletal assessment and interpret findings **S**
k Conduct assessment of the ears, eyes, nose, and throat and interpret findings **S**
o Conduct a geriatric assessment and interpret findings **A**
p Conduct a bariatric assessment and interpret findings **A**

4.4
a Assess pulse **S**
b Assess respiration **S**
d Measure blood pressure by auscultation **S**
c Measure blood pressure by palpation **S**
g Assess skin condition **S**
h Assess pupils **S**
i Assess level of consciousness. **S**

4.5
a Conduct oximetry testing and interpret findings **N**

6.1
a Provide care to patient experiencing signs and symptoms involving cardiovascular system **S**
b Provide care to patient experiencing signs and symptoms involving neurological system **S**
c Provide care to patient experiencing signs and symptoms involving respiratory system **S**
e Provide care to patient experiencing signs and symptoms involving gastrointestinal system **S**

f Provide care to patient experiencing signs and symptoms involving integumentary system **S**

g Provide care to patient experiencing signs and symptoms involving musculoskeletal system **S**

h Provide care to patient experiencing signs and symptoms involving immunological system **S**

j Provide care to patient experiencing signs and symptoms involving the eyes, ears, nose, or throat **S**

l Provide care to patient experiencing non-urgent problem **S**

o Provide care to trauma patient **S**

6.2 c Provide care for geriatric patient **A**

d Provide care for physically-impaired patient **A**

e Provide care for mentally-impaired patient **A**

f Provide care for bariatric patient **A**

6.3 a Conduct ongoing assessments based on patient presentation and interpret findings **S**

REVIEW QUESTIONS

Page references where answers may be found or supported are provided at the end of each question.

SECTION 1

1. What are the components of the patient assessment process? (p. 162)

2. What are the components of the primary assessment? (p. 162)

3. Why would you apply manual stabilization to your patient's head and neck? (p. 171)

4. What are the components of the EMS update? (p. 168)

SECTION 2

5. What are the three basic methods of performing a secondary assessment? (p. 169)

6. What mnemonic helps you to recall the conditions to look for in the secondary assessment? What does each letter in the mnemonic stand for? (p. 170)

7. From which part of the body does a tympanic thermometer take a reading? (p. 176)

8. In which patients is capillary refill used? (p. 177)

9. What is the best reason for using a pulse oximeter? (p. 180)

SECTION 3

10. What mnemonic can help you recall the parts of a patient history? What does each letter in the mnemonic stand for? (p. 181)

SECTION 4

11. What are the components of an ongoing assessment? (pp. 183–184)

SECTION 5

12. What information should be included in the patient hand-off report? (p. 184)

SECTION 6

13. Identify three unique patient groups that require special consideration. (p. 184)

14. Why might it be difficult to obtain a medical history from these unique patients? (p. 185)

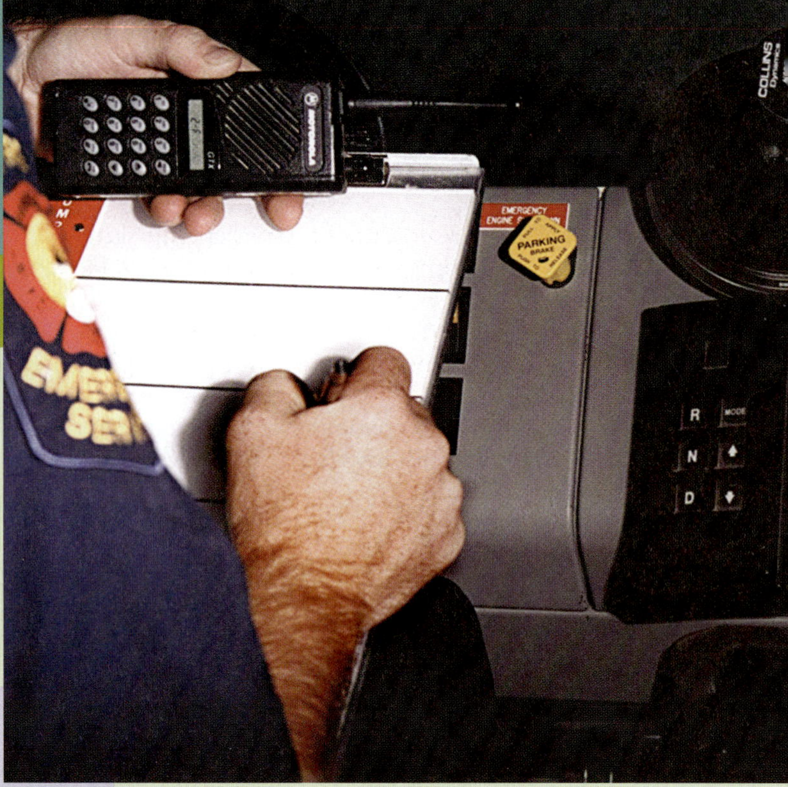
John Mackay

12

Communication and Documentation

1. Explain the importance of effective verbal communication of patient information.

2. Identify five typical components of an EMS radio system.

3. List correct radio procedures.

4. Identify the six essential components of a call to the medical director.

5. Discuss the communication skills that should be used to interact with the patient.

6. List the three components of the written pre-hospital care report and discuss the legalities of the document.

7. Review the special documentation needed concerning patient refusal.

8. List five special EMS reporting situations.

INTRODUCTION

When the stress and confusion of an emergency arise, an EMR must be able to communicate effectively and precisely. You must be able to do so with the patient, family, bystanders, and other EMS personnel by radio, in person, and in writing.

SECTION 1
COMMUNICATION

As an EMR, you must be able to determine a chief complaint, obtain a medical history, and properly reassure and comfort the patient. You must also be able to update incoming EMS units on your patient's status, request help from dispatch, ask the medical director for advice, and provide a hand-off report to the paramedics who take over patient care. All these tasks take skill, including communication skills.

You will have opportunities to communicate with other EMS personnel on the radio or phone, as well as in person. In these situations, it is important for you to be accurate and to speak slowly and clearly. Providing inaccurate information, omitting key information, or speaking in a way that is not clear could result in harm to your patient.

Radio Communication

Radios operate on frequencies that are regulated and licensed by Industry Canada's Spectrum Management. Spectrum Management makes sure that unauthorized persons do not disrupt emergency radio traffic.

There are many components to a radio system. They usually include the following:

- *A base station* (Figure 12–1). This is a stationary radio located in a dispatch centre, station, or hospital.
- *Mobile radios* (Figure 12–2). These are radios mounted in vehicles.
- *Portable radios* (Figure 12–3). These are hand-held radios, which may be carried on your belt or elsewhere on your person.
- *Repeaters.* These devices receive a low-power radio transmission and rebroadcast it with increased power.
- *Cellular phones* (Figure 12–4). These phones may be used to contact the medical director or the dispatcher. They are often used where radio coverage is not available.

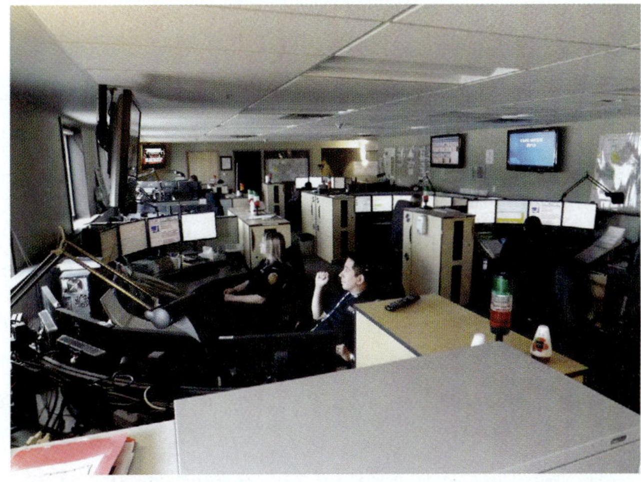

Figure 12–1 Example of an EMS communications centre.

If your EMS system has a dispatch centre and radios, you will need to advise the dispatcher of your activities during an emergency call. You must report the following:

- When you are en route to a call
- When you arrive at the scene of a call
- When you require additional assistance or specialized personnel
- When you return to service and are available for the next call

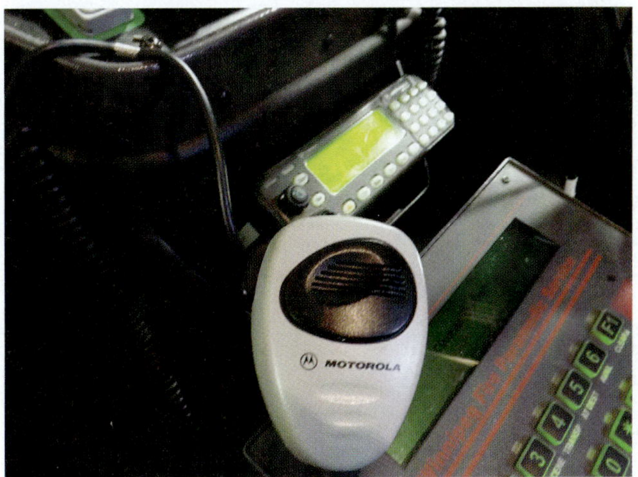

Figure 12–2 A mobile two-way radio.

CASE STUDY

Dispatch

Our EMR unit was sent to the Parkview Place Senior Housing Centre for an 80-year-old female patient who was disoriented and behaving strangely.

Scene Assessment

The outside of the complex was quiet. We were met at the door by the resident aide, who told us that Mrs. Gherson was acting in a most peculiar manner. She brought us up to the apartment. We stayed alert.

Primary Assessment

Mrs. Gherson was sitting at her kitchen table, wondering what all the fuss was about. Two neighbours stood beside her. They told us that Mrs. Gherson had been wandering through the halls babbling incoherently just a short time before. They were amazed that she had suddenly improved.

We found the patient alert. She had no problems with her airway and could speak in full sentences. Her respirations seemed normal. She had no bleeding. Her friends had not witnessed or heard a fall.

Patient History

Mrs. Gherson had no idea why the EMS was called. She didn't remember being out of her apartment. She denied having allergies. She had been on insulin for diabetes and a "heart pill" since her heart attack eight years before. She had eaten dinner and taken her medicines.

Secondary Assessment

Mrs. Gherson had no complaints. We began to do a physical exam, but she stopped us. She said that she really didn't want our help. She felt she was fine. We convinced her to let us take her pulse and respiration. She told us that she would not go to the hospital.

> Patient refusals are challenging calls for any EMS provider. You must make sure you have tried your best to convince the patient to accept your care and that of the paramedics. Consider this patient as you read Chapter 12. How important are communication and documentation in this situation?

You will also use the radio when you update incoming EMS units or need to speak with the medical director.

Using a radio can cause some anxiety, especially the first few times. It is important to remember to speak slowly and clearly. Push the "push to talk" button one second before you begin to speak. Talk with your mouth 5 to 7 cm away from the microphone. It is best to keep a transmission brief to allow others to use the frequency. Listen before you transmit so that you do not disrupt another conversation.

Remember that people with scanners can hear what you say over the radio. Never use a patient's name or say anything over the radio of a personal or confidential

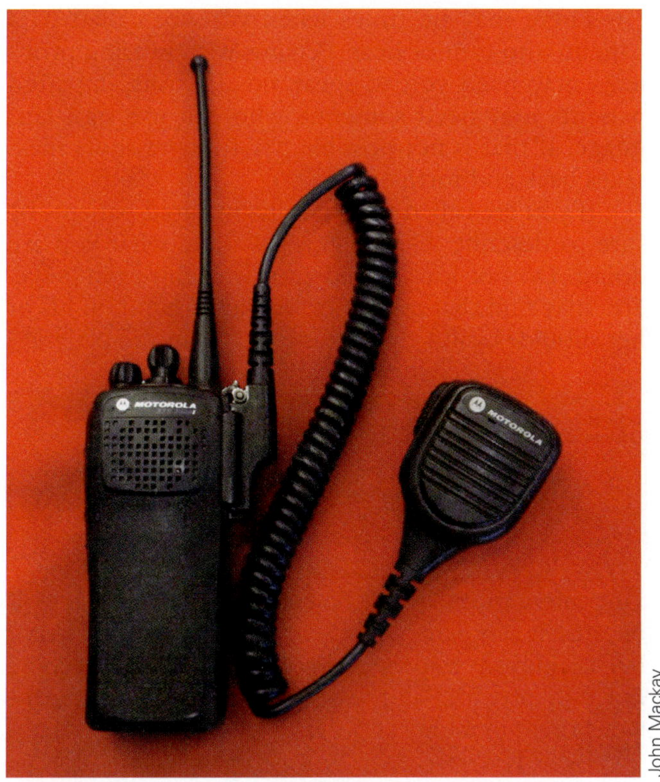

Figure 12–3 A portable hand-held radio.

nature. Of course, you should never use profanities or speak in a less than professional tone of voice.

Communicating with the Medical Director

Consulting with a physician while you are on the scene can help you and your patient. If possible, consult the medical director whenever you have questions that cannot be resolved by protocols.

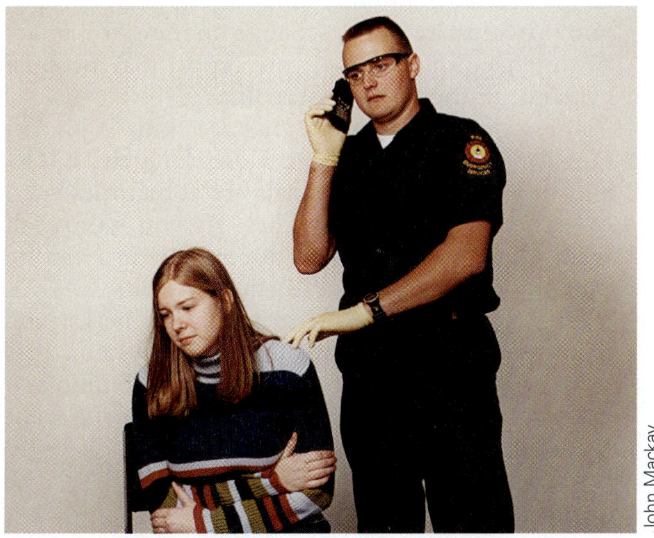

Figure 12–4 Cellular phones are commonly used in EMS.

Since the physician may be many kilometres away, it is up to you to present information clearly and concisely. Be prepared to give a report that includes the following:

- Your unit identifier and the fact that you are an EMR
- Patient's age, gender, and chief complaint
- Brief, pertinent history of the events leading to the injury or illness
- Results of the patient's physical exam, including vital signs
- Care given to the patient and the patient's response to that care
- The reason for calling

If the physician gives you orders, repeat the orders back to verify them. Be sure all orders and advice given to you by the physician are clearly documented. If you have any questions, ask the physician for clarification.

Interpersonal Communication

Medical emergencies can be frightening for patients. Be sure to speak slowly and clearly. Use language that patients and their families can understand. Avoid technical terms that will confuse them.

When speaking to patients, if possible, get down to their level to avoid appearing threatening (Figure 12–5). Make eye contact. Use body language that shows you are open and interested in what patients have to say. Also, address patients by name whenever possible. Note, however, that if your patient is elderly, you should not call him or her by the first name unless you are invited to do so.

Listen carefully to what patients tell you. Observe them when they talk. If a patient appears reluctant to speak about a topic, you may need to reassure him or her. Tell the patient that any information you can get about the problem is important, even if it is upsetting to talk about. Share with them appropriate observations from your assessment and tell them, in advance, everything you plan to do to help them.

Observing patients while they talk can help you identify physical problems. If a patient can speak only a few words before catching a breath, for example, he or she may be in respiratory distress.

Find out why a patient is holding his or her stomach or clutching his or her chest. The patient may not even know he or she is doing it. A patient who winces with pain should be questioned about that pain.

Nothing is more annoying than not being listened to. Consider the last time you had to repeat information to someone several times. It is not a pleasant experience. Listening lets a patient know that you believe he or she is important and conveys that you have empathy. If you ask a patient a question, listen for an answer. Your perceived understanding will convey

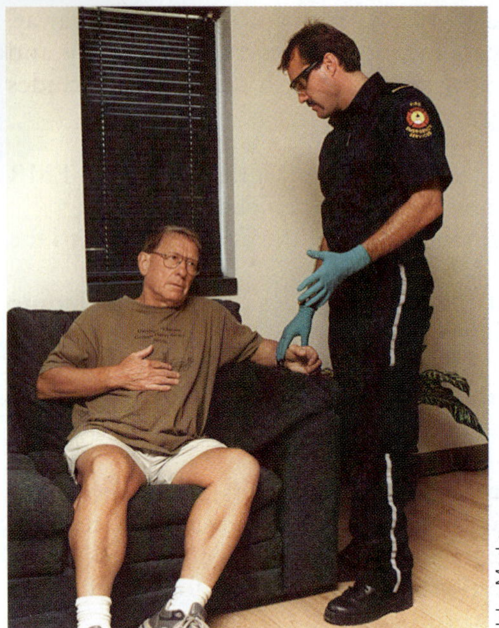

Figure 12–5a You can maintain an attitude of control and authority if you stand above the patient.

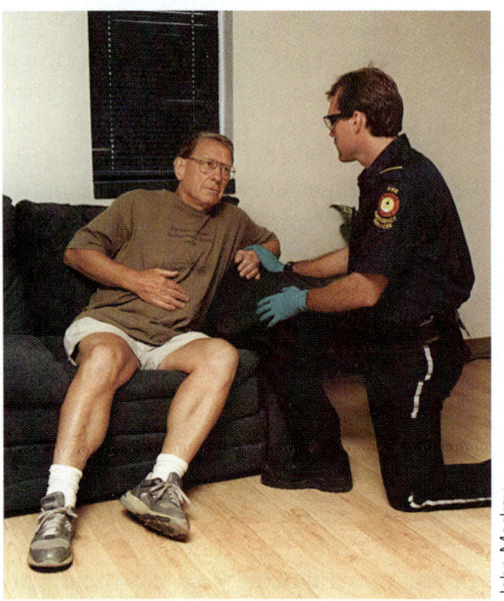

Figure 12–5b If you want to soften your approach, get down to the patient's level.

compassion. Make notes, if necessary, so you do not forget the answers. If you forget too often, the patient will soon stop answering your questions altogether.

Remember that all patients deserve equal care. One patient should be treated with the same respect and dignity afforded to any other. If you are called to a patient who does not speak a language you understand, call for someone who can interpret. A family member or a neighbour, for example, may be able to speak both your language and the patient's.

There may be times when you are called to a patient who cannot hear. Persons with hearing problems may need you to speak up. Hearing-impaired patients may need someone who can use sign language. If that is not possible, try to write short messages back and forth.

If you are called to a visually impaired patient, be sure to describe what is going on and what you are doing. Do not leave a patient alone who cannot see. You may find that talking or keeping a hand on his or her shoulder will help reassure and calm the patient.

SECTION 2
DOCUMENTATION

Documentation should be considered an art. This is because it can paint a picture of the patient and his or her condition. A properly completed written report not only provides all the pertinent facts but also provides them in a logical order.

Pre-Hospital Care Report

A pre-hospital care report is used for all the following reasons:

- *To transfer patient information from one person to another.* Your report is turned over to the EMS personnel who transport your patient. They may turn it over to the hospital staff who will use it to learn the patient's history, including the condition in which he or she was found, what emergency care was provided, and how the patient responded to that care.
- *To provide legal documentation.* A report prepared at the scene of an emergency is a legal record. If you provide care at the scene of an injury or an act of violence, for example, your report may become evidence in the court proceedings.
- *To document the care you provided.* This is important for legal reasons, too. Unfortunately, EMRs and other EMS professionals are sometimes sued by patients and their families. As you will recall from Chapter 3, accurate documentation can be one of your best defences against lawsuits.
- *To improve your EMS system.* Research is performed in many different areas of your EMS system. It is used to improve such factors as response time and the effectiveness of certain procedures. Your accurate reports are vital to that research.

Description

A pre-hospital care report contains three parts (Figure 12–6): run data, patient information, and the narrative.

Date (D/M/Y)	**Emergency Medical Responder Patient Care Report**			

Emergency Medical Responder Patient Care Report

Incident Location		Fire Incident	
Surname	First	Date of Birth (D/M/Y)	Sex : M F
Address	City	Prov	Response Code: 3 4

SCENE ASSESSMENT

Mechanism of Injury

☐ MVA, Plate # _____________   ☐ Medical   Trauma   **Patient Found**

☐ Extrication   ☐ Fire/Smoke   Other:_____________   ☐ Side Lying: L   R

☐ Violence   ☐ MVA/Pedestrian, Plate # _____________   ☐ Sitting   Supine

  Seat Belt: Y   N   ☐ Prone   Ambulatory

Chief Complaint:

History of Chief Complaint:

Past Medical History:

Allergies:

Medications: (Given to Paramedic   Yes ___   No ___)

Comments:

Verbal	Motor	Eye	Pupil Reaction
1 Nil	1 Nil	1 Nil	+ means the pupil reacts to light by constricting
2 Incomplete sounds	2 Extends	2 Pain	- means the pupil does not react to light
3 Inappropriate Words	3 Flexion	3 Voice	**Pupil Size**
4 Confused	4 Withdraws	4 Spontaneous	
5 Oriented/Alert	5 Localizes		•1mm ●2mm ●3mm ●4mm ●5mm ●6mm
	6 Obey		

Time	Resp	Pulse	B/P	Verbal	Motor	Eye	GCS Total	Pupil Size R	Pupil Size L	Pupil React R	(+/-)	Pupil React L	Grip R	Grip L
:			/											☐ **Absent** ☐
:			/											☐ **Normal** ☐
:			/											☐ **Weak** ☐

PATIENT ASSESSMENT

Protocol Code Number: **Assessed By (Primary EMR Regiment Number):**

Patient Care Procedures

Px Code	Patient Care Procedure	Prior to Paramedic arrival	Assist Paramedic	Primary EMR Regiment #	Regiment #	Regiment #

CW781:2000 08

Figure 12–6 An EMR pre-hospital care report form. (Courtesy of the East St. Paul Fire Department)

For the run data, you must fill in the date, time, unit involved, location of the call, and the names of the crew members.

Information on the patient is extensive. It includes the patient's name, address, date of birth, gender, chief complaint, physical exam results, and vital signs, as well as the patient history, changes in the patient's condition, and the care you gave. Some information can be written in specially designated areas of the form. Some can be recorded by way of checking boxes. Some can be in narrative form.

It is important to fill out the report neatly and to spell correctly. Do not draw conclusions or offer opinions. Simply state the facts. Avoid the use of radio codes or abbreviations that others might not understand. Be sure to record your observations of the scene. Noting the mechanism of injury, for example, will help hospital personnel identify the extent of the patient's injuries.

If you must correct an error while you are filling out the report, draw a single horizontal line through the error. Then, write the correct information beside it. If you try to totally cross out or otherwise deface a report, it will appear as if you are trying to hide something.

If you realize that there is an error, or that you omitted information after a report has been submitted, you may still be able to correct it. In general, you may cross out an error as described above and write the correct information. Then, mark your initials and the date next to the new information.

Electronic Patient Care Reporting

Electronic patient care reporting is another form of documentation. Portable laptop computers (Figure 12–7) may be utilized by the EMR for initial documentation that is electronically passed over to a paramedic and ultimately to the hospital receiving the patient.

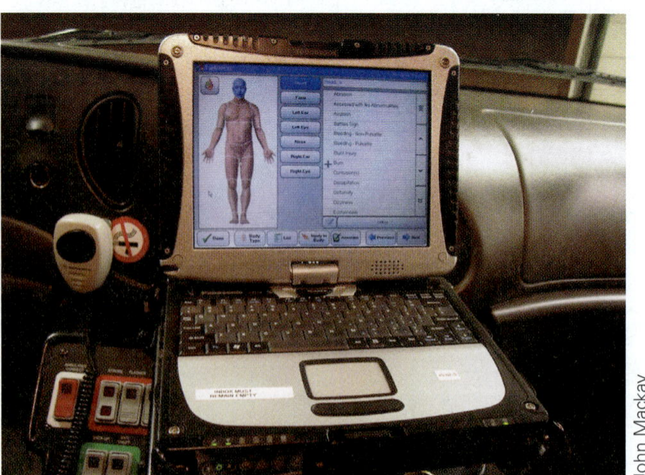

Figure 12–7 Electronic patient care reporting on a laptop computer.

Electronic patient care reports (E-PCRs) can display extensive checklists of patient signs, symptoms, and history (including medication information), which assist the caregiver in compiling pertinent patient information. Other benefits of E-PCRs can include:

- Identification information can be recorded for billing purposes.
- Statistical information for research purposes can be compiled more readily as it is already in an electronic format.
- Spell checkers and typed characters make a document easier to read.
- The need for paper is reduced. (Patient care reports can be printed when necessary.)

The idea of learning to use an E-PCR can be intimidating for an EMR who does not often use computers. However, the specific functions and programming that are set up on a laptop computer used for reporting by EMRs have proven very user friendly. Some medics who have been introduced to electronic patient care reporting have subsequently purchased their own computer system for professional, educational, and other personal use.

Confidentiality

During an emergency call, you will observe how a patient lives, the condition of the home, and his or her relationships with others. You will also be given a personal medical history. Whether the patient is a celebrity or private individual, you must respect his or her privacy. Everything you see, hear, and document at the scene is confidential. It cannot be disclosed to anyone except in very specific circumstances (see Chapter 3).

Patient Refusal

Patient refusal is a major cause of lawsuits against EMS providers. Remember, a competent adult has the right to refuse care and transport. However, it is your responsibility to advise this patient of the risks associated with that refusal.

As described in detail in Chapter 3, before allowing a patient to refuse, take the following steps:

- Make sure the patient is competent and can make a rational, informed decision.
- Try to persuade the patient to accept EMS care and transport.
- Advise the patient of the risks associated with refusing care.
- Consult the medical director, as required by local protocol.

Document each of these points thoroughly. This includes the patient assessment you performed, that you offered care and transport, and that you were willing to respond again at any time the patient desired. Be aware that cancelling a call on the scene or not transporting a patient ("treatment but no transport" call) could constitute abandonment if you cannot provide documentation showing that it was reasonable to do so. Some systems may expect you to have the patient sign a refusal or release from liability form. Other EMS systems prefer to have paramedics respond and speak to the patient. Follow all local protocols.

Special Situations

Special incident reports may be required for infectious disease exposure, injury to EMS personnel, conflicts between agencies, multiple-casualty incidents, and other situations. Since these situations can be very stressful, be sure to stick to the facts when you fill out the reports. They must be accurate and objective accounts in order to serve their purposes well.

One such special situation is the multiple-casualty incident. When there are many patients present in an emergency, there may not be time to provide full documentation on each one. This does not mean that records can be ignored or prepared poorly. Most EMS systems have special tags that are used to record patient information (see Chapter 31). One copy of the tag remains on the patient, while another is kept for EMS records. Your local EMS plan for multiple-casualty incidents should explain the procedure for documentation.

EMR FOCUS

Many of the patients you deal with will not be seriously ill or injured. They will, however, be frightened. This is where your communication skills will be important. Never forget the importance of calming and reassuring the patient. If you have ever been a patient yourself, you will realize the importance of this concept.

Documentation is important for two reasons. First, the documentation you provide follows the patient wherever he or she goes. The information you note and pass on to the paramedics will be relayed to the hospital. Second, proper documentation is a form of legal survival. There is an old saying that is true even today: "If you didn't write it, it didn't happen." This means that if you forget to document the care you gave to a patient, it will appear as if you never gave it. This not only looks bad, but it could also be used against you if you were ever called to court.

While communication and documentation may seem less important than the other parts of a call, they are not. The way you communicate, both verbally and in writing, puts forth an image of you. Make it an image to be proud of.

CASE STUDY FOLLOW-UP

At the beginning of this chapter, you read that EMRs were on the scene with an elderly patient who refused emergency care. To see how the chapter skills apply, read the following account of how the call was completed.

ONGOING ASSESSMENT

We observed Mrs. Gherson as we continued to try to get her to accept care. We were concerned that she had a serious condition. We felt she really needed to go to the hospital. Before we could change her mind, the ambulance arrived.

TRANSFER OF CARE

When the paramedics arrived on the scene, we reported Mrs. Gherson's behaviour, pulse, respirations, medical history, and medication. Then we quickly planned how to explain to her the need to accept care and transport. I called Mrs. Gherson's friends away. This let the paramedics get close to the patient and allowed me to enlist their help in convincing Mrs. Gherson to accept transport. After a while, one of the women, Mrs. Porter, came back in and explained how worried she was. "If you could have seen yourself, Ingrid," she said. She was very convincing. Mrs. Gherson agreed to go. We helped the paramedics and then carefully documented our actions.

During a call a few weeks later, we saw Mrs. Porter. She told us that Mrs. Gherson had had a mini-stroke. She also said that the doctors were watching her more closely now.

Communication and documentation are key elements in every call you make. Be sure you are aware of your EMS system's related rules and regulations.

NOCPs

1.1 a Maintain patient dignity **S**
b Reflect professionalism through use of appropriate language **S**
j Function as patient advocate **A**
1.3 c Include all pertinent and required information on reports and medical records **S**
2.1 a Deliver an organized, accurate, and relevant report utilizing telecommunication devices **S**
b Deliver an organized, accurate, and relevant verbal report **S**
c Deliver an organized, accurate, and relevant patient history **S**
d Provide information to patients about their situation and how they will be cared for **S**

e Interact effectively with the patient, relatives, and bystanders who are in stressful situations **S**
f Speak in language appropriate to the listener **S**
g Use appropriate terminology **S**
2.2 a Record organized, accurate, and relevant patient information **S**
2.3 a Employ effective non-verbal behaviour **A**
b Practise active listening techniques **S**
c Establish trust and rapport with patients and colleagues **A**
2.4 a Treat others with respect **S**
b Employ empathy and compassion while providing care **S**

REVIEW QUESTIONS

Page references where answers may be found or supported are provided at the end of each question.

SECTION 1

1. What are the components of a radio communication system? Describe each one briefly. (p. 189)
2. How can you make sure your radio transmissions are clear? (p. 190)
3. What information should be conveyed when seeking radio medical direction? (p. 191)
4. How should you verify radio medical orders given by a physician? (p. 191)

5. What are some ways you can improve interpersonal communication? (pp. 191–192)

SECTION 2

6. What are the purposes of the pre-hospital care report? (p. 192)
7. What three categories of information does the pre-hospital care report include? (p. 192)
8. List four advantages of an E-PCR. (p. 194)
9. What are the three situations in which you may be required to make a special incident report? (p. 195)

CHAPTER 13

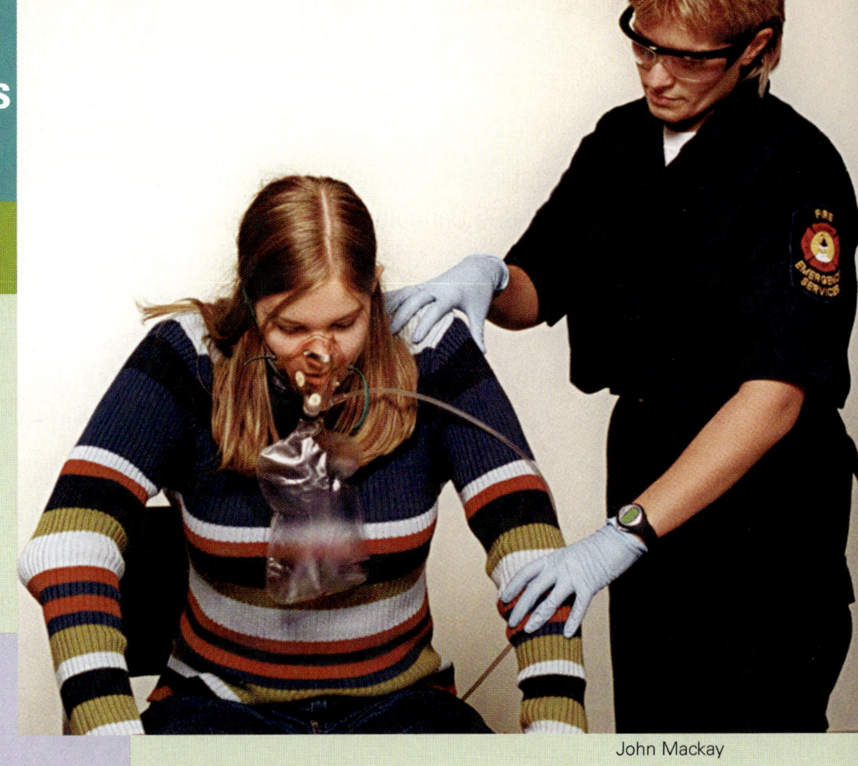

John Mackay

Cardiac and Respiratory Emergencies

OBJECTIVES

1. State seven signs and symptoms of a patient experiencing chest pain or discomfort and describe the emergency care for such a patient.

2. Discuss the cause and the signs and symptoms of the two common causes of chest pain or discomfort: angina pectoris and acute myocardial infarction.

3. List the signs of adequate breathing versus the signs and symptoms of a patient in respiratory distress.

4. Describe the emergency care of a patient in respiratory distress.

5. Discuss the anatomical and physiological aspects of the common causes of breathing difficulty, including chronic obstructive pulmonary disease, asthma, pneumonia, acute pulmonary edema, and hyperventilation.

6. Discuss the signs and symptoms of the five common causes of breathing difficulty.

7. Demonstrate a caring attitude toward the patient and family when dealing with a cardiac or respiratory emergency, while giving priority to the interests of the patient.

INTRODUCTION

Heart attacks and heart disease are the number one killers in Canada today. Each year, approximately 23 000 Canadians die from them.

Illnesses that affect the respiratory system are also very common. According to the Canadian Lung Association, one in five Canadians suffers from a breathing problem, and over 30 000 people die each year from respiratory diseases such as lung cancer, emphysema, and asthma.

Both types of problems—respiratory and cardiac—can be life threatening. When these problems occur, patients can benefit from immediate life-saving care.

SECTION 1
CARDIAC EMERGENCIES

Cardiac emergencies can result from abnormal heart rhythm patterns. They also occur when there is an interruption of oxygen supply to some part of the heart muscle. The reduction of oxygen causes chest pain or discomfort, one of the most common symptoms of a cardiac emergency.

Coronary artery disease affects the inner lining of the arteries that supply the heart with blood. People who have it usually suffer from arteriosclerosis, a condition that causes the walls of the arteries to become thick and hard.

In coronary artery disease, the opening of a coronary artery is narrowed (Figure 13–1). This restricts the amount of blood that can reach and nourish the heart. The rough artery surfaces then cause a buildup of debris, further narrowing the artery. The more the artery narrows, the less oxygen gets to the heart. At some point, the patient may have chest pain. When the artery becomes blocked, the patient may suffer a heart attack that results in death of the heart muscle.

Researchers have identified a number of cardiac risk factors that predispose a person to heart attack. Obviously, some factors cannot be controlled. With awareness and determination, however, a person can change other factors and decrease his or her own risk.

The major risk factors are as follows (Figure 13–2 on p. 200):

- Physical inactivity or a sedentary lifestyle
- Cigarette smoking
- Obesity
- High serum cholesterol and triglycerides
- Diabetes
- Male gender
- Age (incidence increases over 30 years of age)

- Hypertension (blood pressure above 140/84)
- Family history of coronary heart disease under age 60
- Oral contraceptive use in women over 40 years
- Drinking too much alcohol
- Stress
- Prolonged tension, frustration, or hostility

The risk for a patient with high cholesterol, high blood pressure, and a habit of heavy smoking is 10 times that of someone without those risk factors.

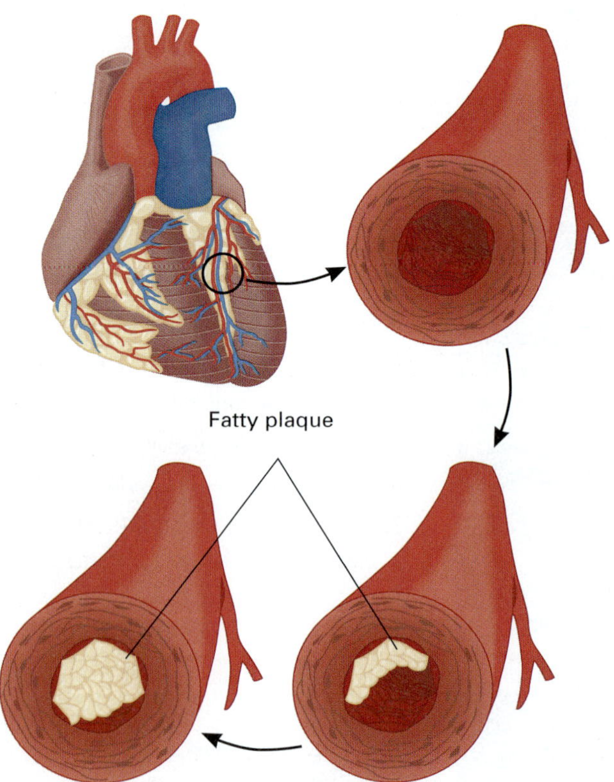

Figure 13–1 Fatty deposits build up in coronary arteries, depriving the heart muscle of blood and oxygen.

CASE STUDY

Dispatch

I was working at the plant during my regular 4 to 12 shift. I was also assigned to the emergency response team (ERT), which is responsible for HazMat problems and medical emergencies. At about 6:30 p.m., I heard our team paged to respond. A man was having chest pain.

Scene Assessment

I approached the scene and looked around. Other than the presence of a few concerned co-workers, everything was quiet. It appeared that there was only one patient. I recognized the man, Harry Nowack, because I used to work with him. He told me that his chest hurt.

Primary Assessment

Harry was alert. His airway was clear. He could speak in full sentences, but his breathing was laboured. He had no obvious external bleeding. Harry told me that he didn't fall or have any injuries. "My chest just hurts," he said. I couldn't help but notice Harry's colour. He looked ashen, which was definitely not normal.

I radioed my findings to the plant office and told them to call 9-1-1. I told them that my general impression was that of an alert 55-year-old man who had chest pain, poor colour, and laboured breathing. The ETA of the ambulance was 10 minutes.

> What do you think this patient's problem may be? What should be done to assess and treat his condition? Consider this patient as you read Chapter 13.

There are many reasons why a patient may develop a condition that leads to a cardiac emergency. An EMR's assessment and treatment of a patient with chest pain will be the same no matter what the actual cause.

Patient Assessment

Signs and Symptoms

The general signs and symptoms of a cardiac emergency are as follows (Figure 13–3):

- Chest pain or discomfort described as heaviness or squeezing, which may radiate to the arms, shoulder, neck, or jaw
- Difficulty breathing, shortness of breath
- Unusual pulse (rapid, weak, slow, or irregular)
- Indigestion, nausea, vomiting
- Sweating
- Pale, grey, or cyanotic skin colour, including mucous membranes
- A feeling of impending doom
- Anxiety or irritability

It is likely that when you gather a medical history, the patient will tell you he or she has a history of heart problems or has had a previous similar experience.

Remember that a patient with chest pain will be very anxious. The patient may feel as if he or she is going to die. This requires compassion and reassurance. Be sure he or she understands that everything that can possibly be done is being done. Advise the patient and family that further help is on the way and that he or she will be transported promptly to a medical facility.

Update incoming EMS units. Request advanced care if it is available in your area. Monitor the patient because he or she may rapidly become unstable.

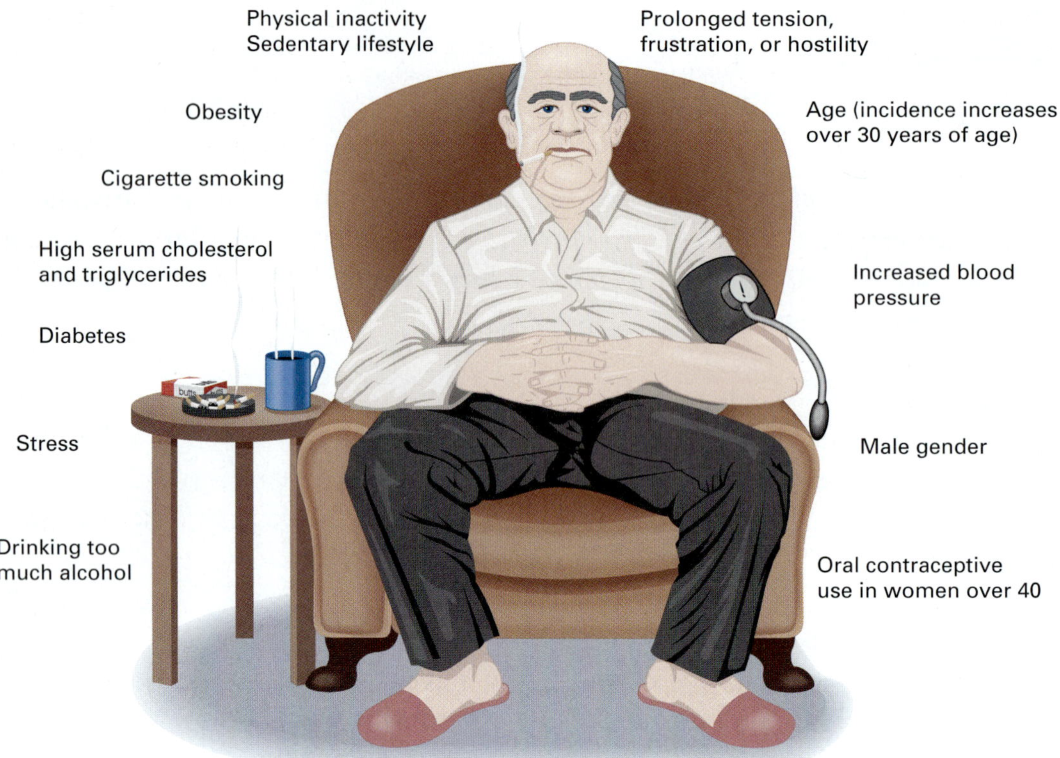

Figure 13–2 Major risk factors for coronary artery disease and heart attack.

Chest Pain and Cardiac Patients

Continue to monitor the patient's airway and breathing during and after the primary assessment. Patients who experience chest pain may need airway maintenance and ventilation. Be alert for changes in the patient's mental status. These patients can lose consciousness rapidly. If the patient becomes unconscious,

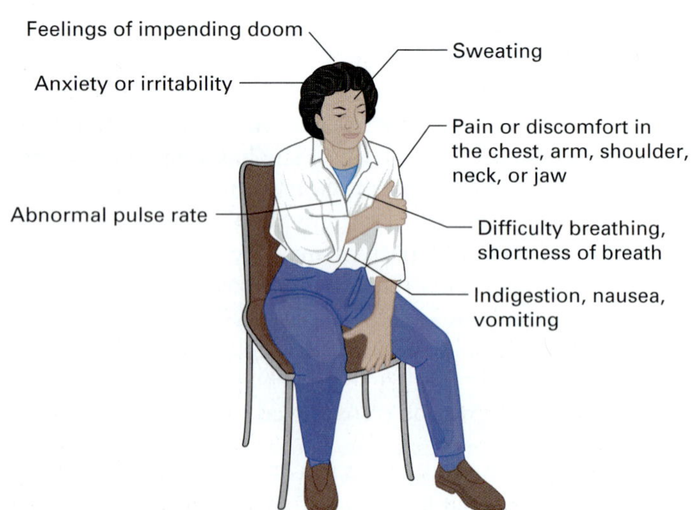

Figure 13-3 Signs and symptoms of a cardiac emergency.

be prepared to perform CPR and, if you are trained, to use an SAED.

When you take a SAMPLE history, you may also want to use the **OPQRRRST** mnemonic to help you get a good description of the pain. Each letter identifies an important area of questioning:

O — Onset. When did the pain begin?

P — Provocation. Did anything cause or start the pain (exercise, an activity)?

Q — Quality. What is the pain like (crushing, stabbing, etc.)?

R — Region. Where is the pain?

R — Radiation. Does the pain begin in one place and then seem to travel somewhere else?

R — Relief. Does anything relieve the pain?

S — Severity. On a scale of 1 to 10, with 10 the worst, how bad is the pain?

T — Time. How long have you had the pain?

When you perform a secondary assessment, palpate the chest for DOTS. Make a note if your touch causes pain. If you are trained to do so, listen to the lungs to determine if air is moving in and out of both sides equally.

General Guidelines for Emergency Care

When the patient's chief complaint is chest pain, be prepared to provide CPR in case he or she becomes pulseless. If possible, you should perform CPR with supplemental oxygen by way of a pocket face mask, or bag-valve-mask device. (See Chapters 7–9 for details on basic life support techniques.)

To provide emergency care, first be sure you have taken BSI precautions. Then proceed as follows:

1. Have the patient cease all movement.
2. Place the conscious patient in a position of comfort. This is usually a semi-reclining or sitting position.
3. Make sure that the airway is open. Administer high-flow oxygen with a non-rebreather mask. (Follow local protocol.) If needed, provide artificial ventilation or CPR.
4. Loosen tight clothing.
5. Maintain body temperature as close to normal as possible.
6. Comfort and reassure the patient.
7. If not done previously, activate the EMS system immediately.

Your patient may tell you that he or she has had heart surgery. Your patient may also tell you he or she has a pacemaker or an implanted defibrillator. (An implanted defibrillator delivers shocks to a patient but at much less voltage than an SAED.) Treat these patients in the same way as described above. Note that a malfunctioning pacemaker may cause a slow heart rhythm. If this occurs, monitor the patient carefully. Provide oxygen and be prepared to administer CPR if necessary.

Specific Cardiac Conditions

Two problems are commonly caused by coronary artery disease—angina pectoris, often called angina, and myocardial infarction, the medical term for heart attack.

The emergency care of patients with angina or myocardial infarction is the same. It is not necessary to differentiate between the two. Taking time to do so might even be harmful. Chest pain patients need prompt care and constant monitoring. Early access to the EMS system and rapid transport to a hospital can literally make the difference between life and death.

Angina Pectoris

The term *angina pectoris* literally means pain in the chest. As you know, the heart relies on a constant supply of oxygen. If it does not get enough because of diseased or narrowed arteries, the patient experiences chest pain or discomfort.

Most often angina occurs as a result of physical activity beyond the patient's limit, emotional stress, or extreme hot or cold weather. Sometimes, though rarely, it has no apparent cause.

Angina is reversible. It does not cause permanent damage to the heart muscle. Generally, the pain is relieved by rest, usually within a few minutes after the patient stops the activity, calms down, moves indoors, or takes nitroglycerin as prescribed by a physician.

Angina can change from a mild ache to a severe crushing pain. It can appear suddenly, but is usually associated with physical exertion. It is usually in the chest, but can radiate to the jaw, neck, left shoulder, left arm, or left hand. It is often mistaken for indigestion. Note that angina does not always manifest itself as pain. It may be a feeling of tightness, gripping, heaviness, squeezing, burning, or a dull constriction.

Other signs and symptoms include the following:

- Shortness of breath
- Profuse sweating
- Light-headedness
- Palpitations (a sensation of throbbing or fluttering of the heart)
- Nausea, vomiting
- Pale, cool, moist skin
- Anxiety
- Denial

It is impossible for you to tell the difference between the pain of angina and the pain of a heart attack. Though angina usually leaves the heart undamaged, if it is left untreated, it may eventually cause a heart attack.

Acute Myocardial Infarction

The term *myocardial infarction* means death of the heart muscle. When blood to a part of the heart is blocked off or greatly reduced, that part dies. Myocardial infarction is most commonly caused by blockage as a result of coronary artery disease.

Myocardial infarction, or heart attack, has four serious consequences:

- *Sudden death.* Of the heart attack patients who die before reaching a hospital, most die within two hours of the first signs and symptoms.
- *Shock.* If 40 percent or more of the left ventricle is damaged after an attack, the heart cannot pump the proper amount of blood to the body. Shock usually occurs within 24 hours, with a mortality rate of about 80 percent.

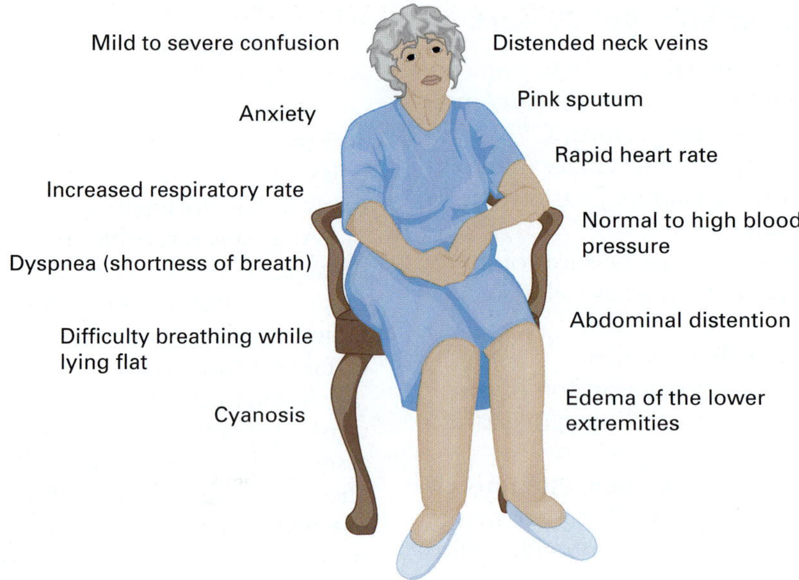

Figure 13–4 Signs and symptoms of congestive heart failure.

- *Congestive heart failure.* This condition may develop after a heart attack. It causes a buildup of fluid, which may accumulate in the lungs (pulmonary edema) and in other parts of the body. This is sometimes observed as swelling in the ankles (Figure 13–4).
- *Cardiac dysrhythmias.* These are the abnormal heart rhythms that follow a heart attack. They are generally caused by injury to the electrical conduction system of the heart.

The most common symptom of a heart attack is a sudden onset of chest pain. About 80 percent of all heart attack patients experience it. Many also have abnormal heart rhythms and may suffer nausea and vomiting. Note that 20 percent of all heart attack patients have no chest pain at all. (This is usually in senior citizens or in patients with diabetes.) A heart attack without pain is called a silent myocardial infarction.

Chest pain associated with a heart attack ranges from mild discomfort to severe pain. The sensation felt by the patient may be described as pain, crushing, tightness, or numbness. It usually lasts longer than 30 minutes. Though the pain can be experienced in a number of ways, the common location is substernal, radiating to the neck, jaw, left shoulder, and left arm (Figure 13–5). It often includes the burning and bloating sensations of indigestion. It can be continuous. It might subside, but do not ignore it even if it does. Any adult with pain or discomfort in the chest, neck, shoulder, arm, or jaw should be suspected of having a heart attack. Treat the patient accordingly.

Other signs and symptoms include the following:

- Sudden onset of weakness, nausea and vomiting, and profuse sweating without a clear cause
- Pain not related to physical exertion and not relieved by rest
- Abnormal pulse, which may be rapid (over 100), slow (below 60), or irregular
- Difficulty breathing or rapid, shallow respirations
- Cool, pale, moist skin and possible cyanosis
- Light-headedness, loss of consciousness
- Frightened appearance, anxiety, feelings of impending doom

SECTION 2
RESPIRATORY EMERGENCIES

Without oxygen, cells such as those in the brain and heart can die within minutes. A variety of diseases and injuries can affect the body's ability to get enough oxygen. The need for rapid treatment in these cases is essential.

Patient Assessment

As you learned in Chapter 7, adequate breathing occurs at a normal rate. For adults, that is 12 to 20 breaths per minute. For children, it is 20 to 40 breaths per minute. For infants, it is 24 to 60 breaths

EARLY SIGNS OF HEART ATTACK

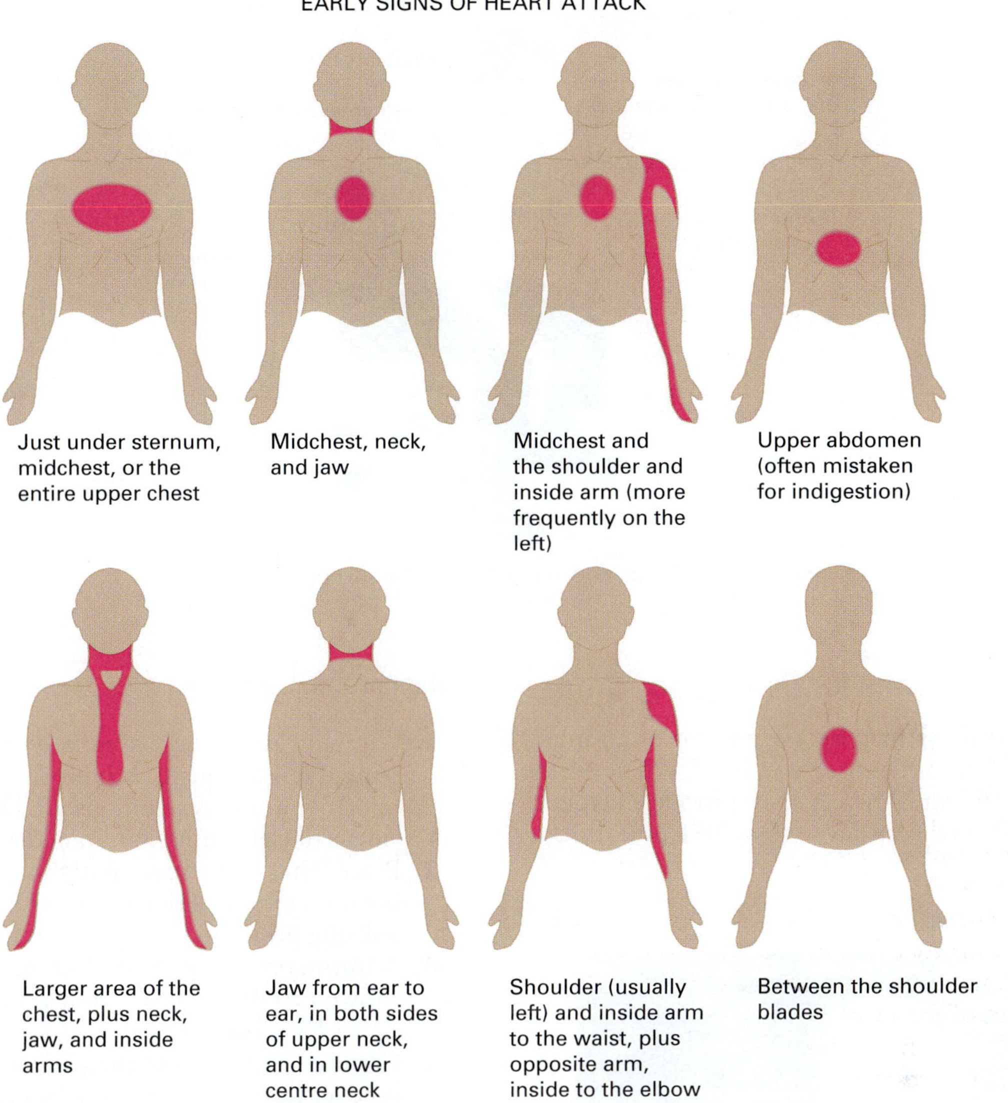

Figure 13–5 Pain or discomfort related to a heart attack can occur in any one location or any combination of locations.

per minute. Adequate breathing is regular in rhythm and free of unusual sounds, such as wheezing or whistling. The chest should expand adequately and equally with each breath. The depth of the breaths should also be adequate. In addition, breathing should be effortless. This means it should be accomplished without the use of accessory muscles in the neck, shoulders, or abdomen.

Respiratory Distress

Respiratory distress is shortness of breath, or a feeling of air hunger, with laboured breathing. It is one of the most common medical complaints. Two circumstances may cause respiratory distress. Either air cannot pass easily into the lungs or air cannot pass easily out of them. Signs and symptoms include the following (Figure 13–6):

- Inability to speak in full sentences without pausing to breathe
- Noisy breathing
- Use of accessory muscles to breathe (muscles in the neck, abdomen, or between the ribs)
- Patient in tripod position (sitting upright, leaning forward) (Figure 13–7)
- Abnormal breathing rate and rhythm
- Increased pulse rate
- Skin colour changes (pale, flushed, or cyanotic)
- Altered mental status

Generally, breathing will be rapid and shallow. Patients may feel short of breath, whether they are breathing rapidly or slowly. Remember, a certain amount of shortness of breath is normal following exercise, fatigue, coughing, or with the production of excessive sputum.

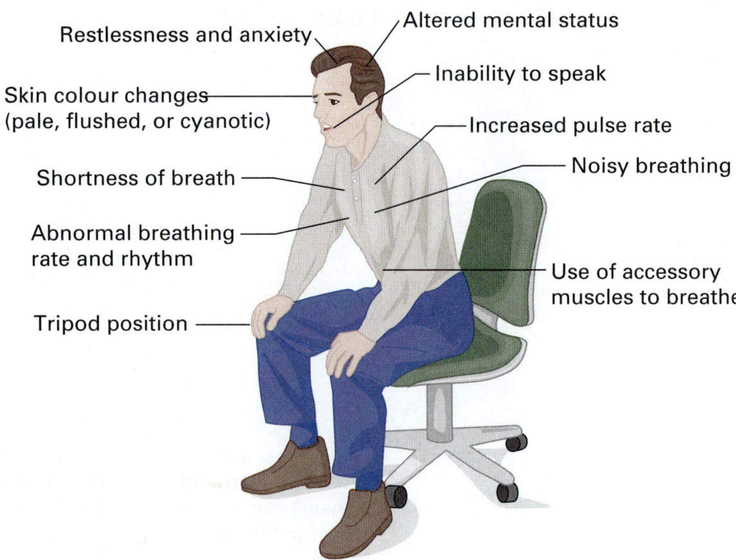

Figure 13–6 Signs and symptoms of breathing difficulty.

General Guidelines for Emergency Care

Respiratory distress may be a symptom of an injury or an illness. It is not a disease in itself. Whatever the cause, the treatment is the same. To provide emergency care, first be sure you have taken BSI precautions.

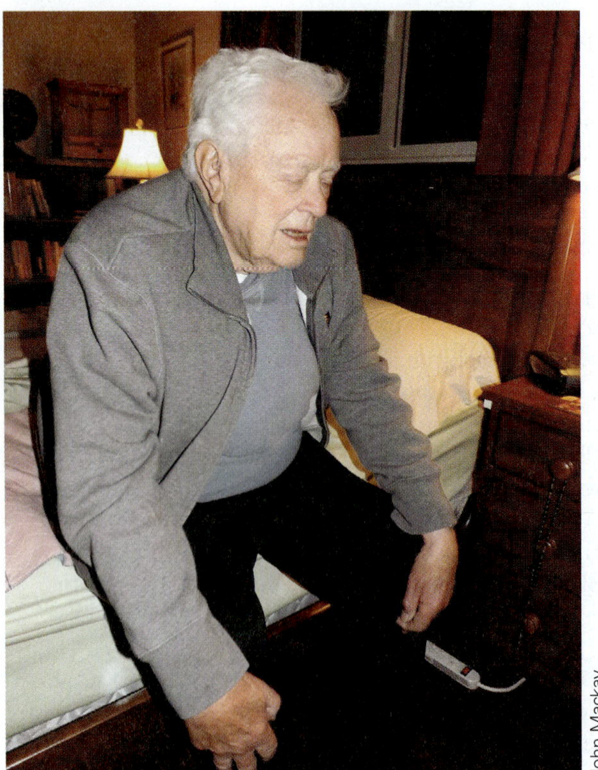

Figure 13–7 Patients with emphysema and chronic bronchitis often lean forward as they breathe.

Then proceed as follows:

1. Carefully assess the patient's breathing to determine if it is adequate. Monitor it throughout the call. If you find respirations are inadequate, provide artificial ventilation immediately.
2. Place the conscious patient with adequate breathing in a position of comfort. This is usually a sitting position.
3. Administer oxygen if you are trained and allowed to do so. Use a non-rebreather mask at 12 to 15 L/min.
4. Comfort and reassure the patient. There are few experiences as terrifying as not being able to breathe. Because of this fear, the patient may become agitated or even angry. Do not take it personally.
5. If not done previously, update en route paramedics.

Specific Respiratory Conditions

The following conditions are among the breathing problems you will commonly see in the field: chronic obstructive pulmonary disease (COPD), asthma, pneumonia, acute pulmonary edema, and hyperventilation syndrome. Remember that although respiratory distress has a variety of causes, EMR treatment is always the same.

Chronic Obstructive Pulmonary Disease

Emphysema and chronic bronchitis are the most common forms of COPD.

In emphysema, the alveoli lose their elasticity, become distended with trapped air, and stop working. As the total number of alveoli decreases, breathing becomes more and more difficult.

Chronic bronchitis is characterized by inflammation, edema, and excessive mucus in the bronchial tree. It features a productive cough that persists for at least three months in one year for two consecutive years. With proper medication and a good exercise program, patients who get medical help early can lead fairly normal lives.

The most important known factor to cause COPD is cigarette smoking. COPD is more common in men than in women. Urban air pollution also plays a role therefore COPD is also more common among city dwellers than among rural populations.

People with COPD usually get colds or the flu often. They also become winded under conditions that do not tax most healthy people (such as walking on a level surface). Other signs and symptoms of COPD include the following:

- Shortness of breath, gasping for air
- Tripod position
- Bulging neck veins
- Coarse rattling sounds in the lungs
- Cyanosis
- Prolonged exhaling through pursed lips
- Barrel-shaped chest (typical with emphysema)
- Presence of home oxygen systems, breathing treatments, medications, and inhaler (puffer) medicines

Both emphysema and chronic bronchitis patients may develop a hypoxic drive to breathe. Healthy people get their drive to breathe from the amount of carbon dioxide in the blood. Patients who have emphysema or chronic bronchitis build up consistently high levels of carbon dioxide. Because of this, the body looks to the level of oxygen, rather than carbon dioxide, to determine the need to breathe. If oxygen levels are low, they breathe faster to get more oxygen.

Giving oxygen to a patient with hypoxic drive can be a problem. After oxygen is administered, its level in the blood increases. In the patient with a true hypoxic drive, increased levels of oxygen may signal the body to slow down or even stop breathing. However, this is rarely encountered in the field.

The general rule is to administer oxygen to all patients who need it. All patients with difficulty breathing, cyanosis, altered mental status, shock, or other signs of a serious condition should be given high-concentration oxygen by a non-rebreather mask. All patients in respiratory or cardiac arrest should receive high concentrations of supplemental oxygen by a pocket face mask, BVM device, or resuscitator.

Asthma

According to the Canadian Lung Association, asthma is the most chronic respiratory disease in children and accounts for one-fourth of all school absenteeism.

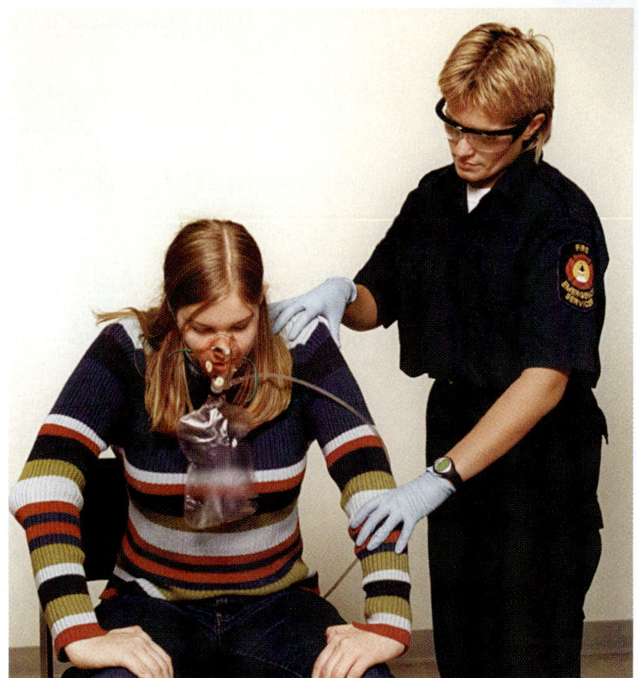

Figure 13–8 Reassure an asthma patient to help reduce stress and fear.

John Mackay

About 500 people die from it every year. Asthma is most common among children and middle-aged women, and it is often present in more than one member of the same family.

Typically, persons with asthma are free of symptoms between attacks. They often do not know what causes the attacks. Many attacks begin while the patient is asleep.

The acute asthma attack varies in duration, intensity, and frequency. It involves airway obstruction due to bronchospasm, swelling of mucous membranes in the bronchial walls, or plugging of the bronchi by thick mucus.

Signs and symptoms of an asthma attack include the following (Figure 13–8):

- Tripod position
- Spasmodic, apparently unproductive cough
- High-pitched wheezing during exhalation (may also occur upon inhalation)
- Very little movement of air during breathing
- Overinflated chest, with air trapped in the lungs
- Rapid, shallow respirations
- Rapid pulse, often exceeding 120
- Fatigue, confusion, agitation, lethargy
- Inability to speak in full sentences without catching breath

Status asthmaticus is a severe, life-threatening, prolonged asthma attack. It is a dire medical emergency (Figure 13–9). The patient may begin shallow breathing or may stop breathing altogether.

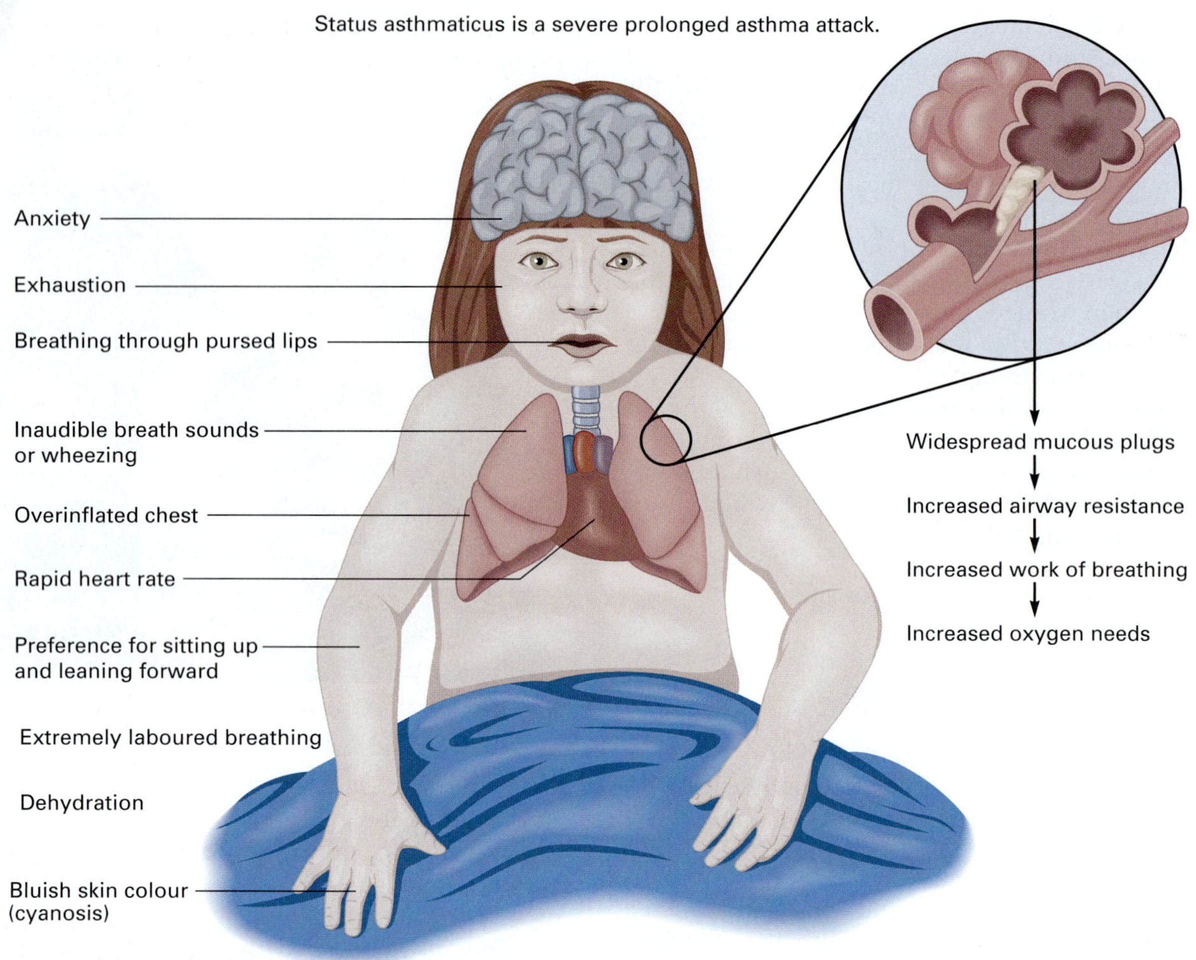

Figure 13–9 Status asthmaticus is a dire medical emergency.

In these cases, the wheezing may stop and it may appear that the patient has improved, but this is not true. Watch all asthma patients carefully for reduced respirations. Be prepared to provide artificial ventilation. Signs and symptoms of status asthmaticus include the following:

- Anxiety, exhaustion
- Breathing through pursed lips
- Wheezing at first, then inaudible breath sounds
- Overinflated chest
- Rapid heart rate
- Tripod position
- Extremely laboured breathing
- Cyanosis
- Walking and talking only with great effort

Caution: All that wheezes is not asthma. Many other diseases and conditions can cause wheezing: acute congestive heart failure, smoke inhalation, chronic bronchitis, anaphylaxis, and acute pulmonary embolism. If they are in respiratory distress, all patients with wheezing should be treated with high-flow oxygen by non-rebreather mask.

Pneumonia

Pneumonia is a term used to describe a group of illnesses characterized by lung infection and fluid- or pus-filled alveoli. Both these conditions lead to inadequately oxygenated blood. Pneumonia is most frequently caused by bacteria or viruses. It may also be caused by inhaled irritants, such as smoke, or by aspirated materials, such as vomit.

Pneumonia patients generally appear ill. Most complain of fever and chills that can produce uncontrollable shaking. Signs and symptoms may be influenced by the area of the lung that is affected. For example, pneumonia of the lower lobes of the lungs may not produce a cough but may cause abdominal pain. In general, look for the following:

- Chest pain, usually made worse with breathing
- Rapid breathing
- Respiratory distress
- Productive cough with pus in the sputum
- Fever, usually exceeding 38°C
- Chills
- Hot, dry skin

Acute Pulmonary Edema

Acute pulmonary edema can be caused by damage to the heart or lungs. It occurs when extra fluids build up in the tissues around the spaces of the lungs. If you know your patient has acute pulmonary edema, and he or she is conscious and in a sitting position, let the legs dangle to encourage blood to pool in the legs. You can also support the back and shoulders with pillows.

Signs and symptoms of acute pulmonary edema include the following:

- Shortness of breath
- Rapid, laboured breathing
- Cyanosis
- Frothy, pink, blood-tinged sputum (a late sign)
- Bulging neck veins
- Rapid pulse
- Cool, clammy skin
- Restlessness
- Anxiety
- Exhaustion

Note that oxygen therapy may be critical to this patient. Be sure to administer oxygen if you are trained and allowed to do so. Also, monitor breathing and other vital signs carefully until medical help arrives.

Hyperventilation Syndrome

Hyperventilation is a condition characterized by breathing too fast. It is normal for most people in certain situations, such as when they are surprised. It is considered normal as long as the rate of breathing quickly returns to normal.

Hyperventilation syndrome is an abnormal state in which rapid breathing persists. It is a common disorder usually associated with anxiety. As the patient becomes more anxious, he or she breathes more rapidly, which in turn makes the patient more anxious, creating a vicious cycle.

The syndrome is characterized by rapid, deep, or abnormal breathing. The lungs overinflate, and the patient blows out too much carbon dioxide. In prolonged cases, the patient may pass out. It typically occurs in young, anxious patients, most of whom are not aware that they are breathing too fast.

Signs and symptoms include the following:

- Air hunger or gulping air
- Deep, sighing, rapid breathing with rapid pulse
- Sensation of choking
- Dryness or bitterness of the mouth
- Tightness or a lump in the throat
- Marked anxiety escalating to panic and a feeling of impending doom
- Dizziness, light-headedness, fainting
- Giddiness or unusual behaviour
- Drawing up the hands at the wrist and knuckles with the fingers flexed
- Blurred vision
- Numbness or tingling of the hands and feet or around the mouth
- Pounding of the heart with stabbing pains in the chest
- Fatigue, great tiredness, or weakness
- A feeling of being in a dream

Not every patient who is breathing rapidly or deeply is hyperventilating. Several serious conditions may be the cause, including diabetes, asthma, or trauma. Hyperventilation may also be related to a medication, such as an ASA overdose. If you are certain that no life-threatening condition exists, then try to calm your patient. Be reassuring and listen carefully to his or her concerns. Try to talk the patient into breathing slowly. If the patient does not respond immediately to your efforts, then administer oxygen. It will not make hyperventilation worse.

You may have heard that having a patient breathe into a paper bag is a cure for hyperventilation. This treatment is dangerous, especially if an underlying medical condition exists. As noted above, calming offers a powerful benefit to the hyperventilating patient. Follow local protocol.

EMR FOCUS

The condition of a patient with respiratory distress or chest pain can deteriorate rapidly. Make sure paramedics have been notified, and be prepared to provide basic life support as soon as it is needed. Also, remember that artificial ventilation is not only for patients in respiratory arrest. Be prepared to provide ventilations if your patient is breathing inadequately. You may want to review Chapters 7, 8, and 9 at this time.

Few things are more frightening than chest pain or not being able to breathe. A patient with either problem may be anxious, argumentative, and scared. Do your best to be calming and reassuring. If the patient yells or snaps at you, realize that he or she is reacting to the situation and not to you personally.

CASE STUDY FOLLOW-UP

At the beginning of this chapter, you read that an EMR was caring for a patient with chest pain, laboured breathing, and poor skin colour. To see how the chapter skills apply to this emergency, read the following. It describes how the call was completed.

SECONDARY ASSESSMENT

Two other members of EMS arrived to help. They performed a head-to-toe exam while I talked to Harry about his history.

PATIENT HISTORY

Harry told me that he was working at his bench when he started having severe pain in his chest. He had never felt anything like it before, and I had never seen Harry that scared. I reassured him and asked a few questions using the OPQRRRST mnemonic.

Harry had been working when the pain came on. He told me it was crushing, like someone sitting right on the centre of his chest. He held his fist there to show me. The pain didn't radiate. Nothing, he said, helped to relieve the pain. On a scale of 1 to 10, he said the pain was an 8. It had started about 10 minutes before.

Harry hadn't seen a doctor in years. He took no medication and had no medical problems or allergies. He had eaten a big spaghetti dinner during his break. When I checked Harry's vital signs—pulse 92 and irregular, respirations 18 and adequate, blood pressure 146/96, with skin that was cool, grey, and moist—I began to wish our plant had an SAED.

ONGOING ASSESSMENT

After helping make Harry comfortable, I continued to talk and to reassure him. We rechecked his ABCs, which remained okay. The chest pain did not diminish. A second assessment of vital signs revealed a pulse of 96 and irregular, and respirations 20 and slightly laboured. Unfortunately, we didn't have oxygen to give him.

TRANSFER OF CARE

The paramedics arrived a short time later. We immediately called their attention to Harry's chief complaint of chest pain and to his poor colour and laboured breathing to let them know how serious we thought his condition was. They agreed. Then we filled them in on the rest:

> "This is Harry Nowack, 55 years old. His chest pain started while he was working. It is in the centre of his chest and is crushing. It is an 8 out of 10 on the scale, and it doesn't radiate. He has no medical problems that he knows of, but he hasn't been to a doctor in years. He has no meds or allergies. He ate a big spaghetti dinner a short time ago. His pulse is 96 and irregular, respirations 20 and slightly laboured, blood pressure 146/96."

The paramedics thanked us, and I helped them put the oxygen on Harry. He wanted me to come with him, and the paramedics didn't mind some help. I made sure that someone called Harry's wife.

It turned out that Harry had had a major heart attack. The word spread around the plant the next day. The way he looked was just as it is described in the books. I always take chest pain seriously. I'm glad we did with Harry.

Problems with cardiac and respiratory systems are frequently the reason why EMRs are summoned. Quickly recognizing these problems as potentially life threatening and making sure the proper medical help is on the way can save your patient's life. Also, keep in mind that these emergencies require compassionate emotional care as well as management of the patient's physical condition.

NOCPs

4.3 c Conduct cardiovascular system assessment and interpret findings **S**

e Conduct respiratory system assessment and interpret findings **S**

6.1 a Provide care to patient experiencing signs and symptoms involving cardiovascular system **S**

c Provide care to patient experiencing signs and symptoms involving respiratory system **S**

6.2 c Provide care for geriatric patient **A**

REVIEW QUESTIONS

Page references where answers may be found or supported are provided at the end of each question.

SECTION 1

1. What are the risk factors for heart disease? (p. 198)
2. What are the signs and symptoms of a cardiac emergency? (p. 199)
3. What is the emergency care for chest pain? (p. 201)

SECTION 2

4. What are four signs and symptoms of respiratory distress in a patient? (p. 203)

5. What is the emergency medical care for respiratory distress? (p. 204)
6. What two conditions are considered the most common types of COPD? (p. 204)
7. What is hypoxic drive? Describe how it works. (p. 205)
8. What is the most common respiratory disease in children? (p. 205)
9. What is the most common cause of hyperventilation syndrome? (p. 207)

14

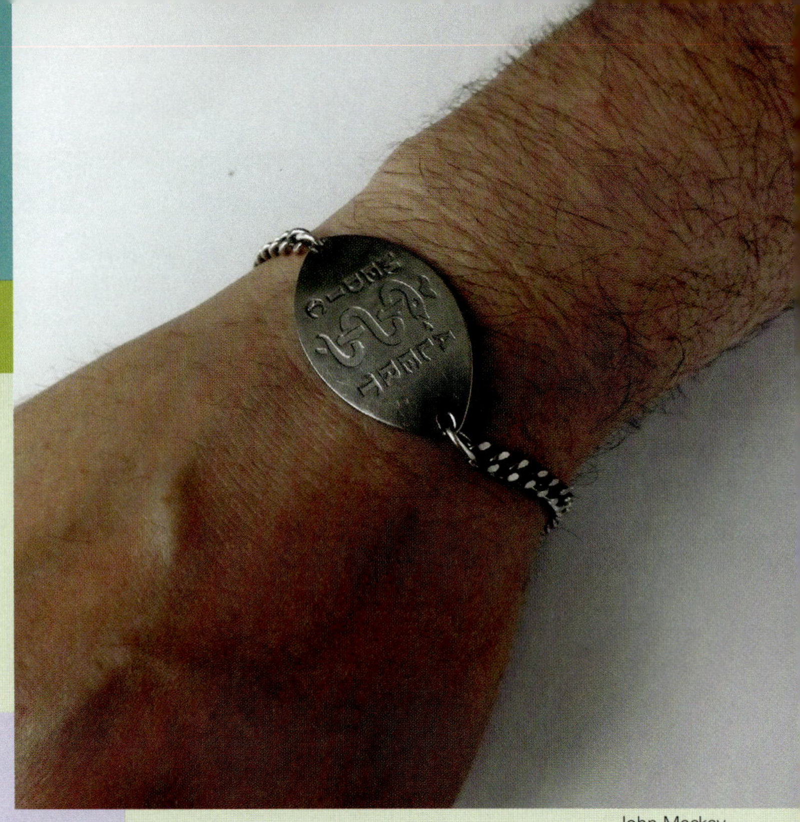

John Mackay

Other Common Medical Complaints

OBJECTIVES

1. Identify the three steps of emergency medical care for a patient with a general medical complaint.
2. List eight possible reasons for altered mental status.
3. Compare hypoglycemia and hyperglycemia, including causes, signs and symptoms, and treatment.
4. List the four routes through which poisons can enter the body and describe the signs and symptoms and treatment of a patient who has been poisoned by each route.
5. Explain how to recognize stroke in a patient.
6. Describe the steps in providing emergency medical care to a patient having a seizure.
7. List the three steps of emergency care for a patient with abdominal pain.
8. Demonstrate a caring attitude toward the patient and family when dealing with a general or specific medical complaint, while giving priority to the interests of the patient.

INTRODUCTION

A medical complaint is any chief complaint that is not caused by trauma. There will be many such calls in your career. They may involve abdominal pain, altered mental status, or even such general complaints as "I don't feel well." As with any patient, your responsibility in the emergency care of these patients is to follow your patient assessment plan from scene assessment to patient hand-off.

SECTION 1
GENERAL MEDICAL COMPLAINTS

As an EMR, you will be called to scenes where patients have specific medical complaints, such as "My chest hurts" or "I can't breathe." Every once in a while, however, your medical patient will have a general complaint, such as "I feel weak" or "I don't feel well."

Handle patients with a general medical complaint the same as you would those with a specific complaint. After your scene assessment, complete a primary assessment and treat any life-threatening conditions you observe. Perform a secondary assessment, as needed, and be especially thorough in gathering the patient's history. It could provide important clues to the underlying problem.

If you are unable to determine a more specific complaint or to obtain a pertinent history, do the following:

1. Monitor the airway and breathing. Be sure there is a patent airway with adequate breathing and circulation.
2. If the patient is conscious and there are no suspected spinal injuries, allow the patient to get into a position of comfort.
3. Perform an ongoing assessment until the incoming paramedics take over patient care. Be sure to report any changes in the patient's condition.

These patients may be just as frightened and worried as patients with more specific problems. Consider their feelings as you assess and care for them. Be gentle and empathetic. If the family is present, they may be very concerned and ask you to tell them what is wrong. Be truthful but kind. For example, you might tell them that although you do not know exactly what the problem is, you are doing all that is possible. Also, reassure them that you have arranged for the patient to be transported to a hospital.

SECTION 2
SPECIFIC MEDICAL COMPLAINTS

Altered Mental Status

A change in a patient's normal level of consciousness and awareness is called altered mental status. It can occur quickly or slowly. It can range from disoriented to combative to unconscious. There are many medical reasons for it. A few examples are as follows:

- **Hypoxia** (decreased levels of oxygen in the blood)
- **Hypoglycemia** (low blood sugar)
- Stroke (loss of blood flow to part of the brain)
- Seizures
- Fever, infection
- Poisoning, including drug and alcohol poisoning
- Head injury
- Psychiatric conditions

As an EMR, you do not need to figure out why your patient has an altered mental status. Your job is to recognize it as soon as possible and to support the patient appropriately. After ensuring scene safety, proceed with patient assessment. Gather an accurate patient history. Do so as soon as appropriate. A patient with altered mental status may deteriorate rapidly. If you wait too long, the history could be lost to the paramedics and hospital staff who take over care. A history of diabetes or seizures, for example, may be important to the paramedics and hospital personnel when they try to determine the cause of the altered mental status.

Emergency care of a patient with altered mental status is as follows:

1. *Assess and monitor the patient's airway and breathing closely.* These patients may not be able to protect their own airway. It is up to you to be aware of this danger. If the patient is unconscious,

CASE STUDY

Dispatch

My partner and I were making rounds on the trails when a group of hikers stopped us. It seemed that an older gentleman was supposed to have packed out that day. Several hikers remarked that he had looked sick. They asked us to check on him. We did.

Scene Assessment

As we approached the man's lean-to, we saw a supine body. We quickly did a scene assessment. There were no mechanisms of injury or obvious dangers, so we put on our gloves and approached the patient.

Primary Assessment

Our general impression was of an elderly male with a medical emergency. He was conscious to verbal stimuli, but his speech was slurred. His airway was patent. His breathing was adequate. Oxygen may have improved his altered mental status, but we didn't carry it on the trail. The patient's radial pulse was slow, strong, and regular. There was no evidence of external bleeding, but he was very pale. We were worried. We radioed our office to request immediate air medical evacuation.

> Consider this scenario as you read Chapter 14. What else may be done to assess and care for this patient?

secure the airway with an adjunct. Suction the airway as needed.

2. *Position the patient.* If there is no reason to suspect head or spinal injury, place the patient in a recovery position. Continue to monitor the patient's breathing closely.

3. *Administer high-flow oxygen.* One of the most common causes of altered mental status is hypoxia. Therefore, if the patient is breathing adequately, apply high-flow oxygen via a nonrebreather mask. If the patient is not breathing adequately, assist with a BVM device attached to an oxygen source. If you cannot provide oxygen, be prepared to assist ventilations.

A patient with altered mental status may be aware of his or her condition. This can be very frightening. If the patient has had a seizure, he or she could lose control of the bowels and bladder, which adds to his or her embarrassment and anxiety. A caring attitude on your part, as well as maintaining the patient's privacy, will help.

The patient's condition may also be very upsetting to the family. Take time, if possible, to make sure they understand that you are caring for the patient and that an ambulance is on the way.

Information on the following conditions that may involve altered mental status will be presented in this section: hyperglycemia and hypoglycemia, poisoning, stroke, and seizures.

Hyperglycemia and Hypoglycemia

The human body needs sugar to produce the energy that sustains it. When blood sugar is too low or too high, the body reacts. The most common reaction is altered mental status.

Hyperglycemia

Patients who have **diabetes** usually have increased blood sugar, or hyperglycemia. This condition is basically one of too much blood sugar and too little **insulin**, a hormone that regulates blood sugar

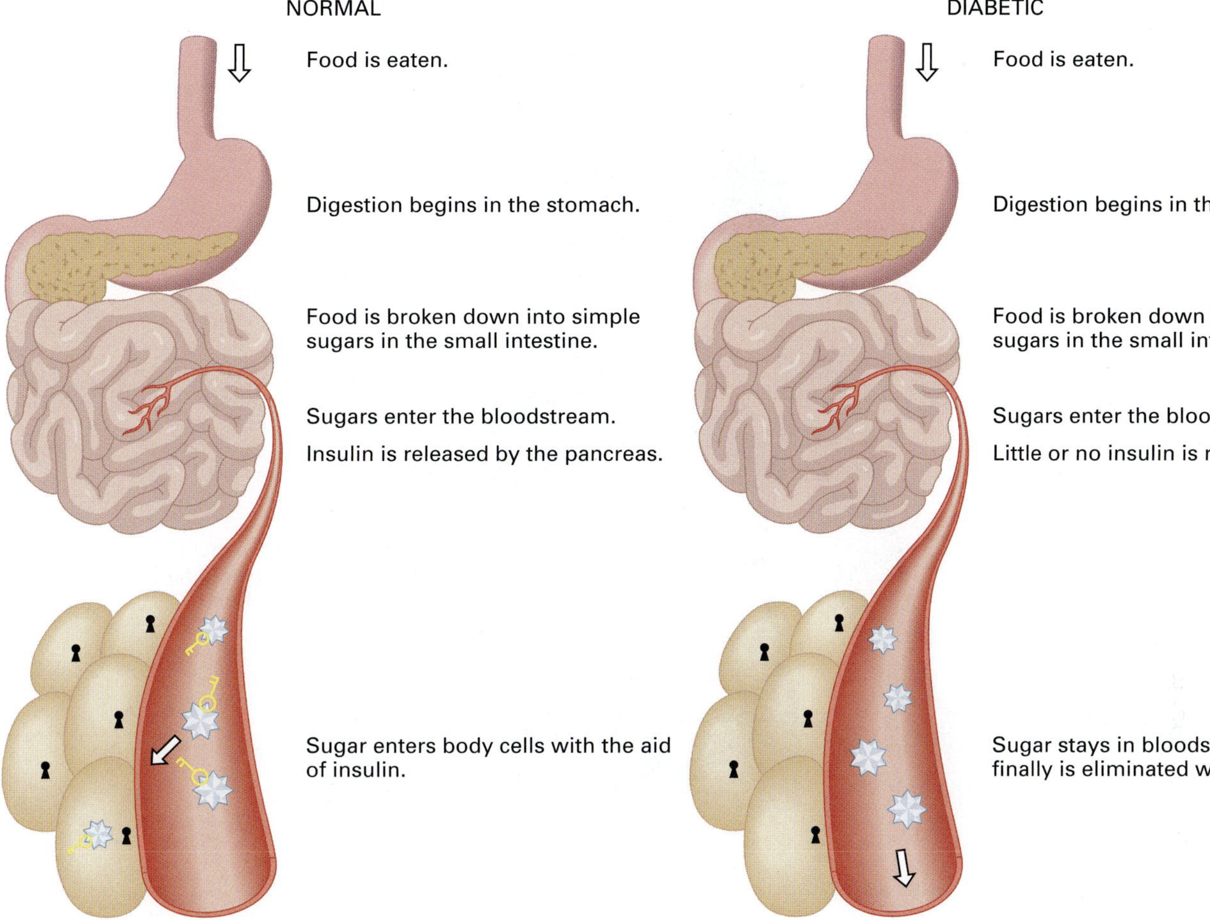

Figure 14–1   Normal versus diabetic use of sugar.

(Figure 14–1). Insulin is also a drug taken by people with diabetes. Common causes of hyperglycemia include the following:

- Infection, such as a respiratory infection
- Failure of the patient to take insulin or to take a sufficient amount
- Eating too much food that contains or produces sugar
- Increased or prolonged stress

Although a hyperglycemia emergency is sometimes called a diabetic coma, the patient is not usually found in a coma. Signs and symptoms may include the following (Figure 14–2):

- Sweet, fruity, or acetone-like breath
- Flushed, dry, warm skin
- Hunger and thirst
- Rapid, weak pulse
- Altered mental status
- Intoxicated appearance, staggering, slurred speech
- Frequent urination
- Reports that the patient has not taken the prescribed diabetes medication

The onset of severe hyperglycemia is gradual. In most cases, it develops over a period of 12 to 48 hours. At first, the patient experiences excessive hunger, thirst, and urination. The patient appears extremely ill and becomes sicker and weaker as the condition progresses. If left untreated, the patient may die. With treatment, improvement is gradual, occurring 6 to 12 hours after insulin and intravenous fluid are administered.

Hypoglycemia

Low blood sugar, or hypoglycemia, is the result of two conditions. One is too much insulin. The other is too little sugar, such as occurs when a patient with diabetes does not eat properly.

People with diabetes are not the only ones who can suffer from low blood sugar. So can alcoholics, people who have ingested certain poisons, and people who are ill. Some common causes of low blood sugar are as follows:

- Skipped meals, particularly for a patient with diabetes
- Vomiting, especially with illness
- Strenuous exercise

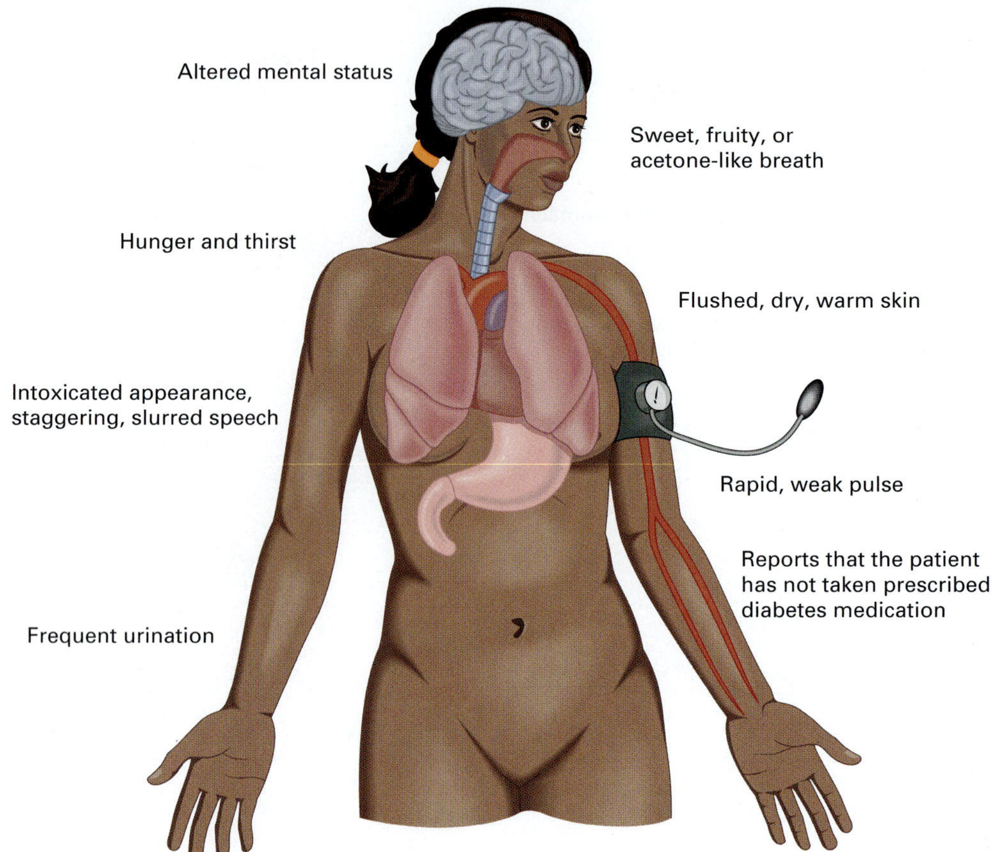

Figure 14–2   Signs and symptoms of hyperglycemia.

- Physical stress from extreme heat or cold
- Emotional stress, such as at weddings or funerals
- Accidental overdose of insulin

The most recognized cause of hypoglycemia is accidental overdose of insulin in a patient with diabetes. After a time, diabetes affects vision and can lead to blindness. This can make it very hard for them to give themselves the proper amount of insulin. This may sometimes be the cause of an insulin overdose and hypoglycemia.

The signs and symptoms of hypoglycemia may include any of the following (Figure 14–3):

- Rapid onset of altered mental status
- Intoxicated appearance, staggering, slurred speech
- Rapid pulse rate
- Cool, clammy skin
- Hunger
- Headache
- Seizures

Patient Assessment

When you gather the SAMPLE history, try to find out about the onset of the emergency. Be sure to ask, "Do you have diabetes?" If the patient says "Yes," ask the following questions: "Have you eaten today? Did you take your insulin? When was the last time you checked your blood sugar?" Also ask about any current illness, stress, and problems with medication.

Look for a medical identification tag during the secondary assessment. If the police are present, ask them to check the patient's wallet. If the patient is at home, check the refrigerator for insulin. Also, check around the house for needles and syringes. Special needle containers are often present in the house of a person with diabetes.

Blood Glucose Determination

In cases of altered mental status due to a medical cause, it is prudent to check a patient's blood glucose level. Glucometers are inexpensive and easy to use. If your service does not sanction this test or provide a glucometer, most diabetic patients will have their own device that can be used by the patient or a family member or caregiver. Many diabetic patients check their own blood glucose level several times a day and may have a log of these readings. Normal blood glucose levels range from 4.0 to 7.0 mmol/L (millimoles per litre).

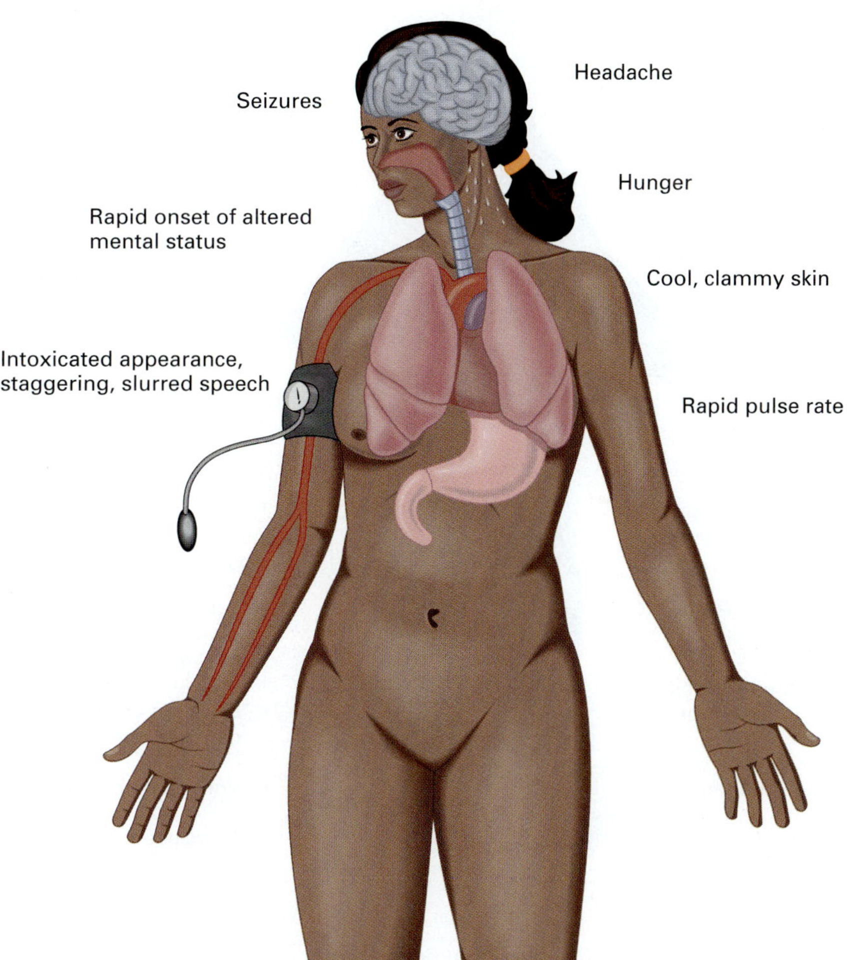

Figure 14–3 Signs and symptoms of hypoglycemia.

To perform this procedure, you will need a glucometer with test strips, finger stick device with sterile lancets, alcohol wipe, and tissue or gauze pad. Clean the patient's finger with the alcohol wipe. Use the lancet to poke the finger and simply place a drop of the patient's capillary blood onto a chemical test strip that has already been inserted into the glucometer (Figure 14–4). The reading will appear on the display screen in half a minute or less. Use the tissue or gauze pad to stop the bleeding.

Since there are many different models of glucometer, you must read the manufacturer's instructions carefully. Any deviation can cause an inaccurate reading. Be sure to allow the finger to dry from the alcohol wipe before you poke it, since alcohol can contaminate the sample. Glucometers are most accurate when they are used properly and calibrated daily.

Emergency Care

Proceed with emergency care as you would for any patient with altered mental status. However, if you suspect hypoglycemia or hyperglycemia, alert the incoming EMS crew immediately. While waiting for them, monitor the airway closely. Note that this

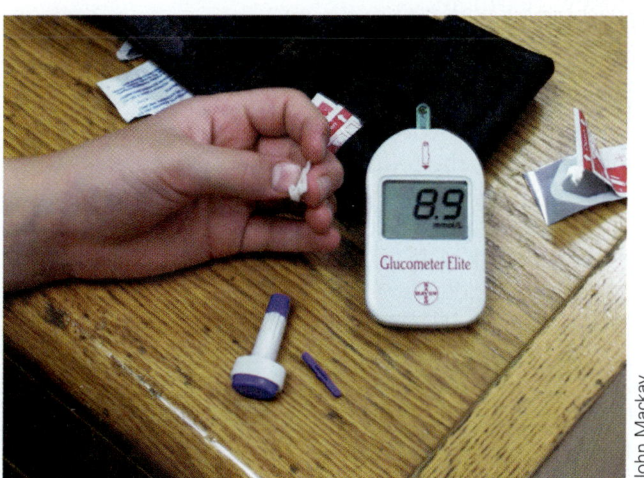

John Mackay

Figure 14–4 A glucometer is used to check a patient's blood sugar.

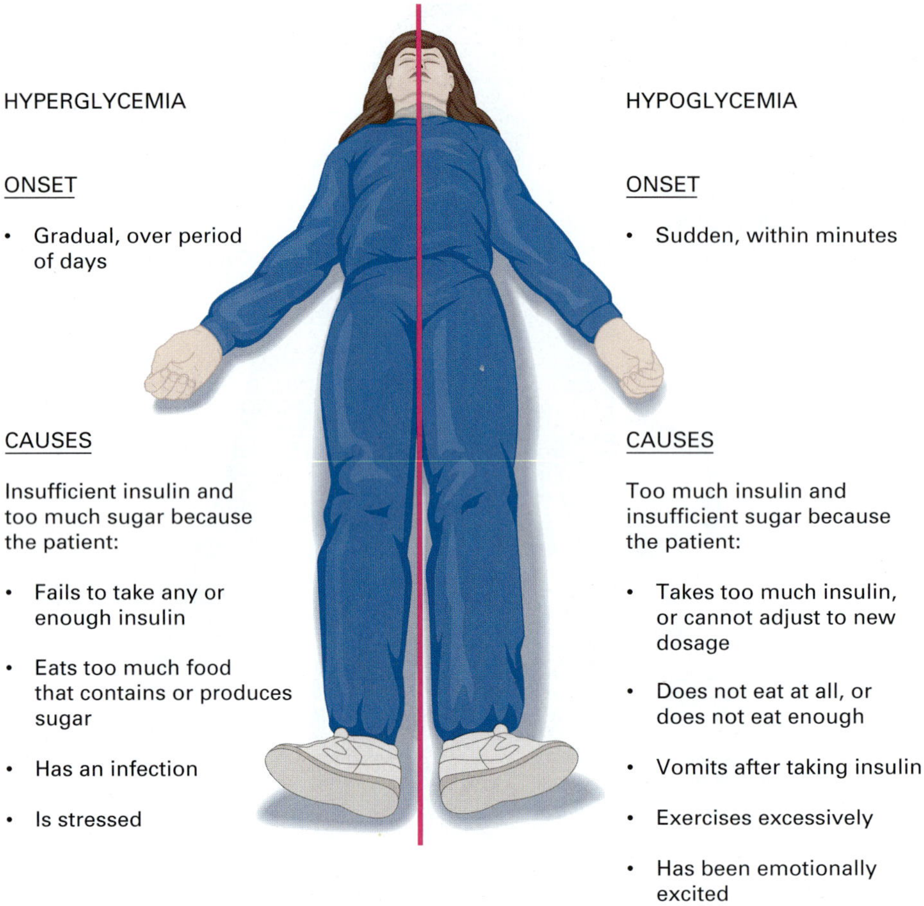

HYPERGLYCEMIA

ONSET

- Gradual, over period of days

CAUSES

Insufficient insulin and too much sugar because the patient:

- Fails to take any or enough insulin

- Eats too much food that contains or produces sugar

- Has an infection

- Is stressed

HYPOGLYCEMIA

ONSET

- Sudden, within minutes

CAUSES

Too much insulin and insufficient sugar because the patient:

- Takes too much insulin, or cannot adjust to new dosage

- Does not eat at all, or does not eat enough

- Vomits after taking insulin

- Exercises excessively

- Has been emotionally excited

Figure 14–5   Onset and causes of hyperglycemia and hypoglycemia.

patient may suddenly have a seizure. Be prepared. (See "Seizures" later in this chapter.)

Remember, patients with diabetes can suffer from either hypoglycemia or hyperglycemia (Figure 14–5). *When in doubt, give sugar.* You will not harm a hyperglycemic patient and you may save the life of a hypoglycemic patient by this emergency treatment.

Your EMS system may permit you to help a patient take some sugar. To do so, the patient must be awake and able to control his or her own airway. Follow local protocols. The patient may benefit from taking one of the following sources of sugar:

- Some sugar dissolved in a glass of water
- A drink that is naturally rich in sugar, such as orange juice
- A commercially prepared glucose paste squeezed onto a tongue depressor (Figure 14–6)

Note that a tube of glucose should be used only for a single patient and then discarded.

Never give anything to eat or drink to patients who cannot control their own airway. They could aspirate the substance into their lungs. This can have grave results, including death. If you are in doubt, call for medical direction. If sugar or glucose is administered, be sure to tell the paramedics who take over care. Also, report any changes in mental status that occurred while the patient was in your care.

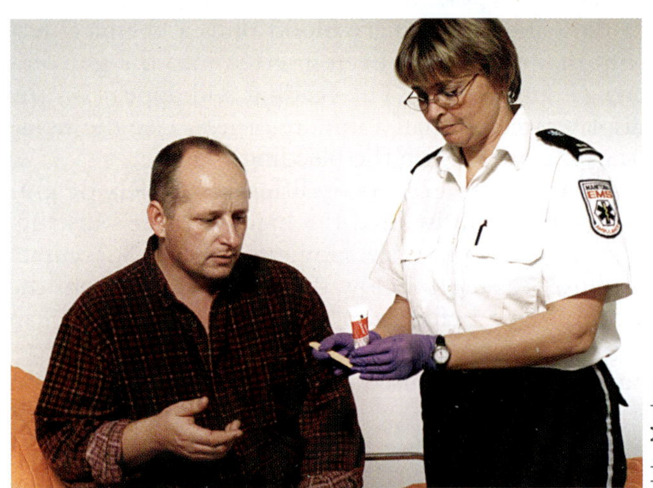

Figure 14–6   Your EMS system may allow you to help a patient self-administer oral glucose.

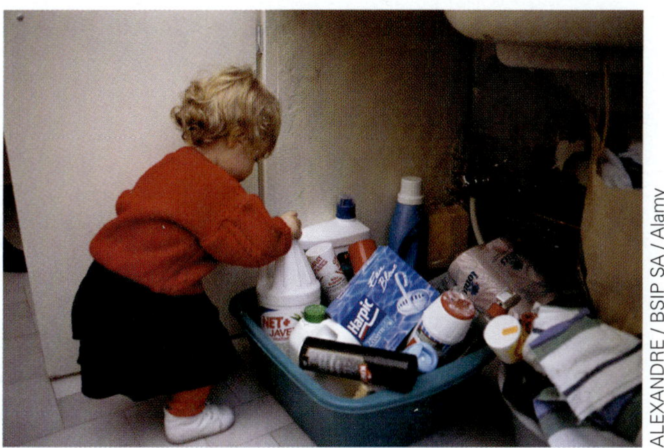

ALEXANDRE / BSIP SA / Alamy

Figure 14–7 Poisoning is a leading cause of injury and accidental death among children.

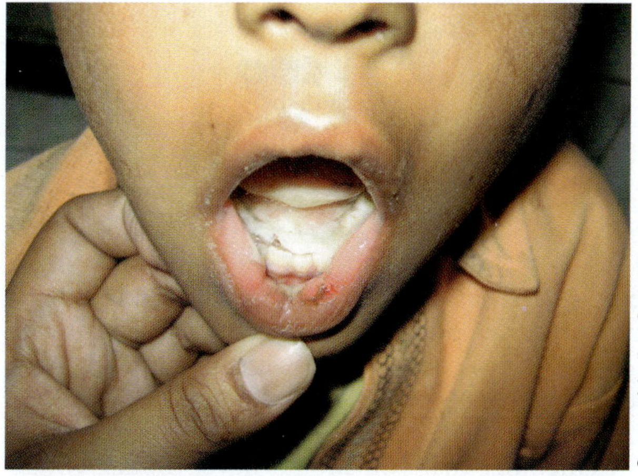

Custom Medical Stock Photo

Figure 14–8 Burns or stains around the mouth may indicate poisoning.

Poisoning

A poison is a substance that can impair health. Poisoning can occur in a variety of settings. However, many poisonings occur in the relative safety of the home (Figure 14–7).

Poisons may be inhaled, ingested, injected, or absorbed. Whenever you suspect a poisoning, try to answer these questions: What substance is involved? How much is involved? When did the poisoning occur? What has the patient done to relieve the symptoms?

Ingested Poisons

An ingested poison is one that is introduced into the digestive tract by way of the mouth. Every year in Canada there are about 800 000 reported ingested poisonings. Drugs such as acetaminophen (Tylenol), alcohol, and tricyclic antidepressants are among the top offenders. Many household plants are also poisonous.

Patient Assessment. Be alert for clues when you first assess the scene, as well as later in the call. A clue to a poisoning may be an overturned or empty pill box, scattered pills, chemical containers, household cleaners, empty alcohol bottles, or overturned plants.

Keep in mind as you do your primary assessment that patients who are poisoned often vomit. Therefore, be alert to airway obstruction and breathing difficulty, which can lead to hypoxia and death.

In addition to altered mental status, the signs and symptoms of poisoning may include the following:

- History of ingesting poisons
- Burns around the mouth
- Odd breath odours
- Nausea, vomiting
- Abdominal pain
- Diarrhea

Note that the symptoms follow a path of ingestion. Start at the mouth. Look for chemical burns around the mouth (Figure 14–8) and smell for a chemical odour on the breath. Then, note if there is or has been any nausea and vomiting. Finally, the patient may complain of abdominal cramps and diarrhea.

Poisons will often affect the central nervous system. You may see dilated or constricted pupils, or you may hear the patient complain of double vision. There may be excessive saliva or foaming at the mouth. There may be excessive tearing or sweating. Finally, the patient may become unconscious or have seizures.

Emergency Care. Your top priority is the patient's airway. With that in mind, proceed as you would with any patient with altered mental status. To help limit the damage a poison can cause, make sure the EMS system is activated. If there will be a delay, call the poison control centre in your area or medical control for instructions. Follow local protocols.

You may be instructed to give the patient **activated charcoal** (Figure 14–9). This is finely ground charcoal that is very absorbent. It binds with the poison in the stomach and then passes through the body harmlessly. It may be effective in reducing the effects of poison for up to four hours after ingestion. Use it only by order of poison control or according to your local protocols. Most activated charcoal is premixed with water. If it is dry, then you must mix two tablespoons of it in a glass of water to make a slurry. Be careful. It stains most clothing easily.

You may be ordered to induce vomiting in the patient. This is usually done with **syrup of ipecac.**

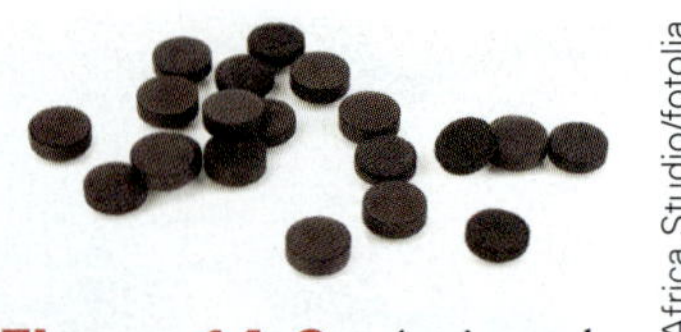

Figure 14–9 Activated charcoal.

Africa Studio/fotolia

Ipecac can have side effects. Use it only on the direct order of either poison control or medical control. In the field, it is never given with activated charcoal unless under direct medical orders. Follow all local protocols.

Remember that you should never induce vomiting in the following circumstances:

- The patient is unconscious.
- The patient cannot maintain his or her airway.
- The ingested poison is an acid, a corrosive (such as lye), or a petroleum product (such as gasoline or furniture polish).
- The patient has a medical condition, such as heart attack, seizures, or pregnancy, that could be complicated by vomiting.

If the patient swallows an acid, a corrosive, or a petroleum product, you may have to dilute it. Use several glasses of either water or milk. Whatever the situation, always follow local protocols. If that means calling poison control, do so, via 911, and follow their instructions exactly.

Inhaled Poisons

A common source of poison gas is fire. The product of incomplete combustion, poison gas may contain carbon monoxide, the most common poison. It may also contain cyanide, a byproduct of burning certain plastics.

Fire is not the only source of poison gas. Large amounts of carbon dioxide can come from sewage treatment plants or industrial sites. Even the chlorine gas from swimming pools can be lethal.

Patient Assessment. Remember, many poison gases are colourless, odourless, and tasteless. You may not know you are in danger until it is too late. Be on the lookout for hazardous materials. Pay constant attention to the nature of the incident and the dangers it might pose. Protect yourself! Also, keep others away from the scene.

It is imperative that you give special attention to the airway of a patient who has inhaled poison gas. Once in a safe location, open the airway. Inspect the mouth and nose. Be careful to note the presence of soot, burns, or singed hair. Other

signs and symptoms of poison inhalation include the following:

- History of inhaling poisons
- Breathing difficulty
- Chest pain
- Cough, hoarseness, burning sensation in the throat
- Cyanosis
- Dizziness, headache
- Seizures, unconsciousness (advanced stage)

Carbon monoxide is a poison gas that is especially lethal. Kerosene heaters, hot water heaters, and car exhaust fumes are some of the most common sources. Be particularly alert to carbon monoxide poisoning if several members of a household have the same signs and symptoms or if they say they are sick only in a certain location in the house. Check to see if the family pet seems sick as well.

The signs and symptoms of carbon monoxide poisoning include the following:

- Throbbing headache and agitation
- Nausea, vomiting
- Confusion, poor judgment
- Diminished vision, blindness
- Breathing difficulty with rapid pulse
- Dizziness, fainting, unconsciousness
- Seizures
- Paleness
- Cherry red colour to skin (very late sign)

Emergency Care. The first rule of EMS is safety. You must protect yourself. Do not enter the scene where a poisonous gas may be present. Call dispatch for specialized rescue teams who will have the appropriate safety equipment, including a self-contained breathing apparatus.

When it is safe to do so, quickly remove the patient from the source of the poison. Then proceed as you would with any patient with altered mental status. Verify that an ambulance is en route. Consider helicopter evacuation if it would be quicker.

Note that all patients who have been exposed to carbon monoxide need medical care, even those who seem to recover.

Absorbed Poisons

An absorbed poison is one that enters the body upon contact with the skin. Examples of natural sources include poison ivy, poison sumac, and poison oak (Figure 14–10). Other sources are corrosives, insecticides, herbicides, and cleaning products.

Patient Assessment. An absorbed poison usually causes harm only to the area of contact.

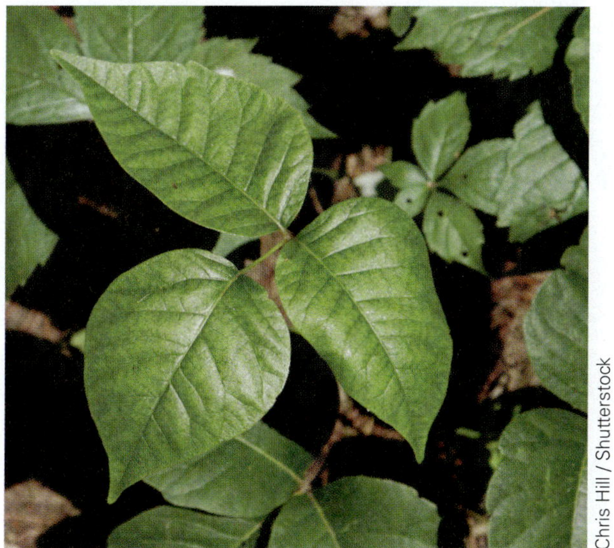

Figure 14–10a Poison ivy.

Chris Hill / Shutterstock

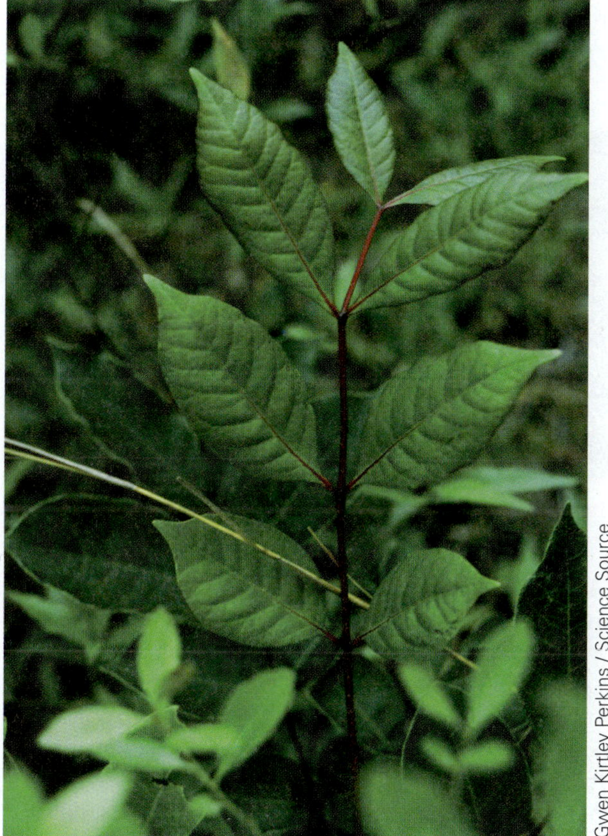

Figure 14–10b Poison sumac.

Gwen Kirtley Perkins / Science Source

In general, the signs and symptoms include the following:

- History of exposures
- Liquid or powder on the skin
- Burns
- Itching, irritation
- Redness, rash, blisters (Figure 14–11)

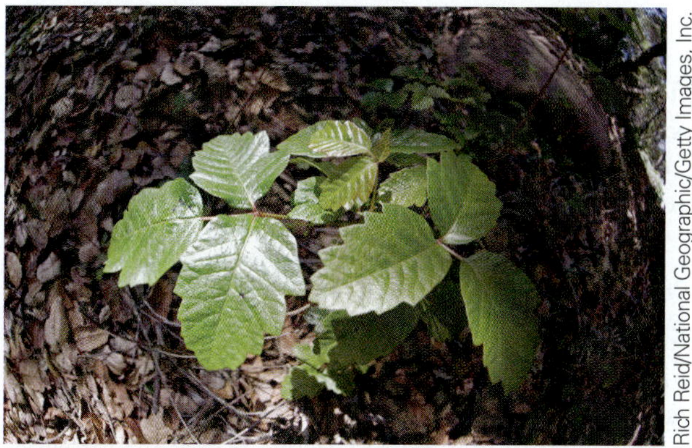

Figure 14–10c Poison oak.

Rich Reid/National Geographic/Getty Images, Inc.

Once a poison is identified, advise the incoming EMS units. If hazardous materials are suspected, follow local protocols. Note that an oil-based poison can spread easily from person to person. Therefore, protect yourself. Gloves are essential. Also consider wearing a gown, mask, and eye protection.

Emergency Care. For emergency care of a patient who has been poisoned by absorption, contact poison control or the medical director. General guidelines for emergency care are as follows:

1. Remove the clothing that came into contact with the poison.
2. Then, with a dry cloth, blot the poison from the skin. If the poison is a dry powder, brush it off.
3. Rinse the area with copious amounts of water. A shower or garden hose is ideal for this purpose. Continue until other EMS units arrive. Note that you may need to use alcohol or vegetable oil with some poisons. Follow instructions from poison control or the medical director.
4. Continually monitor the patient's vital signs. Be alert for sudden changes. Seizures and shock are not uncommon.

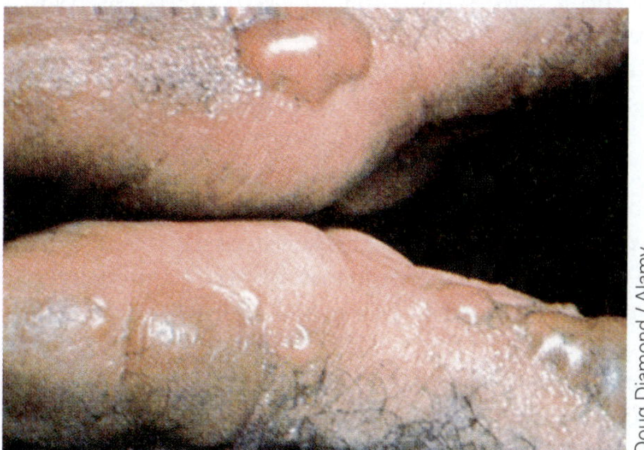

Figure 14–11 Blisters from contact with a poisonous plant.

Doug Diamond / Alamy

The eyes are especially vulnerable to absorbed poisons. If ordered to do so, rinse the eyes with copious amounts of water. If only one eye is affected, be sure to avoid running contaminated water into the other eye. Advise incoming EMS units of the patient's condition. Follow local protocol.

Injected Poisons

An injected poison is one that enters the body by way of an object that pierces the skin. For example, an illegal drug may enter the body by way of a hypodermic needle. An overdose may be the result. For more information on overdose emergencies, see Chapter 18.

Other causes of injected poisoning include bites or stings from insects, spiders, snakes, and marine animals. Venom from these creatures can cause serious allergic reactions, even death. For more information on this type of emergency, see Chapter 17.

Stroke

A patient may suffer a cerebrovascular accident (CVA), or stroke, when an area of the brain is deprived of blood (Figure 14–12). This can occur when a blood clot (thrombus) within the brain blocks an artery, when a blood clot from elsewhere (embolus) lodges in an artery, when an artery is constricted (compression), or when an artery bursts (aneurysm) (Figure 14–13).

According to the Heart and Stroke Foundation of Canada (HSFC), stroke is the leading cause of adult disability in Canada and the fourth leading cause of death. Strokes are more common in people over the age of 65 but can affect anyone.

Patients who are at risk of heart attack may also be in danger of having a stroke. This includes patients with high blood pressure or diabetes and patients who smoke tobacco.

Patient Assessment

The signs and symptoms of stroke are the result of several factors. Among them are the location of the stroke and the amount of brain damage. The signs and symptoms may be mild or life threatening. Sometimes they are temporary. Temporary signs and symptoms indicate a mini-stroke, or transient ischemic attack (TIA). These mini-strokes are a warning sign of an impending larger stroke.

The signs and symptoms of stroke include the following (Figure 14–14 on p. 222):

- *Inability to communicate.* The patient may either fail to speak or fail to understand what is spoken.
- *Impairment in one part of the body.* An example is loss of muscle control on one side of the face or loss of movement on one entire side of the body.

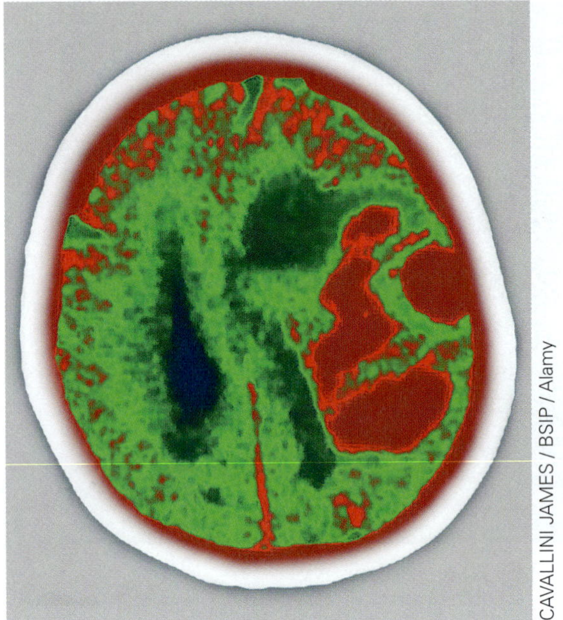

Figure 14–12a   A cerebrovascular accident (CVA), or stroke, from cerebral hemorrhage.

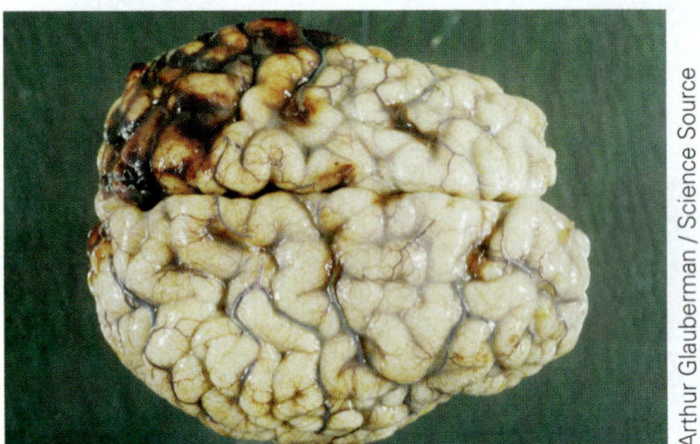

Figure 14–12b   Brain damaged by stroke.

- *Altered mental status.* This can range from a change in personality to seizures and unconsciousness.

About 50 percent of stroke patients have elevated blood pressure during a stroke. However, the combination of elevated blood pressure, slow pulse, and rapid or irregular breathing is a sign of a major stroke. Be prepared for the patient to suddenly start to convulse.

Emergency Care

Proceed as you would with any patient with altered mental status. However, note that as pressure increases in the skull from swelling and bleeding, the patient's breathing will be affected. Be especially alert to the airway of a patient who has slurred speech or difficulty speaking. Never give a suspected stroke patient anything to eat or drink. Be prepared to provide artificial ventilation.

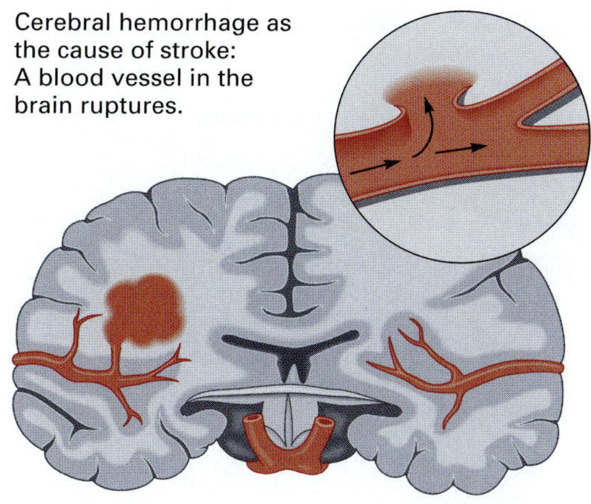

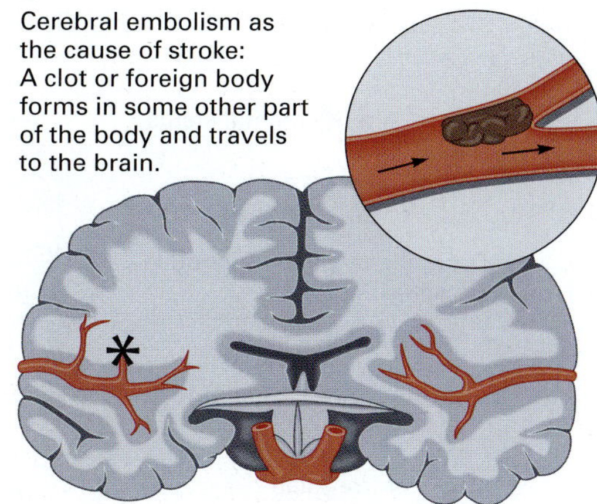

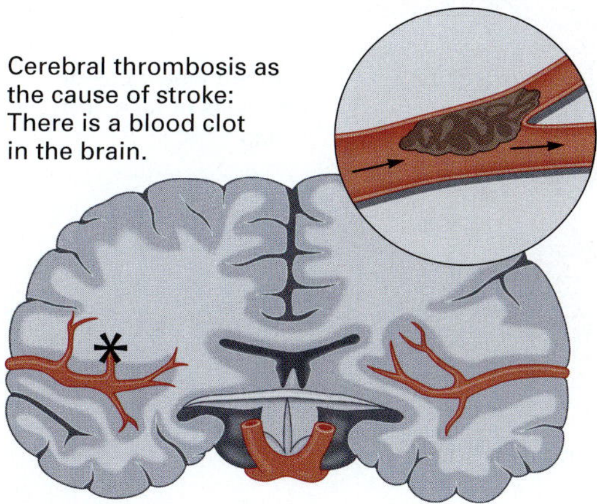

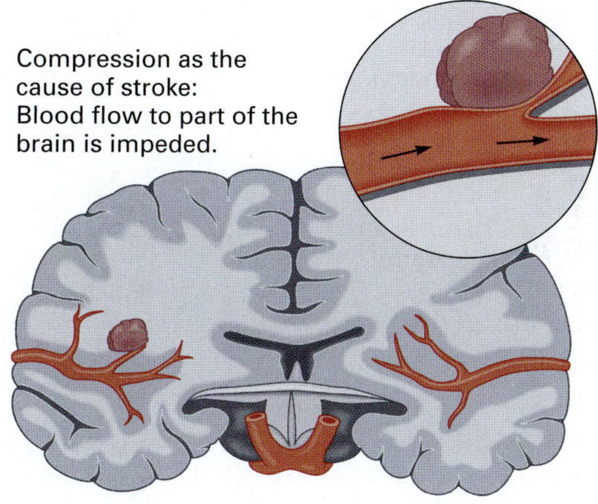

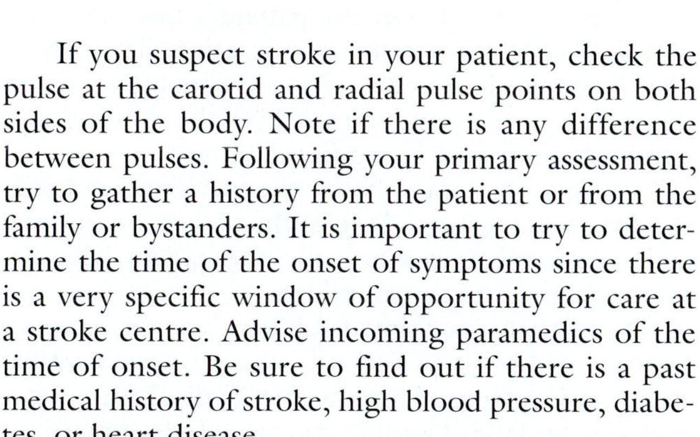

Figure 14–13 Causes of stroke.

If you suspect stroke in your patient, check the pulse at the carotid and radial pulse points on both sides of the body. Note if there is any difference between pulses. Following your primary assessment, try to gather a history from the patient or from the family or bystanders. It is important to try to determine the time of the onset of symptoms since there is a very specific window of opportunity for care at a stroke centre. Advise incoming paramedics of the time of onset. Be sure to find out if there is a past medical history of stroke, high blood pressure, diabetes, or heart disease.

The loss of mental or motor function is a frightening reality for stroke patients. Remain calm, and never make exclamations out loud about abnormal physical findings. Instead, maintain a professional attitude. Reassure the patient. Do not make any statements about long-term disability.

Continue to talk to the patient even if he or she cannot speak. Stroke patients can often hear very well. Explain to them what you are doing. Do not talk down to them or treat them like children.

Handle a patient's paralyzed limbs carefully. There may be no feeling in the limbs, so you could injure them without being aware of it. The patient may also unintentionally cause them to strike an object.

Seizures

There are many causes of seizures. Sometimes the cause is unknown. All the conditions described in this chapter can lead to a seizure. Common causes include the following:

- Chronic medical conditions
- Epilepsy
- Hypoglycemia
- Poisoning, including alcohol and drug poisoning
- Stroke
- Fever (most common in children)
- Infection
- Head injury or brain tumour
- Hypoxia
- Complications of pregnancy

A seizure is the result of nervous system malfunction. It may last five minutes or it may be prolonged. Its symptoms can range from a twitch of a limb to whole-body muscle contractions.

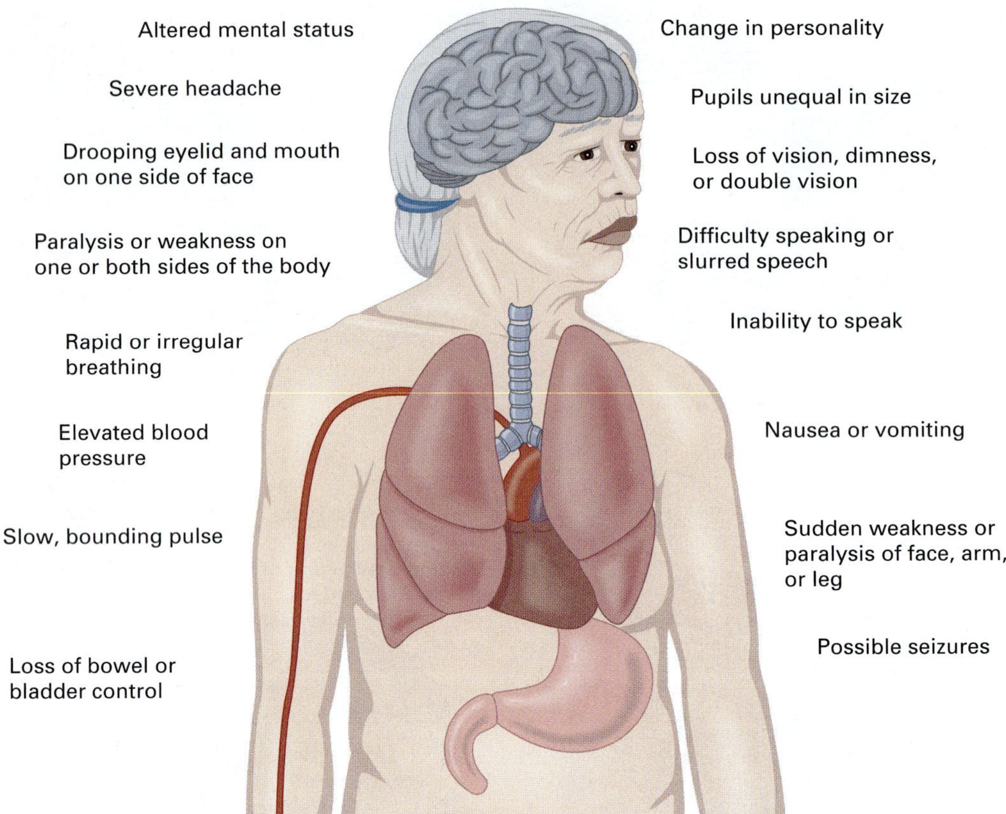

Figure 14–14 One or more signs or symptoms may indicate a stroke.

Most patients become unconscious. Some vomit during the attack. Typically, patients are tired and sleep afterwards. Seizures are rarely life threatening, but they do indicate a very serious condition.

Patient Assessment

You will probably be called most often to a grand mal, or generalized, seizure. There are four phases to this type of seizure. They are (in order) as follows (Figure 14–15):

- Aura phase
- Tonic phase
- Clonic phase
- Postictal phase

In the aura phase, the patient becomes aware that a seizure is coming on. The aura is often described as an unusual smell or a flash of light. It lasts only a split second.

In the tonic phase, the patient becomes unconscious and collapses to the ground. Then, all the muscles of the body contract. This often forces a scream out of the patient. It can also force out sputum, which can look like foam. During this phase, the patient may stop breathing.

In the clonic phase, the patient's muscles alternate between contraction and relaxation. The patient may become incontinent of urine (unable to retain it). Because the patient may bite the tongue and cheek, there may be blood in the mouth.

In the postictal phase, the patient gradually regains consciousness. At first, the patient is confused and even combative. Gradually, the patient becomes aware of his or her surroundings.

Note that a continual seizure, or two or more seizures without a period of consciousness, is called **status epilepticus**. This is a true medical emergency that can be fatal. Complications include aspiration, hypoxia, hyperthermia, and heart problems. If you suspect this type of seizure, advise responding EMS units. Transport of the patient must not be delayed.

Emergency Care

During your scene assessment, ask yourself if the patient was injured when he or she fell to the ground. Pay careful attention to the potential for spinal or head injury. If the patient is still seizing when you arrive on the scene, do the following:

1. Stay calm. Just wait. The seizure will be over in a few minutes.

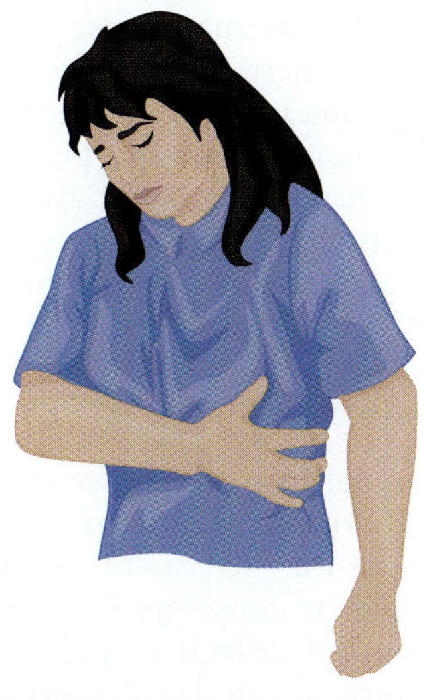

1. AURA PHASE. Often described as unusual smell or flash of light that lasts a split second

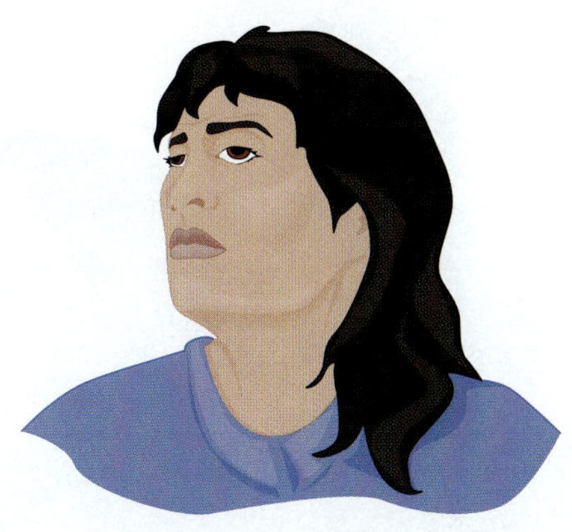

2. TONIC PHASE. 15 to 20 seconds of unconsciousness followed by 5 to 15 seconds of extreme muscle rigidity

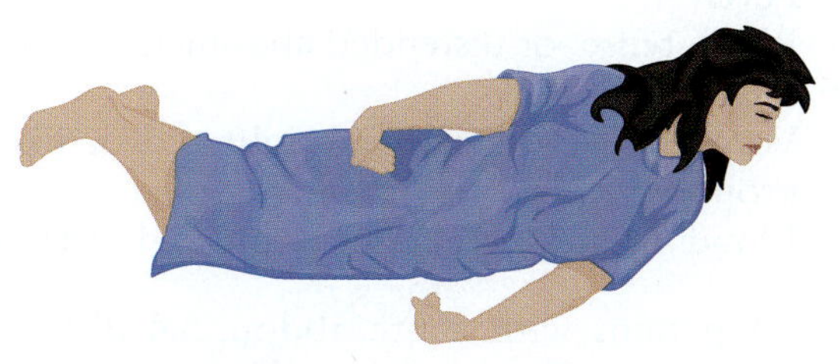

3. CLONIC PHASE. 1 to 5 minutes of seizures

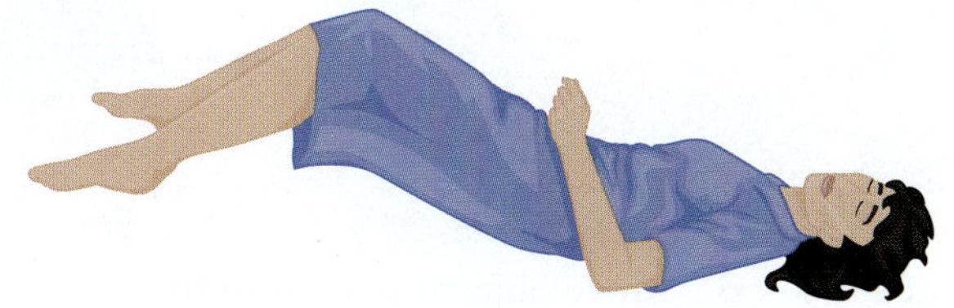

4. POSTICTAL PHASE. 5 to 30 minutes to several hours of deep sleep with gradual recovery

Figure 14–15 Stages of a generalized seizure.

2. Prevent any further injury by moving objects away from the patient (Figure 14–16 on p. 224). If they cannot be moved, then put something between them and the patient. If needed, drag the patient a few feet away from the danger.
3. Place padding, such as a coat or blanket, under the patient's head. Remove the patient's eyeglasses. Do not force anything into the patient's mouth. Do not try to restrain the patient.
4. If you suspect status epilepticus, do your best to prevent aspiration. Position the patient on his or her side or provide suction if possible. Assist ventilations with a BVM device attached to 100 percent oxygen. Notify the incoming EMS unit immediately.

Most often, you will arrive on the scene when a seizure has ceased or when the patient is in the last phase of seizing. When the seizure stops, assess and monitor the patient's airway and breathing closely. If there is no reason to suspect head or spinal injury, place the patient in the recovery position (Figure 14–17 on p. 224). If you are allowed, administer high-flow oxygen. If you suspect the patient was injured during a fall, use a jaw-thrust manoeuvre to open the airway. As the patient recovers, offer comfort and reassurance. Remember that he or she will have muscle soreness as well as fatigue.

While you wait for the paramedics to arrive on the scene, consider the patient's feelings. Often, he or she feels embarrassed. Ask the onlookers to move away to provide the patient with some privacy. Place a sheet or towel over the patient's body if there has been incontinence.

When you give your hand-off report to the paramedics, be sure to include a description of the seizure. It may be important in determining its cause.

Abdominal Pain and Distress

The abdominal cavity contains many different organs and blood vessels. Complaints of pain or discomfort could be caused by a number of problems

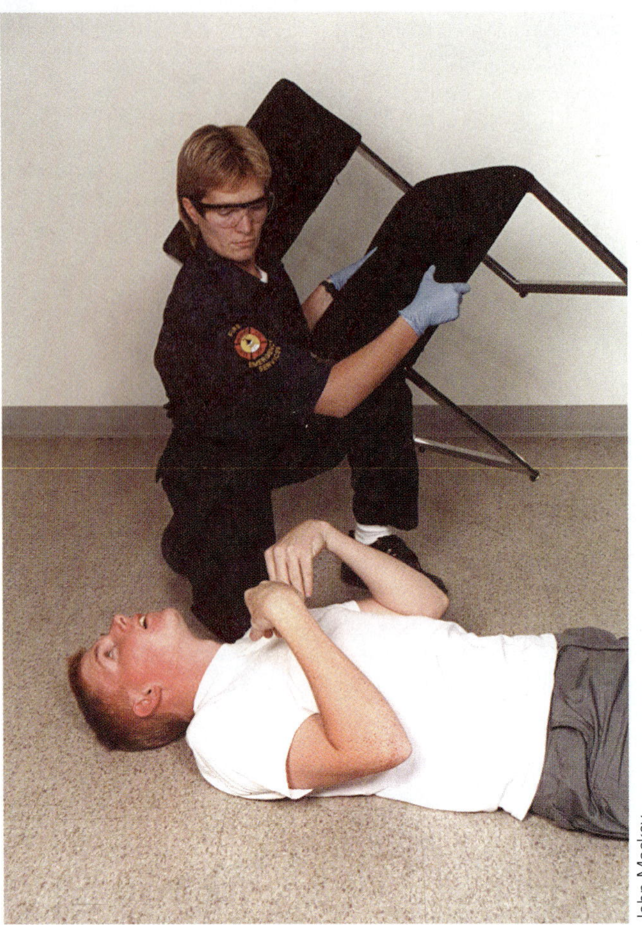

Figure 14–16 Move objects away from the seizure patient.

or conditions. Pain caused by abdominal problems may be located directly over a problem organ in the abdomen, or it may be in a totally different part of the body. This is called referred pain.

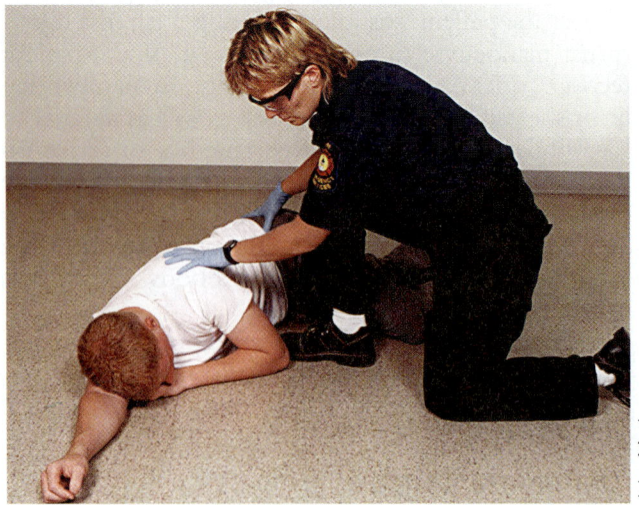

Figure 14–17 When the seizure stops, position the patient to allow drainage of saliva and vomit.

Abdominal problems may cause referred pain in the shoulders and chest. Sometimes, pain begins in the anterior abdomen and radiates to the back. Abdominal emergencies require aggressive care to prevent shock and to save lives. All abdominal pain should be taken seriously. Do not spend time trying to determine its cause. Rather, complete a thorough patient assessment and history.

Patient Assessment

Any severe abdominal pain should be considered an emergency. Any abdominal pain that is persistent or is significant enough for the patient or family to call for assistance should be considered an emergency. A patient with abdominal distress or pain appears very ill. Signs and symptoms include the following:

- Abdominal pain, either local or diffuse
- Colicky pain (cramps that occur in waves)
- Abdominal tenderness, either local or diffuse
- Anxiety, reluctance to move
- Loss of appetite, nausea, vomiting
- Fever
- Rigid, tense, or distended abdomen
- Signs of shock
- Vomiting blood, either bright red or like coffee grounds
- Blood in the stool, either bright red or tarry black

A patient with acute abdominal distress often gets in a **guarding position** (Figure 14–18). In this position, the patient is on his or her side, with the knees drawn up toward the abdomen. This position reduces tension in the muscles of the abdomen, and this, in turn, helps reduce the pain.

In assessing a patient with acute abdominal distress, the primary assessment is the first priority. Even after ensuring the patient's ABCs, stay alert for signs of shock. These include a rapid and thready pulse, restlessness, cold clammy skin, and falling blood

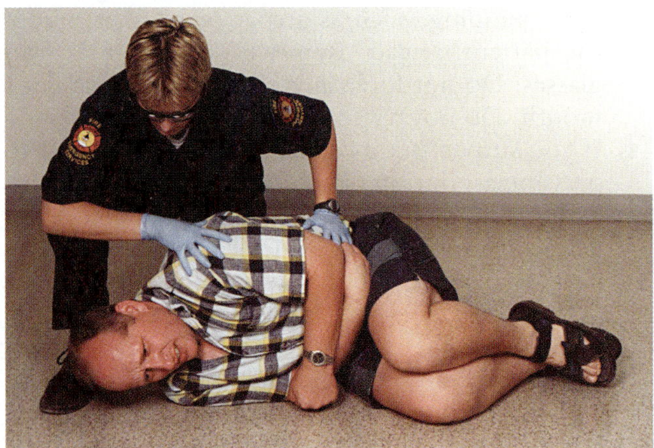

Figure 14–18 Guarding position.

pressure. Shock is common with internal bleeding and continued vomiting and diarrhea.

As with all medical patients, gather a comprehensive patient history. It may identify clues to the patient's condition, such as prior similar problems or factors that may have caused the pain.

During the secondary assessment, determine whether the patient is restless or quiet. Find out if movement causes pain. Check to see if the abdomen is distended and ask the patient to confirm your observation. Note if the patient can relax the abdominal wall when asked to do so. Palpate the abdomen gently to determine if it is rigid or soft. If you know one area is causing pain, examine that area last.

Do not spend too much time on assessment before making sure the paramedics have been updated. Too much palpation can worsen the pain. It can also aggravate the medical condition that caused it.

Emergency Care

The goals of emergency care for acute abdominal distress are to prevent any possible life-threatening complications, to make the patient comfortable, and to arrange for transport as quickly as possible. In addition, do the following:

1. *Maintain an open airway.* Be alert for vomiting and possible aspiration. If the patient is nauseated, position him or her on the left side if it does not cause too much pain.
2. Administer oxygen if you are trained and allowed to do so. Use a non-rebreather mask at 10 to 15 L/min.
3. *Be alert for shock.* If vital signs and other observations point to it, position the patient on his or her back, with the legs elevated. If there are no signs of shock, allow the patient to get into a position of comfort.

Protect the patient from any rough handling. Never give anything by mouth. Do not allow the patient to take any medications. Medications could mask symptoms and complicate the physician's diagnosis and treatment.

EMR FOCUS

Medical complaints will be the most common type of emergency for most EMS calls. The percentage of the population that is elderly is increasing dramatically. This means increased calls for medical problems in the future.

This chapter covered a wide range of medical problems—from stroke to diabetes to poisoning to generalized complaints. Remember that it is not ever necessary to diagnose a patient's medical problem. Sometimes diagnosis even in the hospital is difficult, even with the tests and procedures available to physicians there. It is not practical for you to try to determine the cause of a patient's condition in the field.

There are many things you can do for your medical patients. You must treat any life-threatening problems during the primary assessment. A history is also very important with a medical patient. It will provide the clues to the patient's condition, which will benefit you, the paramedics, and the hospital personnel.

Finally, never jump to conclusions. In this chapter, for example, you learned that under certain conditions a patient who has diabetes may appear to be drunk. Consider all patients who are exhibiting altered mental status or unusual behaviour as having a medical problem. Never assume that the patient is drunk, drugged, or mentally ill.

CASE STUDY FOLLOW-UP

At the beginning of this chapter, you read that EMRs were on the scene with a patient who was experiencing altered mental status. To see how the chapter skills apply to this emergency, read the following. It describes how the call was completed.

PATIENT HISTORY

As nearly as we could tell from the scene, the patient was probably eating breakfast when all this started. In response to questioning, he said he had no allergies and that he was on medication. We found high blood pressure meds in his pack. He denied any other medical conditions. The patient also tried to describe the event. He then indicated that his head hurt, and he suddenly passed out. When he awoke, he could not move the right side of his body.

SECONDARY ASSESSMENT

We quickly performed a head-to-toe exam of the patient. He had definite weakness on the right side of his body. He had no deformities, no open injuries, no signs of tenderness or swelling. We realized quickly that we had limited information because the patient could no longer speak. We took a complete set of vital signs.

ONGOING ASSESSMENT

Our impression was that the patient had had a stroke. Aware that he could get worse, we continued to perform the primary assessment and monitor vital signs. Our patient appeared to be somewhat anxious. Who wouldn't be? We tried to comfort and reassure him. We told him more help was on the way and that he would be in the hospital soon.

TRANSFER OF CARE

When the Medflight team arrived, we gave them a quick hand-off report, including the physical findings and the history we were able to gather. The flight team took it from there. I have to say that this guy was lucky. If he had been left alone much longer, he might have died from exposure.

> Whether or not you know the cause of a medical emergency in your patient, your job is the same. Assess, care for, and monitor the airway until the paramedics arrive to take over. Be prepared to provide basic life support if needed. Try to get a complete patient history from the patient, the family, or bystanders.

NOCPs

4.3 d Conduct neurological system assessment and interpret findings **S**

g Conduct gastrointestinal system assessment and interpret findings **S**

4.5 c Conduct glucometric testing and interpret findings **A**

6.1 b Provide care to patient experiencing signs and symptoms involving neurological system **S**

e Provide care to patient experiencing signs and symptoms involving gastrointestinal system **S**

h Provide care to patient experiencing signs and symptoms involving immunologic system **S**

i Provide care to patient experiencing signs and symptoms involving endocrine system **S**

k Provide care to patient experiencing toxicologic syndromes **S**

l Provide care to patient experiencing non-urgent problem **S**

REVIEW QUESTIONS

Page references where answers may be found or supported are provided at the end of each question.

SECTION 1

1. How would you treat a patient with a general medical complaint? (p. 211)

SECTION 2

2. Why must you monitor the airway and breathing of all patients with altered mental status? (p. 211)

3. What are three common causes of altered mental status in a patient? (p. 212)

4. What are three possible indicators of diabetes in a patient? (p. 214)

5. What is the name of the device often used by patients to check their blood glucose level? (p. 214)

6. What is the normal range of blood glucose in millimoles per litre? (p. 214)

7. List three ways that a poison can enter the body. (p. 217)

8. Why do inhaled poisons pose a risk to EMRs? (p. 218)

9. In addition to altered mental status, what are the signs and symptoms of an ingested poison? An inhaled poison? An absorbed poison? (pp. 217–219)

10. What are the characteristic signs of a stroke? (pp. 220, 222)

11. Why must you be careful with the limbs of a stroke patient? (p. 221)

12. What can you do for a patient who is actively seizing? (pp. 222–223)

13. What should you do for a seizure patient when the seizure has stopped? (p. 223)

14. What signs and symptoms are related to abdominal pain or distress? (p. 224)

15. What are the goals of emergency care of a patient with acute abdominal distress? (p. 225)

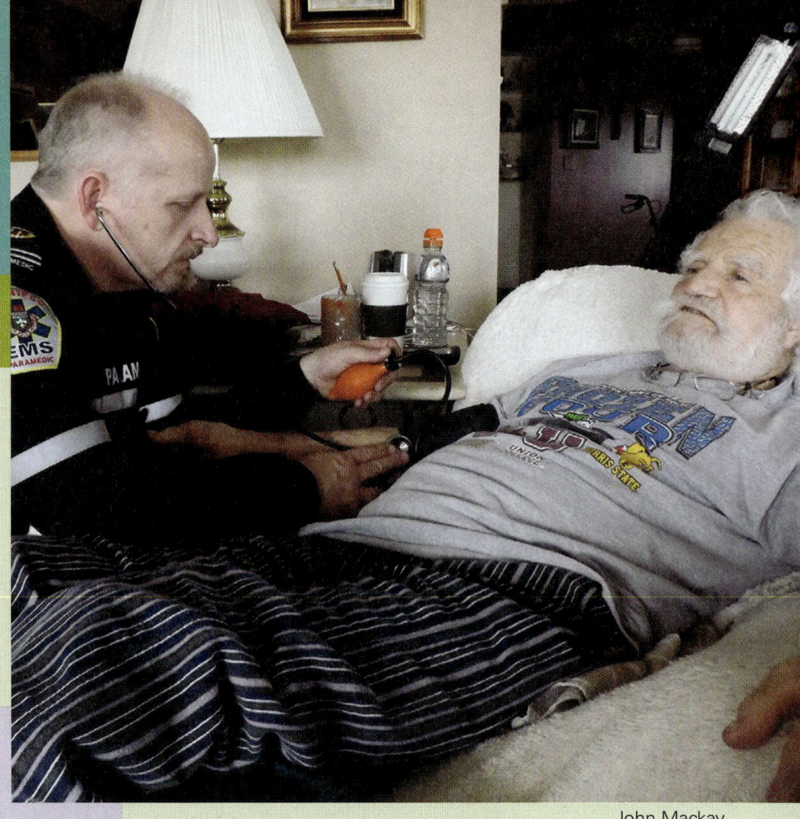
John Mackay

Geriatric Considerations

1. Relate the anatomical and functional changes of aging to illness and injury in older adults for the following body systems: skin, sensory organs, respiratory system, circulatory system, digestive system, urinary system, musculoskeletal system, nervous system, and immune system.

2. Discuss the impact of social, psychological, and financial concerns on the health of older adults.

3. Explain why an older person may be more seriously ill or injured than indicated by signs or symptoms and/or the mechanism of injury.

INTRODUCTION

As an EMR, you are likely to find that the majority of your patients are over the age of 65. Because older adults make up a large segment of our population, it is important to have a clear understanding of the ailments and injuries that these patients frequently experience. Understanding both the anatomical and functional changes, as well as psychological and economic factors related to aging, and applying them to the treatment you render are critical when caring for the older adult patient.

SECTION 1
MISCONCEPTIONS ABOUT OLDER ADULTS

Although Canada's population is rapidly aging, there are still some misconceptions about older people. Often, they are stereotyped as weak, sickly, deaf, blind, and forgetful. In addition, many individuals believe that older adults live only in extended-care facilities. In fact, this is not correct. The majority of older adults live independently and enjoy healthy, active lives (Figure 15–1). To avoid setting the wrong tone when dealing with older patients, remember the following:

- Always treat older adults with respect.
- Never assume that older adults are unable to hear you or answer questions about their own health.
- Be sure to explain who you are and what procedures you may need to do.
- Seek information from family members only after you have already questioned the patient.

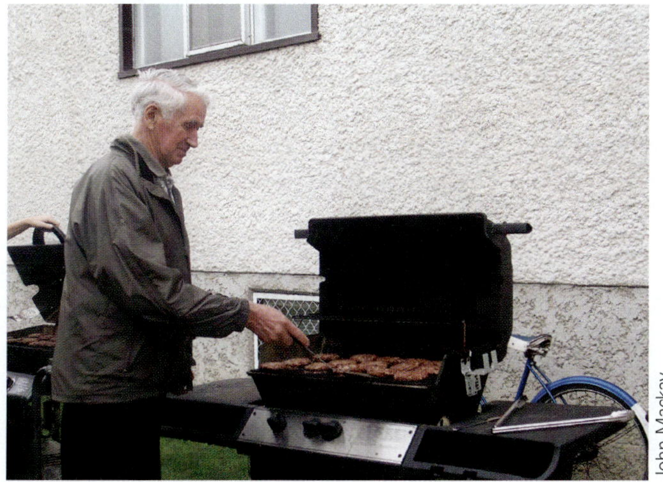
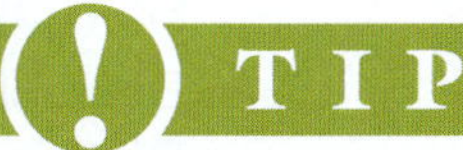

Figure 15–1 Most older adults are healthy, active, and independent.

SECTION 2
CHANGES IN THE OLDER ADULT

Physical Changes and Problems

Scientists often attribute the effects of aging to several causes. Among these are genetic predetermination, environment, and lifestyle. Whatever the actual answer, we know that as time passes, the body's systems begin to decline. The most notable changes can be seen in the following areas (Table 15–1).

Physical and Functional Changes in the Older Adult

The Skin. As individuals age, the skin develops darkly pigmented areas called age spots or liver spots. These spots often appear on the hands, face, and arms and are more noticeable in people with light complexions. In addition, because the skin secretes less oil, dryness and flakiness occur more frequently. This lack of surface moisture contributes to the older body's reduced ability to protect itself against infection. Other secretions, such as perspiration, also decrease, making heat-related emergencies more likely in certain conditions. Medications can also contribute to the patient's inability to exhibit diaphoresis (excessive perspiration) during periods of shock.

With increasing age, the skin also begins to experience a loss of fat and a weakening of its supportive structures, making it looser, thinner, and more fragile. Skin tearing occurs more easily than in the patient's youth, and problems related to restricted movement, like bedsores, occur more frequently.

(!) TIP

When you gently pinch and tug on the skin on the hand of an elderly patient, it may stay in a "tenting" position once you let go. This can be due to dehydration, or it may be normal, as the skin is not as supple as it once was.

CASE STUDY

Dispatch

My partner and I had just gotten into the station when dispatch sent us to the St. Thomas Apartments for a female senior citizen. Although we were given the woman's name and address, we were not told what the nature of her problem was. We had been to this building several times before, so we grabbed our gear and jumped in the truck.

Scene Assessment

Upon arriving at the building, we were met by the superintendent, who led us to the apartment occupied by Mrs. Elizabeth Bourque. We knocked on the door, but there was no response. The superintendent then used his pass key to let us in.

Inside, we saw that the apartment was tidy and well kept. There was no clutter, and the place smelled fresh. After looking around for a few seconds, we found Mrs. Bourque sitting on the edge of her bed. She was well groomed and appeared to have been crying for a while.

Older patients can become emotional for the same reasons that younger adults and children can. Discovering sources of their medical condition can be difficult because there can be so many complicating factors and conditions. As you study Chapter 15, it is important to consider the many common complications that older patients have. Applying what you have learned in the pharmaceutical and communication chapters is key to assessing the older adult patient.

TABLE 15–1
PHYSICAL AND FUNCTIONAL CHANGES IN THE OLDER ADULT

Body System	Changes	Complications
Skin	Decreased perspiration	Heat-related illnesses
	Decreased oil secretion	Masked signs of shock
	Loss of fat and weakening of supportive structures beneath the skin	Decreased resistance to infection
		Thermoregulatory issues
	Reduced adipose	Easily torn skin
	Decreased circulation	Bedsores
Sensory organs	Diminished vision	Falls, motor vehicle crashes
	Diminished hearing	Unable to read directions for medication
	Diminished pain sensation	Unable to hear warnings such as smoke alarms or sirens
	Diminished taste and smell	May be unaware of injury or seriousness of injury
		Decreased appetite, malnutrition
		Unable to smell smoke or leaking gas

(continued)

TABLE 15–1	**Continued**	
Respiratory system	Weakened chest muscles Less lung capacity	Less able to compensate when the body needs oxygen
Circulatory system	Decreased strength of heart contraction High blood pressure Blockage of blood vessels	Cannot meet higher demands for blood flow Heart attack, stroke, poor circulation to extremities Masked signs of shock
Digestive system	Ulcers, tumours Dental problems Dehydration Decreased motility	Gastrointestinal bleeding Malnutrition Choking on poorly chewed food Constipation Bowel obstructions
Urinary system	Incontinence	Catheterization, possibly leading to infection
Musculoskeletal system	Diminished muscle strength Weakened bone structure	Minor falls or bumps, possibly leading to broken bones
Nervous system	Fewer nerve fibres Alteration in chemical balance	Decreased sensory perception Depression Impaired sleep
Immune system	Diminished functioning	Diminished ability to heal Infection Cancer

Sensory Organs. In general, aging is associated with an ongoing reduction in the sharpness (or acuity) of the senses.

With respect to vision, far-sightedness occurs more often, as do cataracts and yellowing of the lens of the eye. Peripheral and night vision, as well as glare tolerance, are all reduced. Because of this, older patients may find it difficult to read instructions on medication bottles or may be unable to distinguish one pill colour from another. Also, unintentional injuries, such as falls or vehicle accidents, can occur.

Hearing, particularly of high-pitched sounds, also suffers. When driving, an older person may fail to hear a siren or horn sound alerting him or her to danger.

The senses of taste, smell, and skin sensation are likewise diminished. It is easy to understand, therefore, how an older adult can fail to detect spoiled food, smell a gas leak, or feel skin trauma. Taste and smell deficits can also contribute to both decreased appetite and nutritional problems.

Respiratory System. As a person ages, breathing becomes more laboured because of chest muscle weakening and because the rib cage cartilage grows stiff. In addition, the ability of the lungs to provide oxygen to the blood is reduced. As a result, the bodies of older persons are less capable of compensating when they require more oxygen as a result of injury or illness. Other lung and immune system changes can also make the older person susceptible to infections like pneumonia.

Circulatory System. The heart's ability to contract with force declines with advancing years. As a result, when the body demands increased blood flow, the heart reacts by contracting more often. If the heart contracts too rapidly, the heart's chambers do not have enough time to fill completely with blood before the next contraction occurs. Therefore, instead of increasing blood flow, this too-rapid heart rate can actually worsen circulation.

In addition, because of the effects of certain medications, it is often more difficult for the body to increase the heart rate in patients with heart disease or high blood pressure. As a result, patients who experience blood loss may actually have a normal pulse rate, even though their condition indicates that it should be rapid.

Older adults with high blood pressure are also at increased risk of both heart attack and stroke. In normal instances, the blood pressure drops as blood loss occurs. However, in a person with high blood pressure, the blood pressure may simply dip into the normal range. Although this is a dip, it may not be recognized as such. The patient may then go into shock.

Shock in the older adult patient may not follow the classic model. Therefore, when assessing the older trauma patient, consider the mechanism of injury and monitor the patient's mental status. A patient on blood thinners, or anti-clotting agents, to reduce the risk of heart attack or stroke, for example ASA (Aspirin) or warfarin (Coumadin), may have increased clotting time and therefore continue to bleed from internal or external injuries. In such instances, the first indication of shock may be a decrease in the level of responsiveness.

Over time, genetic and lifestyle factors may contribute to blood vessel changes, like blockage or a weakening of the arteries to the heart and brain. These problems can lead to heart attack or stroke. In addition, circulation to the extremities is diminished with age, causing the hands and feet to be cold.

Digestive System. The digestive system slows as people get older. Because of this, fewer secretions are available to assist in food breakdown. This can lead to indigestion (heartburn), gas production, and constipation. Because the stomach empties more slowly, vomiting may occur during injury or illness.

Ulcers and intestinal tract disorders that promote bleeding may also plague older adults. Such bleeding can be seen in vomit or in dark, tarry stools. Significant blood loss in this manner can lead to shock.

Malnutrition is another factor to consider when assessing an older patient's health. Decreased ability to taste and smell can lead not only to a decreased interest in food, but also to dental and nutritional problems. Fatigue, depression, and poverty can also lead to the older patient's failure to feed himself or herself properly. When malnutrition is present, medical problems worsen.

Urinary System. A common problem affecting older men involves blockage of urine flow due to prostate gland enlargement. When this occurs, a bladder or kidney infection can result. Older women can also experience urinary tract infections. Frequently, older adults with these infections do not make specific, related complaints. Because of this, overwhelming infection can take hold, leading to septic shock. The EMR should suspect septic shock when shock signs and symptoms are present but no blood loss has occurred. EMR treatment for both types of shock is the same.

Musculoskeletal System. Muscle strength and endurance, as well as bone mass, decrease with age. For an older individual, even minor falls often result in broken bones. A broken hip can lead to a decrease in both mobility and bone stress tolerance. Overall health status can also rapidly decline after a broken hip.

Nervous System. A reduction in the number of nerve fibres and changes in the brain's chemical balance may lead to decreased perception, loss of balance, coordination problems, and altered sleep patterns. These factors contribute to injuries among older patients.

Although it is commonly believed that thinking and memory impairments are normal for the aged, this is not the case. When these events occur, they indicate the presence of an abnormal condition. Sometimes confusion and agitated behaviour are temporary, caused by illness or medication effects. Find out from the patient's family or caregivers if the behaviour related to the emergency is usual or if it occurred suddenly.

Depression is very common among older adults. It can lead to suicide or attempted suicide. Depressed patients may have poor hygiene and eating habits, as well as a disorderly home. In addition, prolonged depression can lead to physical symptoms.

Immune System. Common illnesses like influenza lead to a much higher fatality rate among older adults. Though fever is often a sign of infection, it may not be present in some members of this age group. In addition, the increased risk of infection and decreased ability to heal make injuries and surgery more serious and more often fatal for older adults.

The Aging Body's Response to Medication

The body's ability to respond to and eliminate medications also changes with age. This can result in older patients having exaggerated responses to drugs and more profound side effects compared to younger patients. Medications often need to be introduced, discontinued, or have the dosage adjusted. This can result in repeated visits to a physician. Because older adults tend to be on several different medications, life-threatening drug interactions are more likely.

Psychological and Economic Factors

Many psychological, social, and economic factors affect the lives and health of older adults. Being aware of these possibilities is a step toward developing empathy and compassion for patients of advanced age in your care. These factors include the following:

- Depression
- Substance abuse
- Physical and psychological abuse
- Neglect
- Loneliness
- Poverty

Depression

Depression is common among older adults. It may result from changes in the brain's chemistry or it may be due to a variety of situational factors. Friends or relatives may have died, for example, and the patient may be living alone and feeling isolated. Alternatively, reduced mobility can also lead to depression. Tasks that were once easily accomplished now require daily dependence on another person. Older patients can also feel shame or embarrassment about the loss of certain body functions or about changes in their appearance. Even though depression can be treated with both therapy and medication, for those who are older it is still a contributing factor in suicide.

Substance Abuse

Health care providers often fail to suspect alcohol and other substance abuse as playing a part in the medical conditions of older patients. Abuse may include prescription drugs as well as illegal substances. Substance abuse of any sort can contribute to physical health deterioration, altered mental status, and injuries. While it may seem shocking to think of an older person having a substance abuse problem, it is not unreasonable. After all, many seniors who are now in their 60s or 70s were in their early adult years during the drug heyday of the late 1960s and early 1970s.

Abuse and Neglect

EMS providers are often the first to detect physical and psychological abuse as well as neglect (Figure 15–2). There are several risk factors for the abuse or neglect of older persons. Older adults are most at risk when they meet any of the following conditions:

- Require assistance with daily activities
- Have difficulty sleeping on an ongoing basis
- Have lost bladder control
- Exhibit bizarre behaviour due to altered mental status

The EMR should suspect abuse when an injury seems inconsistent with the description of how it happened or when there are multiple injuries in various stages of healing. Shame or fear of punishment may prevent the patient from being willing to discuss the nature of the injury. It is not unusual for the abused individual to have been denied adequate food, water, or medications. At the same time, basic assistance with activities such as bathing and changing clothes may also be withheld. While it is not recommended that you confront the abuser, it is imperative that you report your suspicions to the incoming EMS crew. Follow local protocol for reporting to other authorities.

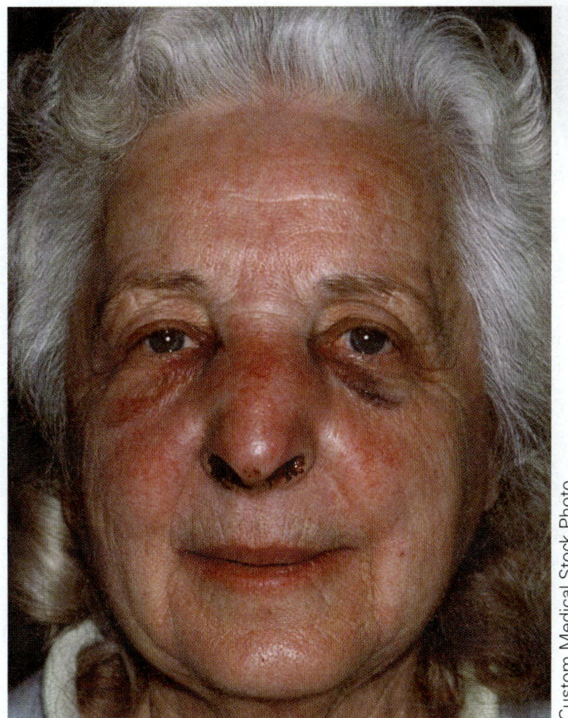

Figure 15–2   Look for signs of abuse or neglect.

Socioeconomic Concerns

Many older people live on fixed and inadequate incomes. As a result, they are often not able to afford proper food, shelter, medication, or safety devices. Homes may be run-down, making the living environment an invitation to injury. Environmental conditions, such as proper heating and cooling, may also be inadequate. In cold weather, this may lead to the use of alternative sources of heat, such as space heaters or an open oven. Improper monitoring of the use of these devices or faulty machines can cause burns, fires, and carbon monoxide poisoning.

SECTION 3
EMR CARE

Illness and Injury in Older Adults

The most common medical complaints in older adults include the following:

- Chest pain
- Breathing difficulty (due to lung or heart problems or airway obstruction) (Figure 15–3)
- Fainting or near fainting (due to heart problems, internal bleeding, medication effects, changes in blood vessels that supply the brain with oxygen)
- Altered mental status

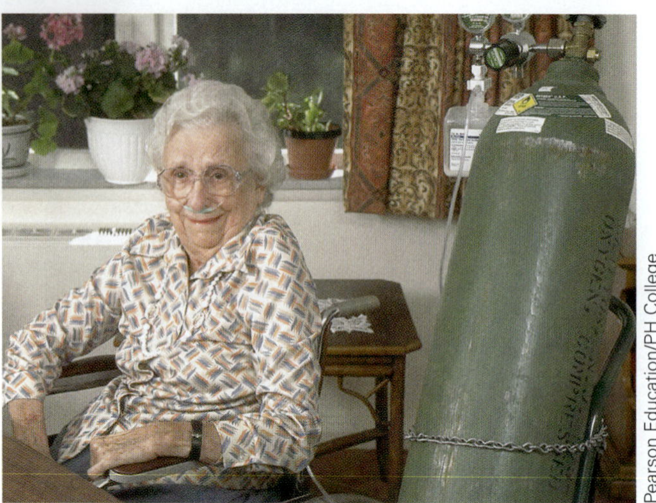

Figure 15–3 Breathing difficulty is a common medical complaint in older adults.

The most common mechanisms of injury in older adults include the following:

- Burns
- Falls
- Vehicle crashes

Many injuries can be attributed to physical aging effects, such as diminished vision, hearing, and pain sensation, as well as a loss of muscular strength, balance, and coordination. However, the physics associated with growing older also plays a role. The force required to produce an injury in an older person is much less than what is needed in someone younger. Also, remember that the medications many seniors take can mask the seriousness of an injury. For example, some high blood pressure medications cause a slower heart rate and can prevent tachycardia during blood loss and shock. Be aware of this and respond accordingly.

Scene Assessment for Older Patients

As with all your calls, your first priority is your own safety and that of your crew. Assess the scene as you would for any other emergency call. Keep in mind the following:

- Substance abuse problems, mental illness, and conditions like Alzheimer disease can produce a violent older patient. Be prepared.
- Stay alert for signs that might suggest abuse, neglect, or a patient's inability to take care of himself or herself.
- Observe any potential hazards, such as home clutter, loose or missing handrails, throw rugs and mats, unstable porches, or loose stairs.

- Look for poor functioning of alternative heat sources to warn you of possible carbon monoxide poisoning.

When approaching older patients, focus your attention on them rather than on family members or caregivers who may be eager to speak on their behalf. This demonstrates respect, and it affords the patients more control over a troubling situation. Make eye contact first and then introduce yourself. Once you have been told a patient's full name, address him or her by the surname preceded by "Mr.," "Mrs.," or "Miss." Use the patient's first name only if instructed to do so by the patient.

Older patients can have communication problems. For example, many older patients have hearing aids but do not always wear them. If your patient has one but is not wearing it, ask him or her to put it on. If your patient has dentures but doesn't wear them due to discomfort, you may have difficulty understanding his or her speech. If this is the case, you may ask the patient to put the dentures in.

After introducing yourself to the patient, position your body at the patient's eye level (Figure 15–4). This stance is less intimidating than one in which you tower over the person. Shake the patient's hand to establish rapport. At the same time, note the patient's skin temperature and ability to move and follow directions. Then ask the patient why EMS was called. Make your questions specific to the information you wish to learn. Otherwise, a general query such as "What is wrong?" can lead to a recitation of medical and many nonmedical complaints. As you begin to collect information, ensure that your face is turned toward the patient, that you speak directly to the patient (Figure 15–5), that you do not raise your voice, and that you let the patient speak at his or her own pace. Use a louder tone only if it is clear that the patient cannot hear you.

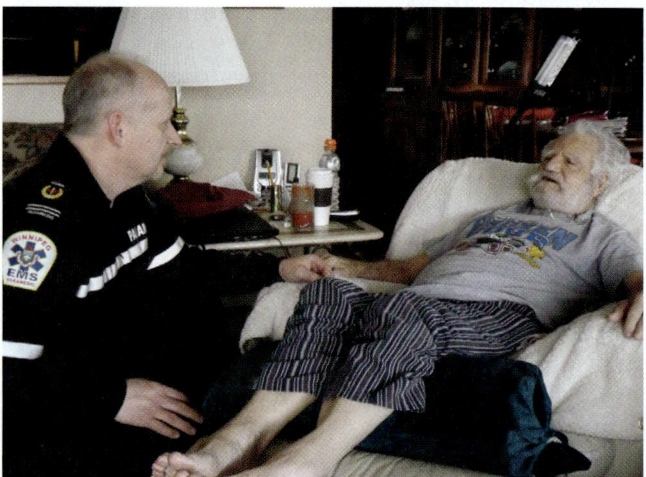

Figure 15–4 Position yourself at the patient's eye level.

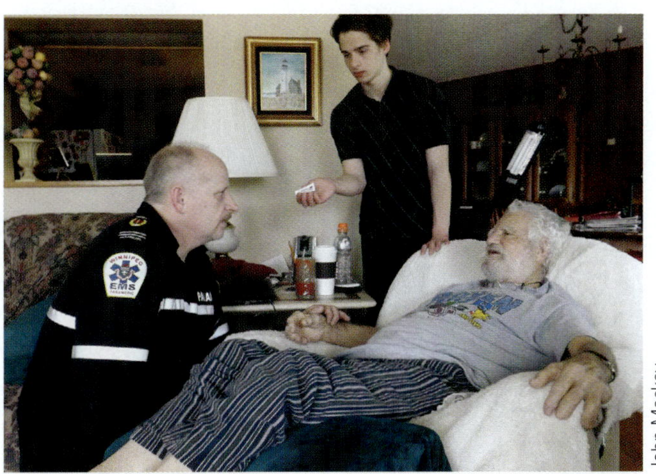

Figure 15–5 Just as with any other patient, speak to older adult patients directly.

> ## TIP
>
> Decreased sensitivity to pain occurs during aging, so maintain a high index of suspicion and treat any complaint of pain in older patients as a symptom of serious illness or injury.

> ## TIP
>
> Anxiety can be raised when the patient can't see properly. If your patient has poor vision, it's a good idea to position yourself directly in front of him or her where the person has the best chance of seeing you.

Primary Assessment of Older Patients

Perform a primary assessment as you would for any other patient. However, keep the following in mind:

- Note whether the patient appears clean and well groomed.
- Observe whether the older patient who has had a stroke has difficulty chewing, swallowing, or clearing the airway of secretions. In the unconscious patient, dentures and other dental devices can cause airway obstruction.
- Correct head and neck positioning for airway care may be challenging because curvature of the spine occurs with aging.
- If you leave a patient's dentures in place, artificial ventilation may be more easily accomplished with a mask.
- If the patient is taking ASA (Aspirin) or blood-thinning medications, controlling bleeding may be more difficult.

Secondary Assessment of Older Patients

Perform a secondary assessment as you would for any other patient. Keep in mind that many older patients wear several layers of clothing, which can make the assessment more difficult to perform.

Patient History for Older Patients

Gather a patient history as you would for any other patient with a similar emergency. Other persons should be questioned only if it becomes apparent that your patient is not a reliable source of information.

It is important to note that older patients may deny illness or injury symptoms. There are many reasons for this, including a fear of leaving home, going to the hospital, and losing their independence. Medical care and ambulance transportation costs, hospital admission worries, and leaving a loved one or pet can also play a part. If at all possible, assist in finding a solution. Sometimes this is as simple as asking if there is someone the patient can phone for help. In some cases, a patient may be more forthcoming with their history and information once friends and family are not present.

Older adult patients may have only vaguely defined complaints, such as nausea or weakness. This can be true even with serious illnesses. Be aware of this and make sure you question appropriately.

Many older patients take several medications (Figure 15–6). Ask where the medications are and then check the labels yourself. This is sometimes easier than asking the patient to remember and recite the name of each one. A list of medications as well as a medical history and the patient's vital information may be affixed to the front of their refrigerator (Figure 15–7).

Treating the Older Patient

When treating, handling, and transporting the elderly patient, the same general principles apply as for all patients. Maintain the patient's dignity at all times and interact in a respectful manner. While the patient may have a lengthy medical history, he or she may be very concise and helpful in conveying it.

When preparing for transport, alert the patient about how and when you plan to move him or her. Await a response so you know if the patient understands and is ready. Handle the patient gently, remembering that fractures have a higher incidence among the elderly as bone density decreases. Make sure the patient is covered and kept warm as

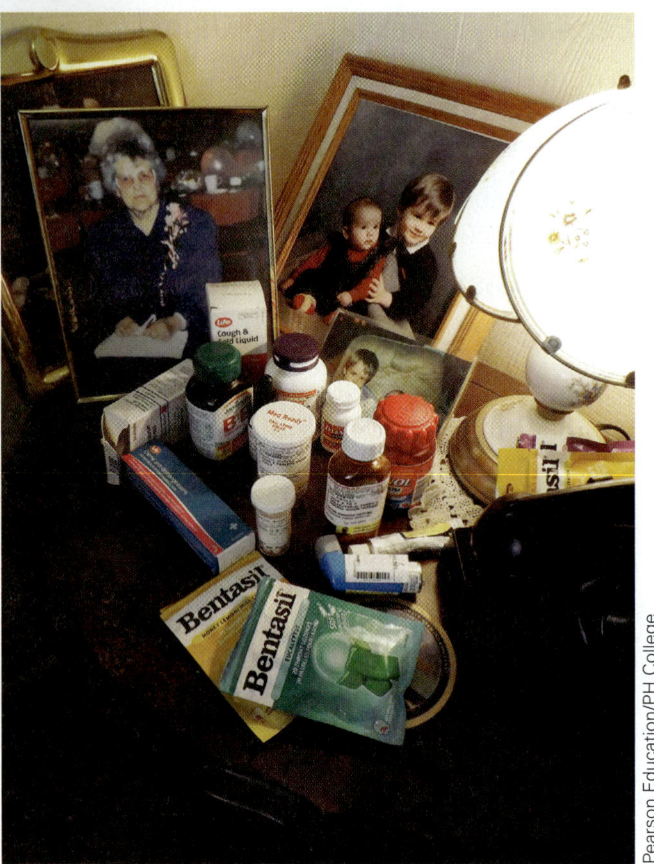

Figure 15–6 Make note of medications when you gather a patient history.

Pearson Education/PH College

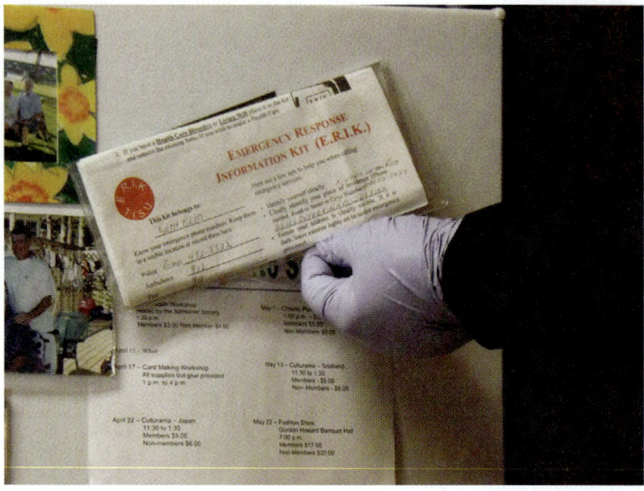

John Mackay

Figure 15–7 Emergency Response Information Kit (ERIK).

the patient may have difficulty preserving his or her own body heat.

Finally, if you must immobilize the elderly patient on a backboard or secure him or her on a stretcher, consider padding natural hollows that are created with curvature of the spine, as skin will break down or tear quickly at pressure points. Treat the elderly patient the same way you would want your own grandparent to be treated.

EMR FOCUS

The priorities for EMR care of older patients are the same as for other patients; however, there are differences in the general approach. Remember that the effects of aging and common medications can make older patients less able to compensate for blood loss and less sensitive to pain. These factors can mask signs usually associated with serious injury or illness. Older people often wait until their condition is criti-cal before calling for assistance. Be sure to continually reassess your patients for changes in mental status and physical condition.

It is essential that you communicate with these patients as you would with any other adult. Make eye contact and speak clearly. Showing respect as you interact with older patients will make them and their family more confident in your ability as a health care provider.

CASE STUDY FOLLOW-UP

At the beginning of this chapter, you read that EMRs were on the scene with a responsive older female with an unknown problem. To see how the chapter skills apply to this emergency, read the following. It describes how the call was completed.

SCENE ASSESSMENT *(Continued)*

I introduced myself to Mrs. Bourque by telling her that my name was John Warkentin and that I was with the fire department. As I leaned down to her side at the bed, I asked her why she had called 9-1-1. Although she was crying, she responded that she was dizzy and could not stand. She looked afraid and told me she could not remember if it was day or night. I told her it was daytime, nine o'clock in the morning. As I answered, I saw 10 pill bottles on the nightstand. I wondered if, perhaps, she had taken either too few pills or too many.

PRIMARY ASSESSMENT

As I continued to reassure her, I checked the ABCs. She was breathing adequately and had a strong pulse. I told her an ambulance was on the way and that we would help her get to the hospital for the care she needed. I also started some oxygen.

SECONDARY ASSESSMENT

I proceeded to take her vital signs and had just begun to perform a head-to-toe exam when the paramedics arrived.

PATIENT HISTORY

Although the paramedics arrived before we could gather a patient history, my partner had found an empty vial of prescription medicine called Synthroid and a home blood glucose testing device in the patient's bathroom.

TRANSFER OF CARE

I conveyed Mrs. Bourque's two major symptoms—dizziness and confusion about the time of day. I reported my assessment findings and made sure that the paramedics saw all the bottles of medication. I also told them that my partner had found an empty Synthroid vial and a home blood glucose testing device.

When the paramedics were ready to leave with Mrs. Bourque, she reached over and asked me to phone her daughter. I wrote down the number she gave me. My partner and I then helped the paramedics wheel her over to the elevator and to the ambulance.

I called the patient's daughter as soon as I could and let her know that her mother had been taken to the hospital. I was glad to hear that she didn't live too far away and would be by her mother's side in a matter of hours.

> When you are called to an emergency involving an older person, stick to your patient assessment plan as you would for any other patient. Try to be especially respectful and compassionate, and keep in mind that a patient's condition may be much more serious than it appears to be.

NOCPs

2.1 e Interact effectively with the patient, relatives, and bystanders who are in stressful situations **S**

f Speak in language appropriate to the listener **S**

g Use appropriate terminology **S**

2.3 a Employ effective non-verbal behaviour **A**

2.4 a Treat others with respect **S**

4.2 b Obtain patient's medication profile **S**

c Obtain chief complaint and/or incident history from patient, family members, and/or bystanders **S**

d Obtain information regarding patient's past medical history **S**

6.2 c Provide care for geriatric patient **A**

REVIEW QUESTIONS

Page references where answers may be found or supported are provided at the end of each question.

SECTION 1

1. When assessing an elderly patient, from whom should you seek information first? (p. 229)

SECTION 2

2. Which one of the following factors does *not* contribute to the risk of injury in older adults? (pp. 230–231)

a. weakened muscles

b. diminished vision

c. increased reaction time

d. diminished coordination

3. Which of the following factors *decreases* an older adult's ability to compensate for bleeding? (pp. 232–235)

a. taking ASA for arthritis pain

b. taking medication for heart problems

c. taking medication for high blood pressure

d. all of the above

4. The older patient may underestimate the seriousness of injury because of which of the following? (p. 234)

   a. diminished pain sensation

   b. specific pain complaints

   c. diminished hearing

   d. high fever with illness

5. Which one of the following is *not* a psychosocial issue of concern for older adults? (pp. 232–233)

   a. substance abuse

   b. loneliness

   c. depression

   d. peer pressure

SECTION 3

6. What are the three most common mechanisms of injury in older patients? (p. 234)

7. List some items that may increase the risk of injury in the home of an older patient. (p. 234)

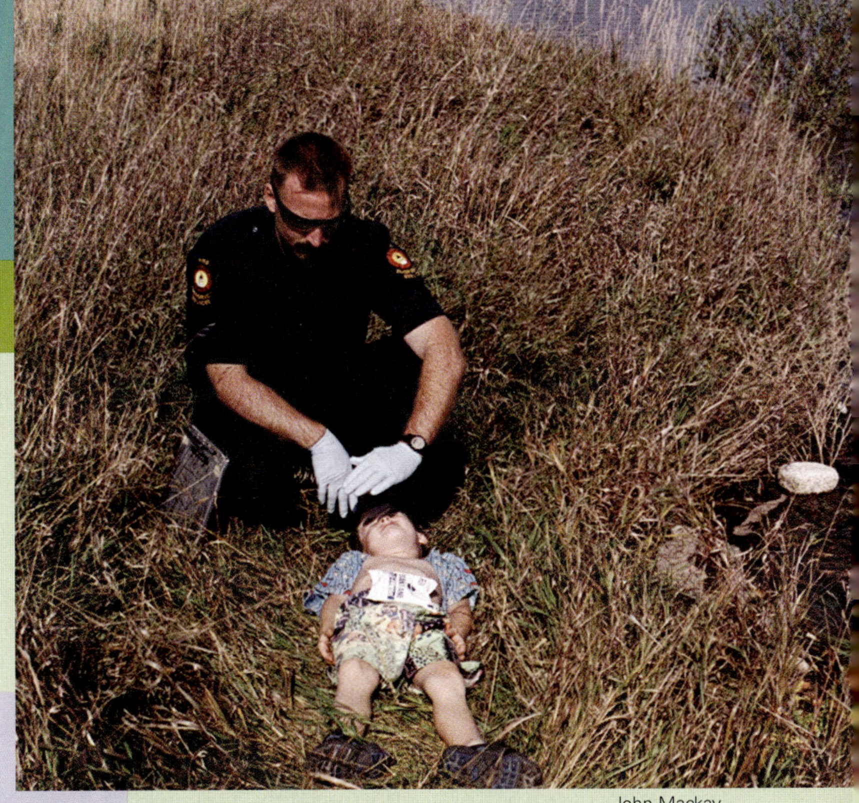
John Mackay

Heat and Cold Emergencies

OBJECTIVES

1. Describe three ways that the body creates heat and two ways it can conserve heat.

2. Describe the five ways in which the body loses heat.

3. Compare the signs and symptoms of mild and severe hypothermia and explain the care of both types of hypothermia.

4. Explain under what conditions rewarming of a local cold injury should be done.

5. List five factors that can contribute to a heat emergency.

6. Describe how to identify a patient with a heat emergency and explain how to cool a patient with hyperthermia.

7. Demonstrate a caring attitude toward the patient and family when dealing with a heat or cold injury, while giving priority to the interests of the patient.

INTRODUCTION

A heat- or cold-related emergency can happen to anyone. Canadian climates can vary dramatically, and temperatures can change by more than 20°C in a matter of hours. Letter carriers, farmers, police officers, and countless others who work or play outdoors are at risk. People may also be at risk indoors, especially the very young and old. Some of these emergencies, such as frostbite, can be minor. Others, like heatstroke, can be life threatening.

SECTION 1
BODY TEMPERATURE

Heat and cold can produce a number of emergencies. To respond to them appropriately, you need a basic understanding of how people adjust to heat and cold.

The body produces heat mainly through the process of metabolism, including the digestion of food. In cold, the body conserves heat by constricting the blood vessels near its surface. Hair also stands erect, thickening the layer of warm air trapped near the skin. The body can produce more heat, if needed, by shivering and by releasing certain hormones such as epinephrine.

In general, the body loses heat in five ways (Figure 16–1):

- *Convection.* This occurs when moving air passes over the body and carries heat away. (See the wind chill calculation chart, Figure 16–2 on p. 242.)
- *Conduction.* This occurs when direct contact with an object carries heat away. For example, a swimmer is in direct contact with water. If it is cooler than the body, the water will take away the swimmer's body heat. It can do so 25 times faster than air.

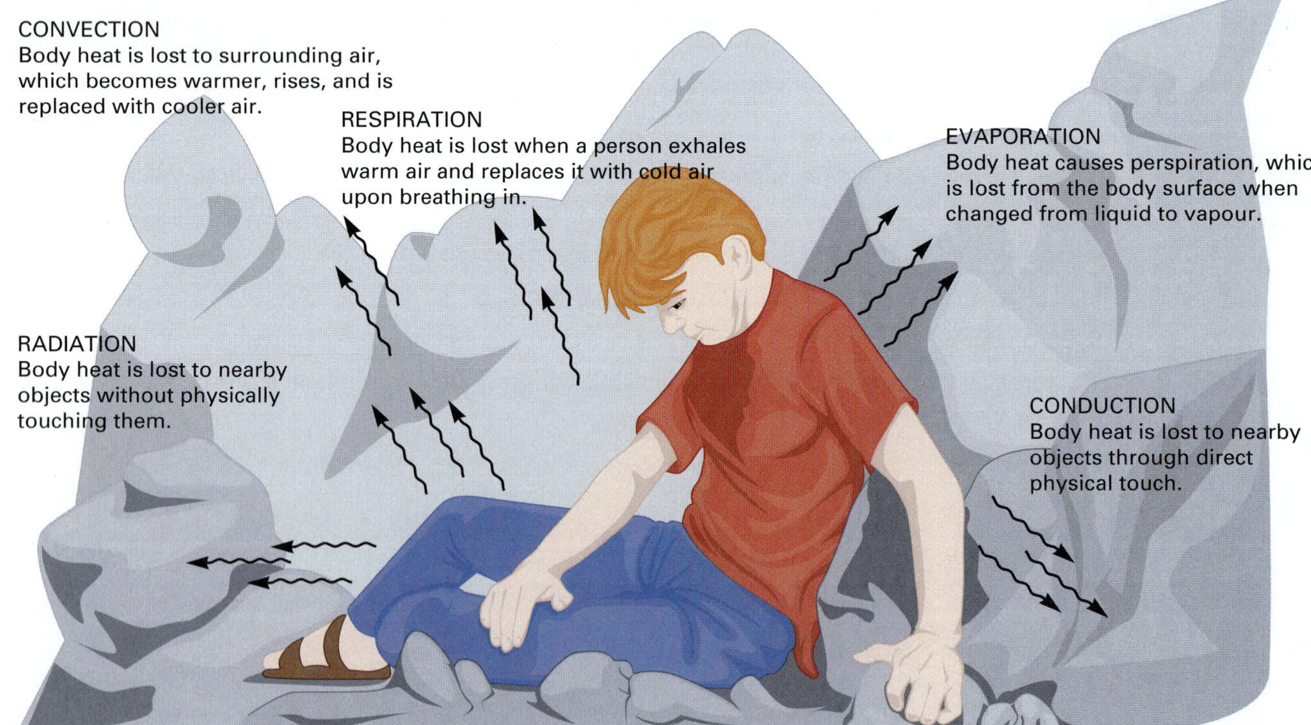

Figure 16–1 Mechanisms of heat loss.

CASE STUDY

Dispatch

It was 9 a.m. and we were on our way to 153 Western Avenue for a woman down. Rescue 3 was dispatched to assist, with an ETA of 15 minutes.

Scene Assessment

The person who called EMS was there to meet us. "Mrs. Gusev and I have tea every morning at 7 a.m.," she told us. "I just know something is wrong." We approached the neat little cottage. I knocked and then yelled through the door, "EMS. Can we help you?" We heard a faint voice from the back of the house.

We entered through the back door and immediately saw the patient. She appeared to be about 80 years old. She was lying supine on the kitchen floor, calling out weakly. The contents of a garbage bag were lying spilled on the floor. We could see dried blood in her hair and under her head.

Primary Assessment

My partner positioned himself and manually stabilized her head. I got down on my knees, introduced myself, and asked her what was wrong. She told us that on the previous night at about 9 p.m. she tripped over her cat and fell. She was sore all over, but her hip hurt the most. I was glad to note that she was awake and alert. Her airway was open, breathing was good, and all bleeding appeared to have stopped.

It appeared at first that Mrs. Gusev was a trauma patient, the fall being her mechanism of injury. However, we found that her skin was ice cold and she was shivering. We reported to dispatch and then continued the assessment.

> Consider this patient as you read Chapter 16. Might she have any problems other than an injured hip?

- *Radiation.* This method involves the transfer of heat to an object without physical contact. Most loss is from the head and neck, areas rich in blood and blood vessels.
- *Evaporation.* The process by which sweat changes to water vapour has a cooling effect on the body. Note that it stops when the relative humidity of the air reaches 75 percent.
- *Respiration.* This occurs when a person breathes in cold air and breathes out air that was warmed inside the body.

SECTION 2
COLD EMERGENCIES

Exposure to cold can cause two kinds of emergencies. One is a generalized cold emergency, or generalized **hypothermia**. It involves an overall reduction of body temperature, which can be deadly. The other kind of emergency is called a **local cold injury**, or damage to body tissues in a specific (local) part of the body.

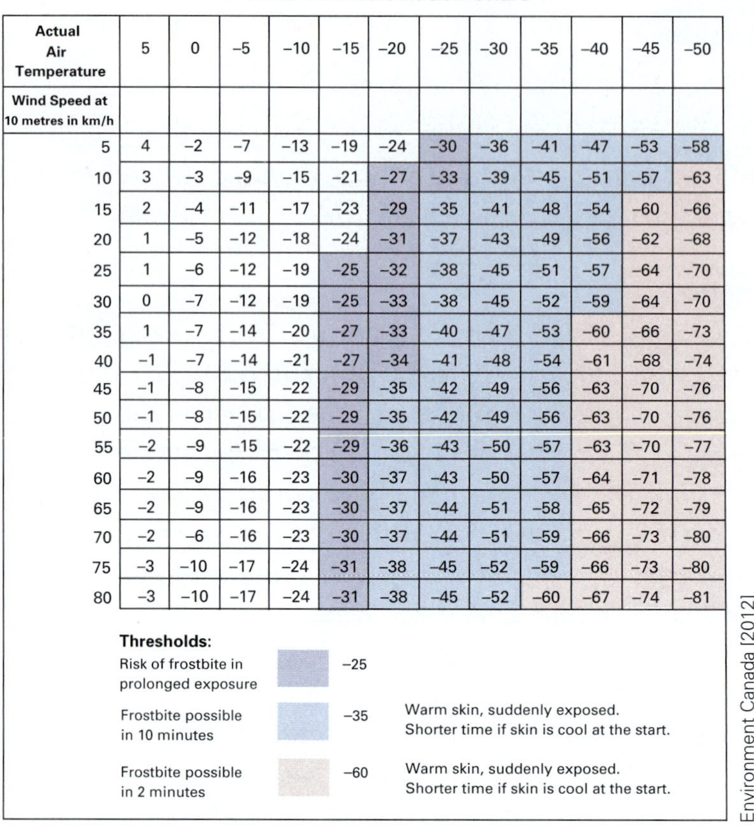

Actual Air Temperature	5	0	−5	−10	−15	−20	−25	−30	−35	−40	−45	−50
Wind Speed at 10 metres in km/h												
5	4	−2	−7	−13	−19	−24	−30	−36	−41	−47	−53	−58
10	3	−3	−9	−15	−21	−27	−33	−39	−45	−51	−57	−63
15	2	−4	−11	−17	−23	−29	−35	−41	−48	−54	−60	−66
20	1	−5	−12	−18	−24	−31	−37	−43	−49	−56	−62	−68
25	1	−6	−12	−19	−25	−32	−38	−45	−51	−57	−64	−70
30	0	−7	−12	−19	−25	−33	−38	−45	−52	−59	−64	−70
35	1	−7	−14	−20	−27	−33	−40	−47	−53	−60	−66	−73
40	−1	−7	−14	−21	−27	−34	−41	−48	−54	−61	−68	−74
45	−1	−8	−15	−22	−29	−35	−42	−49	−56	−63	−70	−76
50	−1	−8	−15	−22	−29	−35	−42	−49	−56	−63	−70	−76
55	−2	−9	−15	−22	−29	−36	−43	−50	−57	−63	−70	−77
60	−2	−9	−16	−23	−30	−37	−43	−50	−57	−64	−71	−78
65	−2	−9	−16	−23	−30	−37	−44	−51	−58	−65	−72	−79
70	−2	−6	−16	−23	−30	−37	−44	−51	−59	−66	−73	−80
75	−3	−10	−17	−24	−31	−38	−45	−52	−59	−66	−73	−80
80	−3	−10	−17	−24	−31	−38	−45	−52	−60	−67	−74	−81

Figure 16–2 Wind chill calculation chart.

Generalized Hypothermia

Exposure to extreme cold for a short time or to moderate cold for a long time can cause hypothermia. Even "warm" temperatures, if they are below body temperature, can cause a decrease in body temperature given time. A child swimming in a 30°C pool or an adult standing in a gentle rain without rain gear can lose a lot of body heat. There are several risk factors you should know about:

- *Medical condition of the patient.* Any underlying problem—such as shock, head or spinal injury, burns, infection, diabetes, and hypoglycemia—can weaken the body's responses to heat and cold.
- *Drugs, alcohol, and poisons.* These also impede the body's ability to maintain body temperature.
- *Age of the patient.* Very young or very old patients are especially at risk.

The anatomy of infants puts them at risk. The head is large in proportion to the body. The body surface is larger compared to their mass. The result is that they lose more heat more rapidly than adults.

Infants also have an immature nervous system. This means that they cannot shiver well enough to warm themselves when needed.

Other people are also at risk, especially older adults. If they are on a fixed low income, for example, they may not be able to afford to properly heat their home. Sudden illness or injury can limit their ability to escape the cold. Impaired judgment due to medication or limited mobility due to a medical condition also contributes to their risk.

Many outdoor clubs and organizations discourage or even ban the use of alcohol. The momentary flush of warmth felt after a drink actually increases heat loss.

Patient Assessment

During scene assessment, note the location of the patient. Ask yourself these questions: Does the environment suggest the possibility of hypothermia? How long has the patient been exposed to those conditions? If scene assessment suggests the possibility of a cold emergency, put your hand on the patient's abdomen during the secondary assessment. If it is cool or cold, treat for hypothermia. That, along with

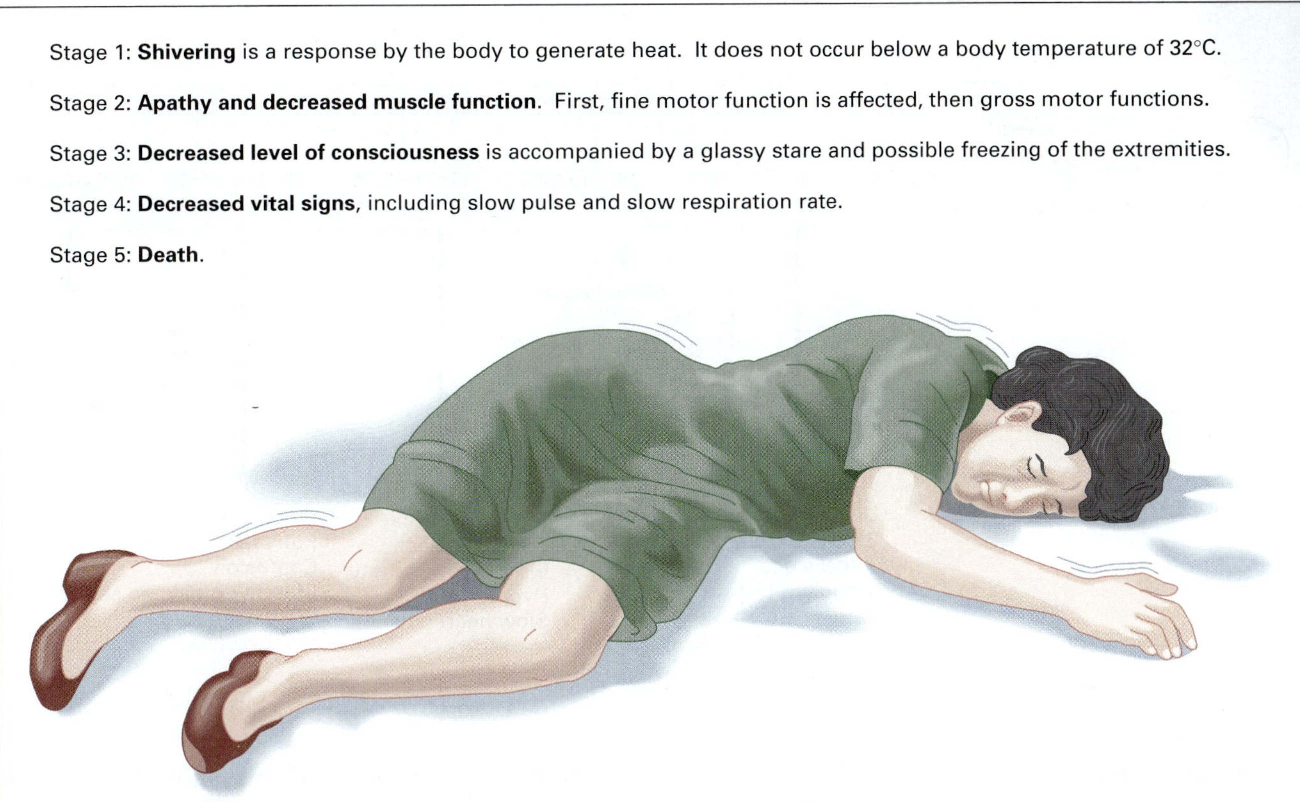

Stage 1: **Shivering** is a response by the body to generate heat. It does not occur below a body temperature of 32°C.

Stage 2: **Apathy and decreased muscle function.** First, fine motor function is affected, then gross motor functions.

Stage 3: **Decreased level of consciousness** is accompanied by a glassy stare and possible freezing of the extremities.

Stage 4: **Decreased vital signs,** including slow pulse and slow respiration rate.

Stage 5: **Death.**

Figure 16–3   Stages of hypothermia.

impaired judgment, can quickly turn a walk in the woods into a deadly excursion.

Note that hypothermia is a progressive condition (Figure 16–3). At first, the patient will shiver. When shivering stops, he or she may appear to be clumsy, confused, and forgetful. He or she may even appear to be intoxicated. Often witnesses will say that the patient had mood swings—one moment calm and the next animated or even combative.

Finally, the patient's level of consciousness decreases. He or she becomes less communicative and is difficult to rouse. The patient may display poor judgment and do things like removing his or her clothing while still in the cold. There may be muscle stiffness, a rigid posture, and loss of sensation. The most ominous sign of a life-threatening condition is unconsciousness. These patients are unstable and need immediate transport.

The signs and symptoms of hypothermia are summarized in Figure 16–4.

Emergency Care

After completing your scene, primary, and secondary assessments, there are several things you can do for your patient. To minimize further injury from cold, do the following:

1. *Remove the patient from the cold environment.* Move the patient to a shelter away from the cold wind or water. If the patient is on the ground, get him or her off it or put a blanket between him or her and the ground.
2. *Administer oxygen if you are allowed to do so.* If possible, it should be warm and humidified.
3. *Remove all wet clothing, and cover the patient with a blanket.* A thin layer of dry clothing or even just a blanket is better than a thick layer of wet clothing (Figure 16–5).
4. *Handle the patient very gently.* Rough handling can make the patient's condition worse and even cause injuries. Do not massage the extremities. Do not allow the patient to walk or exert himself or herself. Do not allow the patient to eat or drink stimulants.
5. *Comfort, calm, and reassure the patient.* Tell him or her that everything that can be done will be done. Communicate with empathy.

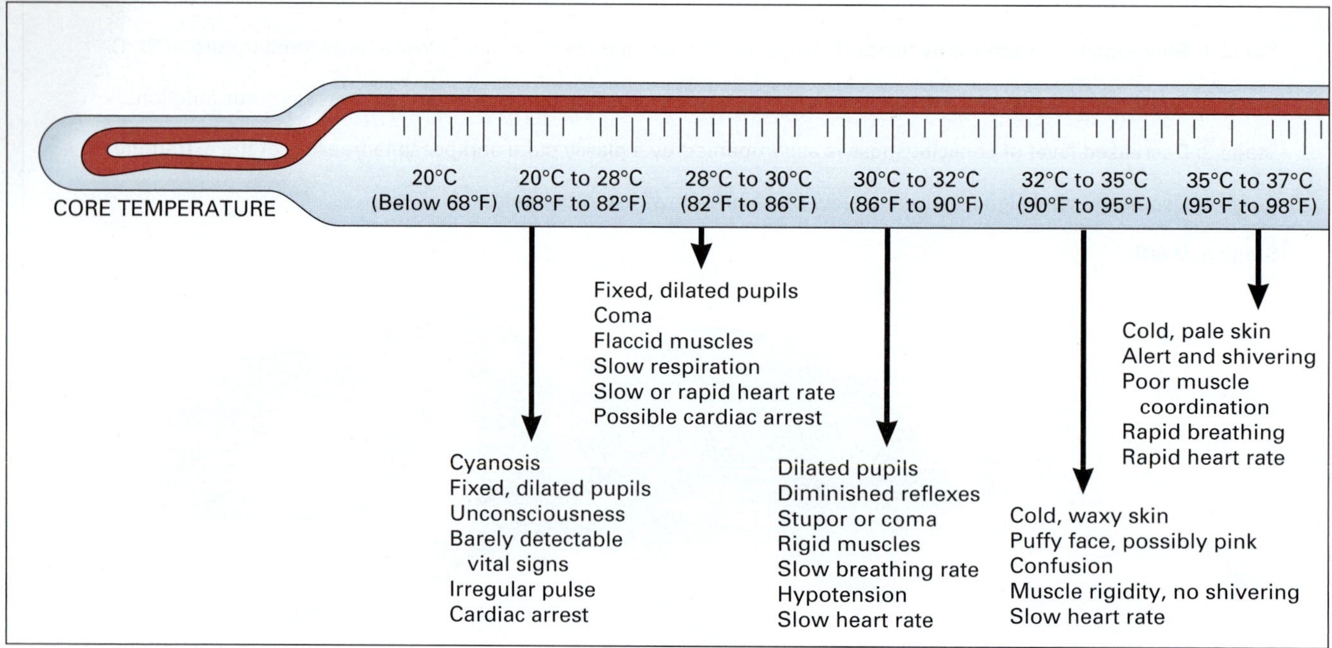

Figure 16–4 Signs and symptoms of hypothermia.

Mild Hypothermia

The patient with mild hypothermia will present with cold skin and shivering and will still be alert and oriented. The signs and symptoms may include the following:

- Increased breathing rate
- Increased pulse rate and blood pressure
- Slow, thick speech
- Staggering walk
- Apathy, drowsiness, incoherence
- Sluggish pupils
- Uncontrollable shivering

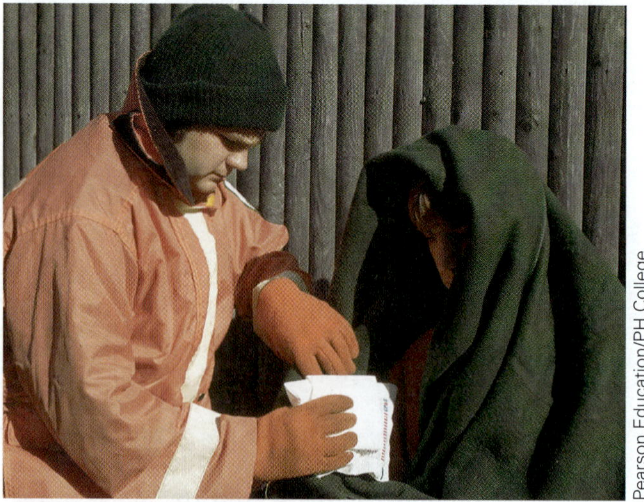

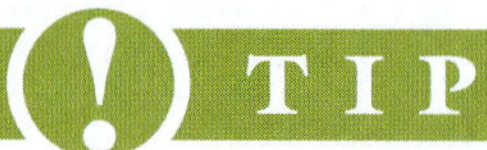

Figure 16–5 A patient with generalized hypothermia needs to be rewarmed.

If the patient is alert and able, allow him or her to drink warm fluids. A good test of the patient's ability to protect the airway is to have him or her hold the cup. If the patient cannot hold the cup or control the drinking, do not allow him or her to drink. Never give a confused or lethargic patient anything to drink. The danger of aspiration is too great. Never give coffee, tea, or other caffeinated drinks such as cola. Do not allow the patient to smoke. Stimulants promote heat loss.

Cover the patient with a warm blanket. Remember that heat loss is greatest from the head and neck—hence, an old sailor's saying, "When your feet are cold, put on a hat." Cover the patient's head with the blanket.

If heat packs are available, consider using them. (Be sure to follow local protocol.) Apply the packs to the patient's neck, armpits, and groin. Remember that the patient may have a decreased sense of touch. Check beneath the heat packs periodically to be sure that they are not burning the skin.

> **① T I P**
>
> Wrapping the heat pack in a small towel or pillow slip may prevent damage to the skin.

Severe Hypothermia

Patients with severe hypothermia may become unconscious. This is a true medical emergency that can lead to death. The signs and symptoms may include the following:

- Extremely slow breathing rate
- Extremely slow pulse rate
- Unconsciousness
- Fixed and dilated pupils
- Rigid extremities
- Absence of shivering

Consider using a nasopharyngeal airway to secure the airway of an unconscious patient. Administer high-concentration oxygen.

When assessing circulation, you may find no pulses in the patient's limbs. Remember that the body is a metabolic icebox at this stage. It does not need normal circulation to sustain life because everything is slowed down. A slow pulse is not deadly and may actually be protective.

Assess the carotid pulse for about one minute before starting CPR. If it is cold outside, remember that your sense of touch may be less than it should be. Consider putting your fingers in your armpits or your groin before taking a pulse. Remember to handle the patient gently. Any rough handling can induce ventricular fibrillation or sudden cardiac death.

If your patient is breathless and pulseless, begin CPR. Note that many of these patients have all the signs of death, including fixed pupils and stiff extremities. The rule of thumb in EMS is "You're not dead until you're warm and dead." Therefore, even with these signs, start CPR.

Rewarming in the field is not recommended for patients with severe hypothermia. They need special attention in a hospital. Arrange for transport to the closest medical facility. Follow local protocols.

Local Cold Injuries

Patient Assessment

Frostbite, or local cold injury, is the freezing or near freezing of a body part. Usually the toes, fingers, face, nose, and ears are most at risk (Figure 16–6).

Frostbitten areas are usually easy to identify. With early or superficial frostbite, light skin will redden, and dark skin will turn pale. When the skin is depressed gently, it will blanch and then return to its normal colour. The patient will often complain of loss of feeling and sensation in the injured area.

In the later stages of frostbite (called late or deep cold injury), the skin may appear waxy. It may also be firm to the touch. As freezing continues, the skin becomes mottled or blotchy. Finally, the area becomes swollen, blistered, and white.

When the injured parts begin to thaw, the skin colour changes. It will appear to be flushed with areas of purple and blanching, or it may be mottled and cyanotic.

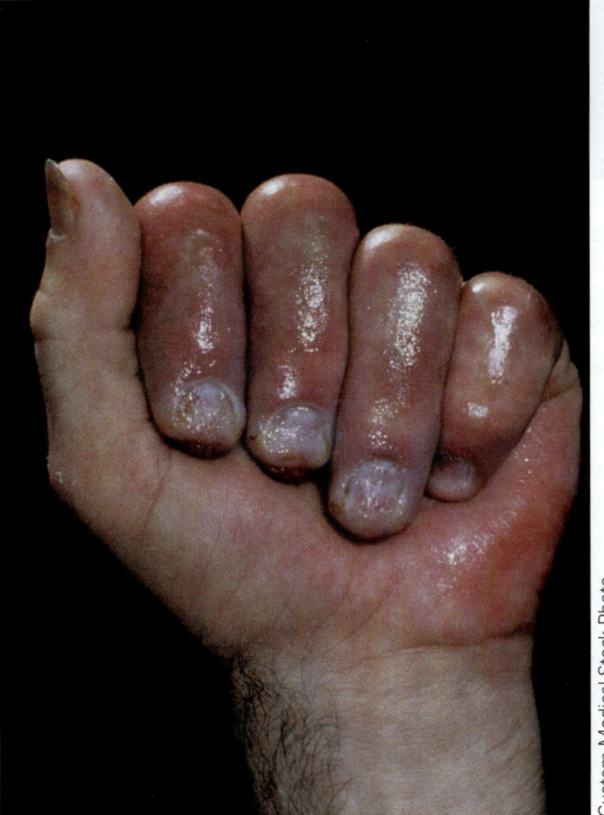

Figure 16–6a   Frostbite, or local cold injury.

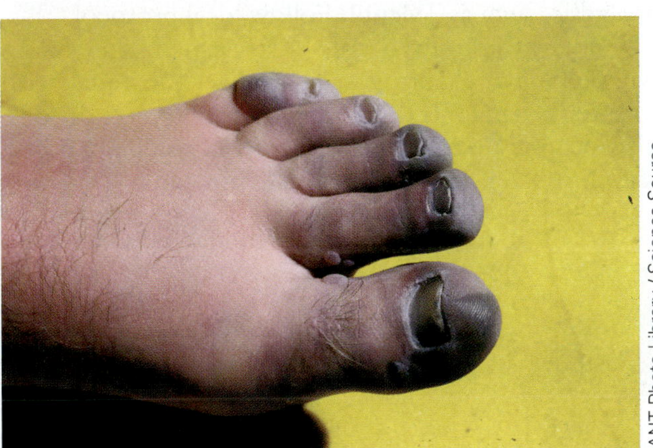

Figure 16–6b   Late or deep frostbite.

Emergency Care

If you suspect hypothermia, treat it before you care for a frostbitten extremity. Emergency care for a local cold injury is as follows:

1. *Remove the patient from the cold environment.* Do not allow the patient to walk on a frostbitten limb.
2. *Administer oxygen if you are allowed to do so.*
3. *Remove all wet clothing.*
4. *Protect the frostbitten area from further injury.* If the injury is to an extremity, manually stabilize it.

If the injury is superficial, cover it with a blanket. If the injury is late or deep, cover it with a dry cloth or dressing. Do not rub or massage the area. Ice crystals under the skin could damage the fragile capillaries and tissues, making the injury worse.

5. *Comfort, calm, and reassure the patient.* Tell him or her that everything that can be done will be done.
6. *Monitor the patient for signs of hypothermia.*

Rewarming

If transport of the patient will be delayed, consider rewarming the affected area if sanctioned by your medical director. Never rewarm an area with late or deep frostbite. Never rewarm an area if there is a chance that it may refreeze. The injury from the second freezing would be much worse than the original one.

Warm the entire frostbitten area in tepid water (about 37.5°C to 40.5°C). The water should feel comfortable to the normal hand. Be sure to pick a container that permits the entire area to be immersed. Continue to support the injured limb during rewarming. Do not allow the injured area to touch the bottom or side of the container. If the water starts to cool, remove the limb from the water. Then, add more warm water. As the area rewarms, the patient may complain of tingling and shooting pains. In this case, some EMS systems allow EMRs to help an alert patient self-administer an analgesic, such as Tylenol. Follow local protocol.

When the injured area is rewarmed, the tissues will be fragile. To protect them, cover the injury with dry sterile gauze. If the injury is to the fingers or toes, also place gauze between them. Consider padding the entire area with a large, bulky dressing.

SECTION 3
HEAT EMERGENCIES

When a person cannot lose excessive heat, hyperthermia develops. Left untreated, hyperthermia can lead to organ damage and death. The stages of hyperthermia are commonly called heat cramps, heat exhaustion, and heatstroke. Heatstroke, the most serious, is life threatening.

Contributing Factors

Factors that contribute to the risk of hyperthermia include the following:

- *Heat and humidity.* High air temperature can reduce the body's ability to lose heat by radiation. High humidity can reduce the ability to lose heat by evaporation.
- *Exercise and strenuous activity.* Each of these can cause a person to lose more than 1 L of sweat (fluid and essential salts) per hour.
- *Age of the patient.* Very young and very old patients may be unable to respond effectively to overheating.
- *Medical condition of the patient.* Any number of conditions, such as heart or lung disease, diabetes, dehydration (fluid loss), obesity, fever, and fatigue, can inhibit heat loss.
- *Certain drugs and medications.* Alcohol, cocaine, barbiturates, hallucinogens, and other substances can affect heat loss in many ways, including through side effects such as dehydration (fluid loss).

Patient Assessment

The general signs and symptoms of a heat emergency include the following:

- Muscle cramps
- Weakness, exhaustion
- Dizziness, faintness
- Rapid pulse rate that is strong at first, but becomes weak as damage progresses
- Headache
- Seizures
- Loss of appetite, nausea, vomiting
- Altered mental status, possibly unconsciousness
- Skin that is moist, pale, and normal to cool in temperature (heat cramps or heat exhaustion)
- Skin that is hot and dry or hot and moist (heatstroke)

Heat cramps involve acute spasms of the muscles of the legs, arms, or abdomen (Figure 16–7). The most common but least serious heat emergency, heat cramps, may be the result of losing too much salt during profuse sweating. Heat cramps usually follow hard work in a hot environment. Hard work in a hot, humid environment can also affect blood flow. This can result in a mild state of shock or heat exhaustion.

If the patient does not stop working, move to a cool environment, and replace lost fluid, the condition will get worse. The result can be heatstroke, which is very serious and life threatening. Heatstroke occurs when the body becomes overheated and, in many patients, sweating stops. If left untreated, the brain cells begin to die, causing permanent disability or death (Figures 16–8 and Figure 16–9).

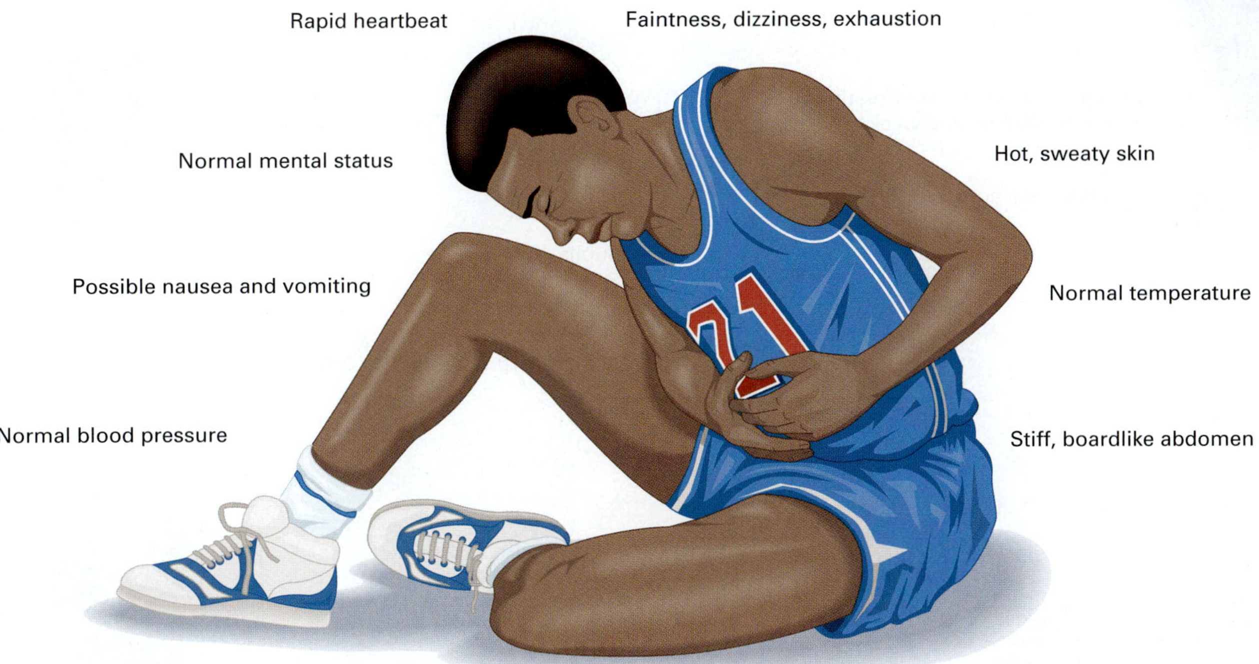

Figure 16–7   Signs and symptoms of heat cramps.

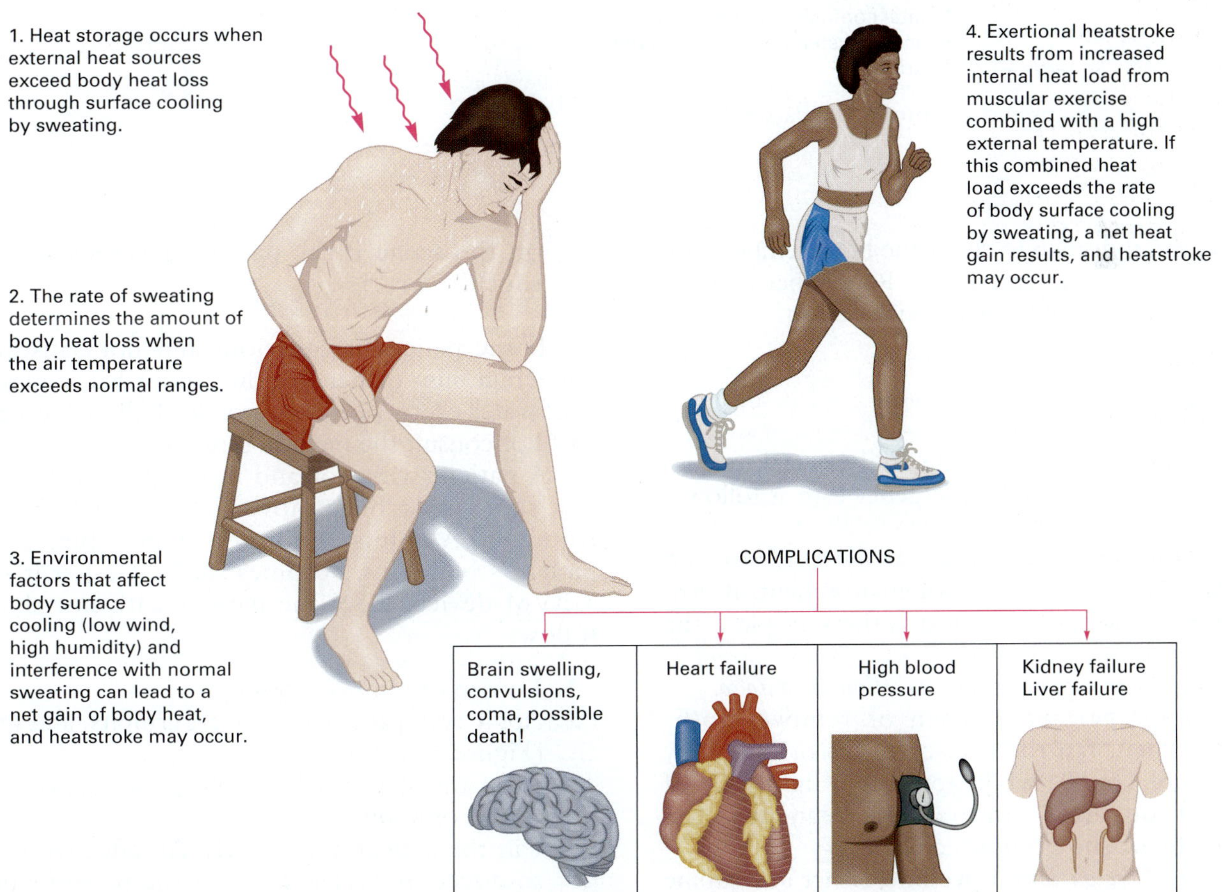

Figure 16–8   Sweating: a defence against heatstroke, which is a life-threatening emergency.

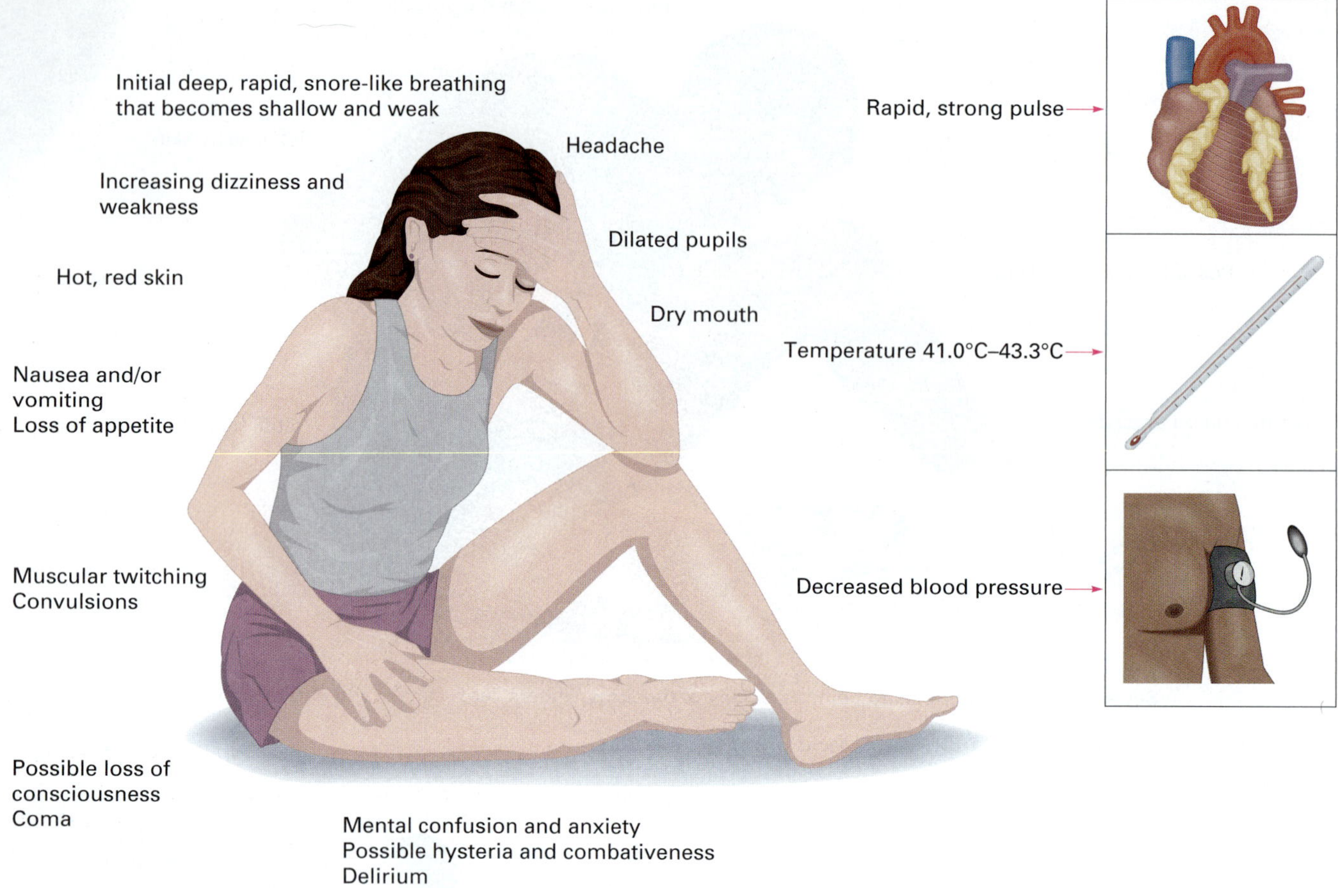

Figure 16–9 Signs and symptoms of heatstroke.

Feel the abdomen to check the body temperature of a patient in a heat emergency. Remember that the chief characteristic of heatstroke is hot skin.

Emergency Care

For a patient with moist, pale, and normal to cool skin temperature, provide emergency care as follows:

1. *Remove the patient from the hot environment.* Place him or her in a cool environment, if possible. If the source of heat is the sun, place the patient in the shade.
2. *Administer oxygen if you are allowed to do so.*
3. *Cool the patient.* Loosen or remove clothing. Then, fan the surface of his or her body (Figure 16–10) while applying a light mist of water. Be careful not to cool the patient so fast that he or she becomes chilled.
4. *Position the patient.* Place him or her in a supine position, with legs elevated 20 to 30 cm.
5. *Monitor the patient.* Take vital signs frequently. Advise incoming units or other EMS personnel on the scene if the patient develops signs of shock.

If the patient is conscious and not nauseated, encourage him or her to drink about half a glass of cool water every 15 minutes or so. Follow local protocol or consult the medical director.

A patient with hot and moist skin, or hot and dry skin, must be removed from the hot environment. Administer oxygen if possible. If the patient's breathing becomes shallow, assist it with a BVM device. Cool the patient with hot skin as follows:

1. Loosen or remove clothing.
2. Apply cold packs to the neck, armpits, and groin (Figure 16–11).
3. Keep the skin wet by applying water with wet towels or a sponge.
4. Fan the patient aggressively. An effective way is to direct an electric fan over the patient's body while you wet the skin.
5. Continually monitor the patient, as appropriate, during your ongoing assessment.

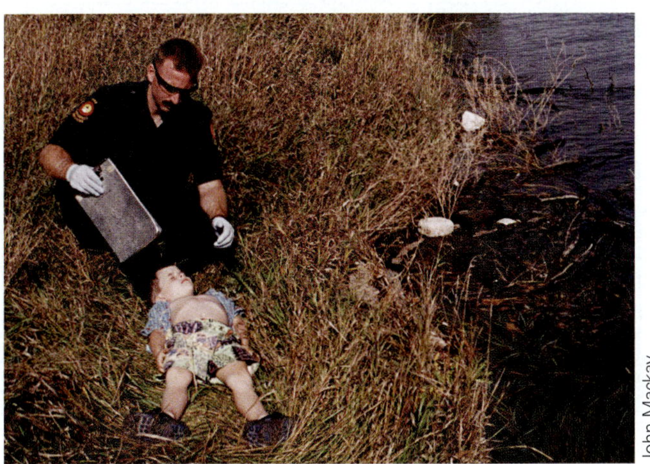

Figure 16–10   Cooling a patient with normal to cool skin temperature.

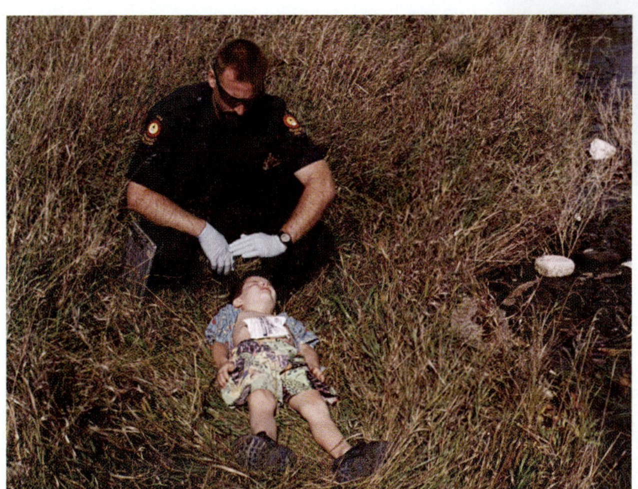

Figure 16–11   Cooling a patient with hot skin temperature.

EMR FOCUS

Conditions resulting from extremes in heat and cold are common in most parts of Canada. Even though many people are aware of the effects of these temperatures, they still fall victim.

Infants and older persons are at increased risk for heat and cold emergencies. Because their temperature control systems are not working optimally, it does not take bitter cold or extreme heat to cause an emergency. People who are exposed to moderate temperatures for long periods of time may also be stricken. Those with wet clothes in the cold and those who do not maintain their fluid levels during hot temperatures will be overcome quickly. Patients may even suffer from these conditions indoors.

The most important concept in this chapter is that the EMR can provide immediate life-saving help. Remove patients from extremes in temperature and begin to treat them. Ensure that you do not become stricken by the same conditions yourself.

CASE STUDY FOLLOW-UP

At the beginning of this chapter, you read that EMRs were on the scene with a woman down. To see how the chapter skills apply to this emergency, read the following. It describes how the call was completed.

SECONDARY ASSESSMENT

I performed a complete physical exam on Mrs. Gusev. My findings included a swollen, painful deformity in her right hip plus a number of bruises to her hips, knees, and ankles. I also noticed that she had been incontinent of urine during the night. Her shivering continued.

Mrs. Gusev had been lying on a cold, wet floor for nearly 12 hours. I suspected hypothermia. After completing the secondary assessment, we placed a warm blanket over her. We didn't want to move her because of both her injuries and the fact that the ambulance was less than five minutes away.

PATIENT HISTORY

Mrs. Gusev told us that she had no allergies and that she was taking several medications, including Aspirin, digitalis, and insulin. She had a long history of circulatory problems. She had not eaten for 12 hours. Unable to get up from the floor, she had been calling out for help until she lost her voice.

ONGOING ASSESSMENT

We monitored Mrs. Gusev's level of consciousness and vital signs. We kept her head stabilized and tried to keep her as warm as possible.

TRANSFER OF CARE

When the Rescue 3 team arrived, we told them what we knew:

"We have an 80-year-old female who fell down 12 hours ago and remained down until we arrived. Her chief complaint is pain in her right hip. Her pulse is 100, respirations 18. We stabilized her head because of the blood we saw. We also felt that she could be hypothermic, so we warmed her with a blanket."

Later that week, I ran into Rescue 3's crew chief. He said that Mrs. Gusev had suffered a broken hip and hypothermia. She was treated successfully at the hospital but would likely go to a nursing home after discharge.

Heat and cold emergencies often occur in isolated areas to such people as campers, hikers, skiers, and mountain climbers. But as you can see, they can also happen in our own neighbourhoods. Always consider the environmental conditions as soon as you get your call. Early recognition and appropriate care can save lives.

NOCPs

5.6 e Treat local cold injury **S**

6.1 n Provide care to patient experiencing signs and symptoms due to exposure to adverse environments **S**

6.2 c Provide care for geriatric patient **S**

REVIEW QUESTIONS

Page references where answers may be found or supported are provided at the end of each question.

SECTION 1

1. What are the five major mechanisms of heat loss? (pp. 240–241)

2. Which will take away a person's body heat faster, air or water? How much faster? (p. 240)

SECTION 2

3. What factors contribute to the possibility that a patient may be at risk of hypothermia? (p. 242)

4. Is hypothermia a progressive condition? Whether your answer is yes or no, describe how a patient with hypothermia may present. (pp. 243–245)

5. How can you minimize the injury your patient experiences from hypothermia? (p. 243)

6. If you find a hypothermic patient breathless and pulseless and with signs of death, should you begin CPR? Explain your answer. (p. 245)

7. For how long should you check for a pulse in a hypothermic patient before starting CPR? (p. 245)

8. Why must you handle a severely hypothermic patient gently? (p. 245)

9. How can you identify a local cold injury? (p. 245)

10. What is the basic emergency care of a local cold injury? (pp. 245–246)

SECTION 3

11. What factors contribute to the possibility that a patient may be at risk of hyperthermia? (p. 246)

12. What are the signs and symptoms of a heat emergency? (p. 246)

13. What is the appropriate emergency care for a patient in a heat emergency? (p. 248)

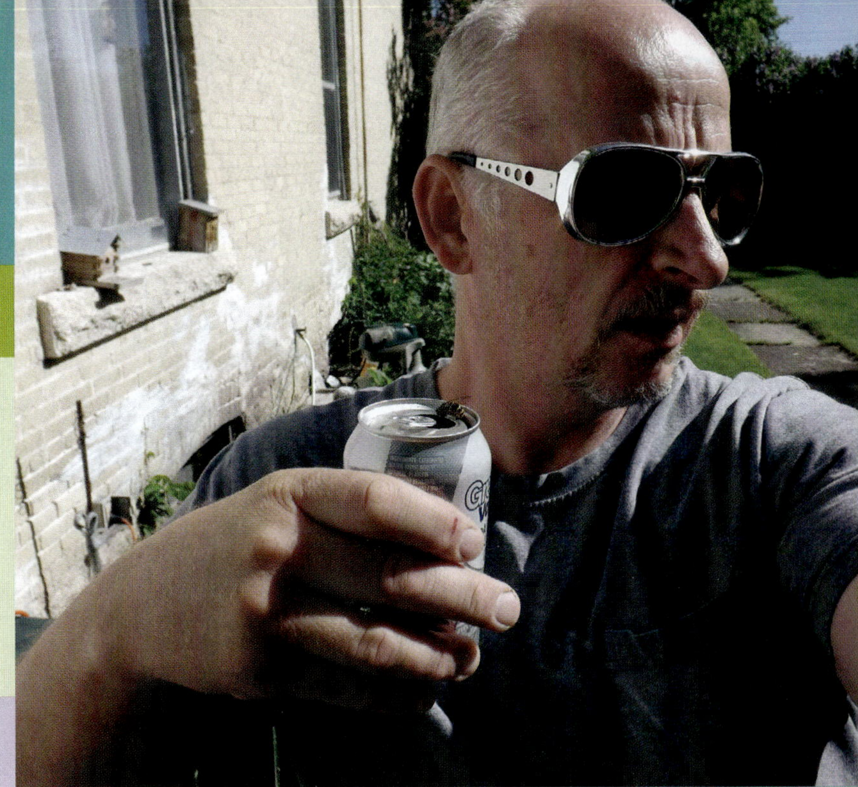

John Mackay

Bites and Stings

OBJECTIVES

1. Recognize the signs and symptoms of an allergic reaction to bites or stings.
2. Describe the eight general guidelines for emergency care of patients with bites or stings, including those who have allergic reactions to them.
3. List five characteristics to distinguish between poisonous and non-poisonous snakes and identify six signs and symptoms of poisonous snakebites.
4. Describe the proper method of applying a constricting band to an extremity.
5. Identify the specific signs and symptoms of bites and stings from the following: black widow spiders, brown recluse spiders, scorpions, fire ants, mites, and ticks.
6. Describe how to remove a stinger from a bee, wasp, or hornet that is embedded in a patient's skin.
7. List the steps in the emergency care of stings and wounds by common marine life.
8. Demonstrate a caring attitude toward the patient and family when dealing with a bite or sting, while giving priority to the interests of the patient.

INTRODUCTION

Insect bites and stings are common and usually minor occurrences in Canada. It is only when the insect is poisonous, or when the patient has an allergic reaction, that the situation becomes an emergency. Under those conditions, prompt emergency care can save lives and prevent permanent tissue damage.

Insects and spiders are not alone in posing a threat to human beings. Snakes and marine animals can also cause life-threatening problems. Though many different kinds of poisonous marine animals live in tropical waters, waders and swimmers have discovered that they can be found in virtually all waters.

SECTION 1
GENERAL GUIDELINES FOR EMERGENCY CARE

For assessment and emergency medical care of a patient with a bite or a sting, follow the general guidelines described below.

Patient Assessment

As always, your priority during scene assessment is to protect yourself. If your patient has been bitten or stung, you could be too. Exercise caution. Do not become a second victim. As you assess the scene, ask yourself the following: Is an insect nest visible nearby in a tree, under the eaves of a house, or in the ground? Are there signs that the patient was engaged in an activity such as clearing underbrush or gardening that might have disturbed snakes or insects? Was the patient working in a garage, basement, attic, or shed where spiders and other insects might nest? Are there dead insects on the ground near the patient?

During your assessment of the patient, be alert to the possibility that insects may have become trapped in your patient's clothing.

Also, keep in mind that some patients will have an allergic reaction to bites and stings. That reaction can lead to **anaphylactic shock**, an emergency that generally has a rapid, life-threatening effect on the airway and breathing.

When you gather the patient history, be sure to ask the patient to identify any allergies he or she may have. Also, if possible and if safe to do so, try to identify what bit or stung your patient.

Signs and Symptoms

General signs and symptoms of bites and stings include the following:

- History of bites or stings
- Bite mark or stinger embedded in the skin
- Immediate pain that is severe or burning
- Numbness at the site after a few hours
- Redness or other discoloration of the skin around the bite or sting
- Swelling around the site, sometimes spreading gradually

If the patient has an allergic reaction, any combination of a range of signs and symptoms may develop. They include the following (Figure 17–1):

- Skin
  - Warm, tingling feeling in the mouth, face, chest, feet, and hands
  - Itching, hives, and flushing
  - Swelling of the tongue, face, neck, hands, and feet
- Respiratory system
  - Tightness in the throat or chest
  - Cough, hoarseness (losing the voice)
  - Rapid or laboured breathing
  - Noisy breathing, stridor, wheezing
- Circulatory system
  - Increased heart rate
  - Decreased blood pressure
- General findings
  - Itchy, watery eyes
  - Headache
  - Runny nose
  - Sense of impending doom
  - Deteriorating mental status

CASE STUDY

Dispatch
My EMR unit was dispatched for a bee sting at a local campground.

Scene Assessment
Everything seemed safe when we arrived. A group was standing around a person who was sitting in a lawn chair. They were frantically waving to us. We put on gloves and approached the scene.

Primary Assessment
The condition of the patient struck us immediately. Our general impression was of an adult female who was having an allergic reaction. The patient was wheezing, pale, and sweaty but breathing adequately—for the moment. If the airway constricted any more, we would have to assist ventilations immediately. We were fortunate to have oxygen and applied it to the patient via a non-rebreather mask. The patient's pulse was rapid. We notified dispatch to alert the paramedics of the patient's condition.

Consider this patient as you read Chapter 17. What more may be done to assess and care for her condition?

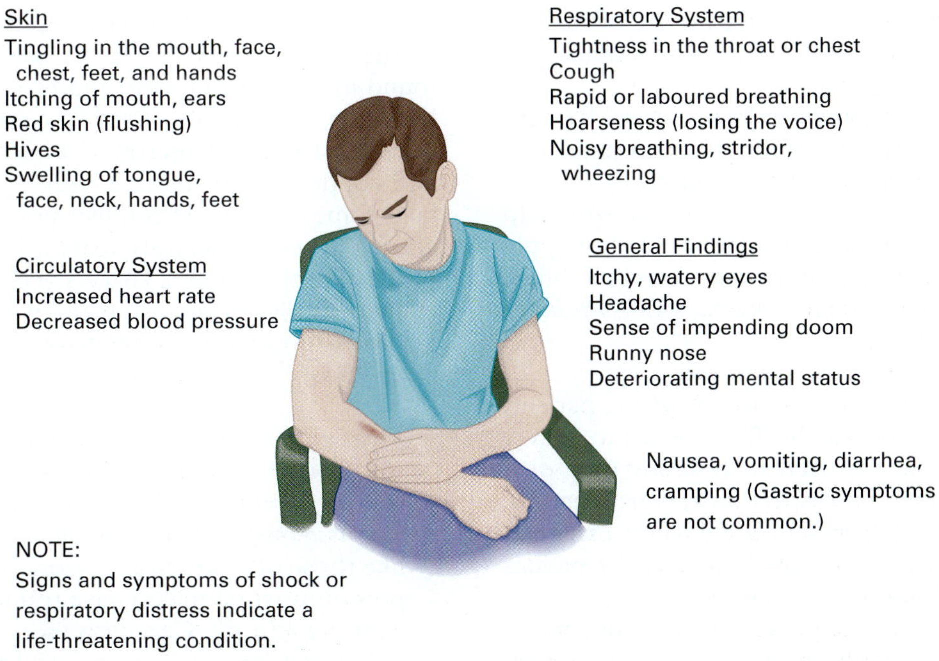

Figure 17–1 Possible signs and symptoms of allergic reactions to bites and stings.

If you suspect an allergic reaction, inform EMS dispatch immediately. Respiratory distress and shock can develop rapidly. (Read more about shock in Chapter 19.)

You may wish to note that allergic reactions are especially common following the stings of wasps, hornets, yellow jackets, and fire ants. Bites or stings from deer flies, gnats, horse flies, mosquitoes, cockroaches, and miller moths can also cause an allergic reaction, as can venom from snakes and spiders.

Emergency Medical Care

Remember to take all appropriate BSI precautions. Then, follow these general guidelines for the emergency care of a patient with a bite or sting:

1. *Perform an initial assessment.* Treat all life threats. If you suspect an allergic reaction, maintain the patient's airway. Insert an airway adjunct if appropriate. Suction as needed.
2. *Administer oxygen if you are equipped and allowed to do so.* If breathing is adequate, deliver oxygen by way of a non-rebreather mask. If the patient needs artificial ventilation, use supplemental oxygen.
3. *Position the site of the bite or sting slightly below the level of the patient's heart.* Manually stabilize a bitten or stung extremity until it can be immobilized.
4. *Remove any constricting objects,* such as jewellery, as soon as possible. Ideally this should happen before swelling begins.
5. *Inspect the bite or sting site.* If a stinger is present, remove it by scraping along the surface of the skin with the edge of a credit card or knife. Make sure you remove the venom sac.
6. *Wash the area around the bite or sting.* Be very gentle. Use soap and water. Then irrigate with clean water. Follow local protocol.
7. *Apply a cold pack* (Figure 17–2). It will help relieve pain, itching, and swelling. Do not apply cold packs to snakebites or marine animal bites.
8. *Keep the patient calm and warm, and limit his or her physical activity.*

During your ongoing assessment of the patient, monitor the ABCs continually. Be prepared to deliver basic life support if it is needed. If at any time during emergency care you suspect an allergic reaction, inform EMS dispatch immediately. (You can read more about the emergency medical care of a patient in anaphylactic shock in Chapter 19.)

Demonstrate a caring attitude toward your patient. Place his or her interests first in any patient care decision. Remember to communicate with empathy when dealing with patients and their family members or friends.

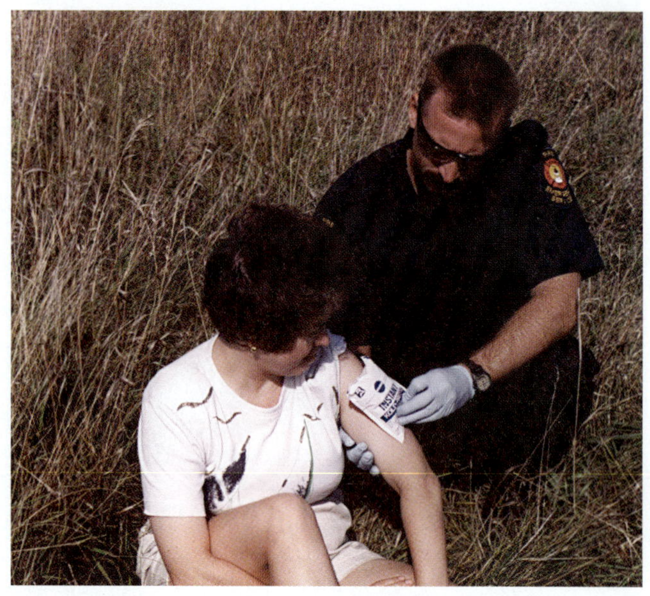

Figure 17–2 Apply a cold pack to an insect bite or sting to help relieve pain and swelling.

SECTION 2
SPECIFIC TYPES OF BITES AND STINGS

Snakebite

While Canada has a number of indigenous species of snake, few are poisonous. However, today's intercontinental travel makes it reasonable for you to know some of the basics about snakebites. Rattlesnakes can be found in southern Ontario and places like the Alberta badlands, but you also need to consider non-indigenous coral snakes, water moccasins or cottonmouths, and copperheads (Figure 17–3). Snake venom contains some of the most complex poisons known. It can affect the central nervous system, heart, kidneys, and blood. Simply stated, a snake's venom is its digestive enzyme. It digests any tissue into which it is injected.

Most poisonous snakes have the following characteristics:

- *Two large, hollow fangs.* These work like a hypodermic needle. Non-poisonous snakes (and the poisonous coral snake) have small teeth.
- *Elliptical pupils.* These look like vertical slits, much like those of a cat. Non-poisonous snakes (and the poisonous coral snake) have round pupils.
- *Presence of a pit.* Certain poisonous snakes have a telltale pit between the eye and the mouth. That is why pit vipers are so named. The pits are heat-sensing organs. They make it possible for the snake

COMMON POISONOUS SNAKES

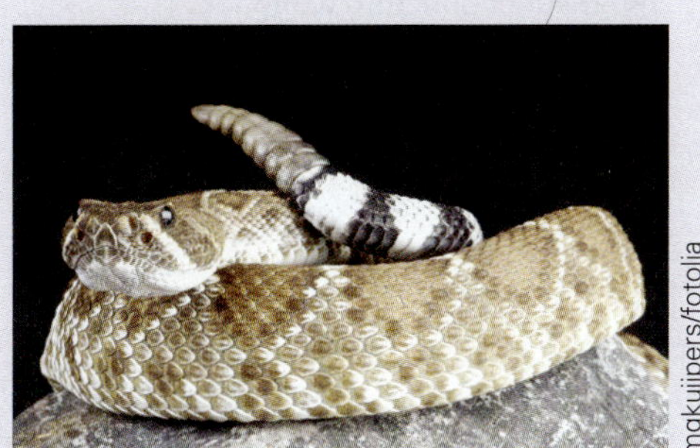

Figure 17–3a Rattlesnake.

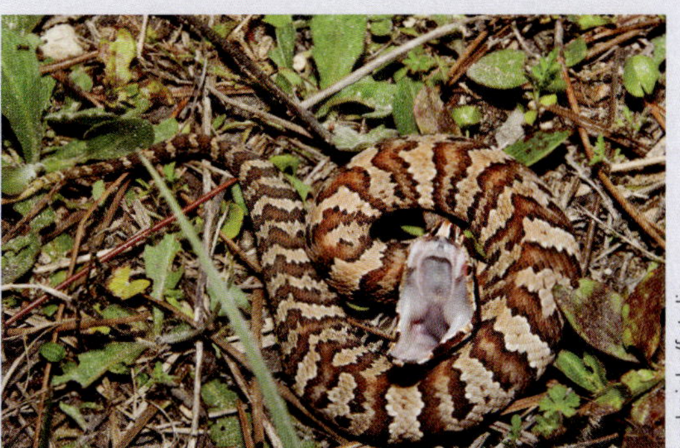

Figure 17–3b Water moccasin or cottonmouth.

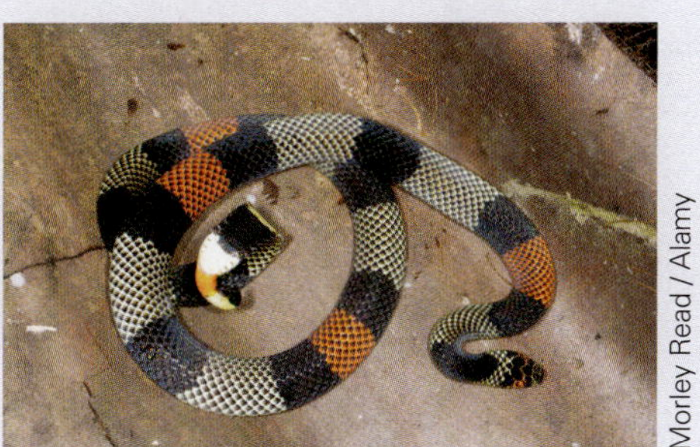

Figure 17–3c Coral snake.

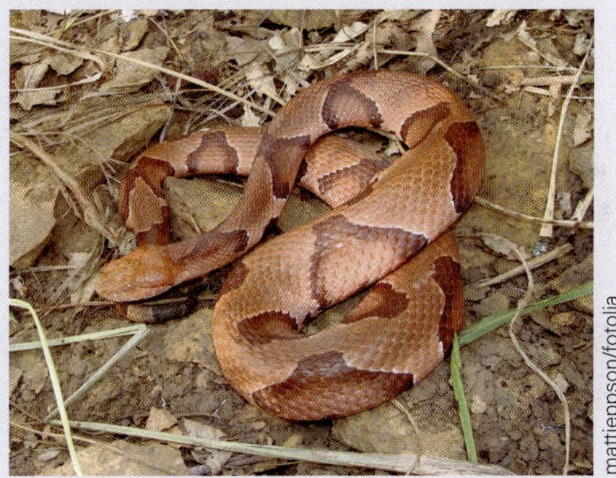

Figure 17–3d Copperhead.

to accurately strike a warm-blooded animal, even if the snake cannot see it.

- *Special markings.* Poisonous snakes are marked with shapes on a background of pink, yellow, tan, grey, or brown skin. The exception is the small coral snake, which is ringed with red, yellow, and black.
- *Triangular head.* It is larger than the neck.

Although many of the world's poisonous snakes are not indigenous to Canada, these characteristics are useful to know if you travel to other regions.

Poisonous snakebites cause medical emergencies. However, only about one-third of all bites cause symptoms. When symptoms do develop, they usually occur immediately after a person is bitten.

Patient Assessment

The signs and symptoms of a poisonous snakebite include puncture wounds, swelling, discoloration, and severe pain and burning at the bite site (Figures 17–4 and 17–5).

In addition, the venom of a coral snake affects the central nervous system. One to eight hours after the bite, the patient will experience symptoms that get progressively worse. The signs and symptoms of a coral snake bite include the following:

- Blurred vision, drooping eyelids
- Drowsiness, slurred speech

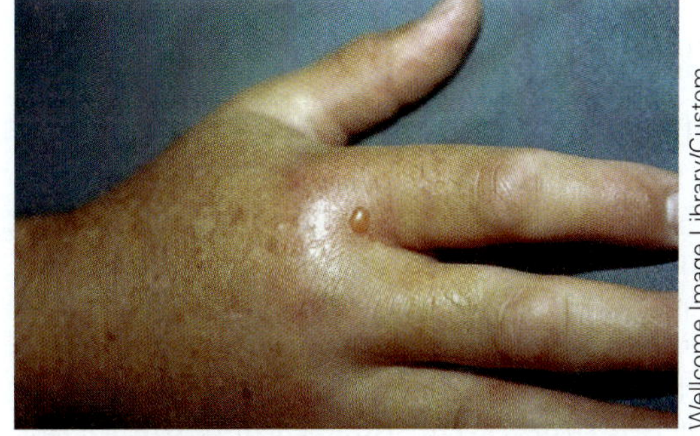

Figure 17–4 Snakebite to the hand.

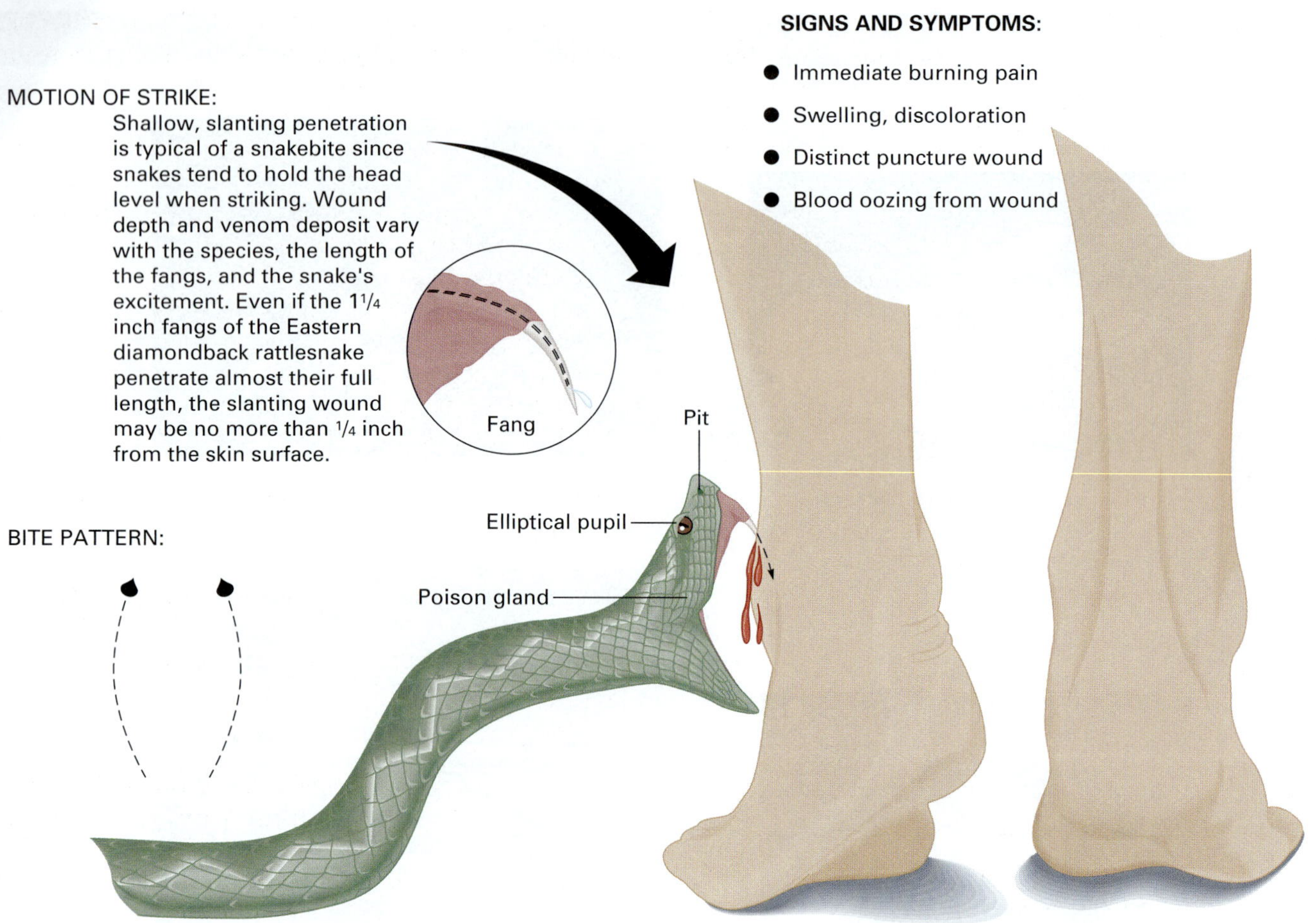

Figure 17–5 Poisonous snakebites.

- Increased salivation and sweating
- Nausea, vomiting
- Weakness, paralysis
- Seizures, unconsciousness

Always make sure the paramedics have been alerted if you suspect any kind of snakebite.

When you gather the patient history, be sure to note how much physical activity the patient engaged in after the bite. (Activity helps to spread the venom.) Also, find out when the patient last had a tetanus vaccination.

Emergency Care

For snakebites, follow the general emergency care guidelines for bites and stings described earlier in this chapter. However, if your EMS system allows you to do so, you might also want to apply a constricting band and suction the wound.

The use of a constricting band is controversial. Some say that they should be used only within 30 minutes of the time of the bite. Others say a constricting band should not be used at all. Constricting bands are used only on extremities. Never place a constricting band around a joint or around the head, neck, or trunk. Follow local protocols.

In order to apply a constricting band, first find the fang marks. Then, wrap a flat band that is about 3 to 5 cm wide around the extremity (Figure 17–6). Place

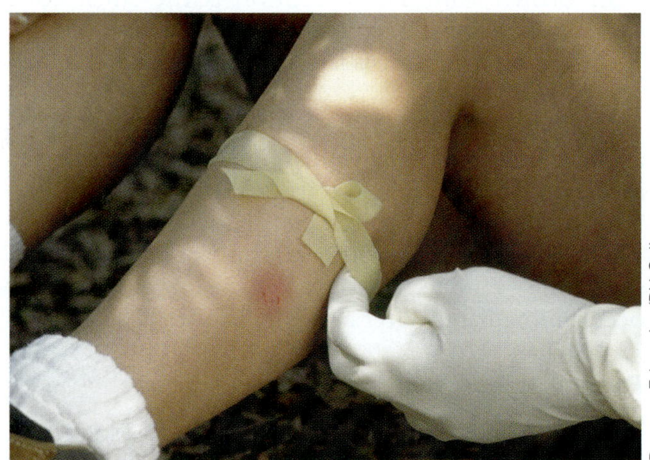

Figure 17–6 Follow local protocol regarding the use of a constricting band.

it 5 to 10 cm above (proximal to) the fang marks. The band should be snug but not too tight. You should be able to slip two fingers between it and the patient's skin. You can adjust the constricting band as swelling occurs so that it does not become too tight. But leave it in place until a physician checks the patient.

The use of suction is also controversial. Some say that it should be used only if the patient is at least two hours from medical help. Follow local protocols. Apply suction to the wound directly over the fang marks. An extractor from a snakebite kit is ideal. Never use your mouth to apply suction. Suction must be strong and must be applied within the first five minutes to be effective. After 30 minutes, the venom is diffused and cannot be removed by suction. *Note:* Never suction coral snake bites.

Insect Bites and Stings

For the assessment and emergency care of insect bites and stings, follow the general guidelines described earlier in this chapter. The discussion below provides details on specific insects and spiders.

Black Widow Spider

The black widow spider is characterized by a shiny black body, thin legs, and a crimson red mark on its abdomen in the shape of an hourglass or two triangles (Figure 17–7). The venom—14 times more toxic than rattlesnake venom—causes pain and muscle spasms within 30 minutes to 3 hours. Severe bites cause respiratory failure and death. Those at highest risk for developing severe symptoms are children under 16 years, people over 60 years, people with chronic diseases, and anyone with hypertension (high blood pressure).

The most serious sign of a black widow spider bite is high blood pressure. Other signs and symptoms, which last for 24 to 48 hours, include the following:

- A brief pinprick sensation at the bite site that becomes a dull ache within 30 to 40 minutes (There is almost never a local reaction, although in some cases there may be some swelling or a raised, round, red mark called a wheal.)
- Flushing, sweating, and grimacing of the face within 10 minutes to 2 hours
- Pain and spasms in the shoulders, back, chest, and abdominal muscles within 30 minutes to 3 hours (These gradually spread over the entire body within 1 to 6 hours.)
- Rigid abdomen with cramping
- Agitation, restlessness, anxiety
- Lack of coordination
- Weakness, headache, both of which may last for months
- Profuse salivation, tearing, or sweating
- Fever, rash
- Nausea, vomiting

The antivenom for the black widow spider bite is generally used only in high-risk patients. If you can do so safely, find the spider. The physician will be able to identify it, even if it is crushed, and will not have to guess about treatment.

Brown Recluse Spider

The brown recluse spider can range in colour from yellow to dark chocolate brown (see Figure 17–7). The characteristic marking is a brown, violin-shaped mark on the upper back. This bite is not often serious. However, about 10 percent of the time the bite

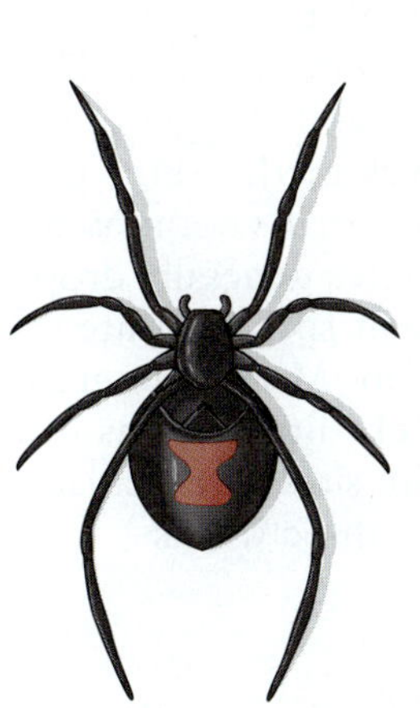

Black widow

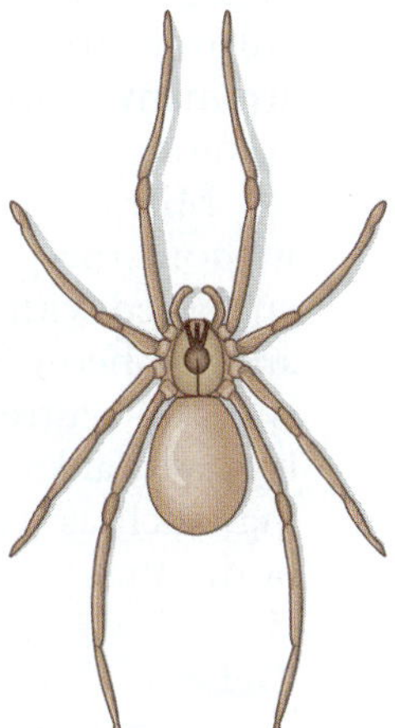

Brown recluse

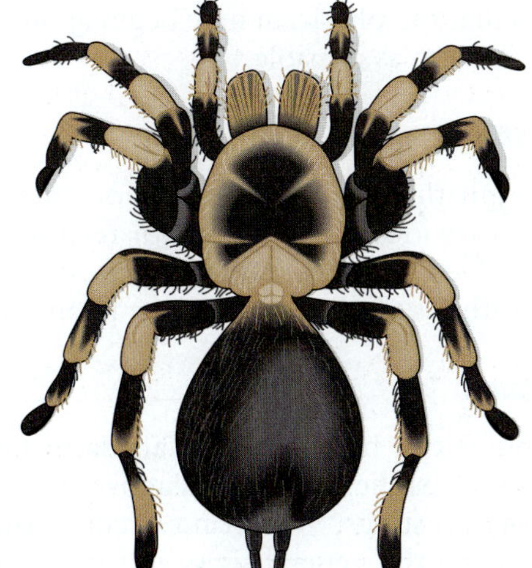

Tarantula

Figure 17–7 Poisonous spiders.

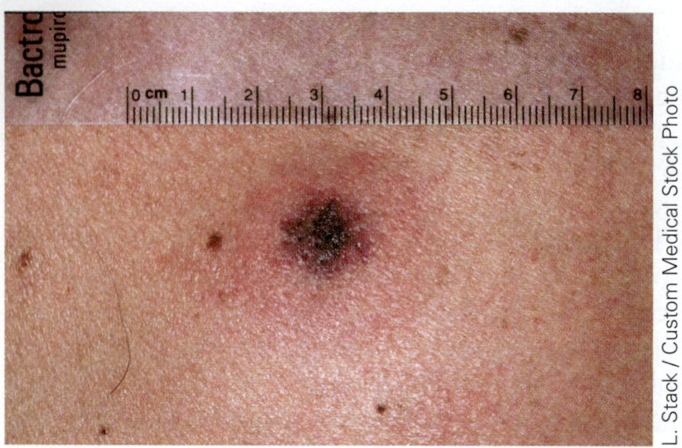

Figure 17–8 Bite mark of a brown recluse spider.

L. Stack / Custom Medical Stock Photo

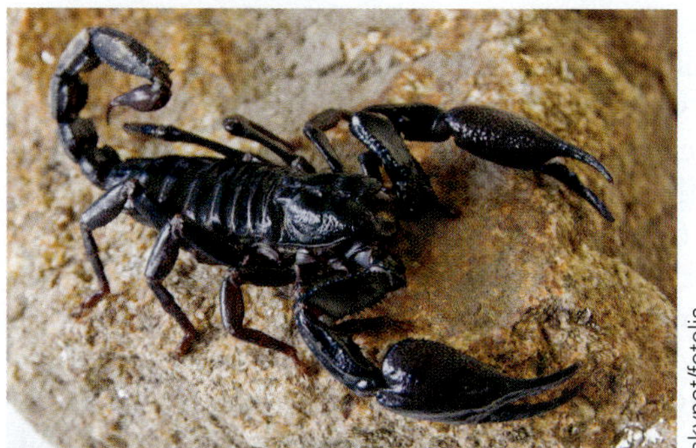

Figure 17–9 Scorpion.

skynet/fotolia

does not heal and the patient needs a skin graft. A small percentage of patients may develop kidney failure and die.

Brown recluse spider bites are rare. They most often occur when spiders are trapped in clothing. Unfortunately, most victims are unaware that they have been bitten since the bite is often initially painless. There may be a slight stinging sensation and itching. The most severe reactions occur in children.

If the patient reacts, the following signs and symptoms may occur:

- Within a few hours, the bite is surrounded by sunken tissue. There is a bluish area with white edges, gradually becoming surrounded by a red halo (a bull's eye pattern). Two tiny puncture marks may be apparent.
- If there is a severe reaction, the bite becomes a large ulcer within 72 hours (Figure 17–8). The following also sometimes occur: a fever of at least 39.5°C, joint pain, nausea, vomiting, and chills.

Again, it is important for you to identify the spider so that the physician may begin appropriate treatment as soon as possible.

Tarantula

Although the tarantula looks more menacing than the black widow and the brown recluse spiders (see Figure 17–7), its bite usually causes only moderate pain. Other symptoms are rare in tarantula bites.

Scorpion

Scorpions can be found in Canada in hot, arid climates such as the Alberta badlands (Figure 17–9). Of all scorpion stings, 90 percent occur to the hands. In addition to the general signs and symptoms of bites and stings, scorpion stings may cause nausea and vomiting, drooling, poor coordination, incontinence, and seizures.

If you are allowed to, apply a flat constricting band to the extremity about 5 cm above the sting. The band should be snug but not too tight. You should be able to slip two fingers between it and the patient's skin. Leave it in place until a physician checks the patient. Follow local protocols.

Fire Ants

Fire ants get their name not from their colour, which ranges from red to black, but from the intense, fiery, burning pain their bites cause.

Fire ants bite and sting downward as they pivot. The result is a characteristic circular pattern of bites, which produce extremely painful vesicles (small blisters). At first the fluid in the vesicles is clear. Later, it becomes cloudy. The bitten extremity usually becomes red, swollen, and painful. Within 24 hours, the bites develop pustules (raised areas filled with pus) on a red, swollen base (Figure 17–10).

Mites

Mites are most common in the southern part of the United States. However, since they feed on tall grasses and grains, they are found in rural and agricultural areas throughout North America. There are many types of mites that bite humans. The most common are the scabies mite and chigger mite.

Mites embed themselves in the skin, generally without the patient realizing it. As soon as they are engorged with blood, the mites generally drop off or are brushed off. If the patient sees the mite at all, it is in the centre of a red lesion. Most bites are on the legs and ankles or under tight-fitting areas of clothing, such as waistbands. Bite sites often enlarge into nodes that persist for two to three weeks.

Ticks

Ticks can cause a serious problem because they can carry tick fever, Rocky Mountain spotted fever, Lyme disease, and other bacterial diseases. A prolonged attachment of a female tick can cause progressive paralysis.

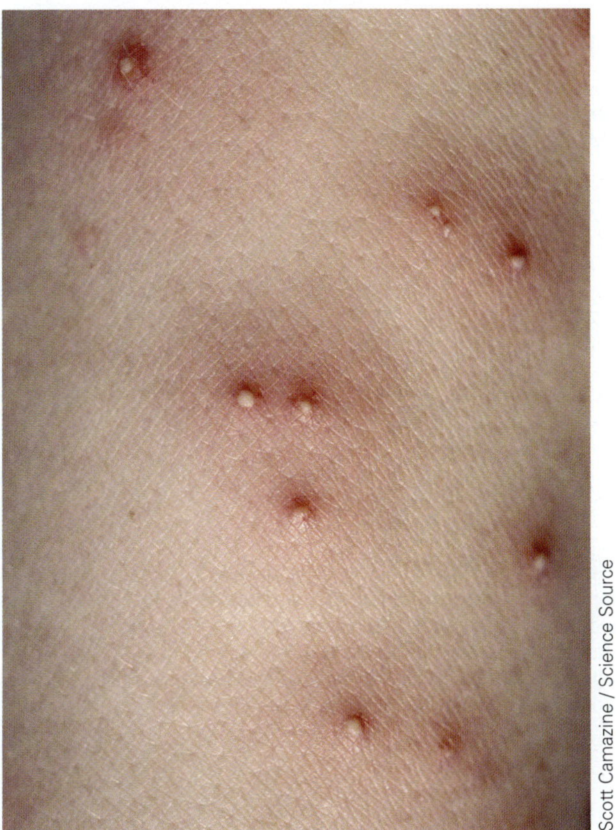

Figure 17–10 Fire ant bites.

Scott Camazine / Science Source

Tick bites are painless. The patient does not notice the bite until he or she finds an engorged tick, which can be as large as a pea (Figure 17–11). Ticks become visible after they have attached themselves to the skin. They often stay attached for more than 10 days. However, since they often choose warm, moist areas, you should carefully inspect the patient's scalp and other hairy areas, such as the armpits, groin, and skin creases. If a tick is brushed off, the mouth parts may stay embedded in the skin, causing infection or an allergic reaction. Never pluck an embedded tick head out of the skin. You may force infected blood into the patient.

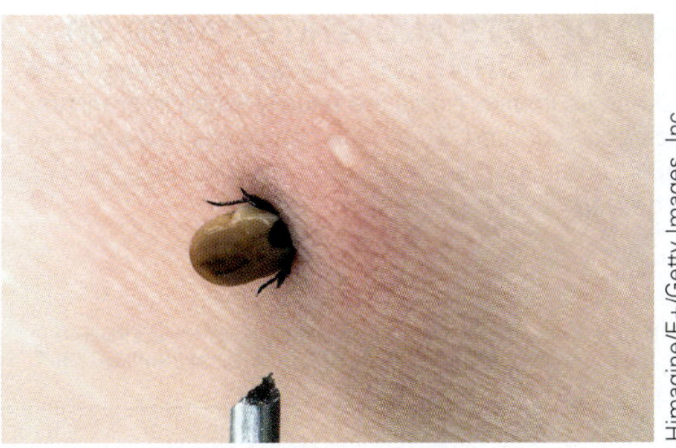

Figure 17–11 Engorged tick.

Himagine/E+/Getty Images, Inc.

If you are providing emergency care in an isolated area, local protocol may permit you to remove a tick. If so, remove it as soon as you discover it. The longer the tick remains attached to the skin, the more likely it is that an infection will result. To remove a tick, first take BSI precautions. Then, follow these guidelines:

1. Use tweezers while wearing protective gloves. If you touch the tick, you may contaminate yourself. If you do not have tweezers and cannot cover your fingers, do not wait to look for an appropriate implement.
2. Grasp the tick as closely as possible to the point where it is attached to the skin. Pull firmly and steadily until the tick is dislodged. Do not twist or jerk the tick since that may result in incomplete removal. Avoid squashing an engorged tick during removal. Infected blood may spurt into your eyes and mouth or into a cut on the surface of your skin.
3. Once the tick is removed, wash your hands and the bite area thoroughly with soap and water. Apply an antiseptic to the bite area to prevent bacterial infection.

Have the patient mark the date on a calendar. This will document the exact time of exposure and will serve as a reminder if he or she needs to seek medical care. If the patient develops fever with chills, headache, or muscle aches after being exposed to a tick, he or she should seek immediate treatment from a physician.

Mosquito Bites

Severe allergic reactions to mosquito bites are uncommon. If they occur, they should be treated as any other anaphylactic reaction. Diseases transmitted by mosquitoes, such as Western equine encephalitis, West Nile fever or encephalitis, and dengue fever, rarely occurred before in Canada, but they are occurring more frequently now. Sticking to your assessment and treatment plan for any medical patient will cover the bases.

Bee, Wasp, or Hornet Stings

A patient with an insect sting (Figure 17–12) should see a physician if the bite is on the face or if there are multiple stings, even if there seems to be no allergic reaction. If there is an allergic reaction, ensure an open airway and adequate breathing and arrange for the patient to be immediately transported to a hospital.

WASPS, BEES, AND FIRE ANTS

The following members of this group commonly attack humans, causing local pain, redness, swelling, and subsequent itching. Always consider the possibility of anaphylaxis.

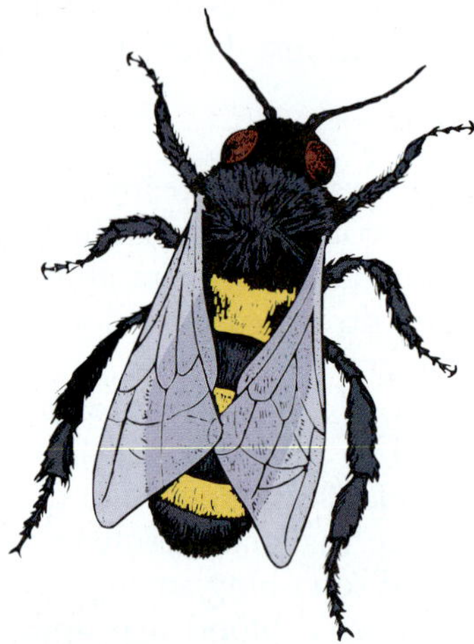

HONEYBEES: They are found throughout Canada, predominantly in warmer seasons. Hives are usually found in hollowed out areas such as dead tree trunks. Honeybees principally ingest the nectar of plants, so they are often seen in the vicinity of flowers. The honeybee, with its barbed stinger, will self-eviscerate after a sting, leaving the venom sac and stinger in place.

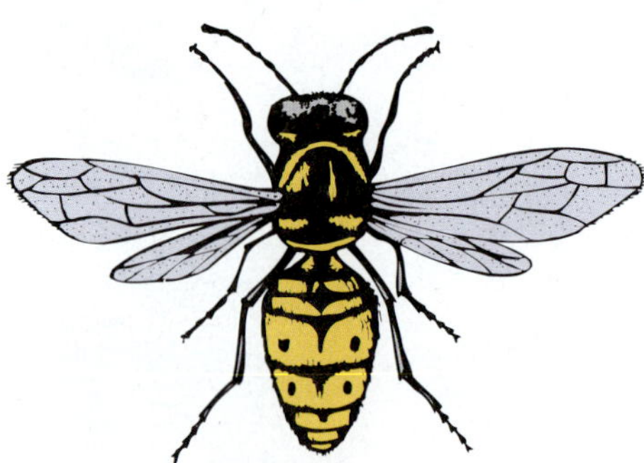

YELLOW JACKETS: Yellow jackets tend to dominate in late summer and fall. Nests are located in the ground. Often seen in picnic areas and garbage cans, yellow jackets are ill-tempered and aggressive and can deliver multiple stings at one time. They will often sting without being provoked.

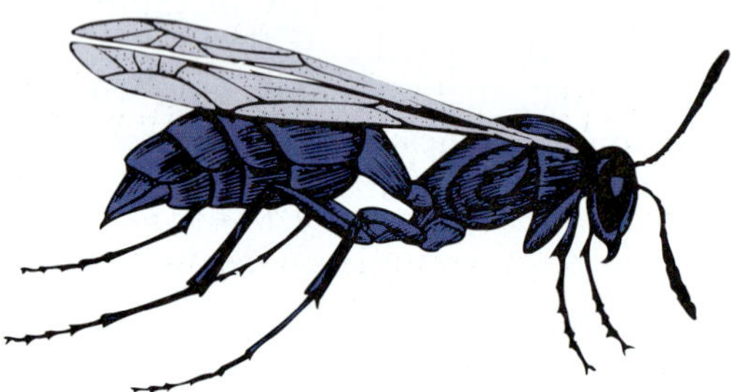

WASPS: Wasps tend to nest in small numbers under the eaves of houses and buildings. These are carnivores that are found in picnic areas, garbage cans, and food stands. They can deliver multiple stings at one time.

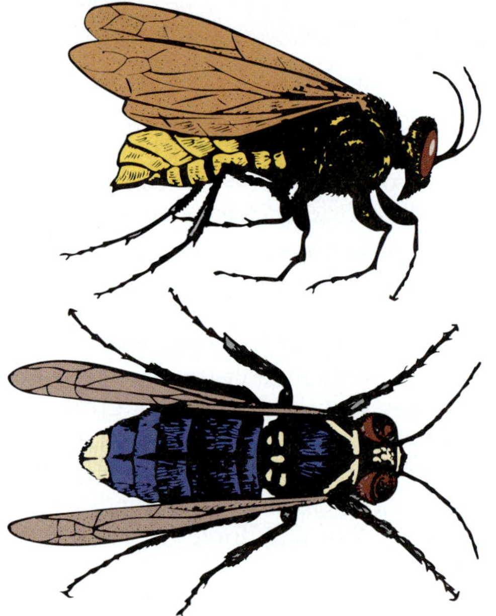

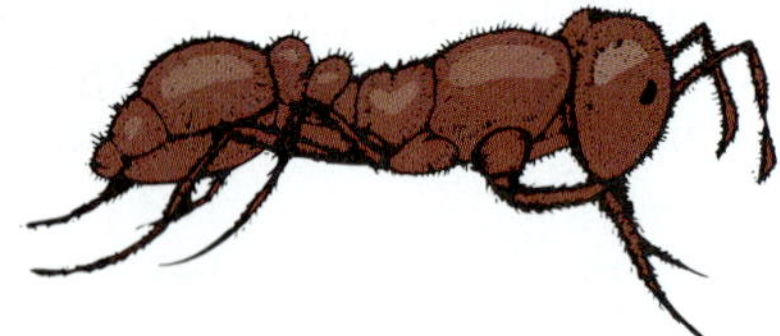

FIRE ANTS: They can range from red to black and live in loose dirt mounds. Fire ant bites may cause serious illness and/or anaphylaxis. The ant attaches itself to the skin by its strong jaws and swivels its tail-positioned stinger about, inflicting repeated stings.

YELLOW HORNETS AND WHITE-FACED OR BALD-FACED HORNETS: They are seen mainly in the spring and early summer. Nests are usually found in branches and bushes above ground. These are carnivores that are seen in picnic areas, garbage cans, and food stands. They can deliver multiple stings at one time.

Adapted with permission from: John W. Georgitis. "Insect Stings – Responding to the Gamut of Allergic Reactions," *Modern Medicine*

Figure 17–12 Wasps, bees, and fire ants.

Emergency care is the same as described for bites and stings at the beginning of this chapter. However, if you are allowed to, proceed with the following:

1. Lower the affected part below the level of the heart.
2. Apply a constricting band above the sting site if it is on an extremity. The band should be snug but not too tight. You should be able to slip two fingers between it and the patient's skin. Remember that the use of a constricting band is controversial. Follow local protocols.
3. If the stinger is still in the skin, remove it. Gently scrape against it with the edge of a knife or credit card (Figure 17–13). Be careful not to squeeze the stinger. If you do, you could inject additional venom into the area. Make sure you remove the venom sac. It can continue to secrete venom for up to 20 minutes.

If you know that the patient is allergic to stings, do not wait for signs or symptoms to develop. Delay can be fatal. If the patient has a history of severe allergic reactions and has an insect sting kit, assist in the administration of the kit's contents. *Follow all local protocols.*

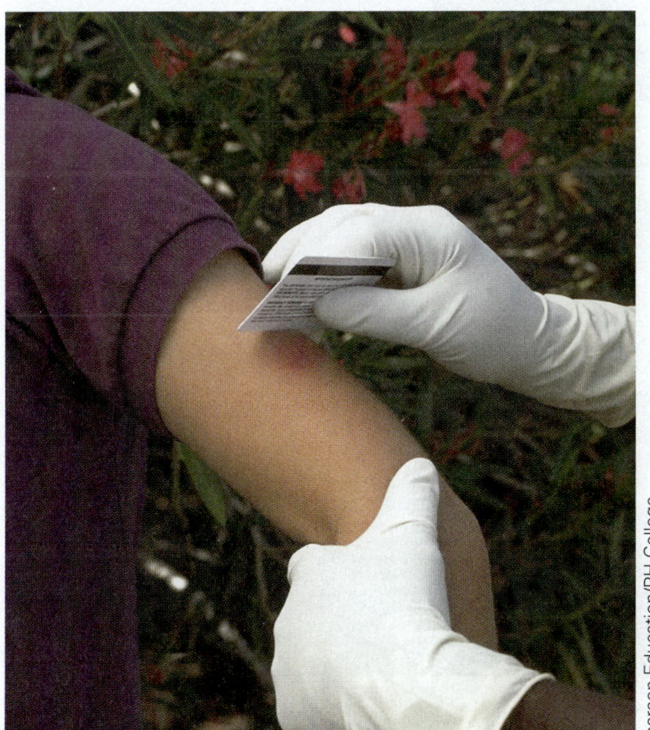

Figure 17–13 If the insect stinger is still present, remove it.

Marine Life Poisoning

See Figure 17–14 for common sources of marine animal stings and wounds. If you are allowed according to local protocol, you may also wish to do the following:

1. Use forceps to remove any material that sticks to the sting site on the surface of the patient's skin.
2. Irrigate the wound thoroughly with water.
3. If the skin is unbroken, wash the wound with an antibacterial agent. Do not scrub the area. Make sure that washings flow away from the body.
4. Remove stingers and barbs the same way you would remove a bee stinger. If you are unable to remove one without excessive force, then bandage it in place. Stabilize the area to keep the venom from spreading.
5. Keep the injured area cool, but do not allow it to freeze, for 30 minutes or until the paramedics take over care. Follow local protocol.
6. Alert incoming paramedics if this has not already been done. Arrange for immediate transport of the patient.

Tentacle Stings

Tentacle stings can be inflicted by jellyfish, corals, hydras, and anemones (Figure 17–15). First, remove the patient from the water. With gloved hands, carefully remove dried tentacles if possible. Immediately rinse the wounds with sea water for 30 minutes until pain is relieved. If possible, pour vinegar on the affected area. Arrange for immediate transport of the patient to a hospital.

Puncture Wounds

To treat puncture wounds caused by stingray spines and spiny fish (Figure 17–16), immediately remove the patient from the water. If a spine is embedded in the skin, treat it as an impaled object and stabilize it in place. Stabilize the injured body part to prevent movement. Apply a sterile dressing and bandage the area. Arrange for immediate transport of the patient to a hospital.

Large Bites

Bites from sharks or other marine life should be treated the same way as any major injury or soft tissue injury from a land animal (see Chapter 20). Perform a primary assessment and treat life threats. Arrange for immediate transport of the patient to a hospital. If possible, try to identify the animal that caused the injury.

COMMON SOURCES OF MARINE LIFE STINGS AND WOUNDS

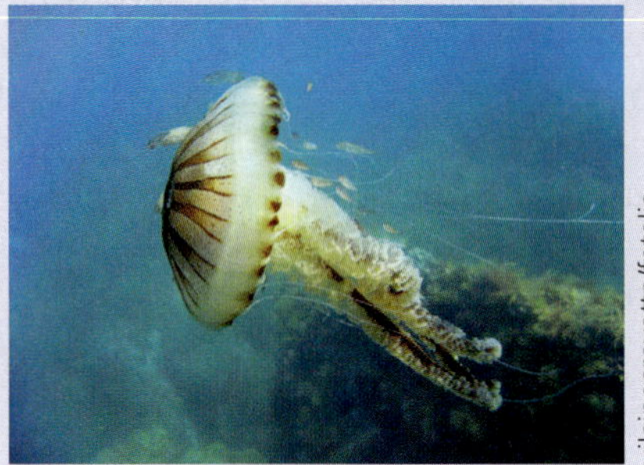

Figure 17–14a Jellyfish.

vilainecrevette/fotolia

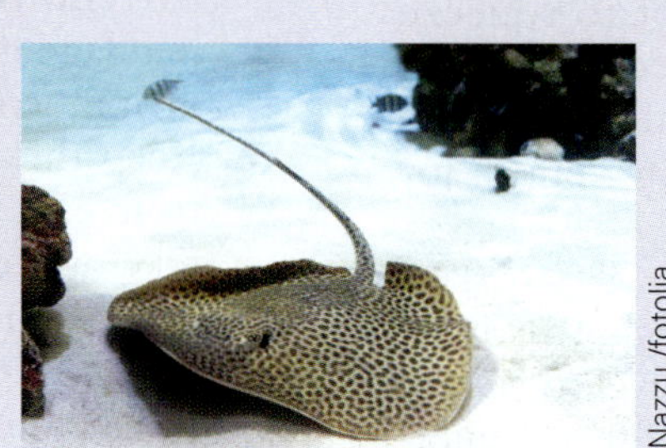

Figure 17–14b Stingray.

Nazzu /fotolia

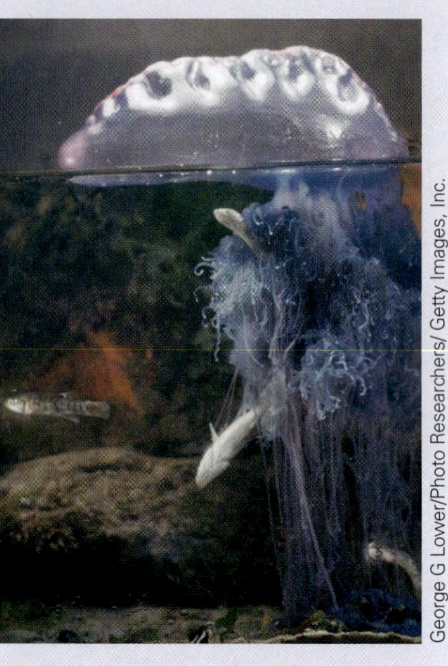

Figure 17–14c Tentacles of the Portuguese man-of-war.

George G Lower/Photo Researchers/ Getty Images, Inc.

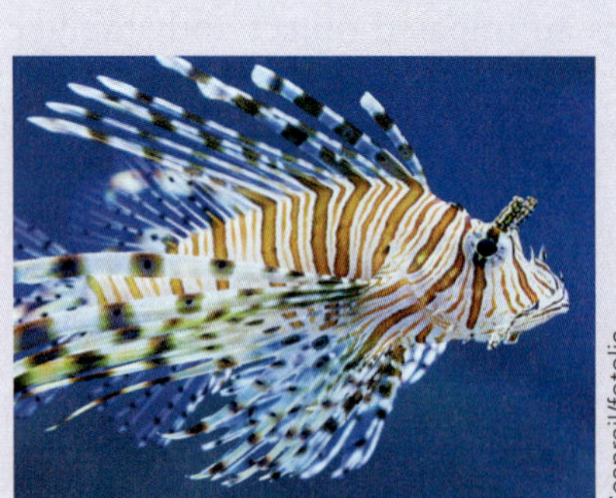

Figure 17–14d Lion fish.

Scanrail/fotolia

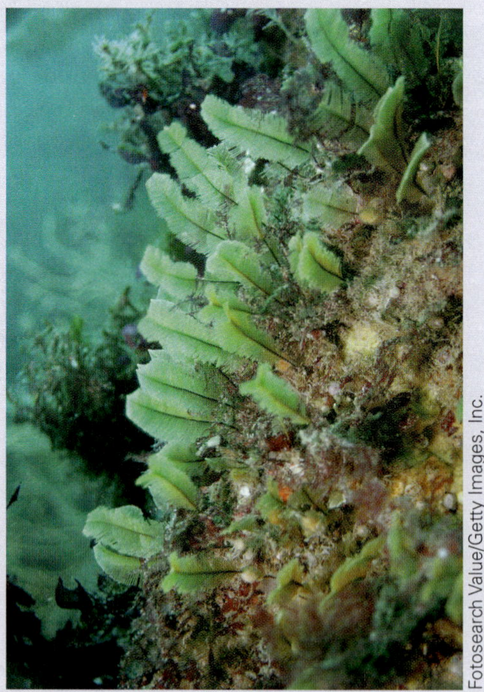

Figure 17–14e Feather hydroid.

Fotosearch Value/Getty Images, Inc.

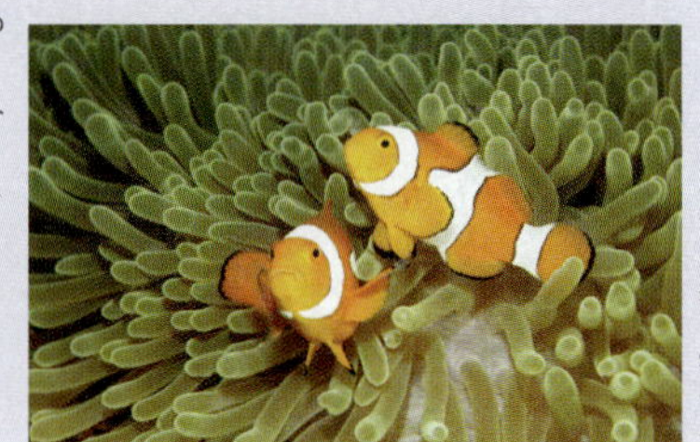

Figure 17–14f Sea anemone and clown fish.

cbpix/fotolia

COMMON SOURCES OF MARINE LIFE STINGS AND WOUNDS *(continued)*

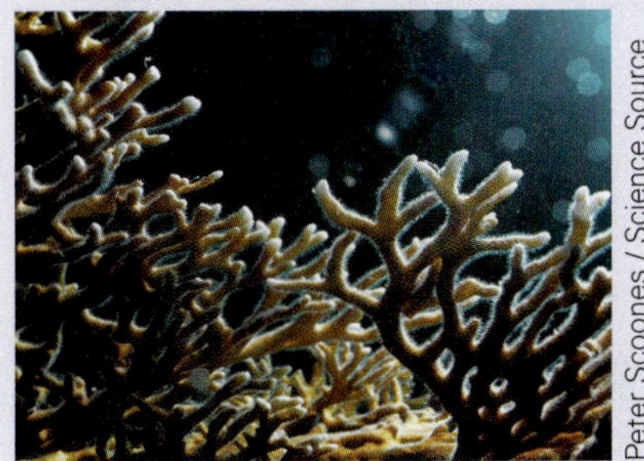

Figure 17–14g Fire coral.

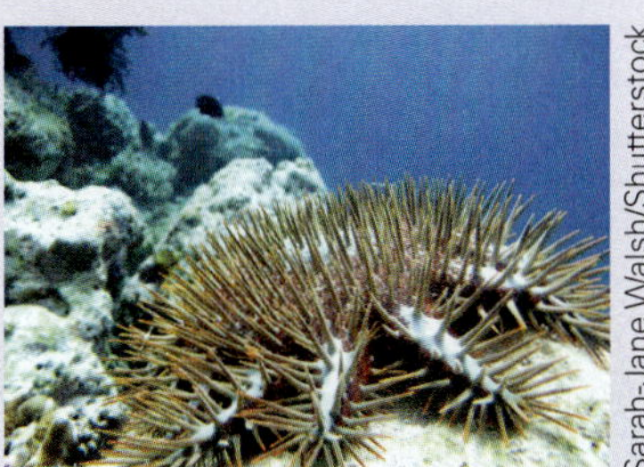

Figure 17–14h Crown-of-thorns starfish.

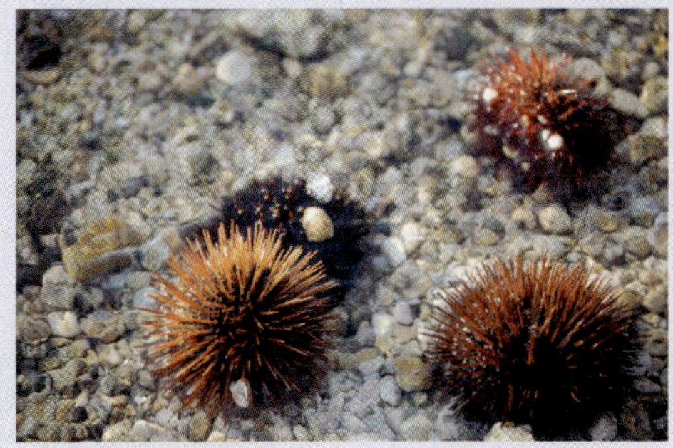

Figure 17–14i Sea urchin.

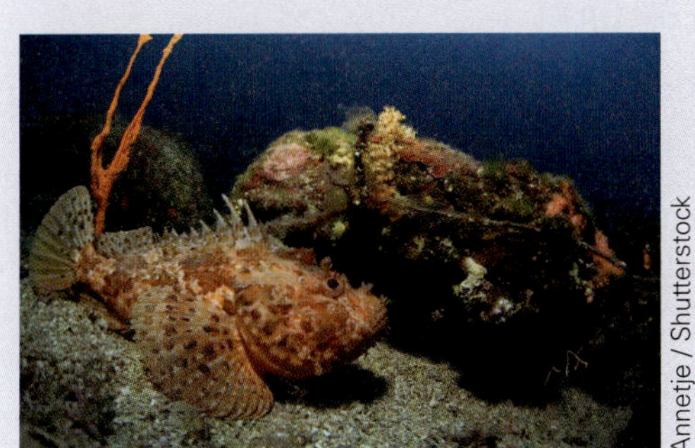

Figure 17–14j Scorpion fish.

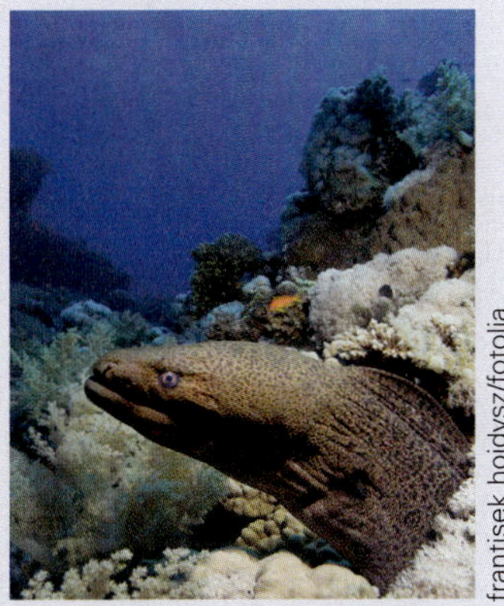

Figure 17–14k Moray eel.

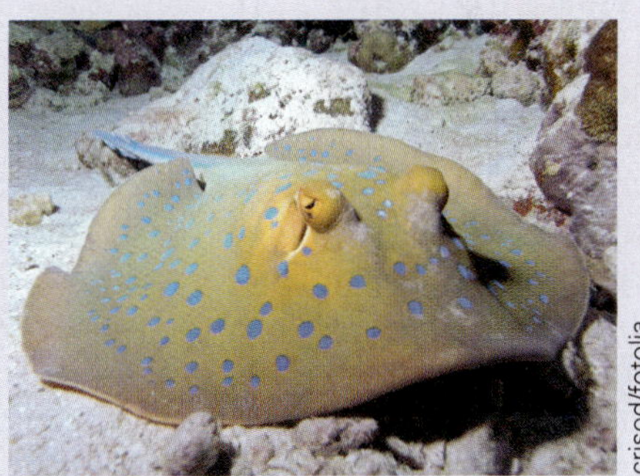

Figure 17–14l Stingray.

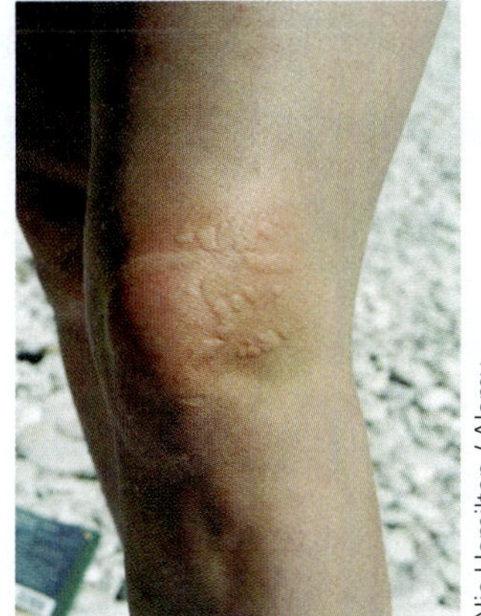

Figure 17–15 Jellyfish sting.

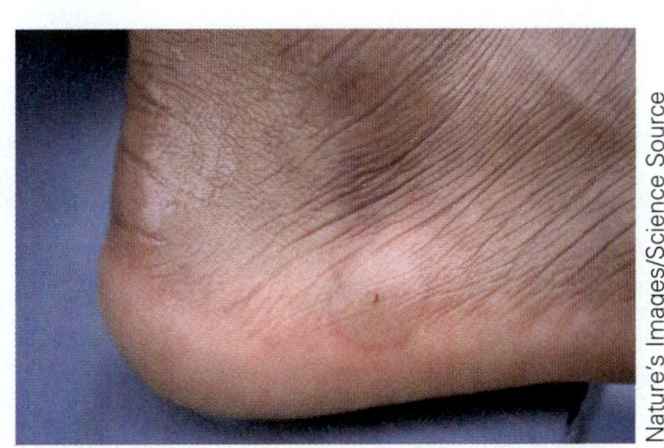

Figure 17–16 Stingray wound.

EMR FOCUS

Bites and stings are a mere annoyance for most people. For others, however, these injuries can cause a severe allergic reaction. As an EMR, you must be alert for the serious—and potentially fatal—reaction called anaphylactic shock.

Some snakebites and marine stings may be deadly to a patient, even without an allergic reaction. If you have poisonous snakes or other dangerous species in your area, be sure to become familiar with local protocols for assessment and treatment. Never forget scene safety. You do not want to be bitten or stung yourself!

CASE STUDY FOLLOW-UP

At the beginning of this chapter, you read that EMRs were on the scene of a female patient who was having an allergic reaction to a bee sting. To see how the chapter skills apply to this emergency, read the following. It describes how the call was completed.

PATIENT HISTORY

The patient's name was Naomi. The people with her told us that she was allergic to bee stings. She got stung by a bee while walking on a path to the lake. We found that she was allergic to nothing else. She had eaten dinner an hour before. She had a device that administered epinephrine for bee stings, but it was at home. She had no past medical history. I found the spot on her neck where she had been stung. I didn't see a stinger in the wound.

SECONDARY ASSESSMENT

My partner spent most of his time trying to keep her calm. I checked her vital signs. Her pulse was 108 and weak. Her respirations were 20 and laboured. Her blood pressure was 100/62. We took her out of the chair and placed her on the ground. She resisted lying flat.

ONGOING ASSESSMENT

We carefully monitored her respirations. It was getting harder for her to breathe. She was becoming increasingly pale and getting sleepy. We decided to place her in the supine position. Then we assisted ventilations. Fortunately, the paramedics arrived quickly.

TRANSFER OF CARE

We made our report quickly. We told the medics about the bee sting, her allergy, her declining condition, and vitals. They went to work immediately. They administered drugs that helped reverse the allergic reaction and shock that had developed. Naomi did fine, but it looked like it was a close one. The medics told us that she stabilized en route, and they gave her their best advice. They made her promise never to leave the house without her medication again.

> It is likely that a bite or sting will make your patient uncomfortable for only a few days. However, the chance that venom has been injected or that a patient may have an allergic reaction is real. Stay alert. Monitor vital signs continually. Be sure EMS has been activated, and be prepared to provide basic life support.

NOCPs

3.3 a Assess scene for safety **S**

4.2 c Obtain chief complaint and/or incident history from patient, family members, and/or bystanders **S**

f Obtain information regarding incident through accurate and complete scene assessment **S**

4.3 c Conduct cardiovascular system assessment and interpret findings **S**

e Conduct respiratory system assessment and interpret findings **S**

i Conduct integumentary system assessment and interpret findings **S**

k Conduct assessment of the ears, eyes, nose, and throat and interpret findings **S**

4.4 g Assess skin condition **S**
6.1 f Provide care to patient experiencing signs and symptoms involving integumentary system **S**

h Provide care to patient experiencing signs and symptoms involving immune system **S**
k Provide care to patient experiencing toxicologic syndromes **S**

REVIEW QUESTIONS

Page references where answers may be found or supported are provided at the end of each question.

SECTION 1

1. What are the general signs and symptoms of bites and stings? (p. 252)
2. What are the signs and symptoms of an allergic reaction in a patient with a bite or sting? Describe those related to the skin, respiratory system, and circulatory system, as well as general findings. (p. 252)
3. What are the general guidelines for the emergency medical care of patients with bites and stings? Include care of a patient who may be having an allergic reaction. (p. 254)

SECTION 2

4. What is the proper method of applying a constricting band to an extremity? (pp. 256–257)
5. How would you remove an engorged tick from a patient's skin? (p. 259)
6. Which common Canadian insect is a carrier of West Nile virus? (p. 259)
7. What is the proper method for removing the barbed stinger of a bee from a patient's skin? (p. 261)
8. How would you treat a large bite from any marine or land animal? (p. 261)

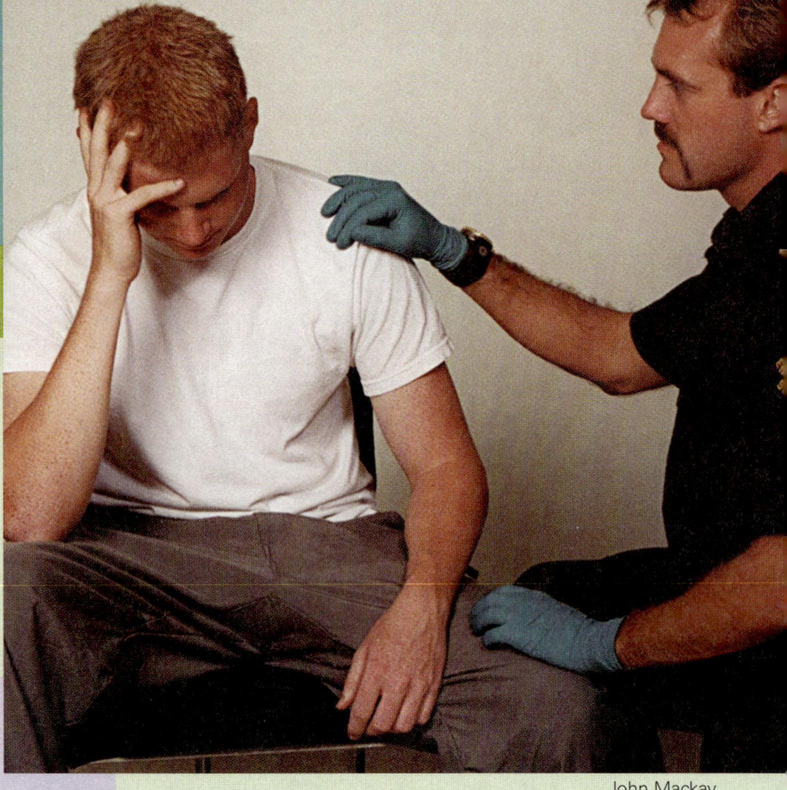
John Mackay

Psychological Emergencies and Crisis Intervention

OBJECTIVES

1. Explain the rationale for modifying your behaviour toward the patient in a behavioural emergency.
2. List five ways to calm a patient in a behavioural emergency.
3. Discuss the guidelines for patient restraint.
4. Describe the legal considerations involved in providing emergency care to a patient in a behavioural emergency.
5. Identify five signs and symptoms of drug or alcohol overdose or withdrawal and six signs and symptoms of a drug or alcohol emergency.
6. Outline the steps of emergency care for a patient suffering from a drug or alcohol overdose.
7. Discuss the four general stages of rape trauma syndrome.
8. Describe the proper management of a rape scene.
9. Demonstrate a caring attitude toward the patient and family when dealing with behavioural emergencies, while giving priority to the interests of the patient.

INTRODUCTION

In emergency care involving physical problems, you can see the wounds you need to treat. You can assess, dress, and bandage them. Often, you also get to see the positive results of your efforts.

Emergency care for behavioural emergencies is different. You cannot easily see the comfort that your presence or your words provide to someone who is panicked or depressed. But the care you give to patients in behavioural emergencies can also save lives.

SECTION 1
BEHAVIOURAL EMERGENCIES

Behaviour is the manner in which a person acts or performs. A **behavioural emergency** is a situation in which a patient exhibits abnormal behaviour or behaviour that is unacceptable or intolerable to the patient, family, or community. Such an emergency may be due to extremes of emotion, a psychological condition such as a mental illness or dementia, or even a physical condition such as lack of oxygen or low blood sugar.

A number of factors can cause a change in a patient's behaviour. They include the following:

- Senile dementia in older adults (from causes such as Alzheimer disease and organic brain syndrome)
- Situational stresses
- Illness or injury, including head trauma, lack of oxygen, inadequate blood flow to the brain, low blood sugar in a person with diabetes, or excessive heat or cold
- Mind-altering substances, such as alcohol, depressants, stimulants, psychedelics, and narcotics
- Psychiatric problems, such as a phobia (irrational fear of specific things), depression, paranoia, or schizophrenia
- Psychological crises, such as panic and bizarre thinking

Patients with behavioural emergencies may act in unusual and unexpected ways. They can pose a danger to themselves through suicide or self-inflicted injuries. They can also pose a danger to others through violence or other actions that they are not able to understand.

Patient Assessment

Consider the need for law enforcement during your scene assessment and throughout the call. If you suspect that the patient may threaten himself, herself, or others, arrange for backup law enforcement at the scene.

The following guidelines may help you determine if your patient is likely to become violent:

- During scene assessment, look around carefully. Locate the patient before approaching (Figure 18–1). Check to see if there are any weapons or items that could be used as weapons, such as a knife or blunt object. If there are any, assume that the patient may use them to hurt you or himself or herself. Overturned furniture or other signs of chaos can also indicate violent behaviour.
- If the patient's family members or friends or any bystanders are at the scene, ask them if the patient has a history of being aggressive or combative. Also, find out if the patient has been violent or has threatened violence at the scene.
- Expect violence if the patient is standing or sitting in a way that threatens anyone (including himself or herself). Clenched fists, even when the patient is holding them at his or her sides, may be a sign.
- Listen to the patient. Expect violence if the patient is yelling, cursing, arguing, or verbally threatening to hurt himself or herself or others.

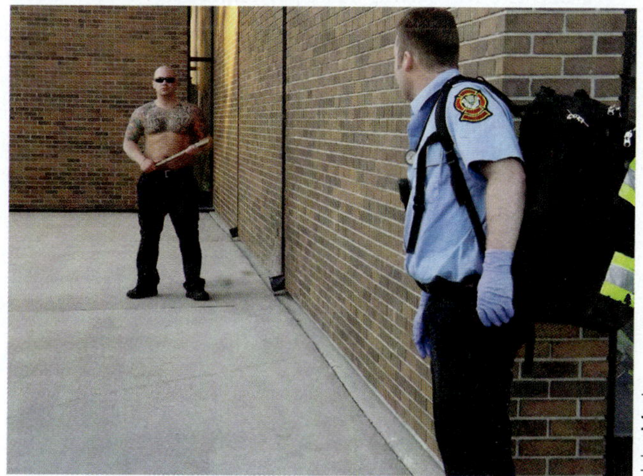

Figure 18–1   Locate the patient before approaching. Check to see if there are any weapons.

CASE STUDY

Dispatch

I was driving home from my shift at the fire department when I saw a man running along the road. He was naked. He stopped every few hundred feet or so to throw punches in the air.

Scene Assessment

I realized this person might be dangerous. So I called the RCMP on my cell phone from my car. I stayed there until they arrived.

Primary Assessment

After the man was restrained by the police, I offered my help. They were careful not to restrict the man's breathing. They also covered him with an emergency blanket to keep him warm. He was screaming at the police officers, so I knew his breathing was adequate. There were no indications of airway problems or external bleeding.

My general impression was that of a patient with altered mental status, possibly from a psychiatric emergency, alcohol, or drugs. We called for an ambulance.

> Consider this patient as you read Chapter 18. What else may be done to assess and treat his condition?

- Watch for signs of possible violence in a patient, including moving toward you, carrying a heavy or threatening object, making quick or irregular movements, and muscle tension.

Keep the following basic principles in mind whenever you are on the scene of a behavioural emergency:

- Identify yourself. Let the patient know you are there to help.
- Inform the patient of exactly what you are doing. Uncertainty will make the patient more anxious and fearful.
- Ask questions in a calm, reassuring voice. Speak directly to the patient. Stay polite. Use good manners. Show respect. Make no unsupported assumptions.
- Without being judgmental, allow the patient to tell you what happened.
- Show you are listening by rephrasing or repeating parts of what is said. Ask questions to show you are paying attention. Also use gestures, such as a nod of the head, or verbal responses such as "I see" or "Go on."

- Acknowledge the patient's feelings. Use phrases such as "I can see that you're very depressed" or "I'm not surprised that you feel frightened."
- Assess the patient's mental status by asking specific questions. Try to determine whether or not the patient is oriented to time, person, and place. Watch the patient's appearance, level of activity, and speech patterns.

General Emergency Care

While caring for a patient in a behavioural emergency, be sure to comfort, calm, and reassure the patient as you proceed.

Never leave the patient alone. All such patients are escape risks, and violence is a real possibility. Once you have responded to a behavioural emergency, the patient's safety is legally your responsibility until someone with more training arrives on the scene. Even if the patient pleads to be left alone for just a few minutes, do not leave. Firmly explain that you could get into trouble if you did.

If you suspect the patient may have overdosed or abused substances, provide emergency medical care as described in Chapter 14 for a poisoning patient. Give any medication or drugs you find on the scene to the transporting EMS personnel.

Methods to Calm Patients in Behavioural Emergencies

The situations presented by behaviourally disturbed patients are often difficult. However, a number of techniques can help:

- Acknowledge that the patient seems upset, and restate that you are there to help.
- Inform the patient of exactly who you are and what you are going to do to help (Figure 18–2).
- Ask questions in a calm, reassuring voice. Speak directly to the patient.
- Always keep a clear path between you and the exit. Do not let the patient be in that path.
- Maintain a comfortable distance between you and the patient. Many patients are threatened by physical contact. Unwanted touching could set off a violent response. After you have established some rapport with the patient, get his or her permission before moving in any closer (Figure 18–3).
- Encourage the patient to tell you what is troubling him or her. Ask the patient to explain the problem.
- Never assume that it is impossible to communicate with the patient until you have tried, even if others insist it cannot be done.
- Do not make any quick movements. Act quietly and slowly. Let the patient see that you are not going to make any sudden moves.
- Respond honestly to the patient's questions. Instead of saying, for example, "You have nothing to worry about," say something like "Even with all your problems, you seem to have lots of people around who really care about you."
- Never threaten, challenge, belittle, or argue with disturbed patients. Remember that the patient is ill. His or her comments are not about you personally.
- Always tell the truth. Never lie to a patient.
- Do not play along with a patient's visual or auditory disturbances. Instead, reassure the patient that they are temporary and will clear up with treatment.
- Involve the patient's family members or friends when you can. Some patients are calmed and reassured by their presence. However, others may be upset or embarrassed. Let the patient decide.
- Be prepared to stay at the scene for a long time.
- Avoid unnecessary physical contact. Enlist the help of law enforcement if you are unable to maintain control on your own.
- Maintain good eye contact with the patient. It communicates your control and confidence. Also, the patient's eyes can reflect emotions. They may tell you if the patient is terrified, confused, struggling, or in pain. The eyes can also indicate the patient's intentions. If a patient is about to reach for a weapon or make a dash, the eyes may alert you.

Just as with any other patient, place the interests of the patient with a behavioural problem first in all patient care decisions. Use empathy when communicating with the patient, as well as with family members and friends.

Restraining Patients

Restraint should be avoided unless the patient poses a danger to himself or herself or to others. Restraints

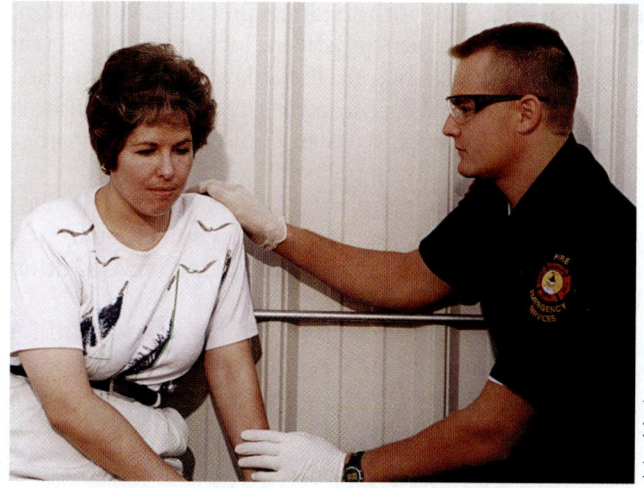

Figure 18–3   With the patient's consent, your touch may be comforting.

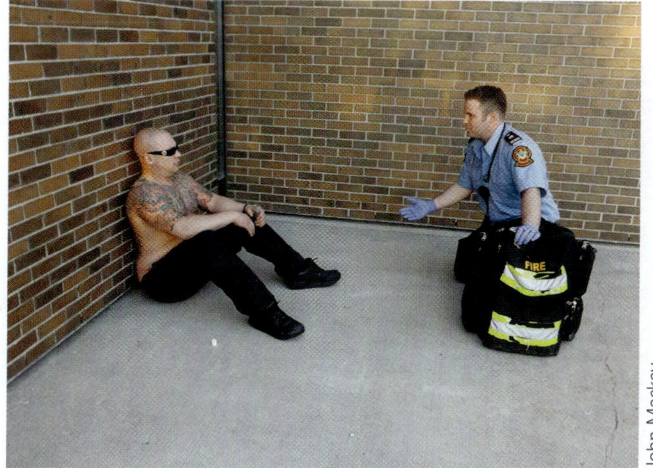

Figure 18–2   Explain who you are and that you are trying to help.

may require police authorization in your EMS system. Seek medical direction and follow local protocol. If you are not authorized by provincial law to use restraints, wait for someone with the authority. If you are authorized to use restraints, work in conjunction with other EMS providers and the police (Figure 18–4).

Be aware that a violent physical struggle is usually brief. However, after a struggle, some apparently calm patients may cause unexpected and sudden injury to themselves and others.

Avoid using unreasonable force. Never inflict pain or use unnecessary force in restraining a patient. Use only as much force as is needed for restraint. **Reasonable force** depends on the amount of force needed to keep a patient from injuring himself or herself or someone else. It depends on the following:

- *The size and strength of the patient.* What may seem reasonable force on a 125 kg athlete may not be reasonable on a 60 kg senior citizen.
- *The type of abnormal behaviour the patient is exhibiting.* You would not expect to use the same kind of force against a frightened patient who is huddling quietly in a corner as you would

THE COMBATIVE PATIENT

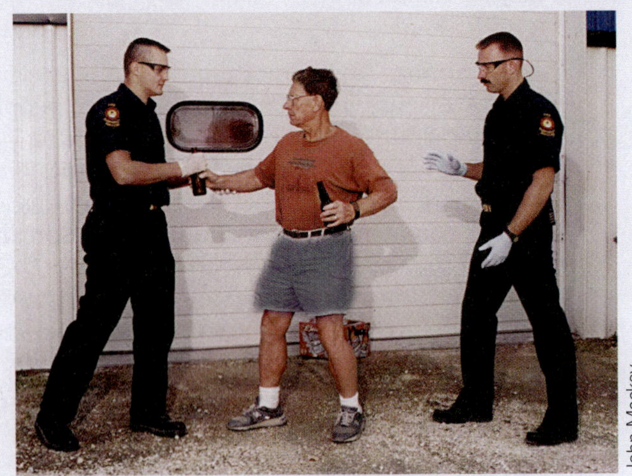

Figure 18–4a If asked to assist other EMS providers, stay beyond the range of the patient's arms and legs.

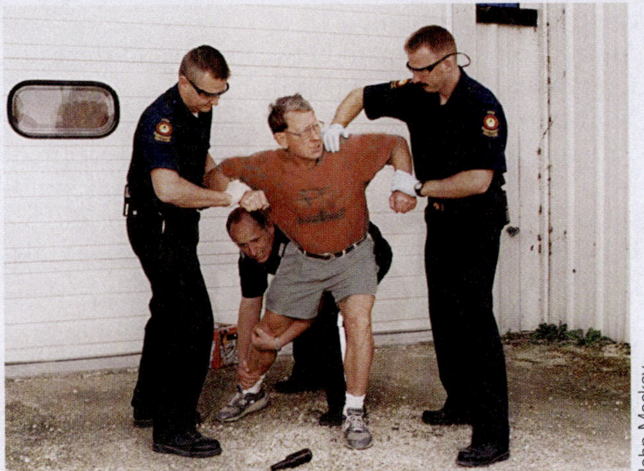

Figure 18–4b If restraints are needed, work in conjunction with an adequate number of other EMS providers.

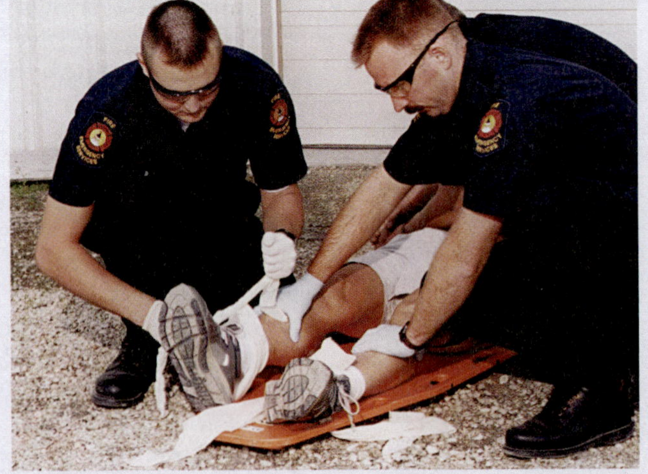

Figure 18–4c You may also be asked to assist the paramedics when they apply the ankle and wrist restraints.

against an angry patient who is loudly threatening to kill you.

- *The mental state of the patient.* It may be reasonable to use more force on a patient who is loud and threatening than on a patient who is quiet and subdued.
- *The method of restraint you are using.* Soft leather or cloth straps are called humane restraints. They are generally considered reasonable. Metal cuffs are not.

In any case, the best way to protect yourself legally is to involve your chain of command. A good rule of thumb is to seek medical direction before you restrain a patient. Follow local protocols.

Remember that law enforcement personnel should also be involved when you need to restrain a patient, when you need to give care without consent, and when there is any threat of violence. If police utilize **Tasers** to subdue a patient, you must call paramedics to the scene, even if the patient will not be transported to a hospital (Figure 18–5a). Do not touch the patient until you are sure that there is no longer any current being transmitted to the patient. Do not remove the Taser darts (Figure 18–5b). Paramedics have specific protocols to follow for Taser dart removal. They will require a complete set of vital signs and the patient's past medical history, as well as information on the time since the patient last had a tetanus shot.

Law enforcement personnel can help protect you from injury, and they can also serve as credible witnesses if a legal case arises. The best way to protect yourself against false accusations by a patient is to carefully and completely document everything that happens during the call. In most

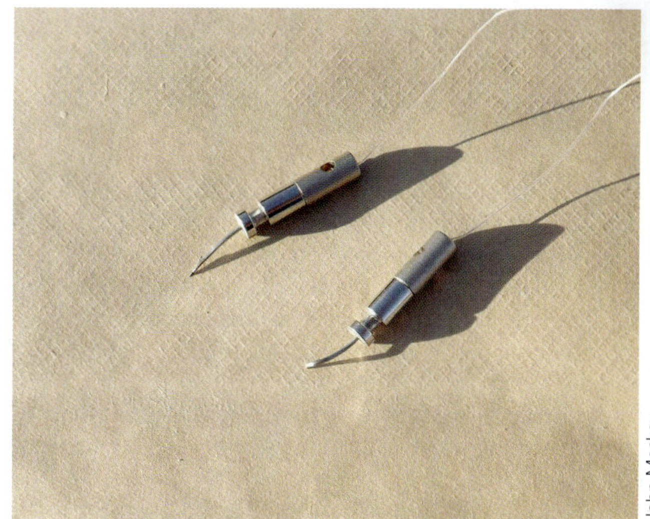

Figure 18–5b   Taser darts.

jurisdictions, anything you document during the call is legally admissible evidence. Anything that is not documented is considered hearsay (not legally admissible).

Another source of protection is witnesses, preferably throughout the entire course of treatment. It is common for emotionally disturbed patients to accuse medical personnel of sexual misconduct. To protect yourself against such allegations, do the following:

- Involve other EMS providers who can testify that there was no misconduct.
- Use EMS providers who are the same gender as the patient.
- Involve third-party witnesses whenever possible.

Legal Considerations

Your legal problems are greatly reduced if an emotionally disturbed patient consents to receive care. However, such patients commonly refuse treatment—especially patients who are intoxicated or who have taken a drug overdose. They may even threaten you or others.

Unless the patient is considered mentally incompetent, legally he or she must provide consent before you can treat. Remember, the patient—not concerned family members—must consent to receive care.

Generally, you may provide care against a patient's will only if the patient threatens to hurt himself or herself or others and only if you can demonstrate reason to believe that the patient's threats are real. A good rule of thumb is to consult with the medical director and involve law enforcement.

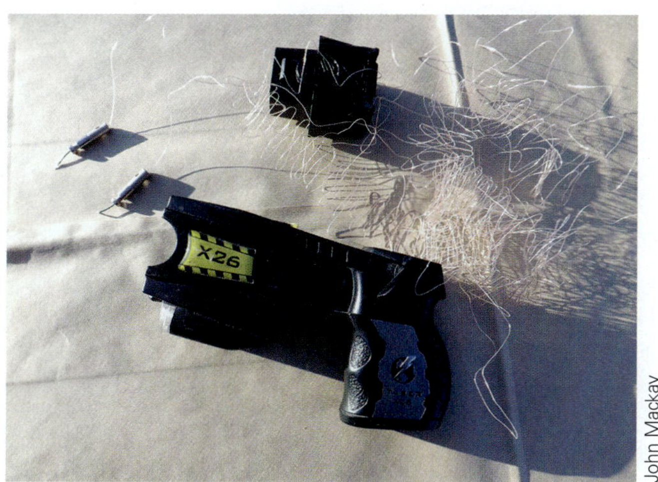

Figure 18–5a   A police Taser for subduing violent patients.

SECTION 2
DRUG AND ALCOHOL EMERGENCIES

Drug abuse is the self-administration of one or more drugs, including alcohol, in a way that is not in accordance with approved medical or social practice. An **overdose** is an emergency that involves poisoning by drugs or alcohol. The term **withdrawal** refers to the effects on the body that occur after a period of abstinence from the drugs or alcohol to which the body has become accustomed. Withdrawal—especially from alcohol—can be as serious as an overdose emergency.

As an EMR you are not required to memorize specific street drug names and their interactions. Reviewing the different classes of drugs used on the street will help you with your assessment. Detection of their use is beneficial as you assess and begin treatment of the patient.

Drugs may be classified as uppers, downers, narcotics, hallucinogens (mind-altering drugs), or volatile chemicals (Figure 18–6). **Uppers** are stimulants that affect the central nervous system (CNS) and excite the user. **Downers** are depressants that relax

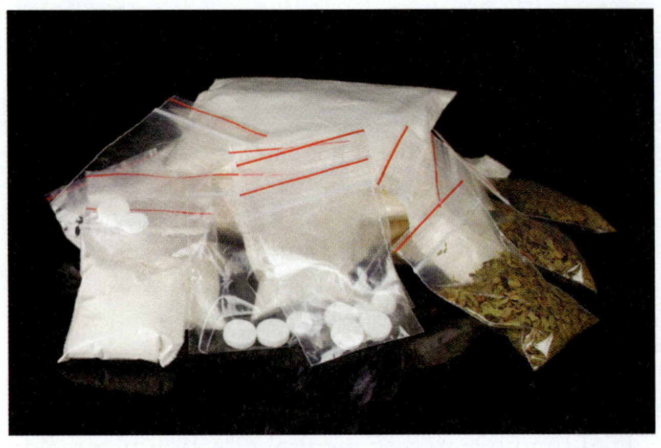

Figure 18–6   Samples of illegal drugs.

the user by affecting the CNS. **Narcotics** affect the CNS and many of the body's normal activities. They can produce an intense state of relaxation and feelings of euphoria. **Hallucinogens** affect the CNS and can produce an intense state of excitement and distort the user's perception of his or her surroundings. **Volatile chemicals** initially stimulate but subsequently depress the CNS. Examples of all these drugs may be found in Table 18–1.

TABLE 18–1
COMMONLY ABUSED SUBSTANCES

Uppers

Aiphetamine (bam)

Amphetamine (Benzedrine, bennies, pep pills, ups, uppers, cartwheels)

Cocaine (coke, snow, crack)

Desoxyephedrine (Desoxyn, black beauties)

Dextroamphetamine (Dexedrine, dexies)

Methamphetamine (Methedrine, speed, crystal meth, diet pills)

Methylphenidate (Ritalin)

Phenmetrazine (Preludin)

Downers

Amobarbital (Amytal, blue devils, downers, barbs)

Barbiturates (downers, dollas, bars, rainbows)

Chloral hydrate (Notec, knockout drops)

Ethchlorvynol (Placidyl)

Glutethimide (Doriden, goofers)

Methaqualone (Quaalude, ludes; Sopor, sopors)

Non-barbiturate sedatives – various tranquilizers and sleeping pills (diazepam [Valium], lorazepam [Ativan], temazepam [Restoril], meprobamate [Miltown, Equanil], chlorpromazine [Thorazine], prochlorperazine [Compazine], chlordiazepoxide [Librium], reserpine, clorazepate [Tranxene], and other benzodiazepines)

TABLE 18–1 Continued

Narcotics

Codeine (often in cough syrup)

Fentanyl

Heroin (H, horse, junk, smack, stuff)

Hydromorphone (Dilaudid)

Methadone (dolly)

Meperidine (Demerol)

Morphine

Opium (op, poppy)

Oxycodone (Oxycocet, OxyContin, Percocet, percs)

Paregoric (tincture of opium)

Hallucinogens

DMT

Hash

LSD (acid, sunshine)

Marijuana (grass, pot, weed, dope)

Mescaline (peyote, mesc)

Methylenedioxymethamphetamine (MDMA, ecstasy) – also has stimulant properties

Morning glory seeds

PCP (angel dust, hog, peace pills)

Psilocybin (magic mushrooms)

STP (serenity, tranquility, peace)

THC

Volatile Chemicals

Amyl nitrate (snappers, poppers)

Cleaning fluid (carbon tetrachloride)

Furniture polish

Gasoline

Glue

Hair spray

Mouthwash

Nail polish remover

Paint thinner

REMEMBER: The most commonly abused substance in Canada is alcohol (ethanol). In addition to its direct effects, alcohol is often mixed with other abused substances, worsening the effects on the body.

Source: Bergeron, J.D., Bizjak, G., Le Baudour, C., Wesley, K., *First Responder*, 8th Edition, © 2009, p. 295. Reprinted by permission of Pearson Education, Inc. Upper Saddle River, N.J.

There are many physical effects of chronic drug abuse (Figure 18–7). Most drug overdoses involve drug abuse by longtime drug users. However, a drug overdose can also be the result of miscalculation, confusion, use of more than one drug, or a suicide attempt.

Various drugs can cause changes in respiration, heart rate, blood pressure, and CNS function. In addition, several major medical problems can result from a drug or alcohol overdose or from sudden withdrawal, including the following:

- Respiratory problems
- Internal injuries
- Seizures
- Cardiac arrest
- Hypothermia or hyperthermia

Patient Assessment

Signs and symptoms that indicate a life-threatening drug or alcohol emergency include the following (Figure 18–8 on p. 275):

- Unconsciousness
- Breathing difficulties or inability to maintain an open airway
- Abnormal or irregular pulse
- Fever
- Vomiting with altered mental status or without a gag reflex
- Seizures

If any of these signs and symptoms are present, your patient is a high priority for transport. Report to

EFFECTS OF ALCOHOL AND DRUG ABUSE

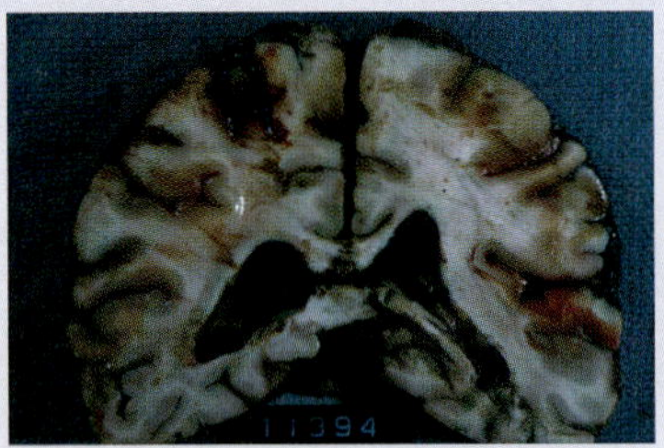

Figure 18–7a Alcohol-related bullet wound to the brain.

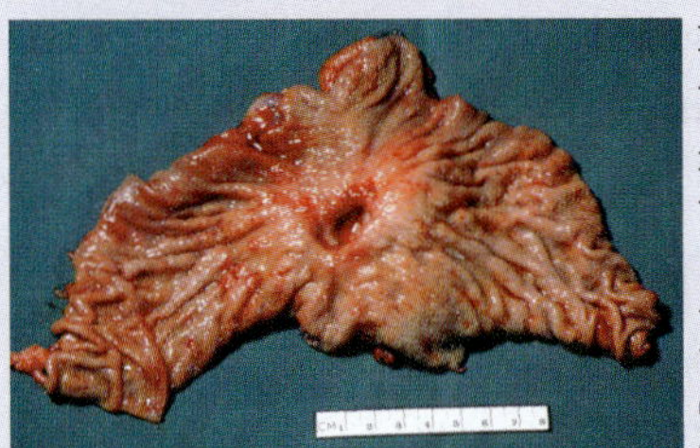

Figure 18–7b Chronic gastric ulcer from alcohol abuse.

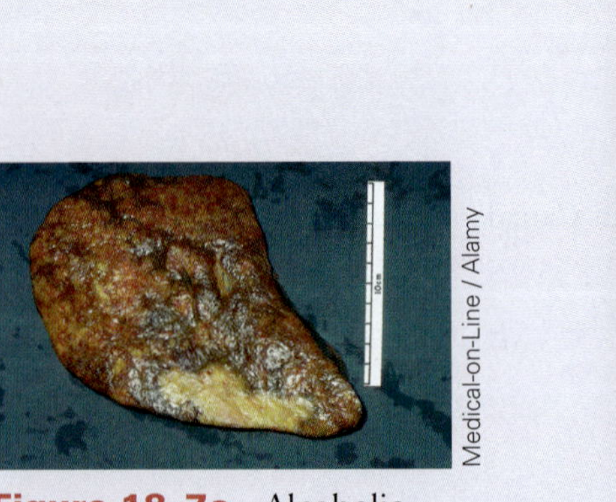

Figure 18–7c Alcoholic cirrhosis of the liver.

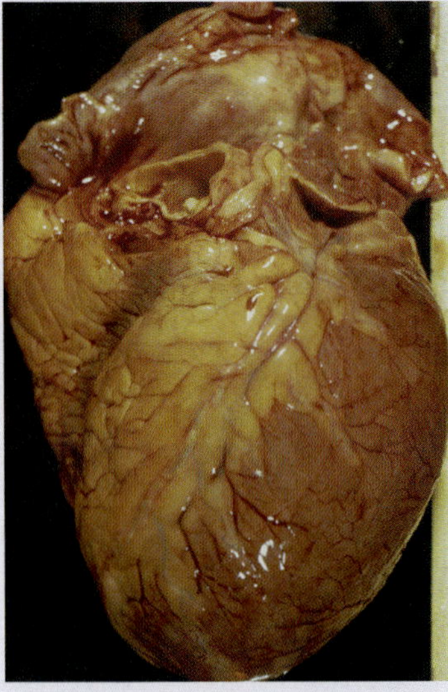

Figure 18–7d Enlarged, weak heart related to alcohol.

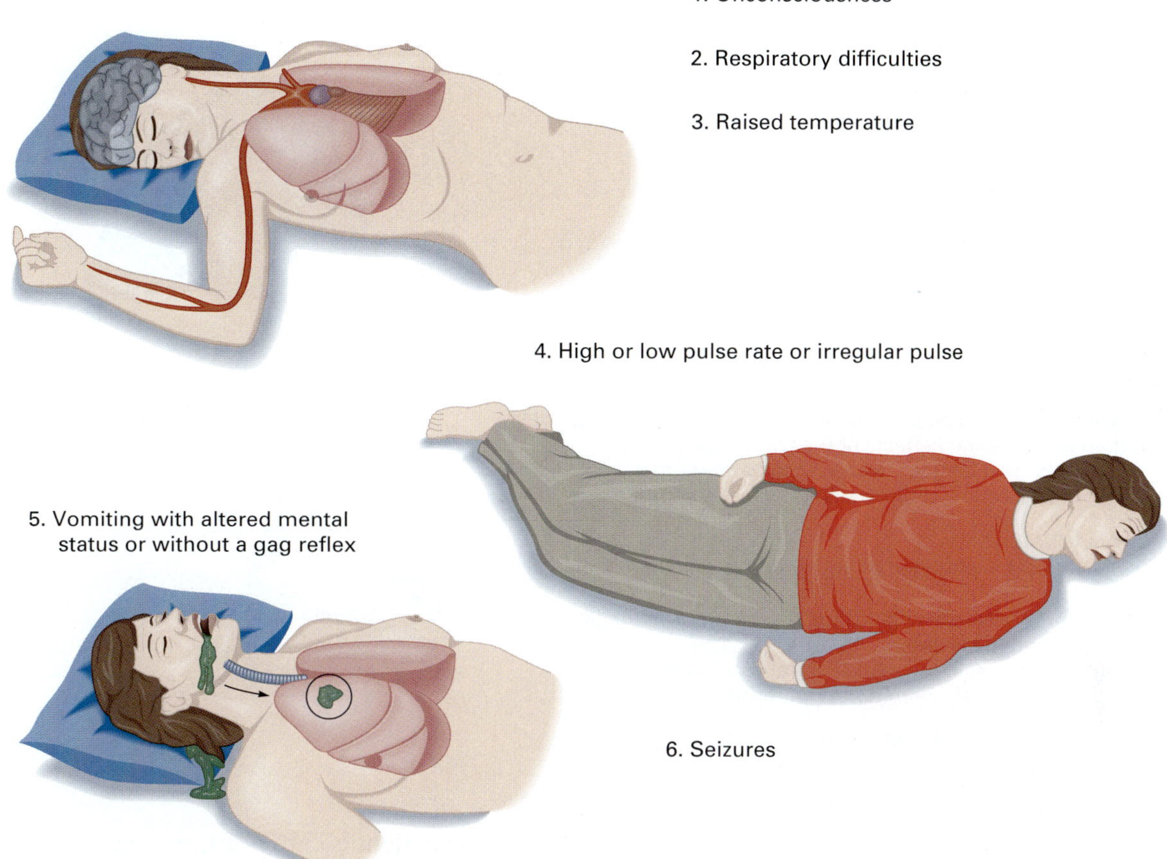

Figure 18–8　Indicators of a drug or alcohol emergency.

dispatch immediately. Additional signs and symptoms will vary widely. They may include the following:

- Altered mental status
- Extremely low or high blood pressure
- Sweating, tremors, and hallucinations (with alcohol withdrawal)
- Digestive problems, including abdominal pain and bleeding
- Visual disturbances, slurred speech, uncoordinated muscle movement
- Lack of interest, loss of memory
- Combativeness
- Paranoia

If your patient is unconscious and you suspect a drug or alcohol emergency, after your primary assessment, proceed with the following:

- With a gloved hand, check the patient's mouth for partially dissolved pills or tablets. If you find any, remove them so that they cannot block the patient's airway.
- Smell the patient's breath for traces of alcohol. Do not confuse the smell of alcohol with musky, fruity,

or acetone odours. These three can indicate an emergency related to diabetes.
- Ask the patient's friends or family members what they know about the incident.

Because signs and symptoms vary so widely and are so similar to many medical conditions, the most reliable indications of a drug- or alcohol-related emergency are likely to come from the scene and the patient history.

Common street drugs may be identified by police or paramedics by their packaging. Always use gloves if you must handle any packaging or paraphernalia. It is a good idea to leave "evidence" where it lies and point it out to police and paramedics.

General Emergency Care

Your immediate goals are to ensure your own safety, maintain the patient's airway, and manage life-threatening conditions (Figure 18–9). If you believe

CAUTION: Do not immediately decide that a patient with apparent alcohol on the breath is drunk. The signs may indicate an illness or injury, such as epilepsy, diabetes, or head injury.

SIGNS OF INTOXICATION
• Odour of alcohol on the breath
• Swaying and unsteadiness
• Slurred speech
• Nausea and vomiting
• Flushed face
• Drowsiness
• Violent, destructive, or erratic behaviour
• Self-injury, usually without realizing it

EFFECTS
• Alcohol is a depressant. It affects judgment, vision, reaction time, and coordination.
• When taken with other depressants, the result can be greater than the combined effects of the two drugs.
• In very large quantities, alcohol can paralyze the respiratory centre of the brain and cause death.

MANAGEMENT
• Give the same attention as you would to any patient with an illness or injury.
• Monitor the patient's vital signs constantly. Provide life support when necessary.
• Position the patient to avoid aspiration of vomit.
• Protect the patient from hurting himself or herself.

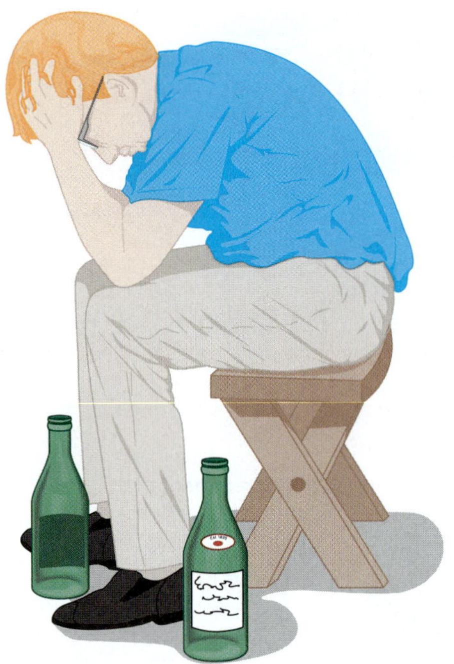

Figure 18–9 Alcohol emergencies.

that the patient has overdosed, follow the emergency care directions offered below and in Chapter 14 for poisoning.

After taking BSI precautions, follow these steps:

1. *Establish and maintain an open airway.* Remove anything from the patient's throat or mouth that might obstruct the airway, including false teeth, blood, or mucus. In case of vomiting, turn the patient's head to the side for drainage unless trauma is suspected. Consider using the recovery position or the HAINES position if spinal injury is suspected.

2. *Monitor the patient's mental status and vital signs frequently.* Overdose patients can be alert one minute and unconscious the next. Be prepared to provide basic life support if needed.

3. *Maintain the patient's body temperature.* If the patient is cold, cover with blankets. If the patient is abnormally hot, sponge with tepid water.

4. *Take measures to prevent shock,* which can result from vomiting, profuse sweating, or inadequate fluid intake. Be alert for allergic reactions.

5. *Care for any behavioural problem.* Follow the guidelines given earlier in this chapter for managing behavioural emergencies.

6. *Support the patient.* Comfort, calm, and reassure him or her while waiting for additional EMS personnel to arrive.

If the patient is conscious, try to get him or her to sit or lie down. Do not restrain a patient unless there is a risk to safety—his or hers, yours, or that of others.

If you suspect trauma in an unconscious patient, begin emergency care by immediately stabilizing the patient's head and neck. If there is vomiting, roll the patient as a unit to facilitate drainage.

SECTION 3
RAPE AND SEXUAL ASSAULT

Rape is one of the most devastating crises that can occur in a person's life. It involves both emotional and physical trauma. **Sexual assault** is defined as any threatened or actual sexual contact that the victim did not initiate or agree to and that is imposed by coercion, threat, deception, or threats of physical violence.

These crimes are often committed by someone the victim knows, such as a relative, friend, classmate, date, neighbour, or friend of the parents.

Rape Trauma Syndrome

An intensely personal experience under forced or terrifying circumstances can destroy a person's inner defences. Most rape victims go into acute emotional shock during or shortly after the attack. Common physical reactions to rape include the following:

- Struggling and screaming to avoid penetration
- Physical and psychological paralysis
- Pain and shock from penetration or physical abuse
- Choking, gagging, nausea, vomiting
- Urinating
- Hyperventilating
- Dazed state, unconsciousness

Following rape, most patients experience a great deal of disorganization in their lives. This emotional trauma follows a pattern described as **rape trauma syndrome**. It involves four general stages:

- Acute (impact) reaction, which takes effect immediately after the rape and continues for several days
- Outward adjustment, which lasts for weeks or months after the rape
- Depression, which is recurrent for days and months after the rape
- Acceptance and resolution, which takes months or years

Rape is a difficult and complex problem. It involves physical and emotional trauma as well as significant legal issues. Supporting the patient is of critical importance, especially during the acute reaction stage. Therefore, when you care for such a patient, remember that his or her coping system has already been stressed to the limit by the attack.

Note that too often the seriousness of rape is equated with physical damage alone. This is a mistake. Even if there are no visible external injuries, the rape victim will suffer profound emotional trauma.

Managing the Rape Scene

Keep the following considerations in mind:

- Be sure the EMS system has been activated.
- Your immediate reaction to the patient is important. Do not impose your own feelings. Instead, try to find out the patient's emotional state.

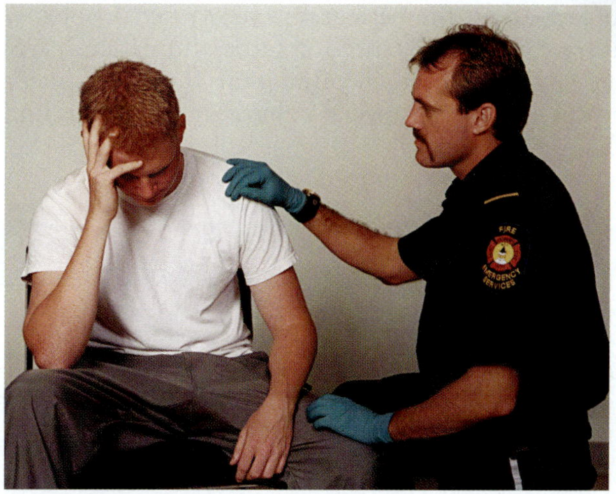

Figure 18–10 It may be best for an EMR of the same gender to assist the rape patient.

- Action can minimize the helplessness the patient may be feeling. Tell the patient what can and should be done immediately.
- The patient might be comforted by a rescuer of his or her own gender (Figure 18–10).
- Perform patient assessment and care as you would for any other patient. Treat all life threats. Check for trauma, especially around the thighs, lower abdomen, and buttocks. If vaginal bleeding is significant, give appropriate care.
- Do not clean the patient. Keep him or her from showering or bathing, brushing teeth, gargling, douching, or urinating. Cleaning could destroy important evidence. Preserve patient dignity by covering them and keeping them warm. This may also help preserve evidence as you offer them discretion.
- Once you have cared for the patient's injuries, check the scene for evidence. Bag each piece separately and transport them with the patient. Follow local protocols.

Note that your documentation of the call should include the patient's chief complaint, information about the incident that relates to your care of injuries, and your objective observations and physical findings. Your notes may be used later as evidence in court.

EMR FOCUS

A psychological crisis can be difficult for any EMS professional to deal with. Medical and trauma emergencies have specific sets of signs and symptoms. Psychological emergencies do not. This can make a psychological emergency awkward for both the patient and the EMR.

Always ensure your personal safety first. Not all patients with psychological emergencies will want to harm you, but you must be cautious.

The best way to care for this patient is to use good people skills. Be empathetic. Listen. Use body language. Usually, if you convey the message that you care about the patient and his or her problems, you have the best chance for successful patient care. Finally, always keep in mind that there are many medical causes for unusual behaviour. Never assume the problem is psychological or alcohol related until medical conditions, such as diabetes, have been ruled out.

CASE STUDY FOLLOW-UP

At the beginning of this chapter, you read that a male patient was in a behavioural emergency. To see how the chapter skills apply, read the following. It describes how the call was completed.

SECONDARY ASSESSMENT

I spoke to the patient. He was beginning to calm down a little. He denied any injuries. Knowing that head injuries or other conditions could affect mental status, I did a head-to-toe exam. It had to be quick since the patient was still quite agitated. Pulse was 88 and bounding. His respirations were 20 and deep.

PATIENT HISTORY

When the patient was quieter, I tried to gather the history. He was talking in a very confused manner. One minute he said he was a god. The next he was crying like a baby. He didn't have any medical identification tags on him. Since he had no clothes, he certainly didn't have a wallet I could check.

One of the officers said he thought he remembered the patient's name from a prior call. The dispatcher checked the RCMP computer and found that the man had done this several times before. He was a frequent patient at the psychiatric centre in the next municipality.

ONGOING ASSESSMENT

While the dispatcher's information answered some questions, I still felt that I should monitor the patient in case there was an underlying medical problem. However, the patient soon became agitated again, so I couldn't recheck his vitals. There was really no other change that I could see.

TRANSFER OF CARE

I told the paramedics what I saw and why I called the RCMP. I told them about the possible psychiatric history, the vitals, and that there were no apparent physical injuries. The paramedics asked the RCMP to ride along with them to the hospital.

I later found out that the local hospital transferred the patient back to the psychiatric centre. It seemed that whenever he stopped taking his medication, incidents like this would occur.

> As an EMR, your patient's well-being is your responsibility. However, your well-being is also important. Call for law enforcement and for additional EMS resources whenever they are needed at the scene. Remember, too, that a patient in a psychological emergency may have a medical problem, such as diabetes or a drug overdose. Monitor these patients carefully.

NOCPs

2.4 a Treat others with respect **S**
b Employ empathy and compassion while providing care **S**
c Recognize and react appropriately to persons having emotional reaction **S**
d Act in a confident manner **S**
e Act assertively as required **S**
f Employ diplomacy, tact, and discretion **S**
g Employ conflict-resolution skills **S**

3.3 a Assess scene for safety **S**
d Exhibit defusing and self-protection behaviours appropriate for use with patients and bystanders **S**
4.3 m Conduct psychiatric assessment and interpret findings **S**
6.1 p Provide care to psychiatric patient **S**

REVIEW QUESTIONS

Page references where answers may be found or supported are provided at the end of each question.

SECTION 1

1. How can you recognize a patient in a behavioural emergency? (p. 267)
2. How can you know if a patient in a behavioural emergency will be violent? (pp. 267–268)
3. What is the general emergency care of a patient in a behavioural emergency? (pp. 268–269)
4. What are some techniques that can help calm a patient in a behavioural emergency? List at least five. (p. 269)
5. Under what conditions would an EMS provider consider using restraints on a patient? (pp. 269–270)
6. What is the definition of reasonable force? What factors does it depend on? (pp. 270–271)

SECTION 2

7. Name five classes by which street drugs may be classified. (p. 272)

8. Name three popular narcotics used as street drugs. (p. 273)
9. What effect do volatile chemicals such as glue, hair spray, paint thinner, or gasoline have on the central nervous system? (p. 272)
10. What are the six signs and symptoms that indicate a life-threatening emergency in a drug or alcohol overdose patient? (p. 274)
11. What are the general guidelines for EMR care of a patient in an alcohol- or drug-related emergency? (pp. 275– 276)

SECTION 3

12. What is the basic management of a scene in which a rape has occurred? (p. 277)

CHAPTER

19

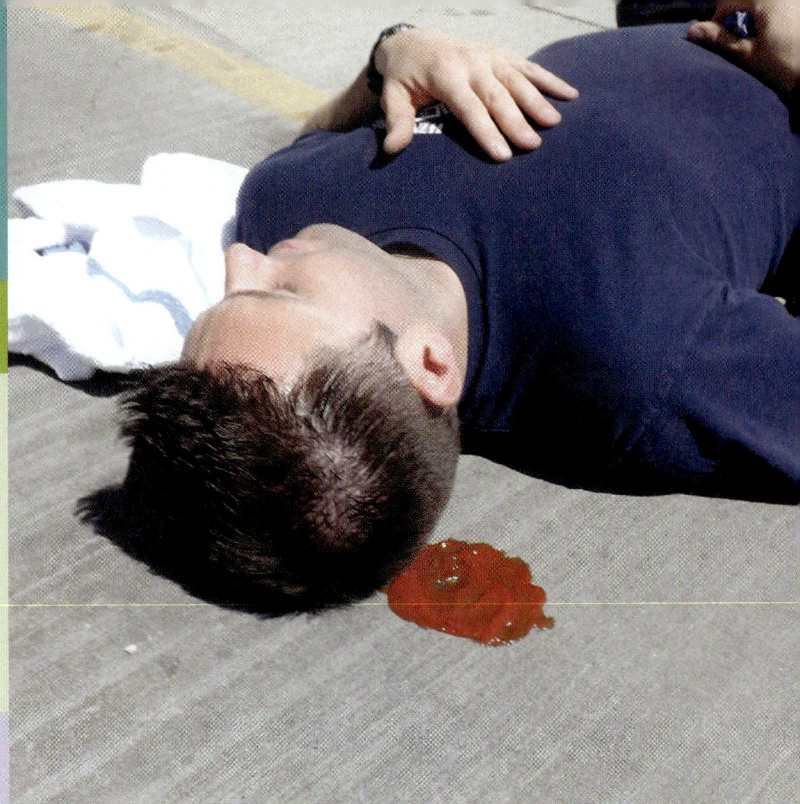

John Mackay

Bleeding and Shock

OBJECTIVES

1. Explain the rationale for BSI precautions when dealing with bleeding and soft-tissue injuries.
2. State the emergency medical care for external arterial, venous, and capillary bleeding, including direct pressure and pressure points.
3. Explain when a splint or tourniquet should be used to stop bleeding.
4. Describe emergency medical care of a patient with a nosebleed.
5. List the nine signs and symptoms of internal bleeding, and describe the steps involved in its emergency medical care.
6. List the three causes of shock and the signs and symptoms of each stage of shock: compensated, decompensated, and irreversible.
7. Outline the emergency medical care of a patient in shock.
8. Identify the signs and symptoms (skin, respiratory, circulatory, and general) of a patient experiencing anaphylactic shock, and describe his or her emergency medical care.
9. Demonstrate a caring attitude toward the patient and family when dealing with bleeding or shock, while giving priority to the interests of the patient.

INTRODUCTION

Bleeding associated with trauma can be a significant, life-threatening emergency. If bleeding is left untreated, your patient can deteriorate rapidly, go into shock, or die. Control of severe external bleeding is performed during the primary assessment. Only airway and breathing have a higher priority. Internal bleeding is more difficult to detect and may be even more deadly than external bleeding. Both internal bleeding and shock are treated immediately following the primary assessment.

SECTION 1
BLEEDING

Protecting Against Infection

Always take steps to protect yourself from diseases that can be transmitted through blood and other body fluids. This is especially urgent when your patient has external bleeding. BSI precautions are your best defence.

This may be a good time to review Chapter 2, Section 2, "Preventing Disease Transmission." Briefly, BSI precautions include the following:

- Keep a barrier between you and the patient's blood and other body fluids. At a minimum, wear a pair of protective latex gloves. Also, use a face mask with a one-way valve if you must provide ventilations.
- Wear approved goggles, mask, and gown if there is spurting or splashing blood or the potential for it.
- Never touch your mouth, nose, or eyes or handle food while you are giving emergency care.
- Keep all of the patient's open wounds covered with dressings.
- Wash your hands properly as soon as you have finished treating the patient.
- Decontaminate or properly dispose of any item that has been in contact with the patient's blood or other body fluids. Follow local protocol.

How the Body Responds to Blood Loss

Blood is part of the body's circulatory system and is distributed throughout the body (Figure 19–1). The natural response of the body to bleeding—external or internal—is blood vessel constriction and blood clotting. When a serious injury prevents that response, uncontrolled bleeding may result.

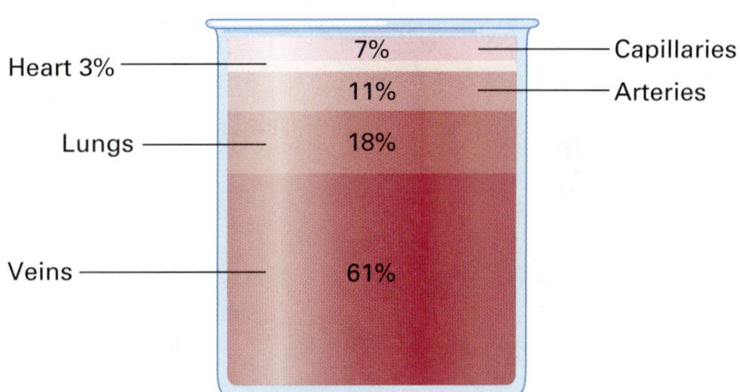

Figure 19–1 Distribution of blood in the body.

The sudden loss of 1 L (1000 mL) of blood in an adult is serious. About one-half litre (500 mL) of blood loss is serious in a child. In an infant, a loss of 100 to 200 mL of blood can be serious. The stages of blood loss and the related effects on the body are summarized in Figure 19–2 on page 283.

Just how severe bleeding is depends on a number of factors:

- The size of the blood vessel and how fast it is bleeding
- Whether the blood is flowing from an artery or a vein (Bleeding from an artery is faster and more profuse.)
- Whether the bleeding is external or internal
- Whether or not the bleeding is a threat to respiration (If the bleeding is in the patient's airway, it could compromise breathing.)
- The patient's age, weight, and general physical condition

In general, bleeding is considered severe when the patient's pulse quickens, level of consciousness falls,

CASE STUDY

Dispatch

Our EMR unit was dispatched to a call for a laceration.

Scene Assessment

When we arrived on the scene, we parked at the curb. A woman opened the door of the house and approached our vehicle. She told us that she had been installing linoleum in her kitchen. The knife slipped and cut her, and she was bleeding badly from her arm. There were no dangers or hazards that we could see, so we exited our vehicle. We put on our gloves and goggles right away.

Primary Assessment

We saw that the woman was holding a blood-soaked towel to her arm. She appeared to be alert and oriented. She had no airway problems and was breathing adequately. Blood was still flowing from beneath the towel.

> What steps would you perform to control this woman's bleeding? How much blood has she lost? At what point could her bleeding become critical? Consider this patient as you read Chapter 19.

breathing rate increases, and blood pressure drops. Uncontrolled bleeding or significant blood loss can lead to shock and possibly death. (Read about shock later in this chapter.)

External Bleeding

There are three types of external bleeding—**arterial**, **venous**, and **capillary bleeding** (Figure 19–3 on p. 284). Each type can be life threatening. Each has its own characteristics:

- *Arterial bleeding*—Bright red blood spurting from a wound usually indicates a severed or damaged artery. The blood is bright red because it is rich in oxygen. Spurting generally coincides with the patient's pulse or contractions of the heart. Because blood in the arteries is under high pressure, this type of bleeding can be more difficult to control than any other. As the patient's blood pressure drops, the arterial spurting may also decrease (a late sign of shock).
- *Venous bleeding*—Dark red blood that flows steadily from a wound usually indicates a severed or damaged vein. The blood is dark red because

it holds little or no oxygen. It flows steadily because it is under less pressure than the blood in the arteries. Venous bleeding may be profuse, but it is usually easier to control than arterial bleeding.

- *Capillary bleeding*—Dark red blood that oozes slowly from a wound usually indicates damaged capillaries. In most cases, this type of bleeding clots spontaneously and is controlled easily. However, if the body surface involved is large, bleeding may be profuse, and the threat of infection may be great.

For emergency medical care of a patient with a bleeding wound, follow the general guidelines described below.

Emergency Medical Care

Remember that management of life-threatening bleeding must occur during the primary assessment. Only emergency care of a patient's airway and breathing takes precedence. In some cases, you may need to care for a patient's airway and breathing at the same time as you control bleeding. Therefore, for a patient

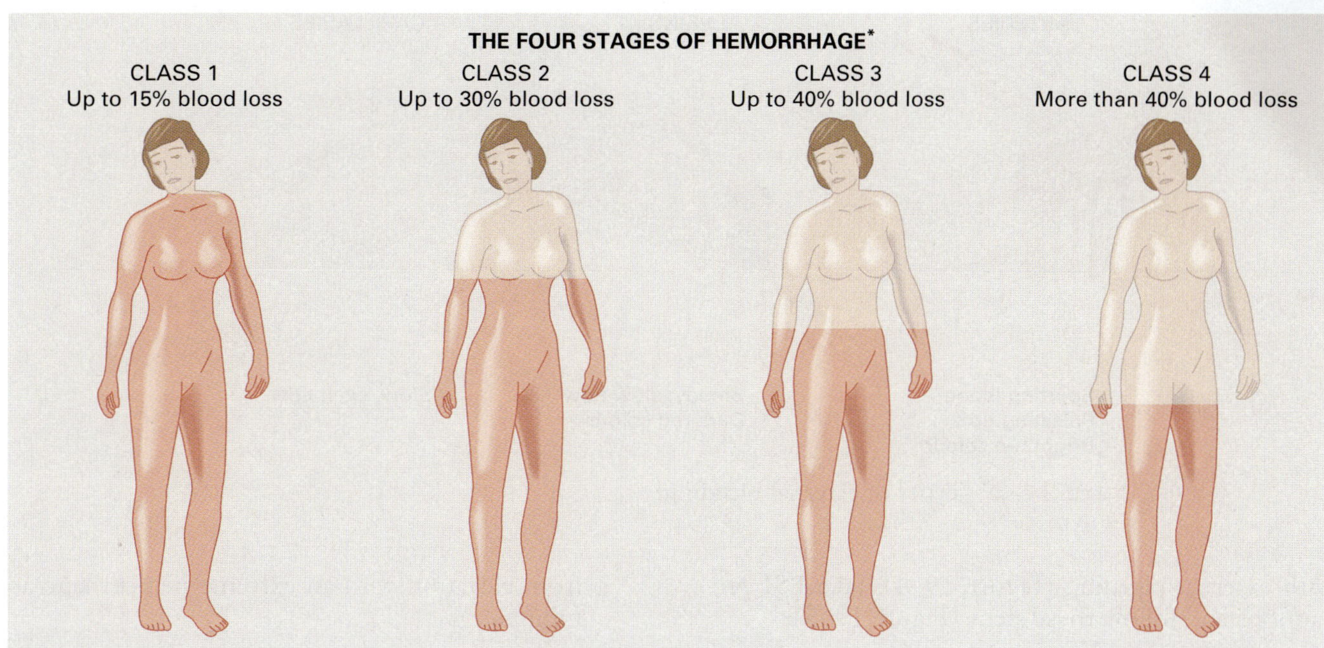

Figure 19–2 The four stages of blood loss.

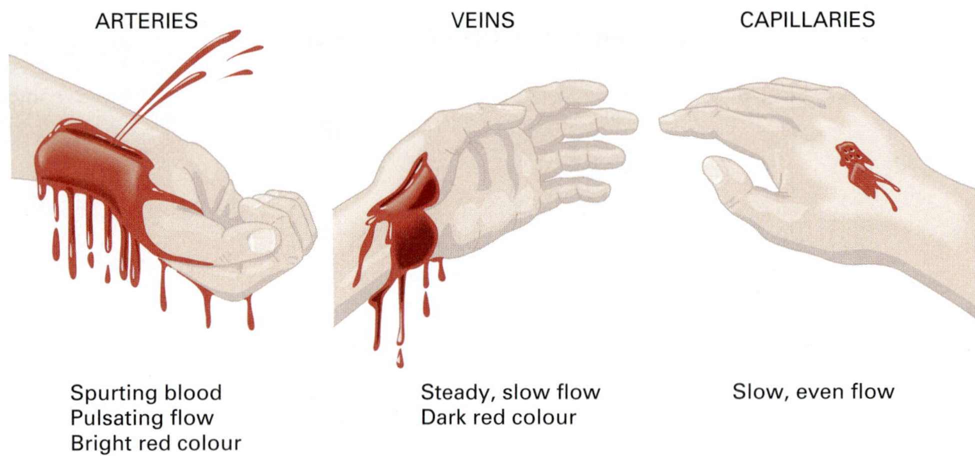

Figure 19–3 Types of external bleeding.

with external bleeding (Figure 19–4), take BSI precautions and follow these steps (Figure 19–5):

1. *Apply direct pressure to the wound.* If profuse bleeding is discovered during the primary assessment, apply pressure to the bleeding site with your gloved hand until dressings can be applied. Then, as soon as possible, place a sterile gauze pad or dressing over the bleeding wound. If it is small, apply pressure directly over the point of bleeding using the flat part of your fingertips. If the wound is large and gaping, pack it with sterile gauze and apply direct hand pressure.
2. *Elevate the bleeding extremity.* As you apply direct pressure, lift the bleeding arm or leg above the level of the heart. This can help slow the flow of blood and aid clotting when the bleeding is minor. *Note:* If you suspect a possible bone or joint injury, do *not* elevate the extremity. In some cases it may be impractical to elevate the site that is bleeding. The chances of the patient benefiting

from elevation with an extreme hemorrhage are minimal.

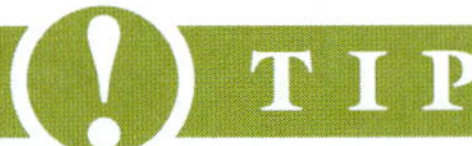

Do not remove a dressing to assess bleeding. Doing so can interrupt the clotting process and promote further bleeding.

3. *Assess bleeding.* If the wound has bled through the dressing, apply another dressing on top of it. Reapply direct pressure.
4. *Use pressure points.* If the bleeding in an extremity persists, and you are allowed to do so by your service protocol, apply pressure to the arterial pulse point to help reduce blood flow (Figures 19–6 and 19–7 on pp. 286 and 287).
   - For bleeding in the arm, find the brachial pulse point. Then use the flat surfaces of your fingers to compress the artery against the bone.
   - For bleeding in the leg, find the femoral pulse point. Use the heel of one hand to compress it.

Because a number of arteries supply each extremity, you may need to use a pressure point at the same time you apply direct pressure to the wound. Always reassess bleeding immediately after using a pressure point to make sure that it has been controlled.

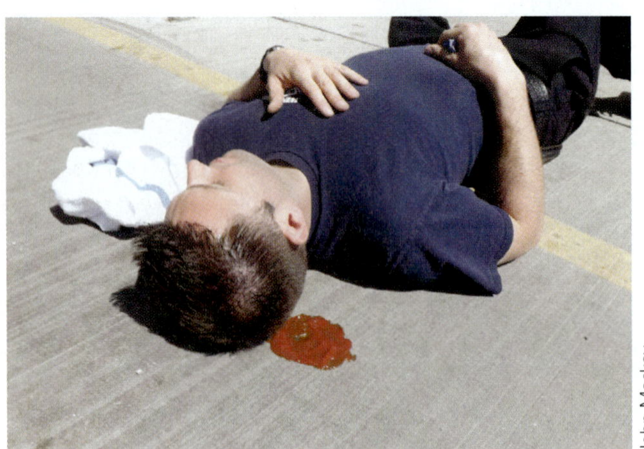

John Mackay

Figure 19–4 Control life-threatening bleeding during the primary assessment of your patient.

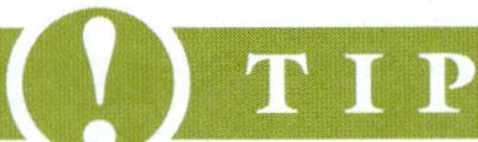

The acronym RED will help you remember how to control bleeding:

R — Rest

E — Elevation

D — Direct Pressure

METHOD OF BLEEDING CONTROL

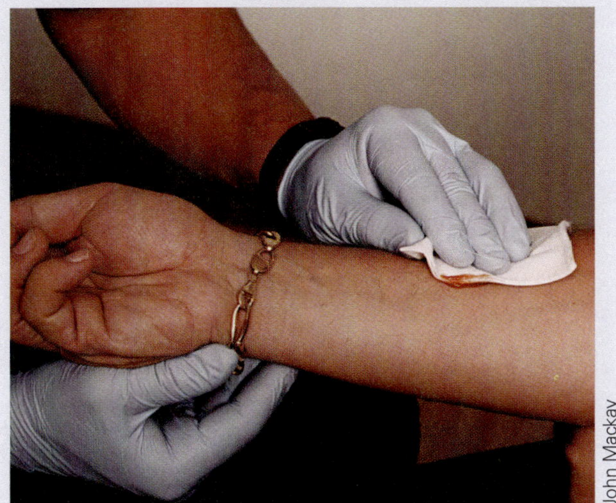

Figure 19–5a   Apply direct pressure.

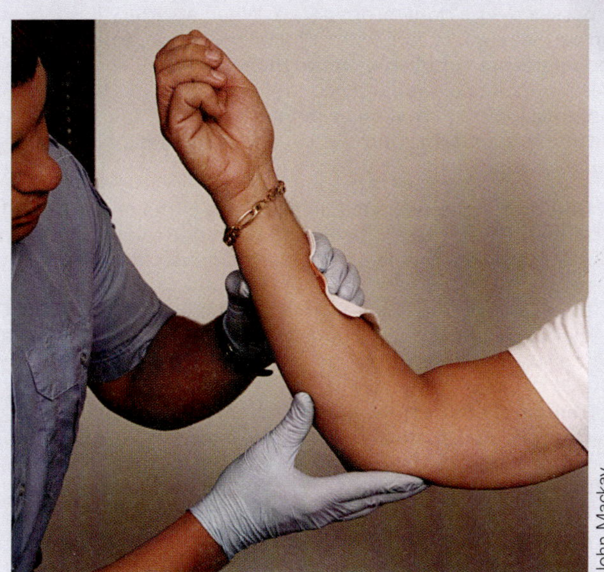

Figure 19–5b   Elevate the extremity.

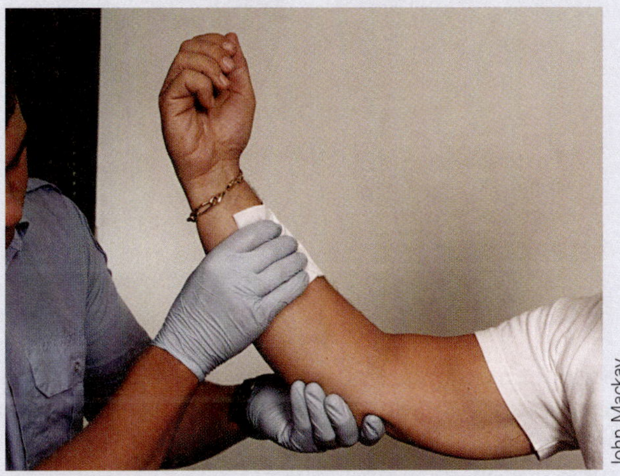

Figure 19–5c   Assess bleeding and apply additional pressure if needed.

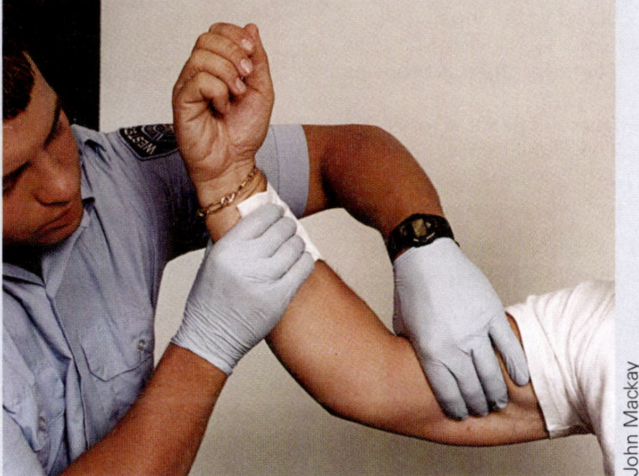

Figure 19–5d   If bleeding persists, compress a pulse point.

Be sure to support your patient while you wait for additional EMS personnel to arrive. Communicate with empathy. Comfort, calm, and reassure him or her. Keep safety and patient care your main priorities.

Note: In some EMS systems, bleeding control procedures are slightly different. When direct pressure and elevation do not work to stop bleeding, these systems dictate that you remove the first dressing to assess the bleeding point. If it is still bleeding, or if there is more than one bleeding point, then you are to apply more pressure directly to the point or points. If this still does not control bleeding, you are to use pressure points as described above. This is a controversial technique. Be sure to follow your own local protocols.

Other Methods of Bleeding Control

Two other methods of bleeding control are the use of splints and the use of a **tourniquet**. Be sure to follow local protocols.

Splints. Bleeding can be life threatening from an open wound to an extremity that also has a bone or joint

Arterial pulse points are places where an artery lies close to the skin or passes over a bony prominence. When an artery is so located, it can be palpated, or felt, with gentle fingertip pressure. Since most body parts are supplied by more than one artery, the use of arterial pressure points alone rarely controls hemorrhage. However, compression of arterial pulse points *in addition to direct pressure* can sometimes help control severe bleeding. Major arterial pulse points include:

- **Carotid arteries**—located on each side of the neck next to the larynx. These two arteries supply blood to the head. *Do not exert pressure on the carotid pulse points.*

- **Maxillary arteries**—supply much of the blood to the face. One can be palpated on each side of the face on the inner surface of the lower jaw.

- **Temporal arteries**—supply part of the blood supply to the scalp. One can be palpated on each side of the face just above the upper portion of the ear.

- **Brachial arteries**—located in the inner arms just above the elbows. These arteries supply blood to the arms.

- **Radial** and **ulnar arteries**—located in the wrist. These arteries also supply blood to the arms and hands.

- **Femoral arteries**—pass through the groin. These arteries supply blood to the legs.

- **Posterior tibial artery**—passes through the ankle.

- **Dorsalis pedis artery**—located on the front surface of the foot. This artery can determine circulation to the feet.

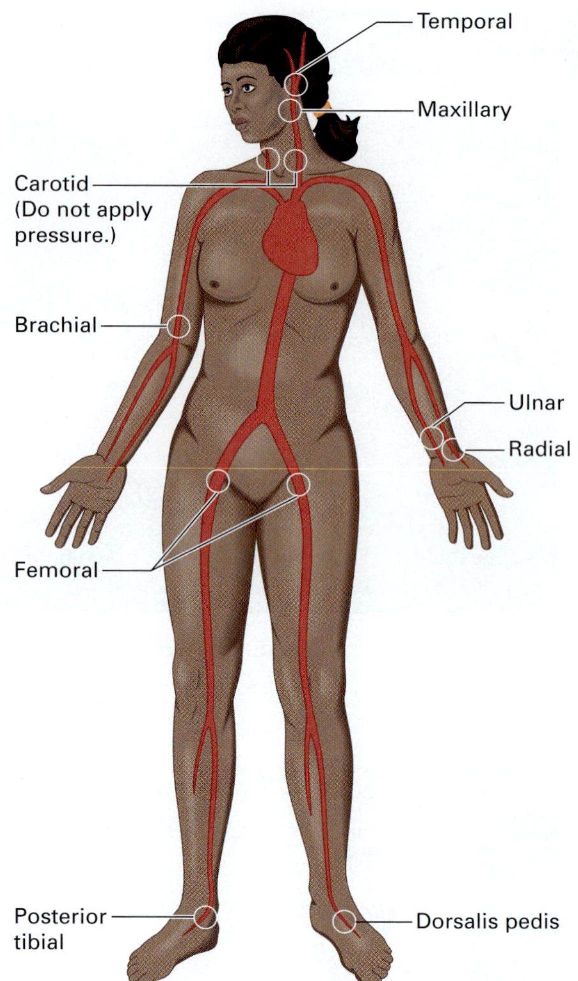

Figure 19–6 Arterial pulse points.

injury. If left unsplinted, the bone ends or bone fragments can move, damaging soft tissues and blood vessels and causing more bleeding. Immobilizing the extremity with a splint can help avoid these problems. (For information on how to apply a splint, see Chapter 26.)

A special splint is used in some EMS systems. An air splint (also called a pressure splint) can exert pressure to an extremity to help provide additional bleeding control. It may be effective over a wound larger than your hand, which would be difficult to control with direct pressure. Note that an air splint will not provide enough pressure to control arterial bleeding or other types of severe bleeding.

To apply pressure to a bleeding wound with an air splint, be sure the wound is dressed and bandaged first. (See Chapter 26 for information on how to apply an air splint.)

Tourniquets. A tourniquet should be used only as a last resort to control life-threatening bleeding when all other methods have failed, because it can stop all blood flow to an extremity. A tourniquet can cause permanent damage to nerves, muscles, and blood vessels, and result in the loss of the affected extremity. Always seek medical direction before using a tourniquet. Follow local protocols.

To apply a tourniquet, do the following (Figure 19–8):

1. Select a bandage 10 cm wide and six to eight layers deep.
2. Wrap it around the extremity twice at a point above, but as close as possible to, the wound.
3. Tie a knot in the bandage material. Then, place a stick or rod on top of it. Tie the ends of the bandage again in a square knot over the stick.
4. Twist the stick until the bleeding stops. Then secure the stick or rod in position.
5. Note the time.
6. Notify the paramedics who take over patient care that you have applied a tourniquet.

In some cases, an inflated blood pressure cuff may be used as a tourniquet until bleeding stops. If you

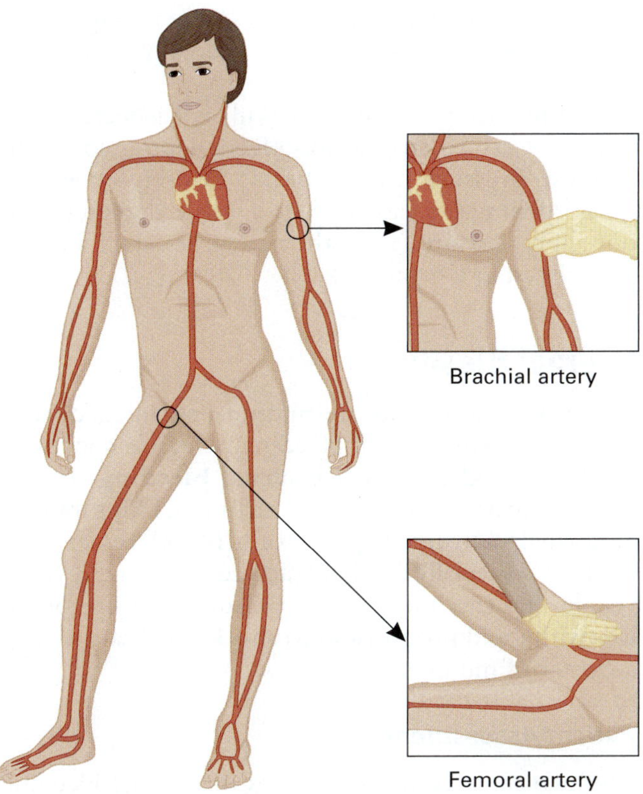

Figure 19–7   Pressure points in the extremities.

choose to do this, you need to monitor the cuff continuously to make sure that pressure is maintained.

When using any type of tourniquet, take the following precautions:

- Always use a wide bandage and secure it tightly. Never use a wire, belt, or any other material that could cut the skin or underlying soft tissues.
- Once applied, never loosen or remove a tourniquet unless you are directed to do so by the medical director.
- Never apply a tourniquet directly over a joint.
- Always make sure the tourniquet is in open view. A tourniquet that is covered by clothing or bandages may be overlooked, resulting in permanent tissue damage.

Nosebleeds

Nosebleeds are a relatively common source of bleeding. They can result from an injury, disease, activity, the environment, or other causes. Generally, they are more annoying than serious. However, enough blood can be lost to cause shock. In an unconscious patient, a nosebleed can also be a serious threat to respiration (Figure 19–9).

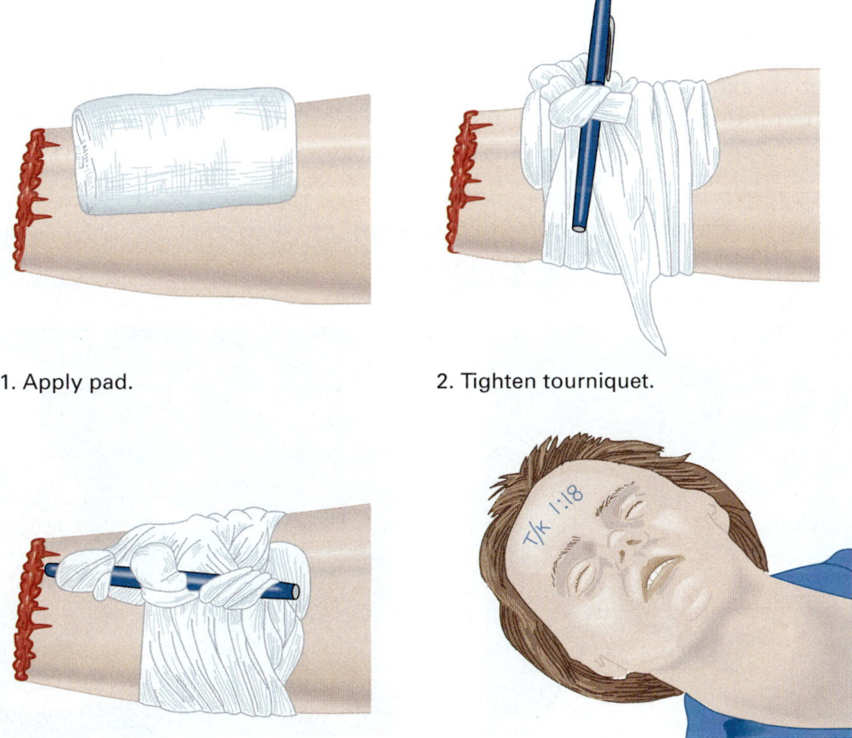

Figure 19–8   Method of applying a tourniquet. (Apply a tourniquet only as a last resort.)

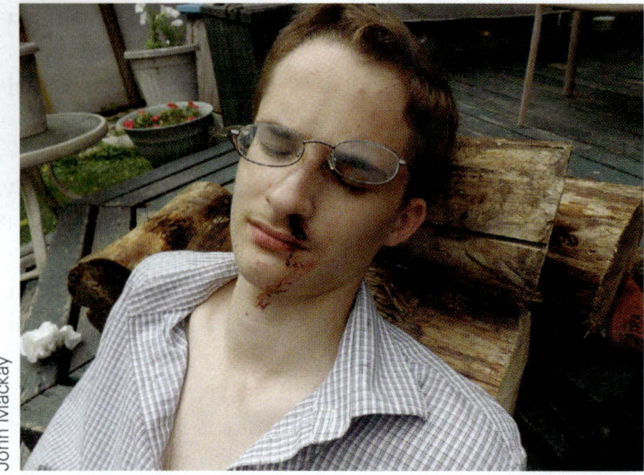

Figure 19–9 A nosebleed in an unconscious patient can be a serious threat to respiration.

In most cases, a nosebleed may be treated as follows (Figure 19–10):

1. Keep the patient still and calm. Have him or her sit leaning forward in order to prevent aspiration of blood into the lungs. (Do not let the patient lean so far forward that the head is below the heart.) If sitting is impossible because of other injuries, have the patient lie down with the head and shoulders elevated.
2. Apply pressure by pinching the nostrils together. Do not pinch the nostrils if you suspect a nasal fracture.
3. Apply cold compresses to the nose and face.
4. Instruct the patient to avoid blowing the nose for several hours. It could dislodge the clot and restart bleeding.

5. If bleeding continues and is severe enough, alert the paramedics if this has not already been done.

Note that if a fractured skull is suspected, you must not try to stop a nosebleed. Doing so might increase pressure on the brain. Loosely cover the nasal opening instead. Use dry, sterile dressings. Do not apply pressure. Treat the patient for skull fracture as outlined in Chapter 24.

Internal Bleeding

When internal organs are injured or damaged, they may bleed. This type of bleeding, which is concealed inside the body, is called **internal bleeding**. It may result from a variety of causes, including blunt trauma, abnormal clotting, rupture of a blood vessel, or a fracture (especially a pelvic fracture). Because it is not visible, internal bleeding can result in severe blood loss with rapid progression to shock and death—all in a matter of minutes.

Patient Assessment

The two most common sources of internal bleeding are injured or damaged internal organs and fractures (especially fractures of the femur and pelvis). The severity of internal bleeding depends on the patient's overall condition, age, and the source of the bleeding.

Suspect internal bleeding if the mechanism of injury suggests it and if there is evidence of scrapes and bruises, swelling, deformity, or impact marks. Always suspect it if there are penetrating wounds to the skull, chest, or abdomen. Always suspect it as well in cases of unexplained shock.

METHOD OF NOSEBLEED CONTROL

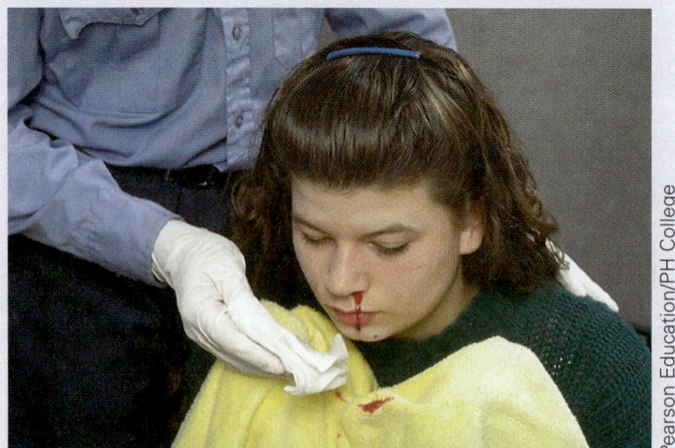

Figure 19–10a Keep the patient quiet and leaning forward in a sitting position.

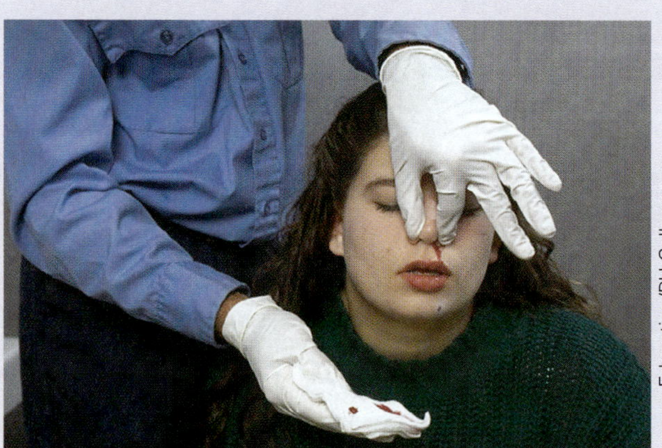

Figure 19–10b Apply pressure by pinching the nostrils.

The signs and symptoms of internal bleeding are as follows:

- Discoloured, tender, swollen, or hard tissue
- Increased respiratory and pulse rates
- Pale, cool, clammy skin
- Nausea and vomiting bright red blood or blood the colour of coffee grounds
- Thirst
- Changes in mental status, including anxiety, restlessness, or combativeness
- Dark, tarry stools or stools that contain bright red blood
- Tender, rigid, or distended abdomen
- Weakness, faintness, or dizziness

Emergency Medical Care

If you suspect internal bleeding in your patient, update the incoming EMS personnel. This patient is a priority for immediate transport. To care for a patient with internal bleeding, be sure you have taken BSI precautions and then follow these steps:

1. Maintain an open airway and adequate breathing. If you are allowed to, apply high-concentration oxygen by way of a non-rebreather mask. Provide artificial ventilation if needed.
2. Control any external bleeding with direct pressure, elevation, and pressure points when necessary.
3. Keep the patient warm, but be careful not to overheat him or her.
4. Treat for shock, as described in the next section.

Always support, comfort, calm, and reassure the patient.

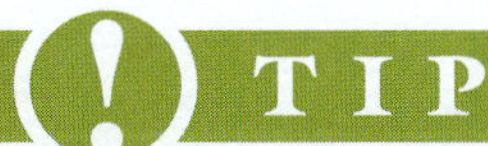

ALL BLEEDING WILL EVENTUALLY STOP!

It is of primary importance that you stop the bleeding before the well runs dry and your patient dies from irreversible shock.

SECTION 2
SHOCK

Perfusion refers to the circulation of blood throughout a body organ or structure. Perfusion delivers oxygen and other nutrients to the body's cells and removes waste products.

When the cells of the body do not receive the oxygen and other nutrients they need, they begin to fail and die. **Shock**, or **hypoperfusion**, is a condition that results from the inadequate supply of oxygenated blood. If the condition persists, cell failure, organ failure, and death will follow. It is therefore imperative to survival that shock be recognized and treated promptly.

Causes of Shock

Shock can be caused by failure of the heart, abnormal dilation of blood vessels, or blood volume loss:

- *Failure of the heart.* Conditions that cause the heart to fail to provide oxygenated blood to the body include heart attack, coronary artery disease, heart valve disease, pulmonary embolism (a blood clot), tension pneumothorax (air leaking from a lung into the chest cavity), and cardiac tamponade (fluid leaking into the sac around the heart).
- *Abnormal dilation of the blood vessels.* This is usually the result of a spinal or head injury that causes the nervous system to lose control over the blood vessels. The blood vessels dilate (enlarge), causing blood pressure to drop and blood to pool in the outer areas of the body, away from vital organs.
- *Blood volume loss.* This is caused either by external or internal bleeding. It may also result from a profound fluid loss that occurs during illness or injury (Figure 19–11). One example is plasma loss due to burns. Another is dehydration due to diarrhea, vomiting, or excessive urination. A patient with a high temperature may have a slightly faster than normal pulse since the body may be compensating for fluid loss associated with infection.

Stages of Shock

Shock passes through three stages: compensated, decompensated, and irreversible (Figure 19–12). As shock progresses, the body works hard to make sure oxygen reaches its cells. However, if shock is severe or prolonged, it may become irreversible and end in death.

Compensated Shock

In the first stage of shock, the body uses its defences to try to maintain normal function. If the injury does not get worse, the body can overcome the condition. The signs and symptoms of shock

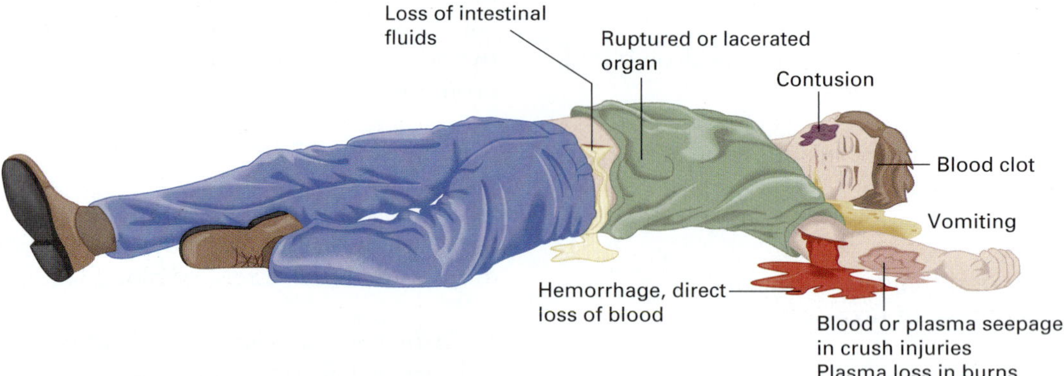

Figure 19–11   Loss of body fluid can be both external and internal.

DEVELOPING SHOCK

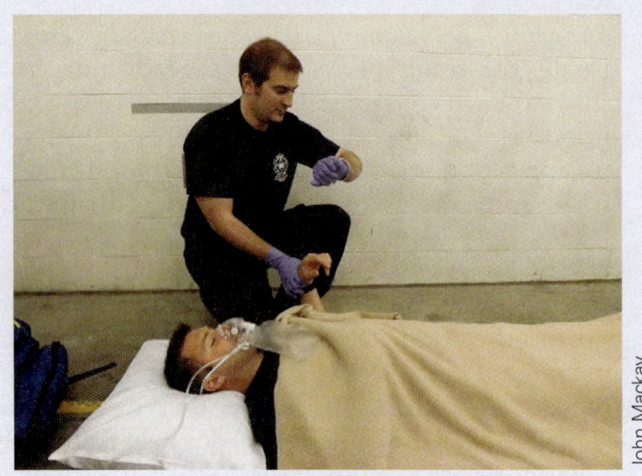

Figure 19–12a   Compensated shock: slight increase in pulse.

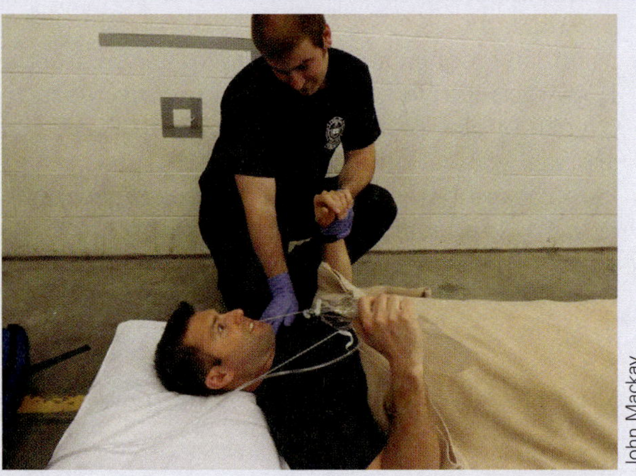

Figure 19–12b   Compensated shock: restlessness or anxiety.

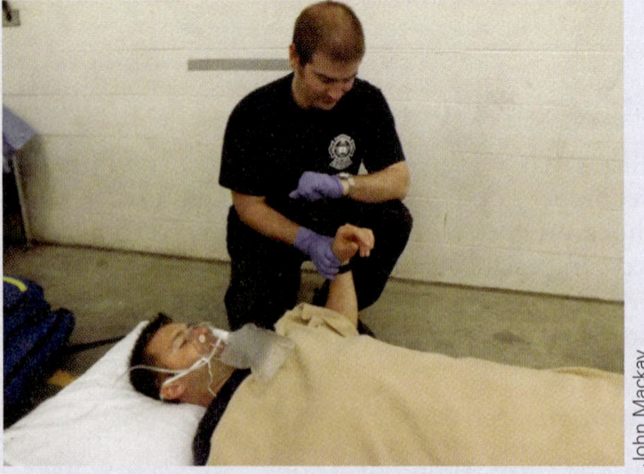

Figure 19–12c   Decompensated shock: rapid, weak pulse.

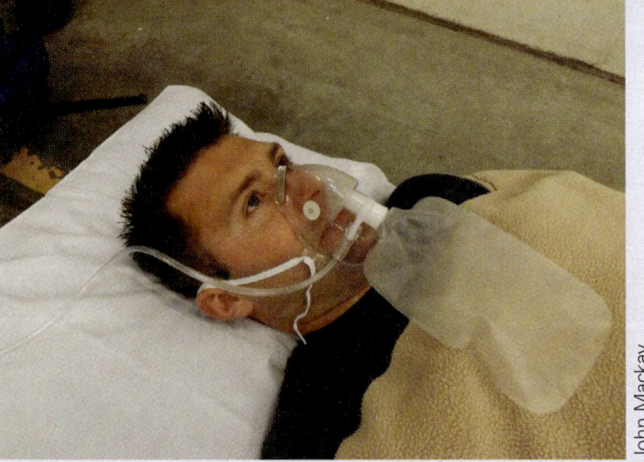

Figure 19–12d   Decompensated shock: skin colour changes and sweating.

(continued)

DEVELOPING SHOCK *(continued)*

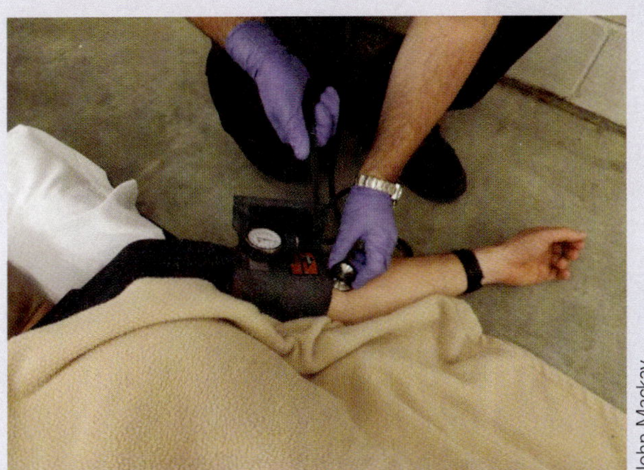

Figure 19–12e Decompensated shock: decreasing blood pressure.

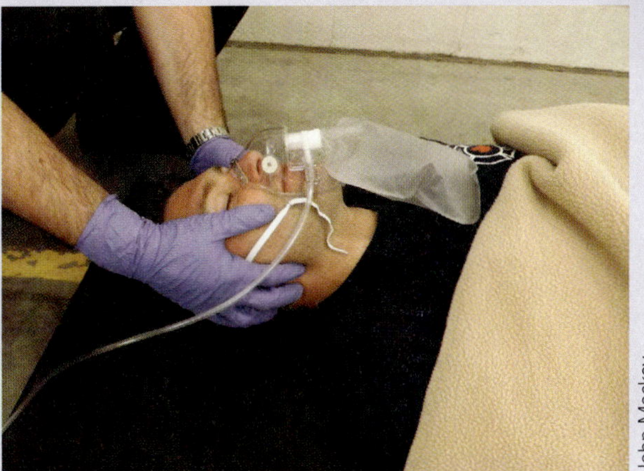

Figure 19–12f Decompensated shock: unconsciousness.

at this stage are very subtle. They include the following:

- Pale skin
- Slightly rapid heart rate
- Blood pressure in the normal range
- Restlessness or anxiety
- Delayed capillary refill in the infant or child

Even though shock is difficult to identify at this stage, it is vital that you recognize and treat it early. You must prevent progression to the next, more serious stage.

Decompensated Shock

At the decompensated stage, the body can no longer make up for reduced perfusion. Without medical intervention, further decline occurs. The body tries to keep vital organs perfused with oxygenated blood. It shunts blood away from the arms, legs, and abdomen and directs it to the brain, heart, and lungs. As a result, tissues in the extremities and abdomen produce toxic byproducts. The signs and symptoms include the following:

- Extreme thirst
- Rapid heart rate
- Decreased blood pressure
- Cool and moist skin that is pale, grey, or bluish and mottled (Figure 19–13)
- Major changes in the patient's mental status

Decreased blood pressure is a very late sign of shock. Note that infants and children can maintain their blood pressure until blood volume is cut almost in half. Their condition then suddenly and rapidly deteriorates. Dropping blood pressure in an infant or child is an ominous sign.

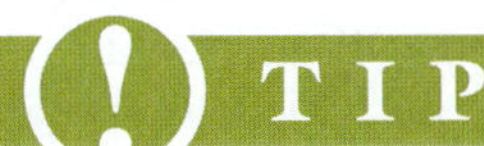

T I P

While there are many causes of shock, there are two types that seem atypical: cardiogenic shock and neurogenic shock. Cardiac dysrhythmias or injuries to the brain or spinal cord can actually result in a slowing of the heart rate, or bradycardia.

Irreversible Shock

In the irreversible stage of shock, blood flow is so low that body cells are dying. The main signs are very low blood pressure and extremely rapid pulse. At this stage, blood is shunted away from the liver and kidneys to the heart and brain. The liver and kidneys then die. Blood vessels are no longer able to sustain pressure. Therefore, blood begins to pool away from the vital organs.

Even with treatment, damage to the vital organs is permanent. The inevitable result of irreversible shock is death.

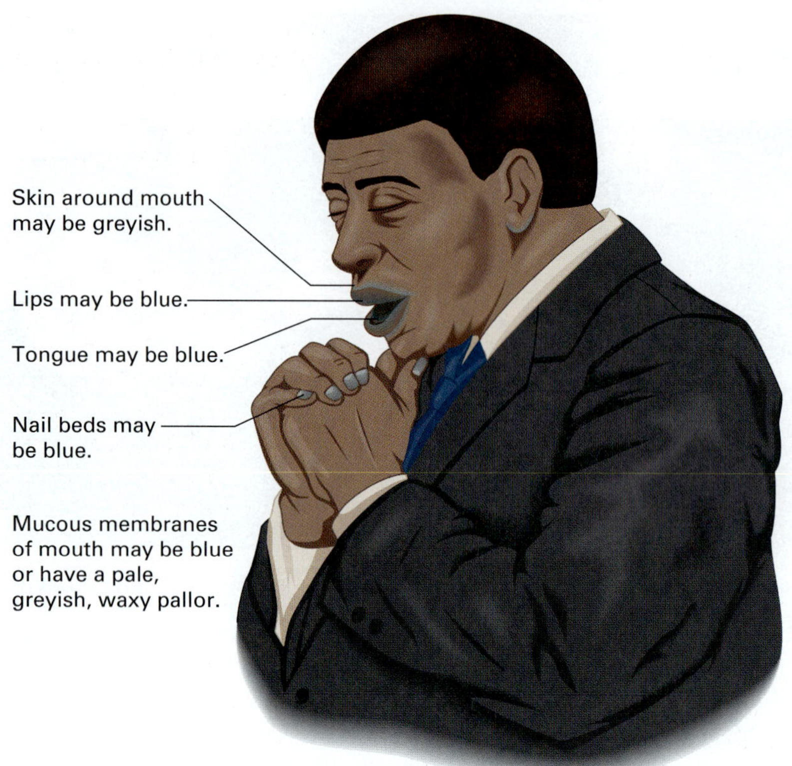

Figure 19–13   Signs of shock in a dark-skinned patient.

Emergency Medical Care

Trauma is a major cause of shock in patients. The term *golden hour* refers to the urgency with which care must be given. It marks the time that elapses from injury until the patient is actually in the operating room.

Your role as an EMR is vital. The general rule is for an ambulance to remain on the scene no longer than 10 minutes. You can help keep time to a minimum by identifying serious trauma patients, performing primary assessments and treatment, and preparing patients for transport.

To provide emergency medical care, make sure you have taken BSI precautions and follow these steps:

1. *Maintain an open airway.* If breathing is adequate, administer oxygen by way of a nonrebreather mask at 15 L/min (Figure 19–14). Be prepared to provide artificial ventilation if needed.
2. *Prevent further blood loss.* Control external bleeding through direct pressure, elevation, and pressure points if necessary.
3. *Elevate the lower extremities about 20 to 30 cm* (Figure 19–15). If there are serious injuries to

the head, neck, spine, chest, abdomen, pelvis, or lower extremities, keep the patient supine.

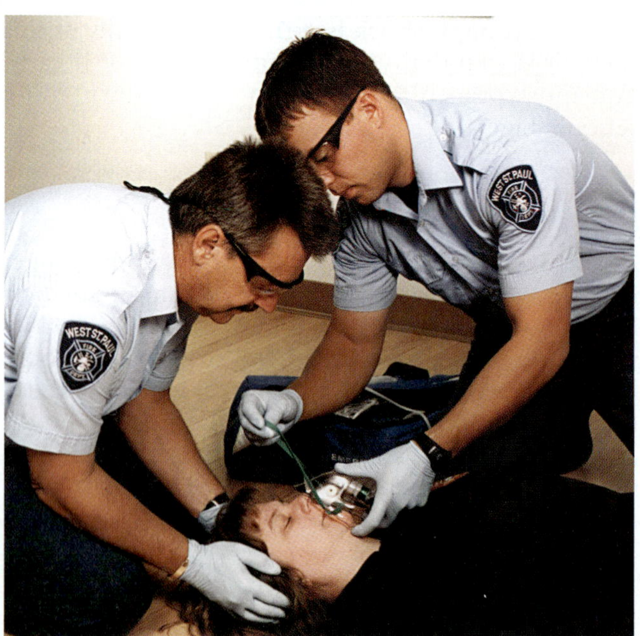

John Mackay

Figure 19–14   Patients in shock have a reduced ability to deliver oxygen to the body. Administer oxygen if you are allowed to do so.

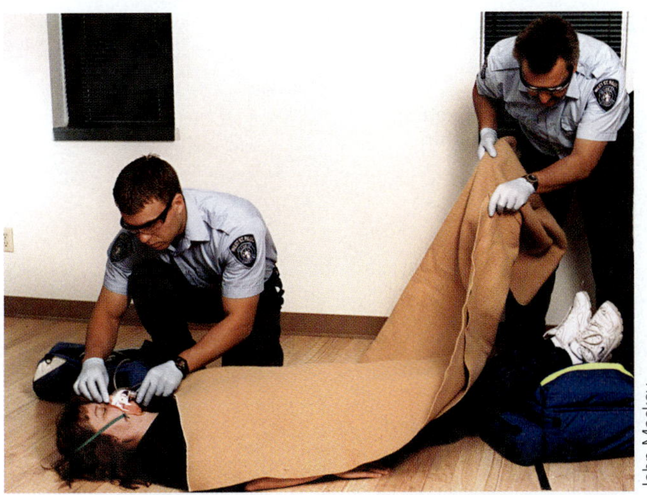

Figure 19–15 When appropriate, elevate the shock patient's feet 20 to 30 cm. Also be sure to keep the patient warm.

4. *Keep the patient warm, but do not overheat him or her.* Try to maintain normal body temperature. If necessary, use a blanket over and under the patient to help prevent loss of body heat.
5. *Provide care for specific injuries while waiting for paramedics to arrive.*

Be sure to comfort, calm, and reassure the patient while you wait for the paramedics to arrive on the scene. Never give the patient anything to eat or drink. During the ongoing assessment, check the patient's vital signs every five minutes and monitor for changes in mental status. Report your observations to the EMS crew when they take over patient care.

Anaphylactic Shock

Anaphylactic shock results from a severe allergic reaction to a foreign protein. It can be caused by an insect sting, food, medicine, pollen, or some other inhaled, ingested, or injected substance. The most common causes of anaphylactic shock are drugs and bee stings. At least one percent of the general population is at risk for developing anaphylactic shock from bee stings alone.

Anaphylactic shock is a life-threatening medical emergency. A reaction can occur within seconds after a sting or other exposure. Immediate treatment is required to prevent death. Note that the shorter the time between the exposure and the appearance of signs and symptoms, the greater the risk of a fatal reaction.

Anaphylactic shock may result in any combination of the following signs and symptoms (Figure 19–16):

- Skin
  - Warm, tingling feeling in the mouth, face, chest, feet, and hands
  - Itching, hives, and flushing
  - Swelling of the tongue, face, neck, hands, and feet
  - Cyanosis
  - Paleness
- Respiratory system
  - Swelling of the mouth, tongue, or throat leading to airway obstruction
  - Painful, squeezing sensation in the chest
  - Cough, hoarseness (losing the voice)
  - Rapid or laboured breathing
  - Noisy breathing, stridor, wheezing
- Circulatory system
  - Increased heart rate
  - Decreased blood pressure
  - Dizziness
  - Restlessness
- General findings
  - Itchy, watery eyes
  - Headache
  - Runny nose
  - Sense of impending doom
  - Deteriorating mental status
  - Nausea, vomiting, abdominal cramping

General guidelines for emergency care of a patient in anaphylactic shock are described below. Be sure that the paramedics have been activated. The patient needs to be quickly transported for further life-saving treatment. Arrange for advanced life support (ALS) care if it is available. Then follow these steps:

1. Perform a primary assessment. Treat all life threats. Be prepared to provide basic life support if it is needed.
2. If you are equipped and allowed to do so, administer 100 percent high-flow oxygen. If breathing is adequate, deliver oxygen by way of a non-rebreather mask. If the patient needs artificial ventilation, use supplemental oxygen.
3. If local protocol allows, assist the patient with his or her medication. Medications may include an epinephrine auto-injector (EpiPen) or antihistamines.

If the reaction is due to an insect sting, local protocol may direct you to place a constricting band between the injection site and the heart. (See Chapter 17 for more specific directions concerning the use of a constricting band.)

During your ongoing assessment of the patient, monitor the patient's ABCs continually. Be prepared to deliver basic life support if it is needed.

ANAPHYLACTIC SHOCK

A grave medical emergency
Anaphylactic shock is a severe allergic reaction to an injected, inhaled, or ingested foreign protein. Onset can occur within minutes, even seconds.

Early signs and symptoms
• Flushing, itching, skin rash
• Sneezing, watery eyes and nose
• Airway swelling
• Cough, "tickle" or "lump" in the throat that cannot be cleared
• Gastrointestinal complaints

The signs and symptoms of anaphylactic shock may swiftly lead to:

Acute Respiratory Obstruction

Circulatory Collapse

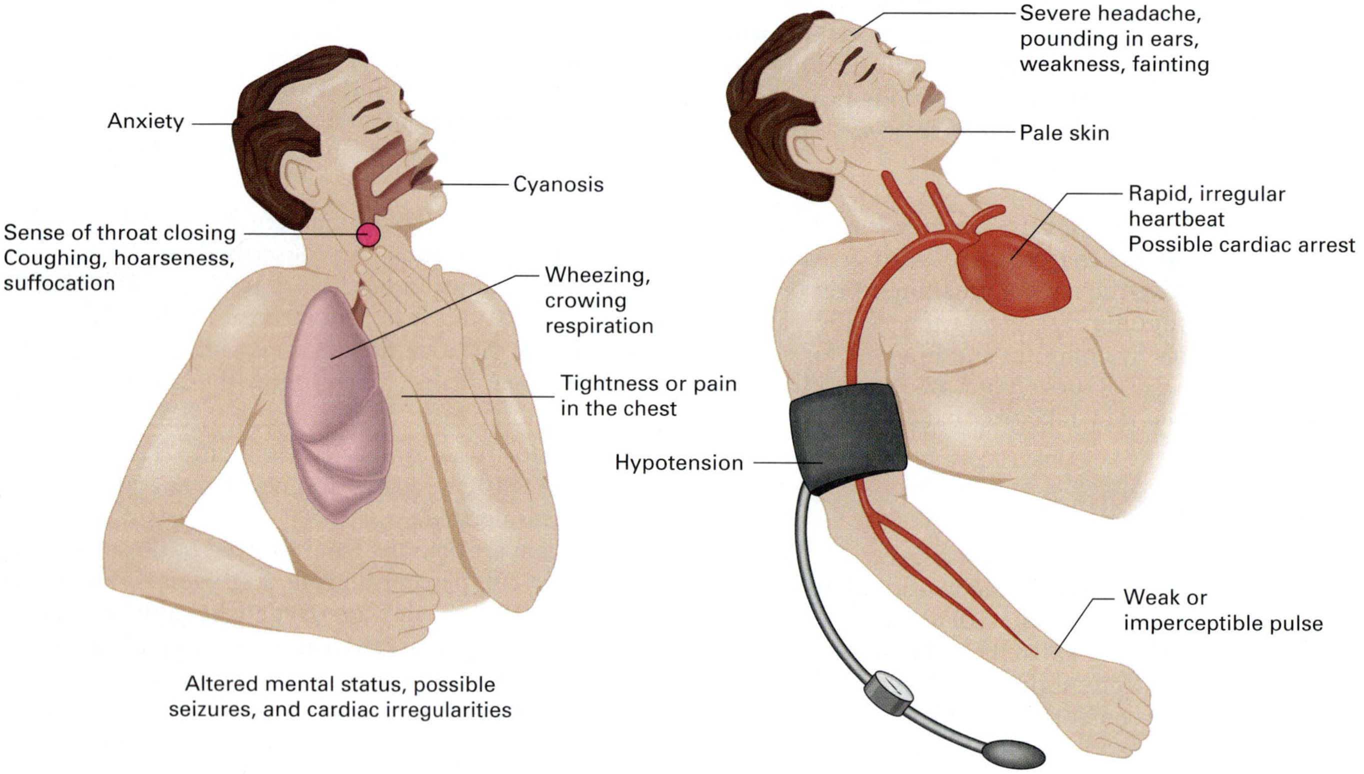

Figure 19–16 The signs and symptoms of anaphylactic shock.

EMR FOCUS

Severe bleeding is controlled during the primary assessment and treatment. The only other problems that take priority concern the airway and breathing. Be assured, however, that even severe bleeding can be controlled by the simple methods described in this chapter—direct pressure, elevation, and pressure points. Rest and supplemental oxygen can slow the progressive nature of shock. Experienced EMRs and paramedics will tell you that these methods work. Use them appropriately and confidently.

CASE STUDY FOLLOW-UP

At the beginning of this chapter, you read that EMRs were on the scene with a woman who was bleeding from her arm. To see how the chapter skills apply to this emergency, read the following. It describes how the call was completed.

PRIMARY ASSESSMENT *(Continued)*

I saw blood flowing steadily from beneath the towel. This, combined with the amount of blood at the scene, indicated severe bleeding. I removed the towel and applied a sterile dressing and direct pressure to the wound. The bleeding stopped in two or three minutes. I kept up the pressure for a bit longer to make sure the bleeding stayed under control. Lian, my partner, updated the paramedics.

SECONDARY ASSESSMENT

The patient claimed to have slipped with her knife. She denied injuring any other part of her body. My partner scanned the patient and confirmed that this appeared to be true. The patient did not fall or lose consciousness. There was no need to do a further assessment. My partner took her vitals. Pulse was 92, strong, and regular. Respirations were 16 and adequate. Blood pressure was 118/84. The patient's skin was cool and dry.

PATIENT HISTORY

The patient claimed to be in good health. She took no medication and said she had no medical problems. She had had a physical examination the previous year. She denied any allergies. She had eaten Chinese food for lunch about two hours before.

ONGOING ASSESSMENT

We took another set of vitals. Pulse was 88, strong, and regular. Respirations were 16 and adequate. Blood pressure was 120/78. Her skin was cool and dry.

We rechecked the status of our bleeding control. The bleeding had been stopped for several minutes. We applied a pressure bandage to maintain pressure over the wound. We were careful not to cut off the patient's circulation. The paramedics arrived shortly after.

TRANSFER OF CARE

We advised the paramedics that the bleeding was under control and gave them the report:

"This is Jill Romano, a 27-year-old woman who slipped with her knife while installing linoleum. The knife caused a laceration of about 10 cm to her left arm. The blood was flowing steadily on our arrival, but the bleeding was quickly brought under control by direct pressure. She did not lose consciousness or suffer any further injuries. Jill has no past medical history, no meds, no allergies. Her vitals are pulse 88, strong, and regular; respirations 16; blood pressure 120/78; skin cool and dry. Jill had Chinese food for lunch about two hours ago. We applied a pressure bandage. The bleeding is controlled, and there is good circulation distal to the bandage."

The paramedics took over care and applied oxygen to the patient. They transported her to the hospital. It was one of the worst cases of bleeding I had seen. I was glad to get it under control. We saw the paramedics later. They told us that the patient's wound required a lot of stitches. They also told us she had sliced open her leg on another home repair project three months before. She was considering another hobby.

A patient's blood can be an unnerving sight, especially if the bleeding is profuse. While the volume of external hemorrhage is often overestimated, compensated shock can begin rather quickly. One way to stay clear-headed is to stick to your patient assessment plan. Always start with scene assessment. Move to primary assessment and treatment. Continue, if you can, with a secondary assessment, patient history, ongoing assessment, and patient hand-off. Remember, your patient's well-being depends on it.

NOCPs

5.5 b Control external hemorrhage through use of direct pressure and patient positioning **S**

6.1 f Provide care to patient experiencing signs and symptoms involving integumentary system **S**

o Provide care to trauma patient **S**

6.3 a Conduct ongoing assessments based on patient presentation and interpret findings **S**

b Re-direct priorities based on assessment findings **S**

REVIEW QUESTIONS

Page references where answers may be found or supported are provided at the end of each question.

SECTION 1

1. How can you identify arterial, venous, and capillary bleeding? (p. 282)

2. What is the emergency medical care for external bleeding? Describe each step briefly. (pp. 282, 284)

3. What are the two most common sources of internal bleeding? (p. 288)

4. What is the emergency medical care for a patient with internal bleeding? (p. 289)

SECTION 2

5. What are the signs and symptoms of shock (hypoperfusion)? (pp. 289–291)

6. Where would you look to see signs and symptoms of shock in a dark-skinned patient? (p. 292)

7. How should you care for a patient in shock? (pp. 292–293)

8. What are the two most common causes of anaphylactic shock? (p. 293)

20

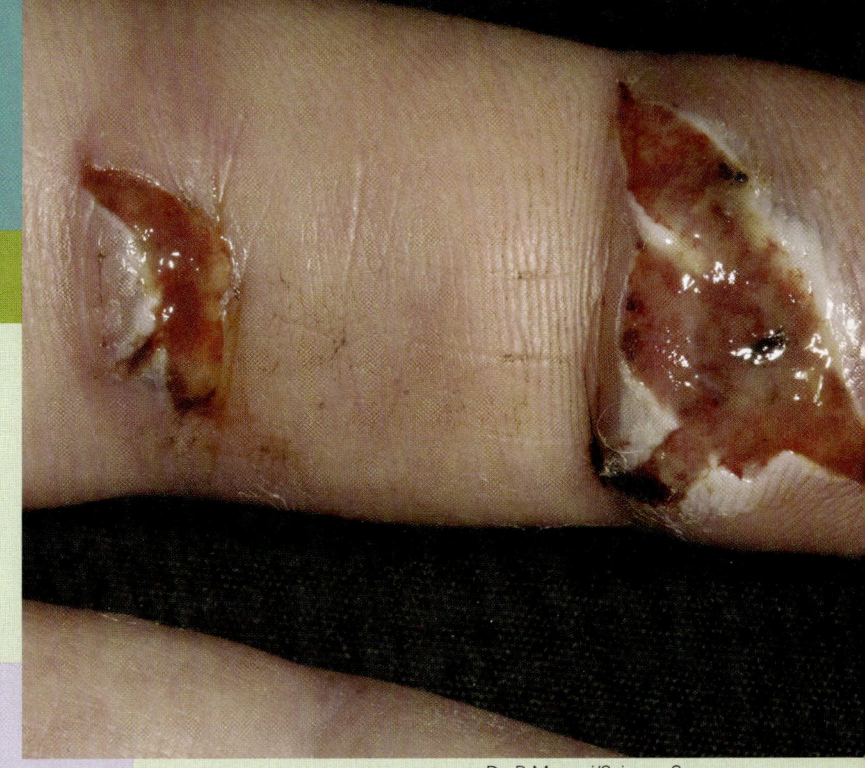

Dr. P. Marazzi/Science Source

Soft-Tissue Injuries

OBJECTIVES

1. State the types of open soft-tissue injury.
2. Explain the relationship between BSI precautions and soft-tissue injuries.
3. Describe the general emergency medical care of the patient with a soft-tissue injury.
4. Describe the emergency medical care of open wounds that require special consideration, including chest injuries, impaled objects, large and open neck wounds, eviscerations, amputations, avulsions, and bites.
5. List the four basic functions of dressing and bandaging.
6. State the 12 principles of applying dressings and bandages.
7. Demonstrate a caring attitude toward the patient and family when dealing with a soft-tissue injury, while giving priority to the interests of the patient.

INTRODUCTION

Injuries to a patient's skin, muscles, nerves, and blood vessels are among the most common for which you will care. Some will be minor cuts, scrapes, and bruises. Others may be life threatening. Whatever your patient's soft-tissue injuries may be, your priorities will include controlling bleeding, preventing further injury, and reducing the risk of infection.

SECTION 1
SOFT-TISSUE INJURIES

Soft-tissue injuries are injuries to the skin, muscles, nerves, and blood vessels. They are often dramatic, but they are rarely life threatening. They can be serious, however, if they lead to airway or breathing problems, uncontrolled bleeding, or shock.

A soft-tissue injury is commonly referred to as a **wound**. Wounds may be classified as open or closed, single or multiple. They are also classified by location (head wounds or chest wounds, for example).

In general, emergency medical care focuses on controlling bleeding, preventing further injury, and reducing the risk of infection. Unless it is a life threat, a soft-tissue injury is usually attended to after the primary assessment.

Closed Wounds

In a **closed wound**, soft tissues beneath the skin are damaged (Figure 20–1). The skin itself is not broken. There are three general types of closed wound. They are a **contusion** (bruise), a **clamping injury**, and a **crushing injury**.

Generally, contusions are characterized by swelling and pain at the injury site. If small blood vessels have been broken, the patient will also have **ecchymosis** (black-and-blue discoloration). If large blood vessels have been torn, a **hematoma** (a collection of blood beneath the skin) is evident as a lump with bluish discoloration.

A clamping injury usually involves a finger or limb stuck in an area smaller than itself. This type of injury occurs when a patient reaches into a space and gets the body part stuck there. The body part can swell rapidly, making the condition worse. Another type of clamping injury occurs when an object, such as a ring, strangles a body part that was previously injured.

Blunt trauma is caused by a sudden blow or force that has a crushing impact. A crushing injury may be open or closed. Either way, it can be treacherous. Blunt trauma can cause serious internal injuries, including organ rupture, with few external signs. A patient may look fine at first and then very quickly slip into shock. The result can be decompensated shock and death. For this reason, always suspect internal damage in patients with injuries involving blunt force.

General Guidelines for Emergency Care

Small contusions generally do not need treatment. Cold compresses help relieve pain and reduce swelling in larger contusions.

In a clamping injury, a lubricant, such as green soap, may help free the body part. If not, then it may need to be freed at the hospital. Apply a cold pack to help reduce swelling. Since circulation to the body part may be reduced, do not cool it for longer than 15 to 30 minutes at a time. Elevate the injured part above the level of the heart. Keep it well supported.

Large areas of discoloration of the skin can indicate serious internal bleeding. A bruise the size of a fist, for example, could mean a 10 percent blood loss. If the patient has a large contusion, or if the mechanism of injury suggests a crushing injury caused by blunt trauma, treat the patient for internal bleeding. Be sure to assess carefully for broken bones, especially when swelling or deformity is present.

If you are ever in doubt about the seriousness of a closed wound, treat the patient for internal bleeding.

Note: Always take BSI precautions when there is any possibility that you will come into contact with a patient's blood or other body fluids. When caring for a patient with closed wounds, at a minimum, wear protective latex gloves.

CASE STUDY

Dispatch

I work as a lathe operator at the mill. I'm also an EMR. One day, the emergency signal broke into the noise of the machines. I called in and was told to report to Building B.

Scene Assessment

My partner and I arrived at the main entrance, where a guard directed us to the injury site. He advised us that there were no dangers. A worker had a piece of wood impaled in one hand. We put on protective gloves and glasses and approached the scene.

Primary Assessment

The patient was standing near a workbench. We saw that her mental status, airway, and breathing were okay because she was swearing quite loudly about her injury. We approached her and identified ourselves. There was surprisingly little bleeding coming from the wound. We calmed her down and asked her to sit down while we assessed the injury.

We reported the patient's status and the nature of the injury to the incoming paramedics. Their ETA was 10 minutes.

> Consider this patient as you read Chapter 20. What may be done to treat her condition?

Open Wounds

When the skin breaks as a result of an injury, the wound is referred to as an **open injury** (or open wound) (Figure 20–2 on p. 301). Open injuries place the patient at risk of contamination with microorganisms, which can lead to infection. An open injury may also be the first indicator of a deeper, more serious injury, like a fracture.

Abrasions

An **abrasion** is an open wound caused by scraping, rubbing, or shearing away of the epidermis (outermost layer of skin) (Figure 20–3 on p. 302). Even though an abrasion is considered a superficial injury, it is often very painful because of exposed nerve endings. Although there may be no bleeding at all from an abrasion, there is usually capillary bleeding.

Small abrasions are not usually life threatening. Large ones, however, may be cause for concern. For example, a motorcycle rider who is thrown and slides across the pavement may sustain head-to-toe abrasions (road rash). Bleeding in such a case may not be serious, but contamination, infection, and the potential for underlying injuries may be.

Lacerations

A **laceration** is a break of varying depth in the skin. It may occur in isolation. It may also occur with other types of soft-tissue injury (Figure 20–3 on p. 302). Lacerations are caused by forceful impact with a sharp object. Bleeding may be severe, especially if an artery is involved.

The edges of a laceration may be regular or irregular. Regular lacerations are usually caused by a knife or razor. They may heal better because their edges are smoother. Irregular lacerations are commonly caused by a blunt object, serrated knife, or broken bottle. The edges of the wound are jagged, and healing is usually prolonged.

Penetration/Puncture Wounds

A **penetration/puncture wound** is usually the result of a sharp, pointed object being pushed or driven into the soft tissues. This type of injury may have both an entry wound and an exit wound.

The entry wound may be small, and there may be little or no external bleeding (Figure 20–4 on p. 303). However, such injuries may be deep and damaging and cause severe internal bleeding. A gunshot injury is a good example (Figure 20–5 on

CLOSED WOUNDS

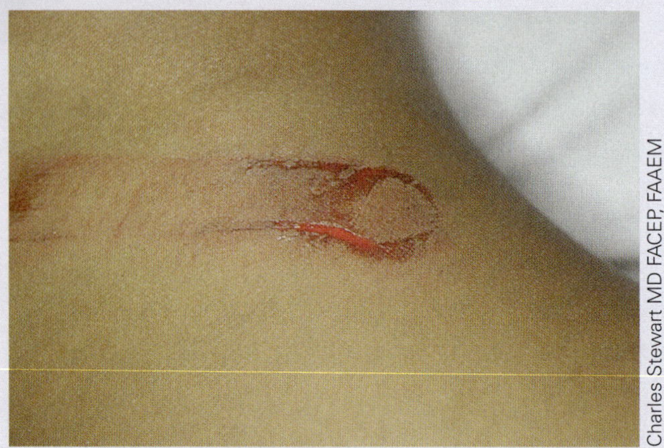

Figure 20–1a Contusion.

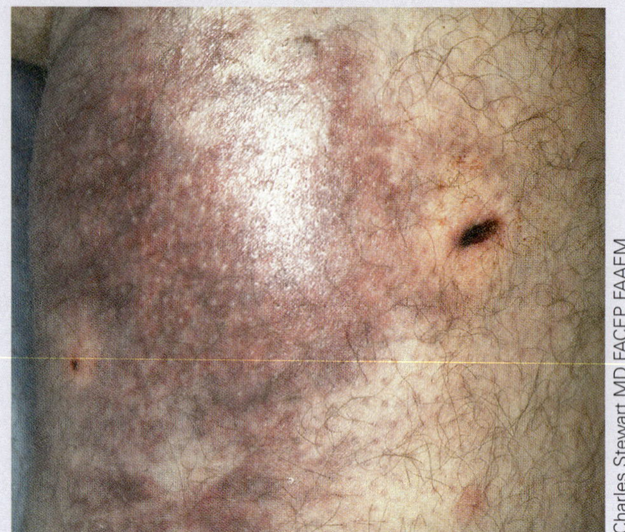

Figure 20–1b Hematoma.

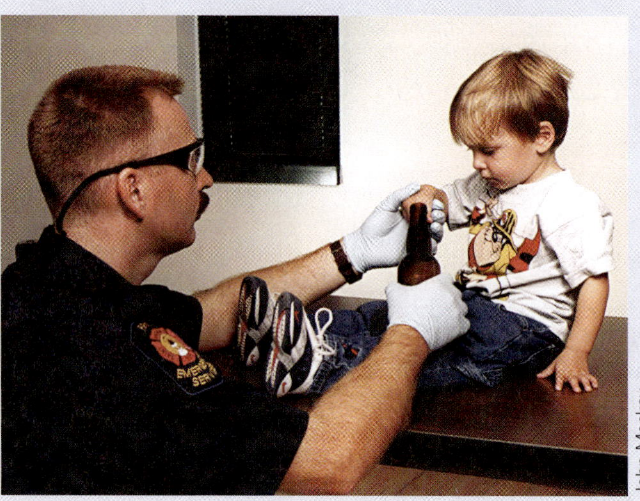

Figure 20–1c Clamping injury.

p. 303). The entry wound in many cases is smaller than the exit wound. If the patient was shot at close range, the entry wound may be surrounded by powder burns. The larger exit wound generally bleeds more profusely.

The overall severity of a penetration/puncture wound depends on the following factors:

- The location of the injury
- The size of the penetrating object
- The forces involved in creating the injury

It can be difficult to determine the extent of these injuries only on the basis of external signs.

Therefore, treat penetration/puncture wounds with great caution.

General Guidelines for Emergency Care

Since it is likely that you will be exposed to your patient's blood and other body fluids, take all appropriate BSI precautions. Wear protective latex gloves. Protect your face and eyes, and wear a disposable gown as necessary. After patient care, wash your hands—even if you wore gloves. Handwashing is still the single most important thing you can do to prevent the spread of infection.

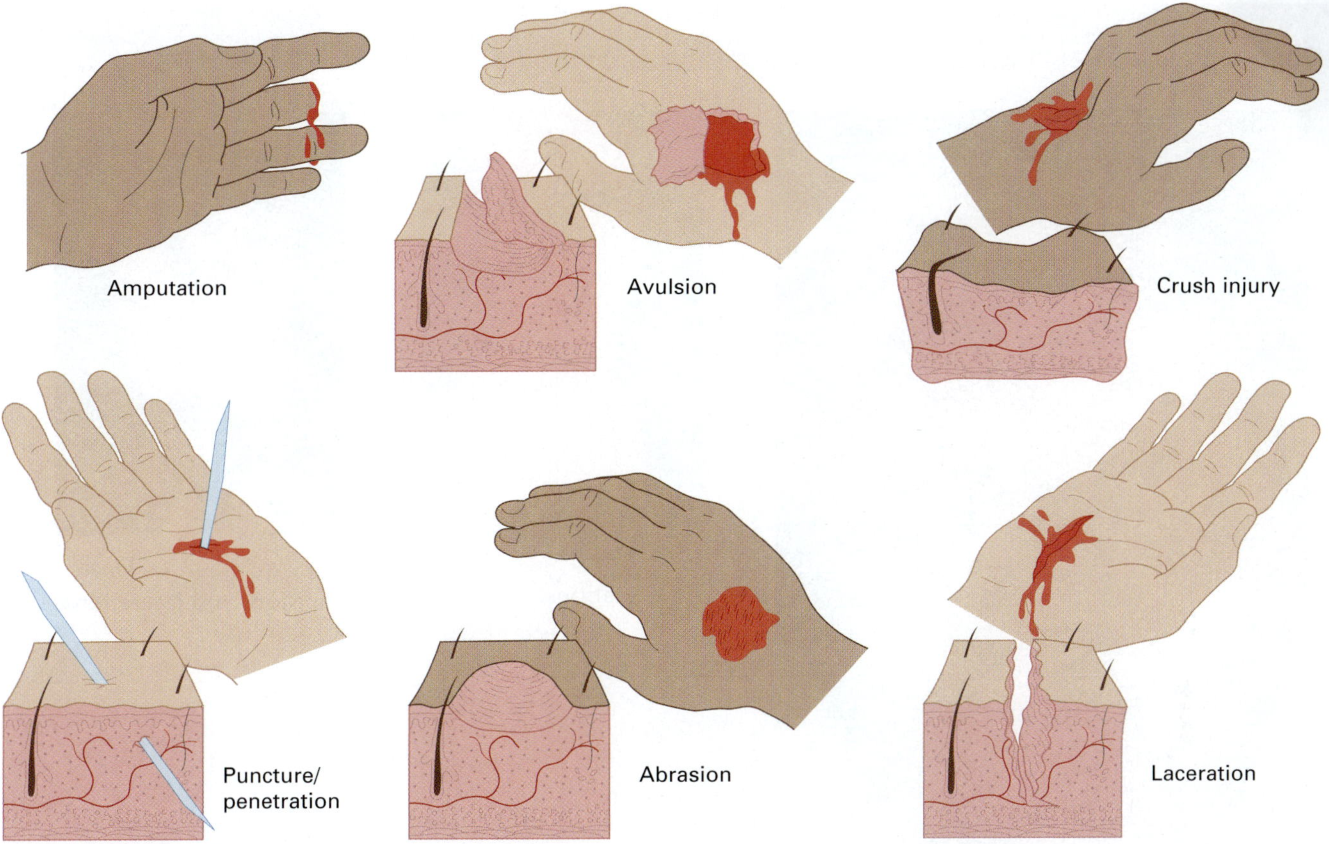

Figure 20–2 Open wounds.

To care for a patient with an open soft-tissue injury, follow these guidelines:

1. *Assess and treat all life threats*. Maintain a patent airway and adequate breathing. Administer oxygen by way of a non-rebreather mask. If the patient's breathing is inadequate, provide ventilations with supplemental oxygen if allowed.
2. *Expose the entire injury site*. If needed, cut away clothing. Clear the area of blood and debris with sterile gauze or the cleanest material available. Remember to look for additional wounds or injuries, especially in the case of a gunshot wound. (Often, multiple gunshot wounds are involved.)
3. *Control bleeding*. Begin with direct pressure and elevation. If bleeding is still not controlled, then use a pressure point.
4. *Prevent further contamination*. Keep the wound as clean as possible. If there are loose particles of foreign matter around the wound, wipe them away from the wound. Never wipe toward it. Never try to pick embedded particles or debris out of the wound.
5. *Dress and bandage the wound*. Apply a dry sterile dressing. Then secure it with a bandage. Check distal pulses both before and after applying the bandage to make sure it is not cutting off circulation.

As you care for a patient's soft-tissue injuries—especially when they are open, bleeding ones—be careful about what you say and do. Do not alarm the patient by your reaction to the wounds. In fact, it will help the patient significantly if you do your best to be comforting, calming, and reassuring. If possible, also keep the patient's on-scene family members informed and reassured.

Special Considerations

Some open wounds need special consideration. Basic emergency medical care is the same as for all other open wounds, but there are certain exceptions described below. In all these cases, administer oxygen by way of a non-rebreather mask, or if breathing is inadequate, provide ventilations with supplemental oxygen.

Chest Injuries

A penetrating chest wound can prevent a patient from breathing adequately. In this case, apply an occlusive dressing. (This is a special type of dressing used to form an airtight seal.)

Secure the dressing with tape on three sides (Figure 20–6 on p. 304). Leave one side untaped to allow air to escape as the patient exhales. This

ABRASIONS AND LACERATIONS

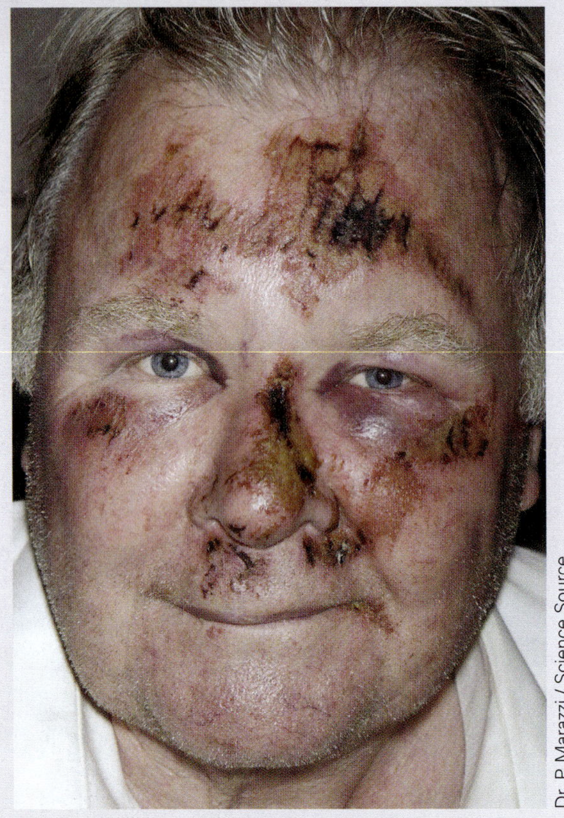

Figure 20–3a   Abrasions.

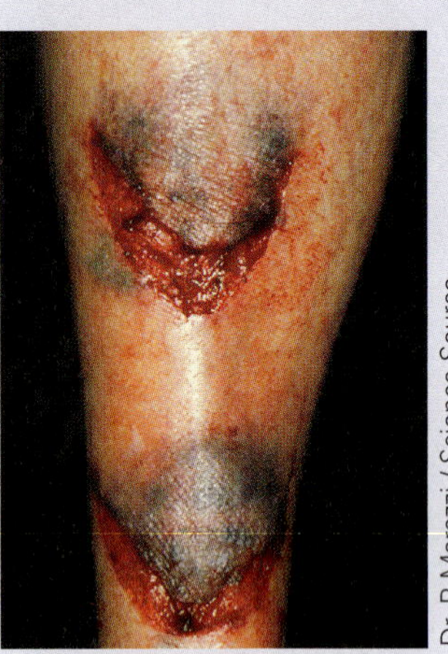

Figure 20–3b   Irregular lacerations.

Figure 20–3c   Deep abrasions and lacerations.

will help prevent a condition called tension pneumothorax, a severe buildup of air that compresses the lungs and heart toward the uninjured side of the chest.

Let the patient assume a position of comfort if you do not suspect spinal injury. Generally, the patient will favour the position that allows for the greatest chest expansion. Assume spinal injury if there is any significant mechanism of injury to the chest, including a gunshot wound.

Impaled Objects

An **impaled object** is an object that is embedded in an open wound. It should never be removed in the field unless it is through the patient's cheek or interferes with airway management or CPR. To provide emergency care to a patient with an impaled object, follow these guidelines:

1. Manually secure the object to prevent any movement. Movement of the object could cause further damage and bleeding.
2. Expose the wound area. Remove clothing from around the wound. Remember to take care not to move the object at all.
3. Control the bleeding. Apply direct pressure to the edges of the wound. Avoid putting pressure directly on the impaled object.
4. Use a bulky dressing to help stabilize the object (Figure 20–7 on p. 304). Surround the entire object with dressings. Pack them around the object and tape securely in place. A rolled-up cravat may be used to stabilize the object (Figure 20–8).

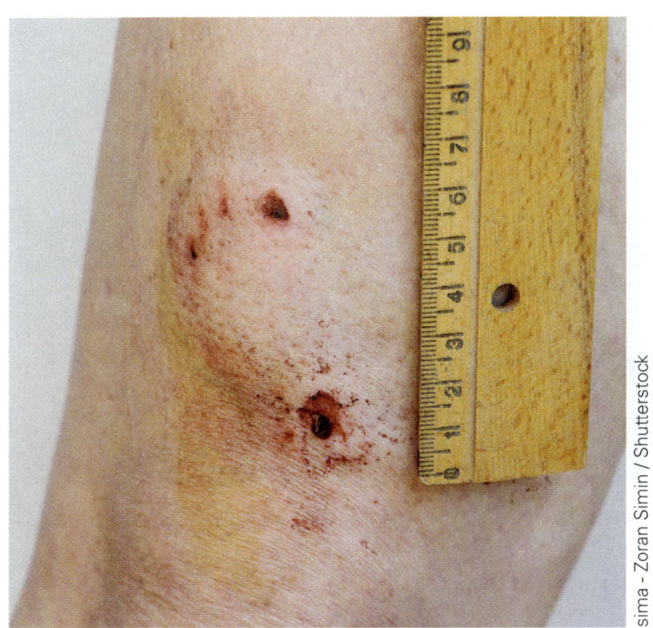

Figure 20–4   Puncture wound to the knee.

sima - Zoran Simin / Shutterstock

When an object is impaled in a patient's cheek, bleeding can interfere with breathing. If this is the case, then remove the object as follows (Figure 20–9):

1. While maintaining an open airway, feel inside the patient's mouth with gloved fingers. Find out if the object has penetrated the cheek completely.
2. Remove the object in the direction in which it entered.
3. Control the bleeding from outside the cheek. Then dress the wound.
4. If the object penetrated the cheek completely, pack sterile gauze between the cheek wall and the teeth.
5. Continue to monitor the airway. Suction when necessary.

You may encounter resistance when you try to remove the object from the cheek. If so, maintain an open airway and suction as needed. Stabilize the object while you wait for the paramedics to arrive on

GUNSHOT WOUNDS

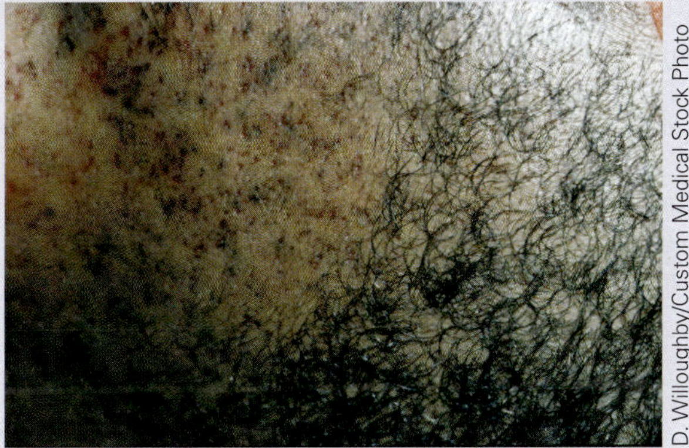

D. Willoughby/Custom Medical Stock Photo

Figure 20–5a   Powder burn from a gunshot.

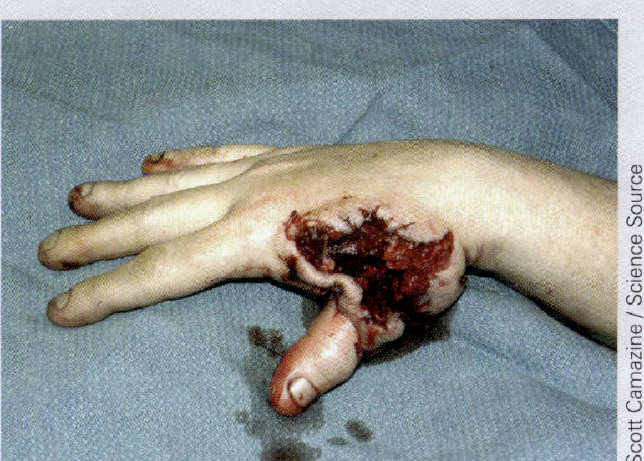

Scott Camazine / Science Source

Figure 20–5b   Gunshot wound to the hand.

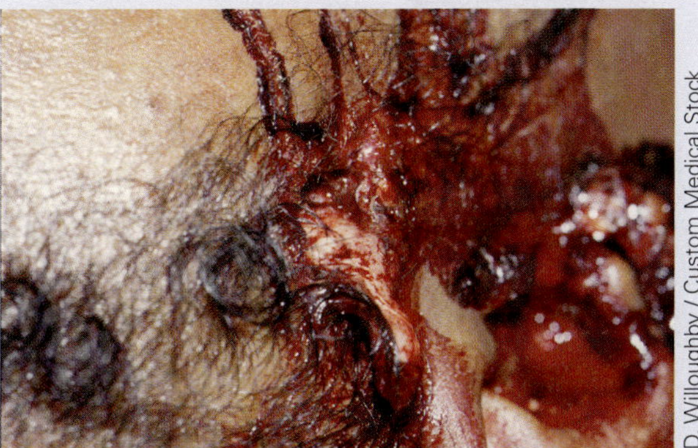

D. Willoughby / Custom Medical Stock Photo

Figure 20–5c   Entrance and exit wound.

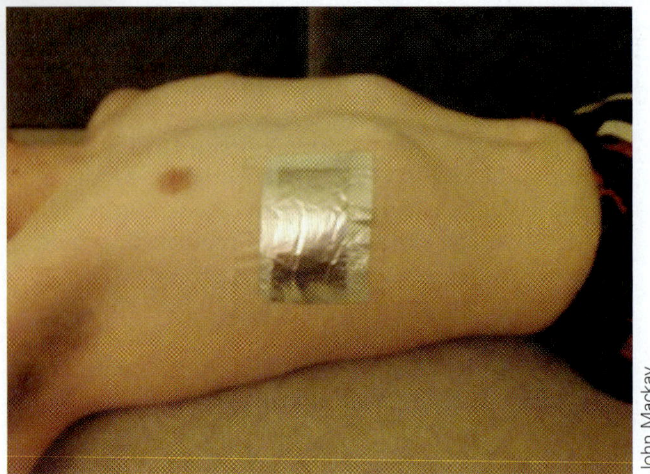

Figure 20–6 Occlusive dressing, taped on three sides, for a chest injury.

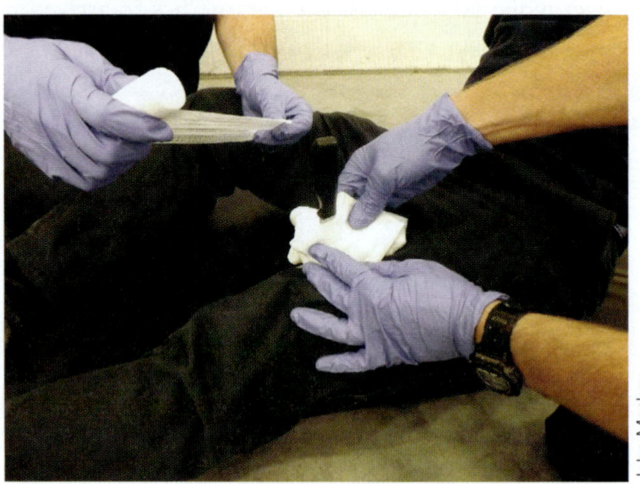

Figure 20–7 Bulky dressings can help stabilize an impaled object.

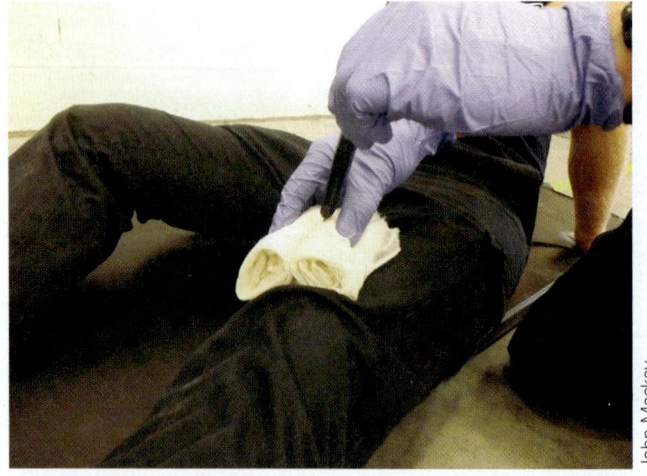

Figure 20–8 A cravat roll for stabilizing an object.

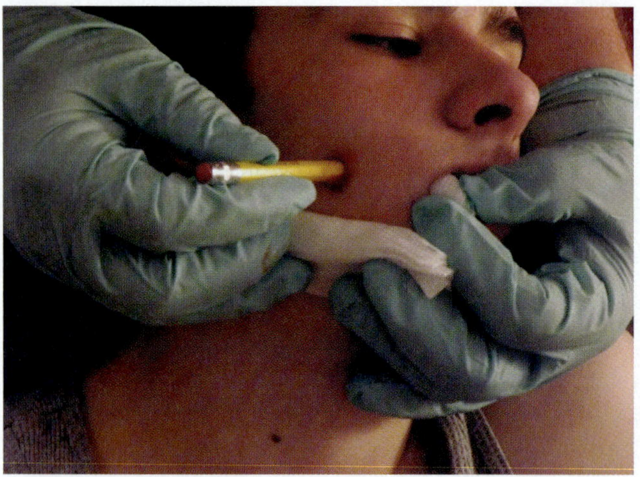

Figure 20–9 An impaled object in the cheek.

the scene. Position the patient on his or her side for drainage.

Large, Open Neck Wounds

Severe bleeding from a wound involving a major blood vessel of the neck is a serious emergency. In addition to the possible loss of a great deal of blood, there is the danger of air being sucked into a neck vein and carried to the heart. This can be lethal. Also suspect spinal injury with any significant injury to the neck.

In this case, control of bleeding and prevention of an air embolism (air bubble) are your major goals. Follow these steps:

1. Immediately place a gloved hand over the wound to control the bleeding.
2. Apply an occlusive dressing. Make sure it extends beyond the wound on all sides to prevent it from being sucked in. Tape the dressing on all four sides.
3. Cover the occlusive dressing with a regular one. Then apply enough pressure to control the bleeding. Compress the carotid artery only if it is severed.
4. Once the bleeding is controlled, apply a pressure dressing. Do not restrict air flow or compress major blood vessels. Do not apply a dressing that encircles the neck. Dressing may be held firmly in place by a cervical collar even when a spinal injury is not suspected.

Eviscerations

An **evisceration** occurs when internal organs protrude through an open wound. This most commonly occurs with abdominal wounds.

When you care for a patient with an evisceration, never try to reposition the protruding organs and never touch them. You could cause further damage

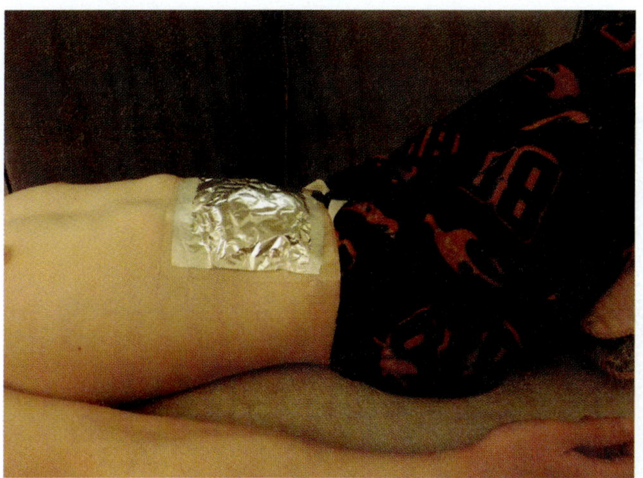

Figure 20–10 Abdominal evisceration protected with a thick, moist, sterile dressing and an occlusive covering.

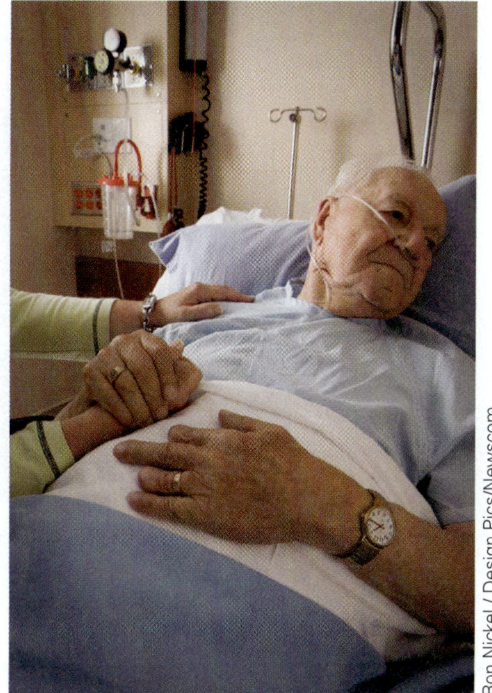

Figure 20–11 Finger amputations.

and contaminate both the organs and the cavity from which they protrude.

Cover the exposed organs with a thick, moist, sterile dressing. You can moisten the dressing with sterile water or saline. The dressing should be large enough to cover all the protruding organs. Sterile gauze is preferred. Never use absorbent materials, such as toilet tissue or paper towels, which can shred and cling to the organs. Loosely cover the moistened dressing with an occlusive dressing (Figure 20–10).

Maintain the temperature of the wound area by covering the dressing with layers of a more bulky dressing, such as a particle-free bath blanket or towel. The dressings may be held loosely in place with a bandage or clean sheet.

Amputations

In an **amputation**, a body part has been completely severed from the body (Figure 20–11). This is the result of ripping or tearing forces, often from an industrial accident or MVA. Massive bleeding is usually present. In some cases, however, the elasticity of the blood vessels helps them contract and bleeding is minimal. Care for an amputation in the same way you care for all open injuries.

With amputations, you must also care for the amputated part. First provide emergency care to the patient. Do not spend time looking for the amputated body part. If possible, have other EMRs or support personnel search for it. Once the body part is found, follow these guidelines (Figure 20–12):

1. Wrap the amputated part in sterile gauze that is moistened with sterile saline.

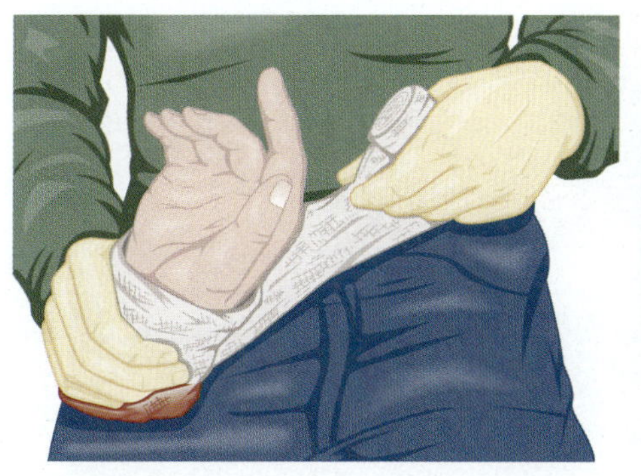
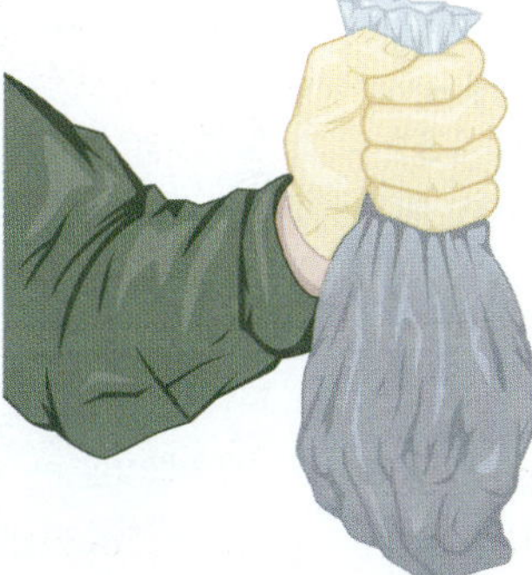
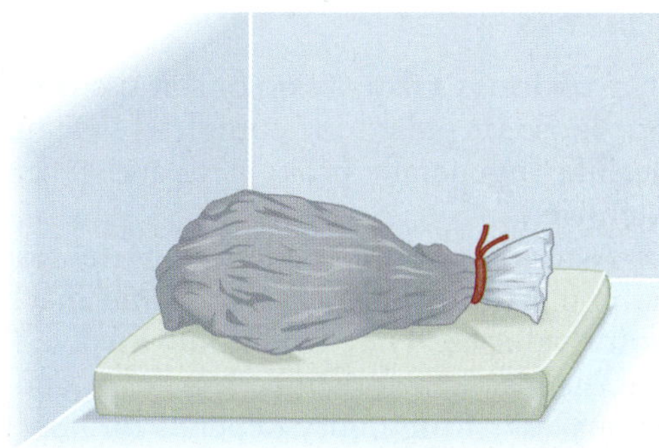

(1) Wrap it completely in saline-moistened sterile dressings.

(2) Place it in a plastic bag and seal the bag shut.

(3) Place the sealed bag on top of a cold pack or another sealed bag of ice. Do not allow the tissue to freeze.

Figure 20–12 Emergency care for an amputated body part.

AVULSIONS

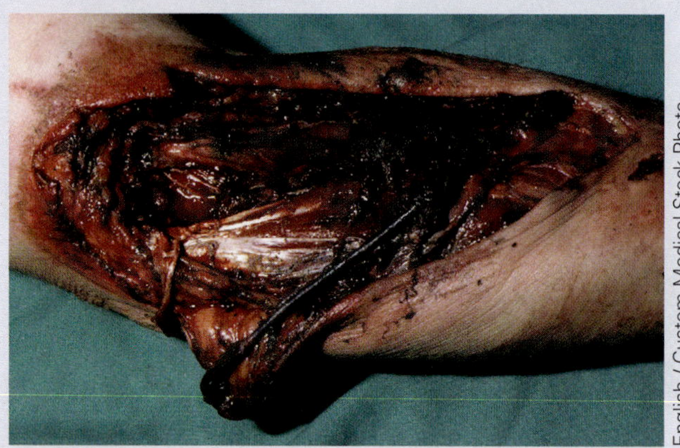

Figure 20–13 Avulsion to the forearm.

2. Place the amputated part in a plastic bag. Label the bag with the patient's name, the date, and time the part was bagged. Never immerse the part in water.

3. Keep the amputated part cool. Place the bagged part in a larger bag or container of ice and water. Do not use ice alone. Never use dry ice. Never place the part directly on ice. Mark the container with the patient's name, date, and body part.

4. Give the packed part to arriving EMS personnel so that they can transport it with the patient to the hospital.

Note that if the amputation is partial, you should never complete it. Care for the injury as you would any other soft-tissue injury. Make sure that the partially amputated part is not twisted or constricted.

Avulsions

An **avulsion** is a flap of skin or soft tissue that has been torn loose or pulled off completely (Figure 20–13). Healing is generally prolonged, and scarring may be extensive.

Avulsions are most commonly the result of accidents involving industrial or home machinery and motor vehicles. They commonly involve the fingers, toes, hands, feet, forearms, legs, ears, and nose. The seriousness of the injury depends on how well blood can circulate to the avulsed skin. If it is still attached but the flap is folded back, circulation may be compromised severely. If this is the case, emergency care includes making sure the flap is lying flat and aligned in its normal position.

Bites

Bite wounds can be quite serious (Figure 20–14). Even when they look minor, soft tissues may be badly lacerated. The threat of infection is usually high. During emergency care, wash a bite wound with plenty of warm, soapy water. Check it for any teeth fragments as well.

Note that you should not kill the animal that bit your patient unless it is absolutely necessary to stop an attack. If you do kill the animal, call an animal control officer and request that the corpse be examined for rabies, a viral infection that affects the nervous system. If you do not kill the animal, try to trap it in some kind of enclosure so that it can be examined for rabies. Take care not to injure the animal's head. Remember to protect yourself from any danger.

If the animal is not present, find out where it can be located. If getting an address is not possible, obtain

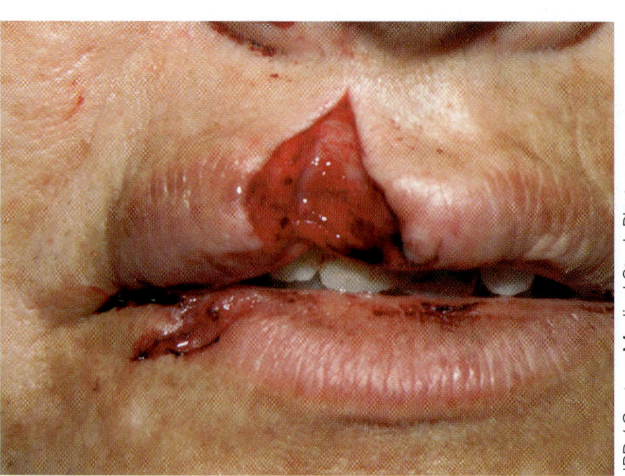

Figure 20–14 Dog bite.

a description of the animal, where it was encountered, and whether or not the attack might have been provoked. Follow local protocols on reporting requirements.

SECTION 2
DRESSING AND BANDAGING WOUNDS

The basic purposes of dressing and bandaging are to control bleeding, prevent further contamination and damage to the wound, keep the wound dry, and immobilize the wound site. Proper wound care also enhances healing. It adds to the comfort of the patient, and promotes more rapid recovery. Improper wound care can cause infection, severe discomfort, and, in rare cases, loss of a limb.

Dressings

A **dressing** is a covering for a wound (Figure 20–15). It should be **sterile** (free of all microorganisms and spores). Ideally, a dressing is layered and consists of coarse mesh gauze. It should also be absorbent and large enough to protect the entire wound from contamination. In an emergency, you can use clean handkerchiefs, towels, sheets, cloth, or sanitary napkins as dressings. Never use elastic bandages, which have a tourniquet effect. Never use toilet tissue, paper towels, or other materials that can shred and cling to a wound.

DRESSINGS

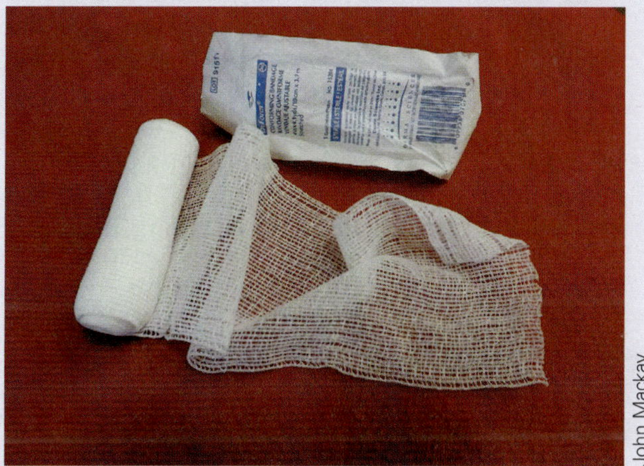

Figure 20–15a Non-elastic, self-adhering dressing and roller bandage.

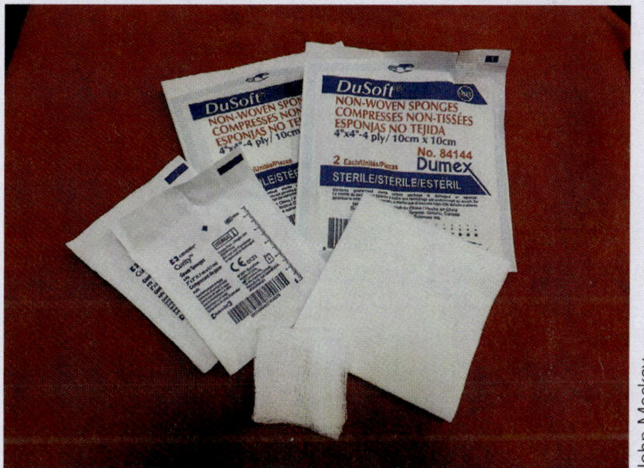

Figure 20–15b Sterile gauze pads.

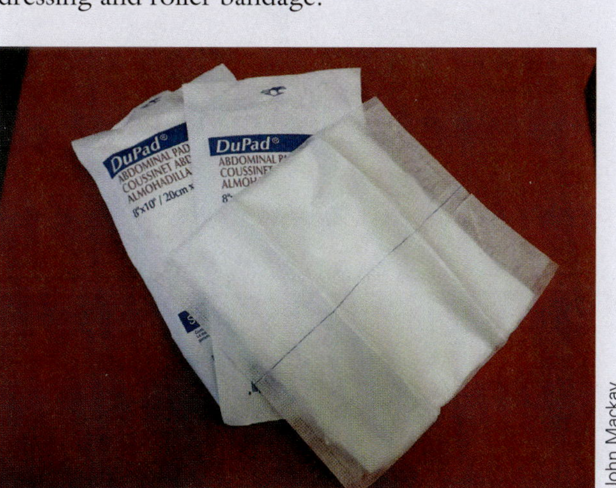

Figure 20–15c Multi-trauma dressing.

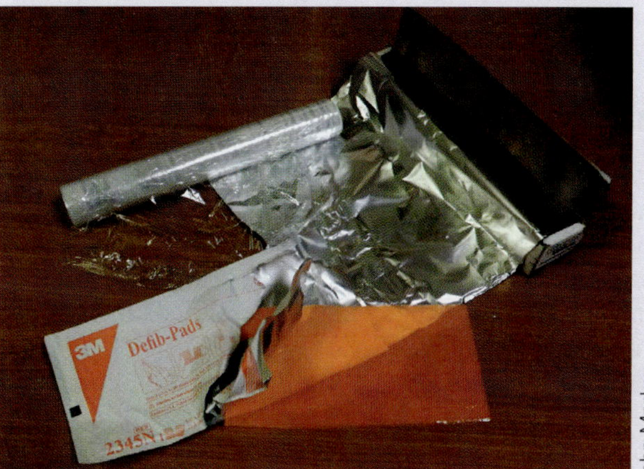

Figure 20–15d Occlusive dressings.

The types of dressings include the following:

- *Gauze pads*—These are usually individually wrapped and sealed to prevent contamination. Take care not to touch the portion of the gauze that is to make contact with the wound. Unless otherwise specified, all gauze dressings should be covered with open triangular, cravat, or roller bandages.
- *Trauma dressing*—Large and absorbent, this type of dressing is used on larger injuries and when maximum absorbency is needed.
- *Bandage compress*—This is a gauze pad that is attached to the middle of a strip of bandaging material. The pad can be applied directly to an open wound with virtually no exposure to the air or your fingers. The strips of bandage can be folded back and used to tie it in place. When necessary, the sterile pad may be extended to twice its normal size by continued unfolding.
- *Occlusive dressing*—Made of plastic wrap, aluminum foil, petroleum gauze, or other material, this dressing is used to form an airtight, moisture-proof seal over a wound.
- *Petroleum gauze*—This is a sterile gauze saturated with petroleum jelly to prevent it from sticking to a wound.

Large, thick, layered, bulky pads (some with waterproof surfaces) are also available. They come in several sizes for quick application to an extremity or to a large area of the trunk. They are used to help control the bleeding and to stabilize impaled objects. These pads are also referred to as bulky dressings, multi-trauma dressings, trauma packs, general purpose dressings, burn pads, or ABD pad dressings.

If a commercial bulky dressing is not available, you can improvise one with a sanitary napkin. If purchased in individual wrappers, sanitary napkins have the added advantage of sterility.

Bandages

A bandage does not make contact with a wound. It is used to hold a dressing in place, create pressure to help control the bleeding, or provide support for an injured body part. Properly applied, a bandage promotes healing. It also helps the patient to remain comfortable during transport.

Bandages should be applied firmly and fastened securely. They should not be so tight as to stop circulation, but they should not be so loose as to let the dressings slip. If a bandage becomes unfastened, the wound could bleed or become infected.

Before bandaging, remove the patient's jewellery and other potentially restricting materials, such as tape that the patient may have applied as a bandage. In case of swelling, these items can restrict circulation. Loosen bandages if the skin around them becomes pale or cyanotic, if pain develops, or if the skin is cold, tingly, or numb distal to the bandage.

Even if the pain or discomfort caused by a bandage disappears after several hours, severe damage may have already occurred. Permanent muscle paralysis may result. Please note that improper bandaging can be defined in a court of law as negligence.

The types of bandages include the following:

- *Triangular bandage*—This is used to support injured limbs, secure splints, form slings, and make improvised tourniquets. It can also be used to bandage the forehead or scalp (Figure 20–16). The standard triangular bandage is made from a piece of unbleached cotton about 1 m square, which is folded diagonally and cut along the fold. It can be handled and applied easily. If applied correctly, it usually remains secure. In an emergency, one can be improvised from a clean handkerchief or clean piece of shirt.
- *Cravat*—This is a triangular bandage that has been folded lengthwise (Figure 20–17). For a wide cravat, make a 3 cm fold along the base of

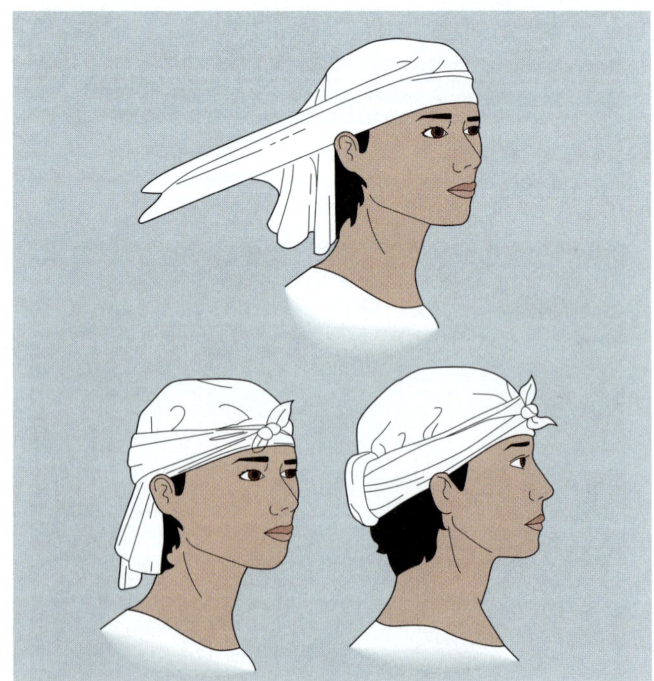

Figure 20–16 Triangular bandage for the forehead or scalp.

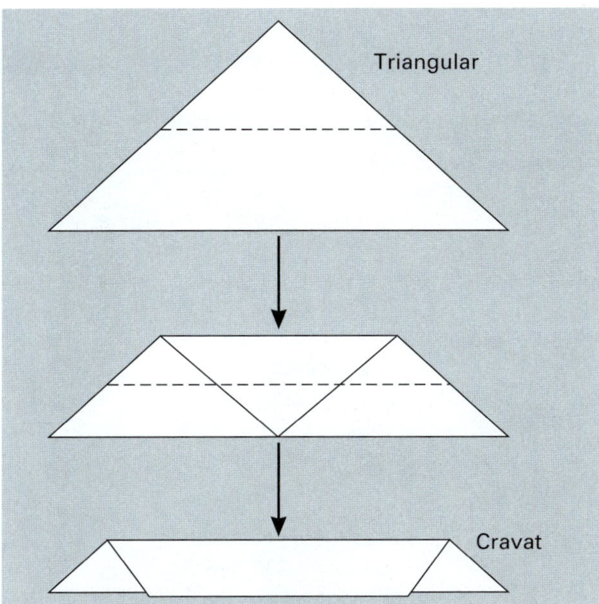

Figure 20–17 Triangular and cravat bandages.

the triangle. Bring the point to the centre of the folded base, placing the point under the fold. For a medium cravat, fold lengthwise along a line midway between the base and the new top of the bandage. For a narrow cravat, folding is repeated. To complete the procedure, the ends of the bandage are tied securely.

- *Roller bandage*—The self-adhering, form-fitting, non-elastic roller bandage is the most popular and easy to use. Overlapping wraps cling together and can be cut and tied or taped in place (Figure 20–18).

Elastic roller bandages should not be used because a tourniquet effect may result.

To apply a pressure dressing to a bleeding wound, follow these steps:

1. Cover the wound with a sterile bulky dressing.
2. Apply hand pressure over the wound until the bleeding stops.
3. Apply a firm roller bandage, preferably the self-adhering type. The pressure dressing may also be used to hold some manual pressure while you use a pressure point to stop the bleeding.

Principles of Application

There are no hard and fast rules for dressing and bandaging wounds. Often, adaptability and creativity are far more important. In dressing and bandaging, use materials you have on hand but be sure to meet the general conditions listed below (Figure 20–19):

- The material used for dressings should be sterile. If sterile items are not available, use the cleanest cloth available.
- Make sure that the sterile dressing is opened carefully. Avoid contaminating it before it reaches the wound surface.
- The dressing should adequately cover the entire wound.
- Do not bandage a dressing in place until the bleeding has stopped. The exception is a pressure dressing, which is meant to stop the bleeding.

ROLLER BANDAGE

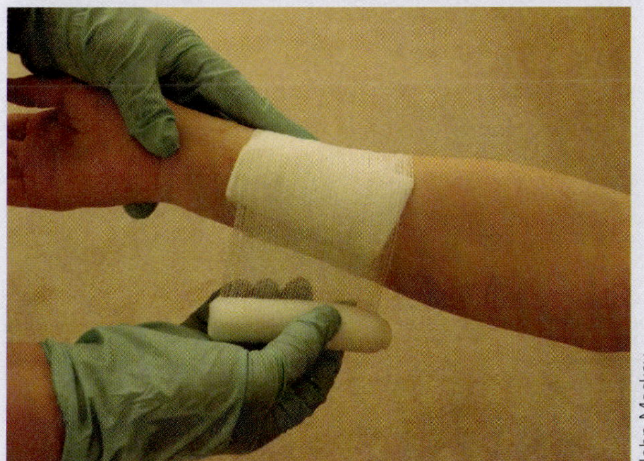

Figure 20–18a Secure the bandage with several overlapping wraps.

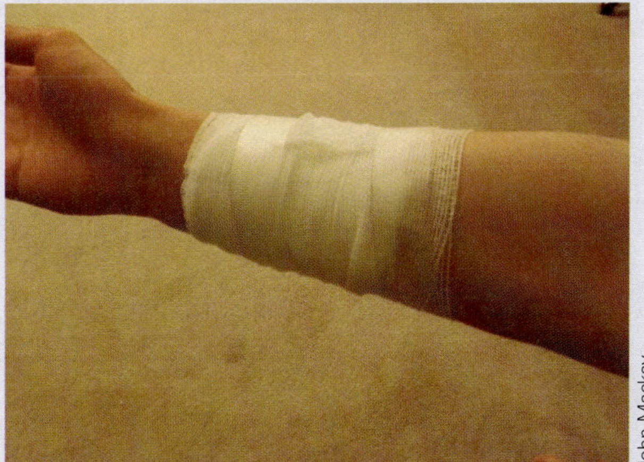

Figure 20–18b When the bandage covers an area larger than the wound, secure it with tape or tie it in place.

BANDAGES

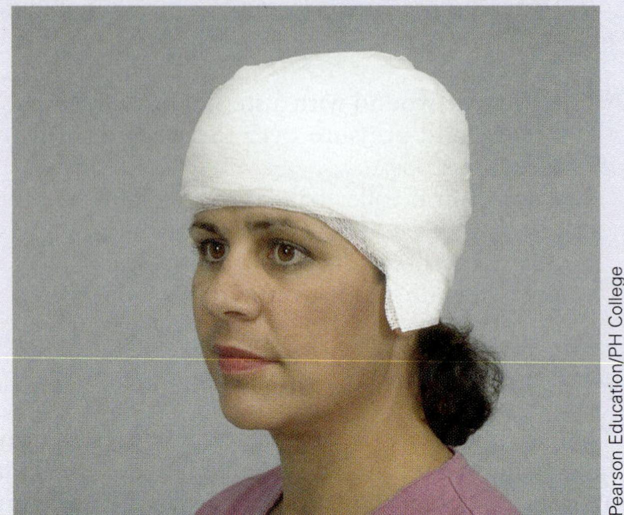

Figure 20–19a Head or ear bandage.

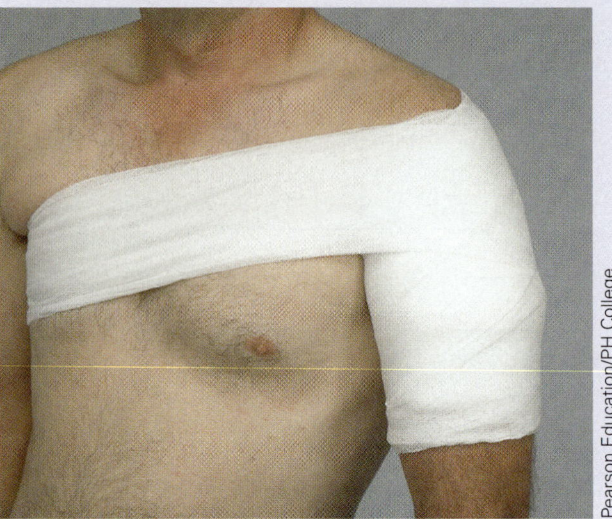

Figure 20–19b Shoulder bandage.

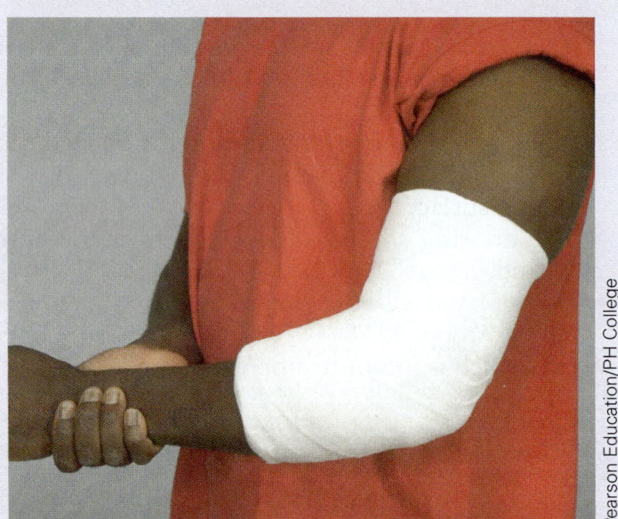

Figure 20–19c Elbow bandage.

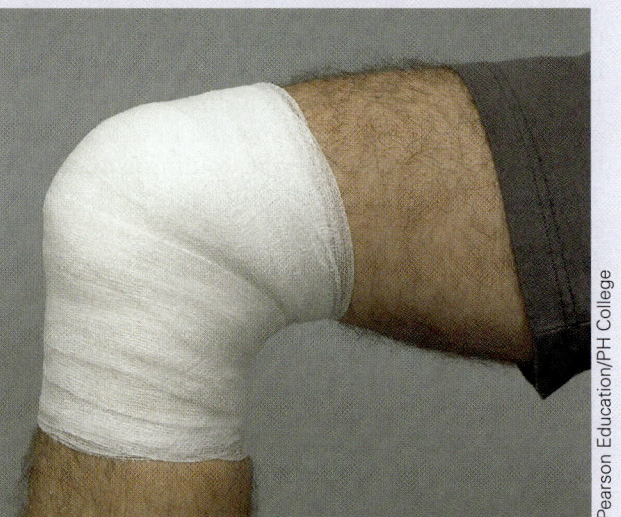

Figure 20–19d Knee bandage.

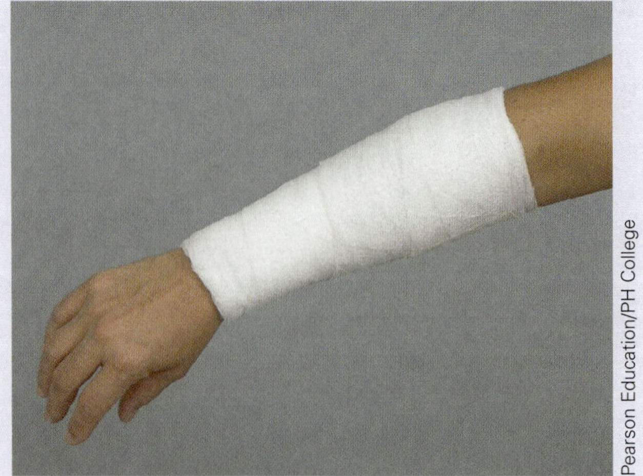

Figure 20–19e Lower arm bandage.

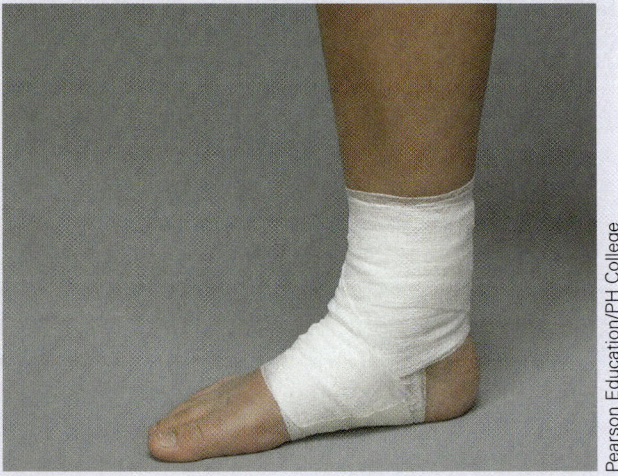

Figure 20–19f Foot or ankle bandage.

- All the edges of a dressing should be covered by the bandage. There should also be no loose ends of cloth or tape.
- Do not bandage a wound too loosely. Bandages should not slip, shift, or allow the dressings beneath to slip or shift.
- Bandage wounds snugly, but not too tightly. Be sure to ask the patient how the bandage feels. Be careful not to interfere with circulation.
- If you are bandaging a small wound on an extremity, cover a larger area with the bandage. This will help avoid creating a pressure point and will distribute pressure more evenly.
- Always place the body part to be bandaged in the position in which it is to remain. You can bandage across a joint but do not try bending a joint after the bandage has been applied to it.
- Tape bandages in place or tie them by using a square knot (Figure 20–20).
- Leave the fingers and toes exposed when the arms and legs are bandaged so that you can check for problems with circulation.
- Keep the bandage neat in appearance. You will be perceived as more professional, which can result in easier patient management.

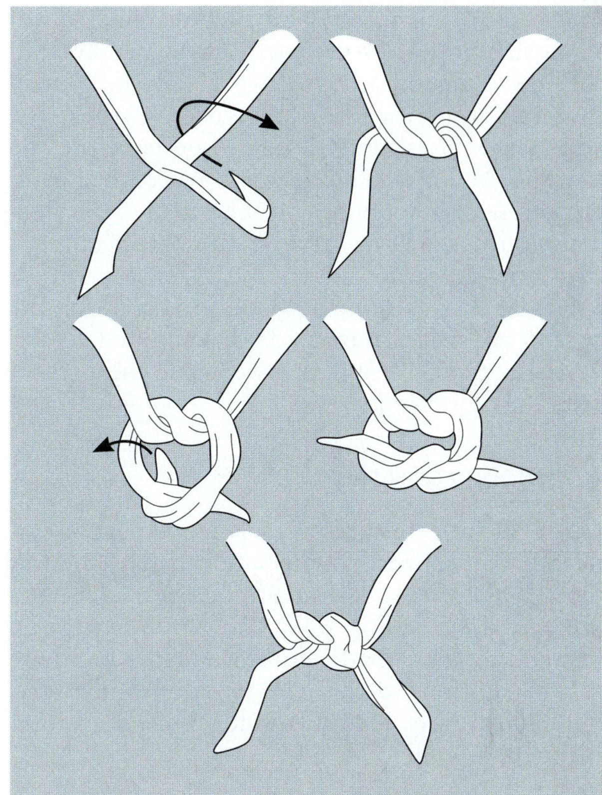

Figure 20–20 Tying a square knot.

In your experience as an EMR, you will come across many patients with soft-tissue injuries. Some injuries will be minor. Others will be large and gaping. Keep your evaluation of these wounds in perspective with the patient's overall condition. If the patient has a laceration that is not bleeding profusely, then it is not your first priority. You must not neglect life-saving care for an obvious but non-life-threatening wound.

This does not mean that care for soft-tissue injuries is unimportant. It is. You must control the bleeding, as necessary, and bandage a wound to keep it clean. Your patient will be very aware of these injuries. Offer reassurance as you provide care.

CASE STUDY FOLLOW-UP

At the beginning of this chapter, you read that EMRs were on the scene with a female patient with an impaled object in one hand. To see how the chapter skills apply to this emergency, read the following. It describes how the call was completed.

SECONDARY ASSESSMENT

A sliver of wood about 15 cm long had penetrated the palm of the patient's hand. About 6 cm of wood protruded from each side. The patient's name was Victoria Mashot. Vicky hadn't passed out or fallen after the injury. She had sensation in her fingers distal to the injury. There was no numbness or tingling. I didn't ask her to move her fingers because I didn't want to take the chance of causing further problems. Vicky's pulse was 88, strong, and regular. Her respirations were 20 and adequate. Her skin was cool and dry.

My partner stabilized the impaled object while I obtained the patient history.

PATIENT HISTORY

Vicky was still upset that she was so careless as to let this happen. We were able to find out that she had no drug or environmental allergies. She was in good health and took no medication. Vicky told us she never missed a day of work. She had eaten a doughnut and coffee from the vending truck that came to the mill grounds about an hour before the injury. She confirmed that she had placed her hand where she wasn't supposed to. She denied any loss of consciousness before or after the object entered her hand.

My partner was doing a good job of securing the piece of wood with gauze pads. I continued to stabilize the patient's arm and hand while my partner secured the object in place.

ONGOING ASSESSMENT

We kept Vicky calm and performed our reassessment. She had calmed down some by then. She was still alert. Her airway and breathing were adequate. There was no bleeding from her wound through the bandage. We made sure that the bandage wasn't too tight and that the impaled object was being held securely. Her pulse and respirations were unchanged.

TRANSFER OF CARE

When the paramedics arrived, we told them what we had:

> "This is Victoria Mashot. She is 34 years old and has a 15 cm sliver of wood impaled in her left hand. She never lost consciousness and hasn't fallen or suffered any other injury. We applied some bulky dressings and then bandaged around the object so it wouldn't move. Vicky has no allergies and is not on any medication. She tells us that she has no medical problems. She had a doughnut and coffee an hour ago. Her pulse is 88, strong, and regular. Her respirations are 18 and adequate."

The paramedics took Vicky to the hospital. A plastic surgeon removed the wood from her hand. Fortunately, there was no permanent damage. I heard that Vicky now keeps that sliver of wood over her workbench as a reminder to be more careful.

> Whatever your patient's soft-tissue injuries may be, remember that your priorities will always be control of bleeding, preventing further injury, and reducing the risk of infection.

NOCPs

5.6 a Treat soft-tissue injuries **S**
     d Treat penetration wound **S**
6.1 f Provide care to patient experiencing signs and symptoms involving integumentary system **S**

6.3 a Conduct ongoing assessments based on patient presentation and interpret findings **S**
     b Re-direct priorities based on assessment findings. **S**

REVIEW QUESTIONS

Page references where answers may be found or supported are provided at the end of each question.

SECTION 1

1. How are soft-tissue injuries classified? Name the different types. (pp. 298–299)
2. What is the recommended emergency care for closed wounds? (p. 298)
3. In general, how would you care for a patient's open wounds? (pp. 300–301)
4. What special considerations are made in caring for open chest injuries? Impaled objects? Eviscerations? Amputated body parts? (pp. 301–306)

5. What are two reasons for identifying and locating an animal that has inflicted a bite injury on a patient? (pp. 306–307)

SECTION 2

6. What are the functions of dressing and bandaging? (pp. 307–308)
7. What are the five basic types of dressing? What are the special characteristics of each? (p. 308)
8. What are the three types of bandage? (pp. 308–309)
9. What are the five or more general principles of dressing and bandaging? (pp. 309–311)

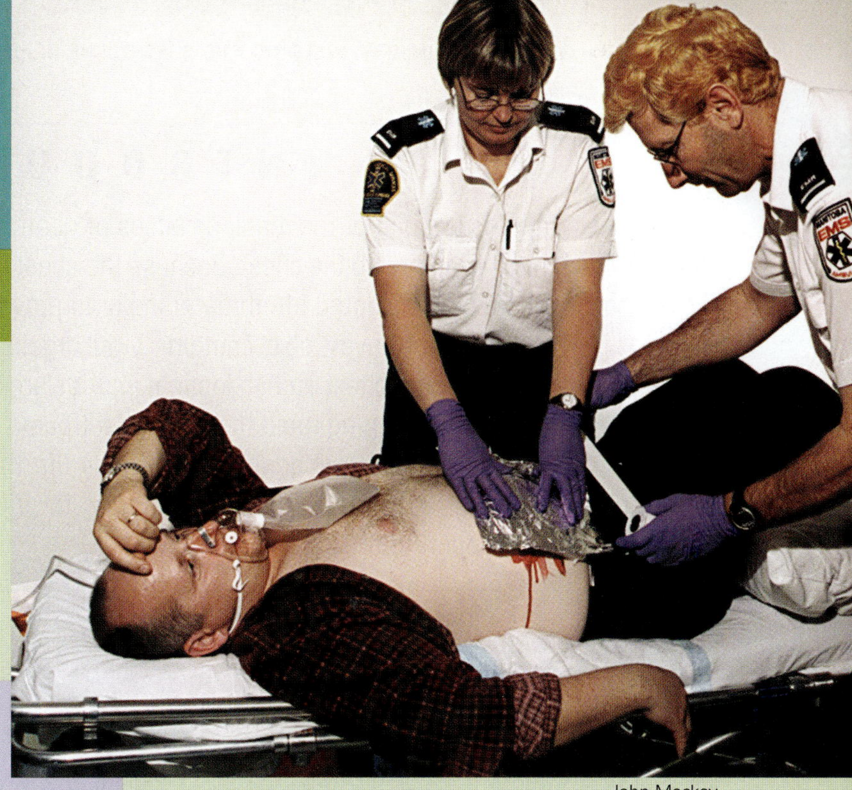

John Mackay

Injuries to the Chest, Abdomen, and Genitalia

OBJECTIVES

1. List the 12 major signs and symptoms of a chest injury.
2. Discuss the emergency medical care considerations for a patient with a closed chest injury, including blunt injuries, compression injuries, broken ribs, and flail chest.
3. Discuss the emergency medical care considerations for a patient with a sucking chest wound.
4. Describe the three common complications of an open chest injury: hemothorax, pneumothorax, and tension pneumothorax.
5. List the 16 general signs and symptoms of an abdominal injury.
6. State the emergency medical care considerations for a patient with an injury to the abdomen, and explain how to dress an abdominal evisceration.
7. Describe emergency care of a male patient with injuries to the genitalia, including avulsion, amputation, and blunt trauma.
8. Describe emergency care of a female patient with injuries to the genitalia.
9. Explain the special considerations concerning sexual assault and the preservation of evidence.
10. Demonstrate a caring attitude toward the patient and family when dealing with injuries to the chest, abdomen, or genitalia, while giving priority to the interests of the patient.

INTRODUCTION

Chest injuries are one of the leading causes of death from trauma. Many of the deaths caused by MVAs involve injuries to the chest. Because the chest contains organs vital to life, all injuries to the chest should be considered life threatening until proven otherwise.

The abdominal cavity also contains vital organs. Injuries to them can be life threatening. Remember that both chest and abdominal injuries are serious emergencies that require immediate emergency care, including rapid transport to a trauma centre.

Injuries to the external genitalia are rarely life threatening, but they can cause considerable pain and embarrassment. In addition to caring for injuries to the genitalia, remember to provide emotional support to the patient.

SECTION 1
INJURIES TO THE CHEST

For a quick review of the anatomy of the chest, see Figure 21–1. In addition, now is a good time to review the respiratory and circulatory systems as described in Chapter 4.

Patient Assessment

There are two categories of chest injuries—open and closed. As you would expect, an open chest wound occurs when an object passes through the chest wall. A closed injury is one in which the skin of the chest is not broken. The main types of chest injury include blunt trauma, penetrating injury, and compression injury.

Whether the injury is open or closed, certain signs and symptoms will occur in chest trauma. Many of them may occur simultaneously. The major signs and symptoms include the following (Figure 21–2):

- Shortness of breath or difficulty breathing
- Pain during breathing
- Failure of the chest to expand normally during inhalation
- Cyanosis
- Coughing up blood
- Distended neck veins
- Rapid, weak pulse
- Falling blood pressure
- Bruising to the chest
- Chest wall deformity
- Pain at injury site
- Shock

Two of the most important signs are the patient's respiratory rate and change in the normal breathing pattern. In general, a normal breathing rate is from 12 to 20 breaths per minute. Breathing is also done without strain, pain, or difficulty. If a patient breathes more than 20 times per minute, experiences pain with breathing, or finds it difficult to take a deep breath, the patient probably has a chest injury.

If the chest is injured, suspect serious underlying damage, even if the skin is not broken. Always assume cardiac damage until it is ruled out. Assume spinal injury if there is any significant mechanism of injury to the chest, including a gunshot wound.

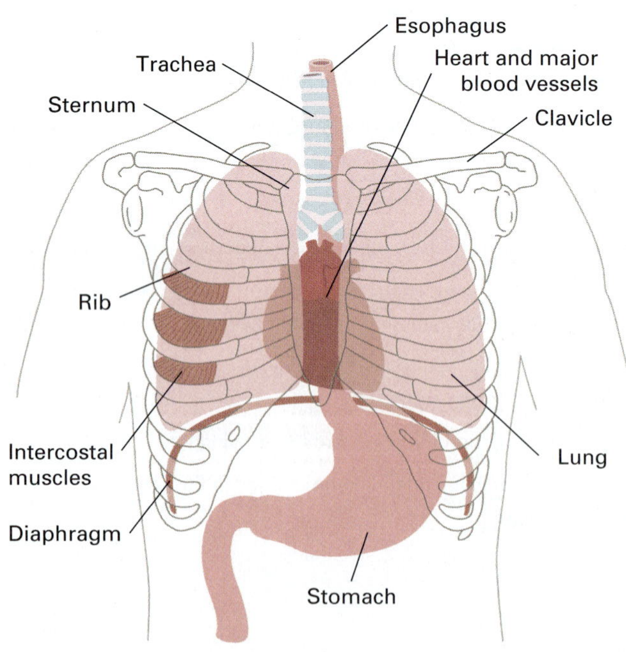

Figure 21–1 Chest cavity.

CASE STUDY

Dispatch
My EMR unit was called to a woman down at the corner of Hamilton and Lake Shore Drive.

Scene Assessment
Before we approached, we turned off the lights and sirens to prevent a crowd from being drawn to the scene. The police on the scene waved us in. We were still cautious as we pulled up and put on our gloves and eyewear. There was a woman lying on the ground. An officer was leaning over her.

Primary Assessment
The police officer reported that the woman had been stabbed, probably during a robbery. I saw a hole in the patient's shirt just below the nipple level on the right side of her chest. The woman was moaning and moving around.

Consider this patient as you read Chapter 21. What else may be done to assess and treat her condition?

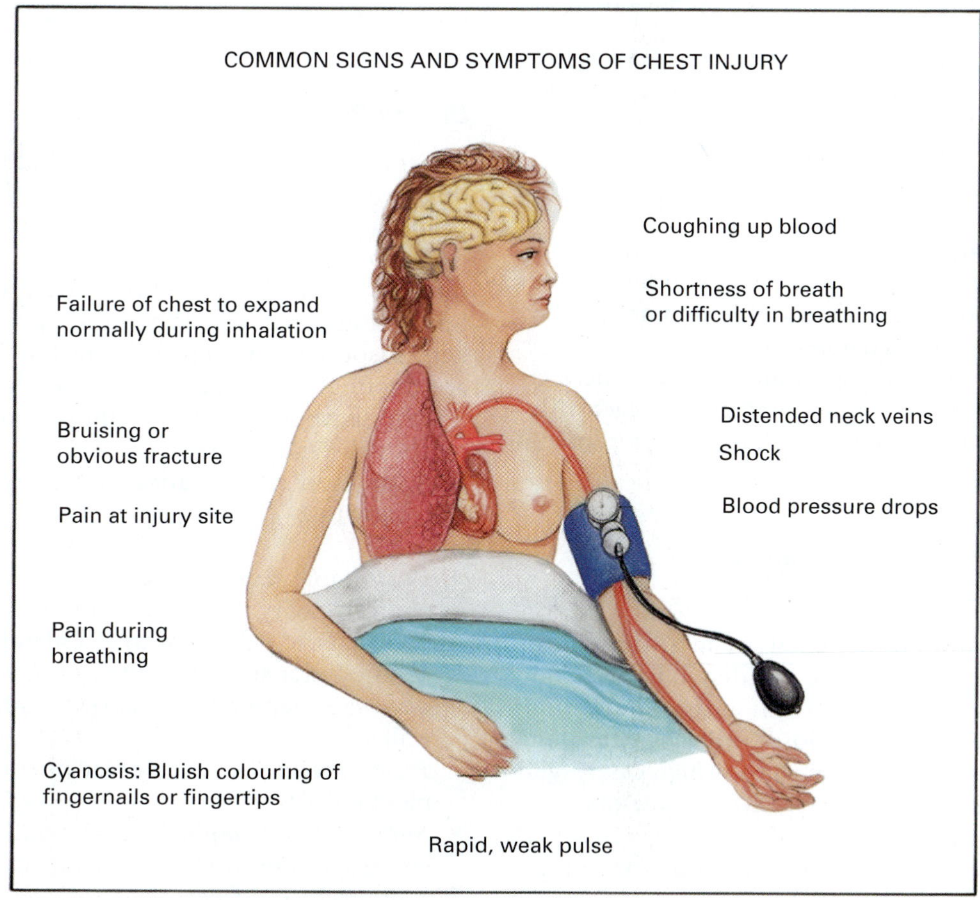

Figure 21–2 Common signs and symptoms of chest injury.

Remember, there is nothing quite as frightening to a patient as a breathing problem. Be sure to stay calm. Your demeanour will encourage the patient to stay calm as well. Demonstrate a caring, professional attitude to both the patient and the patient's family.

Closed Chest Injuries

Guidelines for Emergency Care

In case of any chest injury, update or activate the EMS system immediately. The patient must be stabilized and transported as quickly as possible to a trauma centre or other appropriate medical facility. To provide emergency care for a patient with a closed chest injury, follow the guidelines outlined below:

1. *Maintain an open airway.* Watch for airway obstruction from foreign objects, blood, mucus, and swelling. Suction when needed.
2. *Ensure adequate ventilations.* If possible, administer high-concentration oxygen. Be prepared to provide artificial ventilation or CPR if needed. Follow local protocol.
3. *Control any external bleeding.* It is likely for a patient who has a chest injury to have multiple injuries. Perform a quick assessment to detect any source of external bleeding. If appropriate, treat for shock.
4. *Allow the patient to get into a position of comfort if there is no suspected spinal injury.* Generally, the patient will favour the position that allows for the greatest chest expansion.
5. *Monitor vital signs regularly.*

More information on specific types of closed chest injury is provided below. Emergency medical care is basically the same for any closed injury to the chest. Any exceptions are noted below.

Note: Always take BSI precautions when there is any possibility that you might come into contact with a patient's blood or other body fluids. Wear protective latex gloves.

Blunt Injuries, Compression Injuries, and Traumatic Asphyxia

Severe blunt injuries to the chest are life-threatening emergencies. These include sudden compression of the chest due to being thrown against a steering wheel in an MVA. These closed injuries cause an increase in pressure inside the chest, which can result in *pulmonary contusions, myocardial contusions,* or *traumatic asphyxia.*

The signs and symptoms of pulmonary (lung) contusions are as follows:

- Severe shortness of breath
- Rapid pulse
- Extensive, obvious bruising of the chest wall

The signs and symptoms of myocardial (heart) contusions are as follows:

- Generalized chest pain
- Obvious bruising of the chest wall
- Rapid, sometimes irregular, pulse

When traumatic asphyxia occurs, blood is forced the wrong way out of the heart—from the right side instead of the left. It is then forced back into the veins, particularly the veins of the head and shoulders. The signs and symptoms include:

- Shock
- Distended neck veins
- Bloodshot, protruding eyes
- Cyanotic tongue and lips
- Coughing up or vomiting blood
- Swollen, cyanotic appearance of the head, neck, and shoulders

Guidelines for emergency care are the same as described earlier in the chapter. Note that these conditions are dire emergencies. Time is critical. Be sure the paramedics have been notified and updated.

Broken Ribs

Rib fractures are not common in children. In adults, direct blows and blunt trauma to the chest often result in broken ribs. The ribs most often broken are those in the middle of the rib cage. Upper ribs are difficult to break because they are protected by the bony shoulder girdle. When the upper ribs are broken, suspect severe internal injuries. The lower ribs are floating. They are not attached to the sternum. So, they have more ability to move and a greater ability to withstand impact.

Common complications of rib fracture include the following:

- *Pneumothorax*—an accumulation of air in the pleural cavity (The pleural cavity is the space between the *visceral pleura,* a membrane that covers the outer surface of the lungs, and the *parietal pleura,* a membrane that covers the internal chest wall.)
- *Hemothorax*—an accumulation of blood in the pleural cavity
- *Subcutaneous emphysema*—a condition in which air escapes into body tissues, especially in the chest wall, neck, and face

- *Lacerated intercostal vessels*—torn and cut blood vessels that surround the ribs
- *Lung contusions*
- *Injuries to the liver or spleen*

The most common symptom of a broken rib is pain at the fracture site. It usually hurts the patient to move, cough, or breathe deeply. The patient will likely want to hold a hand over the area since stabilization often offers some pain relief (Figure 21–3). Other signs and symptoms may include the following (Figure 21–4):

- Grating sound upon palpation
- Chest deformity
- Shallow, irregular breathing
- Crackling sensation near the suspected fracture site (subcutaneous emphysema)
- Bruising or lacerations at the suspected fracture site
- Frothy blood at the nose or mouth, indicating that a rib may have punctured a lung

The greatest priority of emergency care is to make sure the patient can breathe adequately. Give the patient a pillow or blanket to hold against the broken ribs for support. Apply a sling and swath to hold the patient's arm against the injured side of the chest.

If the patient is alert, allow him or her to assume a position of comfort. Some EMS systems recommend placing the patient on the injured side. Do not bind, tape, or use other methods that encircle the chest. They may impair breathing.

Flail Chest

Flail chest, a closed chest injury, results when the chest wall becomes unstable due to fractures of the

BROKEN RIBS

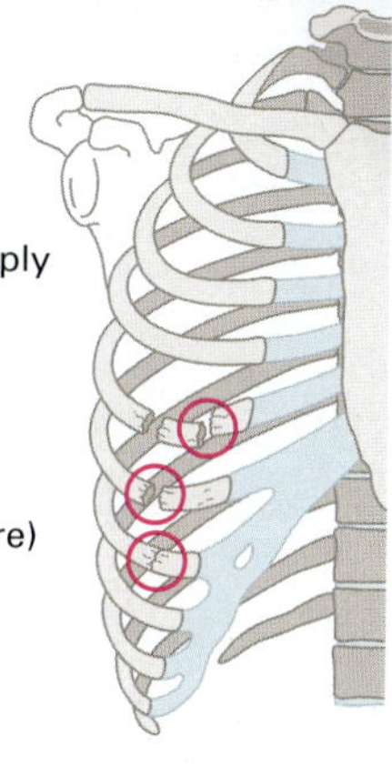

Figure 21–4 Signs and symptoms of broken ribs.

sternum, fractures of the cartilage connecting the ribs to the sternum, or fractures of the ribs. Flail chest can affect the front, back, or sides of the rib cage. It most often occurs when two or more adjacent ribs are broken, each in two or more places (Figure 21–5).

In flail chest, an area of chest wall between the broken ribs becomes free floating. This area is referred to as the **flail segment**. Its motion is opposite the motion of the rest of the chest (Figure 21–6). When the patient inhales, the flail segment collapses or does not expand. When the patient exhales, the flail segment protrudes while the rest of the chest wall contracts. This condition is called **paradoxical breathing**. (You may not notice paradoxical breathing since the chest muscles may spasm and splint the chest.)

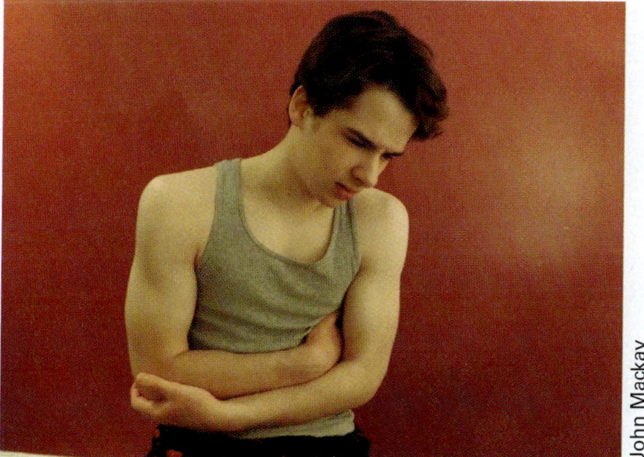

Figure 21–3 Typical upright guarding position for broken ribs.

John Mackay

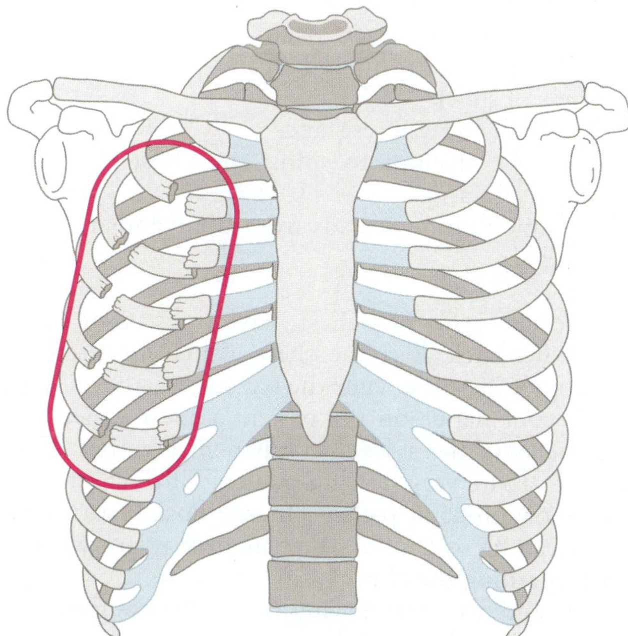

Figure 21–5 In flail chest, two or more ribs are fractured, each in two or more places.

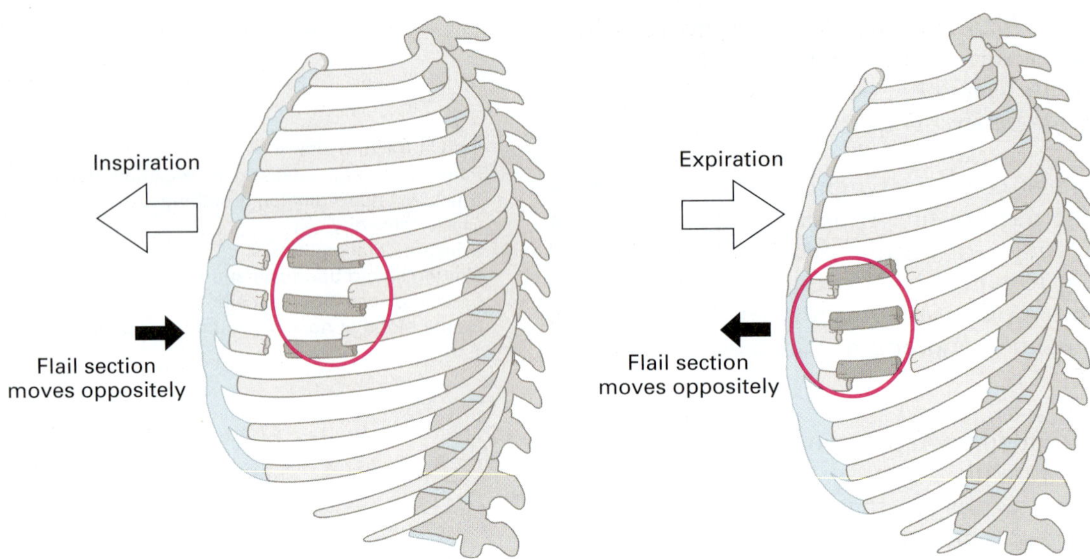

Figure 21–6 In flail chest, a free-floating segment of the chest wall moves in the opposite direction to the rest of the chest.

Flail chest can be a life-threatening injury. It usually involves bruising of the lung tissues beneath the flail segment and can lead to inadequate oxygenation of the heart. Fractured ribs can also puncture a lung. Flail chest may involve serious bleeding within the thorax from the arteries and veins between the ribs. This can lead to shock.

The signs and symptoms of flail chest include the following:

- Shortness of breath
- Paradoxical breathing, which is almost always accompanied by severe pain
- Swelling over the injured area
- Signs of shock
- Increasing airway resistance
- Patient's attempt to splint the chest wall with hands and arms
- Possible grating sounds from bone ends rubbing together

To check for flail chest, have the patient lie on his or her back. Bare the chest. Watch for a see-saw motion of the chest while the patient breathes. Gently place your hands on the patient's chest. Check for symmetry of the sides as the patient breathes. Note that it can be very difficult to detect flail chest in an obese or muscular patient. In addition, because flail chest can be so painful, the patient may not want to stop guarding the chest.

In addition to following the guidelines for emergency care of chest injuries described above, you must try to splint the chest. It will help improve respirations. First, remove all clothing from the chest area. Then, tape a small pillow or thick, heavy dressing over the injury site. The dressing should weigh less than 2 kg (Figure 21–7).

If you suspect internal bleeding or if there is increased pain and discomfort, have the patient lie on the injured side. However, do so only if there is no possibility of spinal injury.

Open Chest Injuries

All chest injuries are serious. However, open chest injuries pose an additional problem because they upset the delicate balance of pressure between the inside and outside of the chest. It is vital for you to identify and treat open chest injuries immediately. Remember that the chest cavity has a front, side, and back. Injuries to the back may also penetrate the chest cavity.

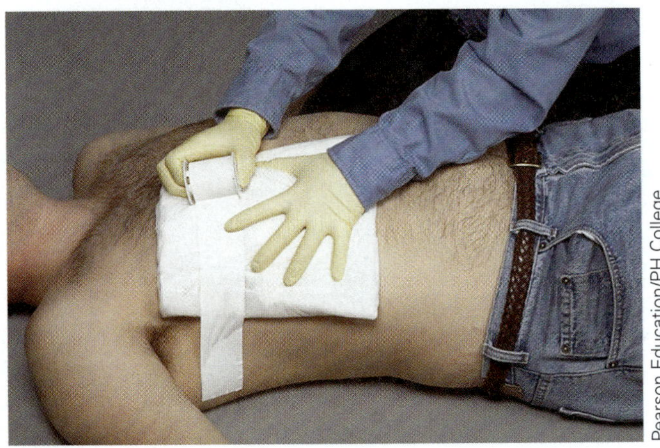

Pearson Education/PH College

Figure 21–7 Stabilize flail chest by applying a pillow or bulky dressing.

Sometimes an open wound to the chest or back bubbles or makes a sucking noise. Such a wound is typically called a **sucking chest wound**. However, even if a chest wound does not bubble or make a sucking noise, treat it as if it has penetrated the chest cavity.

> ## (!) T I P
>
> Closely monitor breathing in a patient with an open chest wound and remember that a patient with an entrance wound may also have an exit wound requiring your attention.

Guidelines for Emergency Care

Treatment for both an open chest injury and a closed one are basically the same. However, there is one very important difference. You must apply an occlusive dressing to a sucking chest wound (Figure 21–8). The dressing should be at least 5 cm larger than the wound on all sides and should be large enough not to be sucked into the wound. Seal the dressing on three sides, leaving the fourth side unsealed. The open side of the dressing acts as a relief valve, which allows air to escape but prevents air from entering the chest cavity (Figure 21–9).

If you have to improvise an occlusive dressing, do not use household plastic wrap. It is not strong enough. If necessary, use material such as a plastic

DRESSING A SUCKING CHEST WOUND

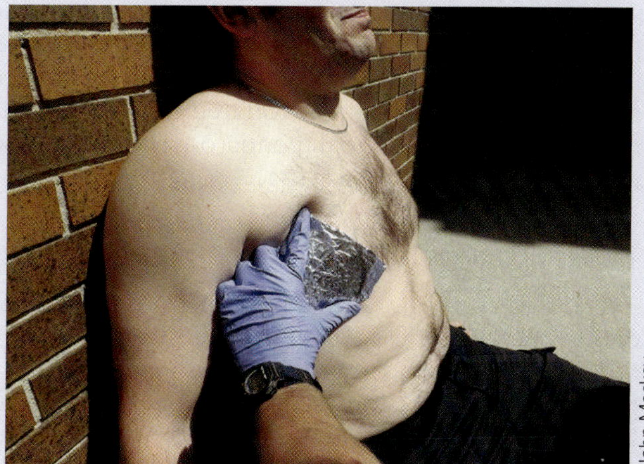

Figure 21–8a Position an occlusive dressing in direct contact with the chest wall.

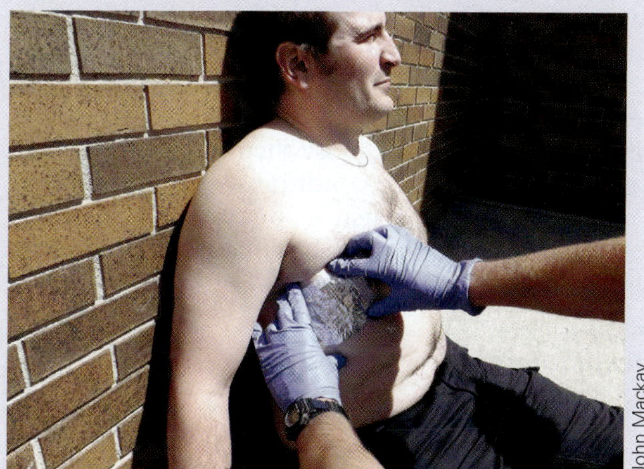

Figure 21–8b Tape the occlusive dressing on three sides.

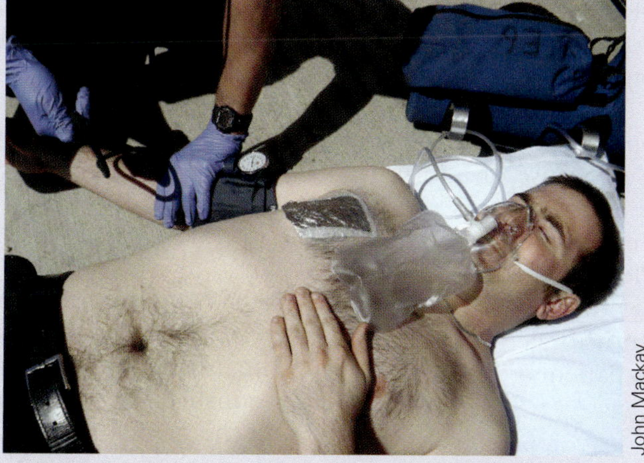

Figure 21–8c Position the patient to help ease breathing.

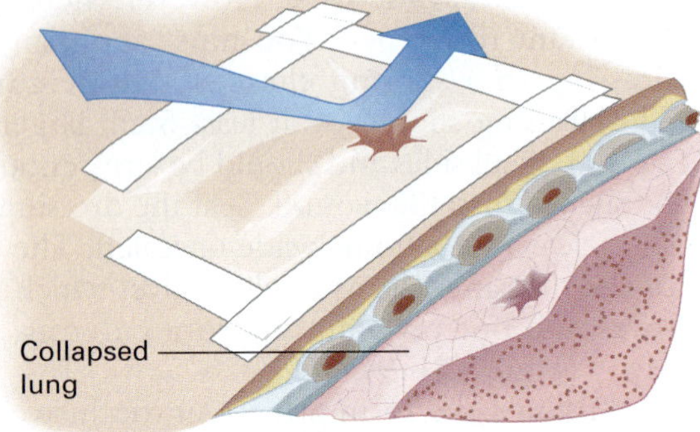

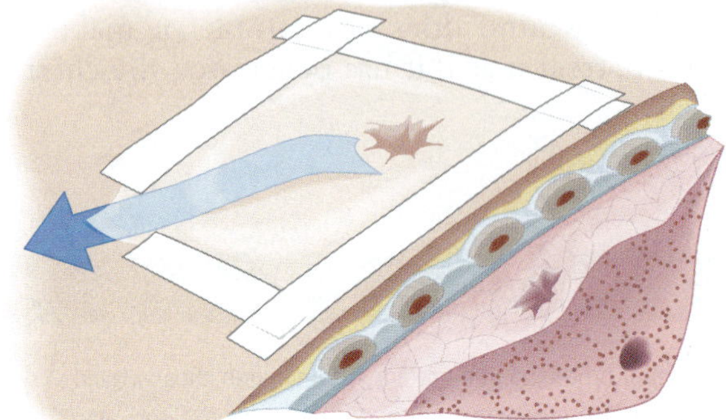

Figure 21–9 Occlusive dressing with a relief valve for a sucking chest wound.

bag. If you have no other choice, use aluminum foil or Vaseline gauze held in place with a pressure dressing.

If the patient develops increased respiratory distress after application of an occlusive dressing, release the seal immediately. The increased distress usually means pressure is building up within the chest cavity.

There are three conditions that occur inside the chest cavity as a result of an open or closed chest injury. It is not necessary to diagnose them. EMR care is the same for all. The three conditions—pneumothorax, hemothorax, and tension pneumothorax—are presented below to improve your understanding of chest injuries (Figure 21–10).

Pneumothorax

Pneumothorax occurs when air from a wound site enters the chest cavity but not the lungs. The pressure of the air in the chest presses against a lung, separating it from the chest wall and causing it to collapse. The volume of the lung is reduced, resulting in respiratory distress.

Air can enter the chest cavity in one of two ways. It can enter from a sucking chest wound that allows air to enter from the outside, or air can leak out of a lung laceration. Once the lung is ruptured, it does not expand properly.

In some cases, called spontaneous pneumothorax, the lung does not collapse because of injury. It collapses because the patient has a weak area on the surface of the lung that ruptures. The weakened lung loses its ability to expand. The patient then experiences sharp chest pain and mild to severe respiratory distress. Spontaneous pneumothorax is common among smokers or emphysema patients.

Hemothorax

Hemothorax occurs when the pleural space fills with blood, creating pressure on the heart and lungs. The lungs cannot expand, and the same process occurs as

with pneumothorax. In addition, severe bleeding can cause shock.

Hemothorax is the result of blunt or penetrating trauma to the chest. It can occur with closed chest wounds as well as open ones. It often accompanies pneumothorax. The blood usually originates from lacerated blood vessels in the chest wall or cavity. In rare cases, it results from a lacerated lung. The severity of the hemothorax depends on the amount of blood lost into the pleural space.

Tension Pneumothorax

Tension pneumothorax is one of the most life threatening chest injuries. Air continuously leaks out of a lung and becomes trapped in the pleural space. A process of compression starts and worsens with each breath, until the lung on the affected side is reduced to the size of a small ball, sometimes only a few centimetres in diameter.

Even after the lung is as compressed as it can be, air continues to leak into the pleural space potentially causing the trachea to shift toward the uninjured side. Pressure continues to rise and may then compress major blood vessels, the heart, or the opposite lung. The extreme pressure in the chest cavity prevents blood from returning to the heart through the veins, and blood is no longer pumped out. Death can occur rapidly.

Penetrating Injury

Penetrating injuries are open chest wounds in which the chest wall is torn, typically by a foreign object. The most common injuries are caused by stabbing or a gunshot. In addition to the possibility of lacerating the great vessels in the chest, penetrating injuries can result in massive bleeding, sucking chest wounds, pneumothorax, hemothorax, or laceration of the heart and lungs. A penetrating injury can be fatal. Surgery is generally required.

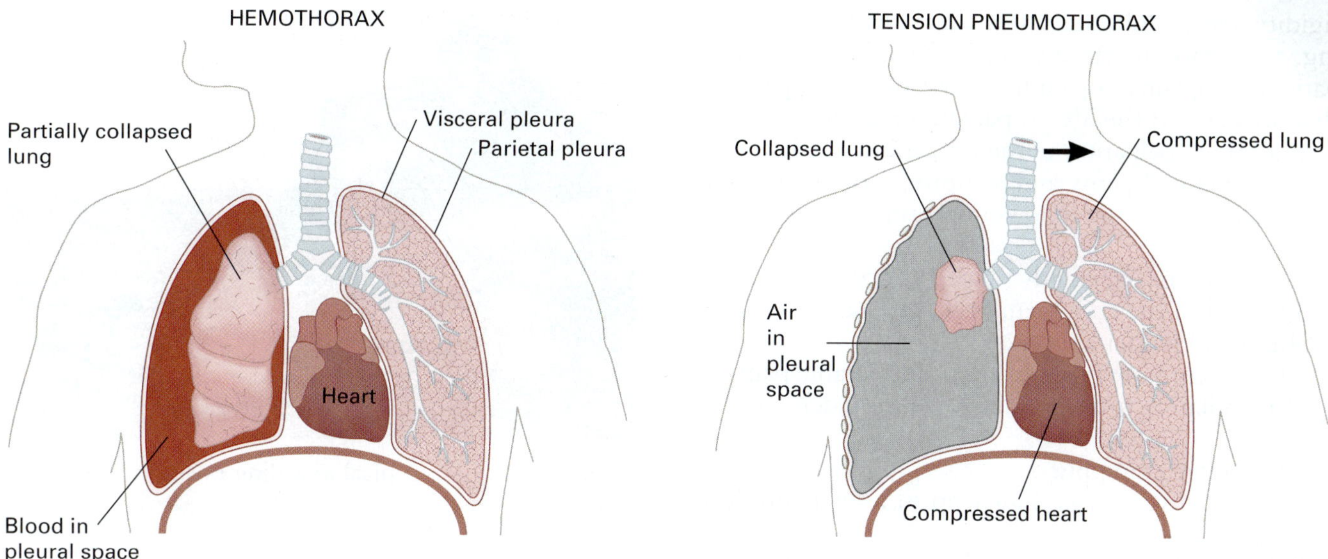

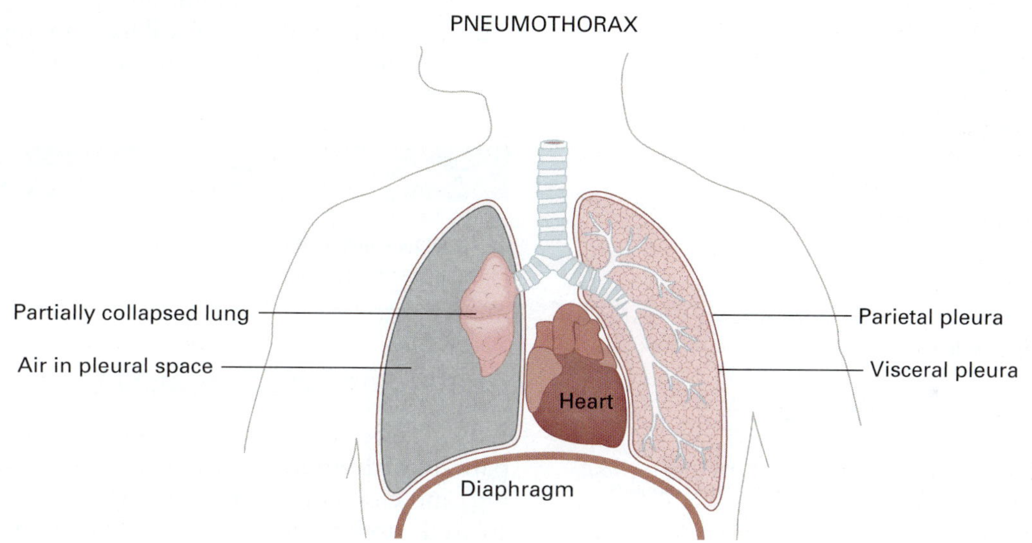

Figure 21–10   Complications of chest injuries.

To provide emergency care, follow the guidelines already discussed for open chest wounds.

SECTION 2
INJURIES TO THE ABDOMEN

Now is a good time to review the four quadrants of the abdomen as described in Chapter 4.

Patient Assessment

Suspect abdominal injury in patients involved in fights, falls, and MVAs. Injuries can range from severe bleeding and shock to evisceration. Look for the most common symptom of abdominal injury—pain.

A wound that penetrates the skin and abdominal cavity is dangerous. Internal bleeding may occur. Bacteria may be introduced into the abdomen from the outside and from a penetrated intestine. In the presence of open wounds in the abdomen, assume that organs have been damaged.

In closed abdominal injuries, a severe blow or crushing injury does not break the skin. Such wounds may be extremely dangerous. Serious injury to the internal organs, internal bleeding, and shock may occur.

To assess for a closed abdominal injury, have the patient lie down on his or her back. The knees should be flexed and supported. Remove or loosen clothing over the abdomen. Then look and feel for signs of injury. Look for bruising, lacerations and other open wounds, impaled objects, and protruding organs. Watch how the abdomen moves as the patient breathes. Gently feel all four quadrants. Note rigidity, pain, and tenderness. Also note any guarding, a common reaction to a painful abdomen. If the patient complains of pain in a particular area, palpate that area last. If the area is palpated first, it may prevent accurate palpation of the remaining quadrants.

The general signs and symptoms of an injured abdomen include the following (Figure 21–11):

- Distended or irregularly shaped abdomen
- Bruising of the abdomen, back, or flanks
- Rigid and tender abdomen
- Mild discomfort progressing to intolerable pain
- Pain radiating to a shoulder, both shoulders, or the back
- Abdominal cramping
- Lying still with legs drawn up in a fetal position (Figure 21–12)
- Rapid, shallow breathing
- Rapid pulse, low blood pressure
- Open wounds, penetrating wounds
- Nausea, vomiting
- Evisceration
- Blood in the urine, vomiting of blood
- Shock
- Weakness
- Thirst

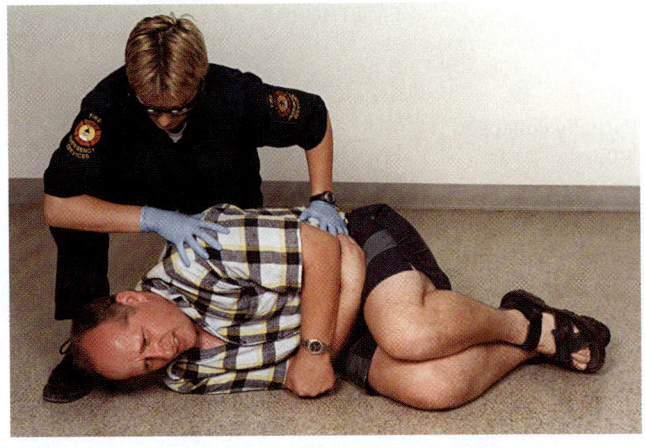

Figure 21–12   Typical guarding position when lying.

Remember to communicate with empathy. Your attitude toward the patient will have an impact, so put his or her needs first. Stay calm, cool, and sympathetic.

> (!) **T I P**
>
> Maintain a high index of suspicion so as not to be fooled by the subtle morbidity of a closed abdominal injury.

Guidelines for Emergency Care

As with any other patient, your top priorities for a patient with abdominal injuries are airway, breathing, and circulation. Once the ABCs are assessed and treated, update or activate the paramedics immediately to arrange for transport.

Provide the following emergency medical care:

1. *Maintain an open airway.* Be alert for vomiting. Position the patient for adequate drainage. Be prepared to suction. Do not give the patient anything to eat or drink.
2. *Expose the abdomen.* Remove all clothing from the abdominal area to allow proper assessment.
3. *Suspect and treat for shock.* Work diligently to prevent it. Keep the patient warm, but do not overdo it. Administer high-concentration oxygen if you are allowed to.
4. *Control external bleeding.* Dress open wounds with dry, sterile dressings or follow local protocol.
5. *Position the patient.* The patient is usually most comfortable lying on his or her back with the knees flexed. If possible, elevate the feet. If you suspect a pelvic fracture, prevent movement. Immobilize the patient on a long backboard if possible.

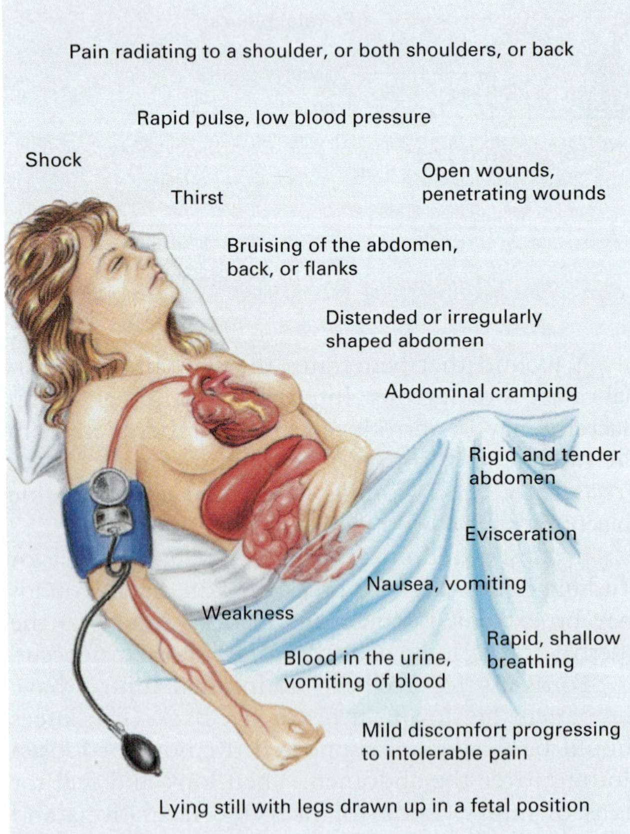

Figure 21–11   Signs and symptoms of abdominal injury.

If there is abdominal evisceration, you must cover the exposed organs (Figure 21–13). Never touch the exposed organs. Never try to reposition them. Instead, use a thick, moist, sterile dressing to cover them completely. You can moisten the dressing with sterile saline. Never use as dressings absorbent materials such as toilet tissue or paper towels, which can shred and cling to the organs.

Gently and loosely tape the moist dressing in place. Then loosely cover it with an occlusive dressing, such as plastic wrap or aluminum foil. If you use foil, make sure the edges do not cut exposed organs. Tape down the edges to help keep the first dressing moist and warm.

Maintain the temperature of the wound area by covering the dressing with layers of dressings, such as a particle-free bath blanket or towel. They may be held loosely in place with a bandage or clean sheet.

SECTION 3
INJURIES TO THE GENITALIA

While assessing injuries to the male or female genitalia, act in a calm, professional way. Protect the patient from onlookers. Use sheets, towels, or other material as a drape over the area. Provide the same emergency care as for any other soft-tissue injury, with a few exceptions described below. (Now is a good time to review the reproductive systems as described in Chapter 4.)

Male Genitalia

Injuries to the external genitalia of a male can cause severe pain, though they are not usually life threatening.

DRESSING AN ABDOMINAL EVISCERATION

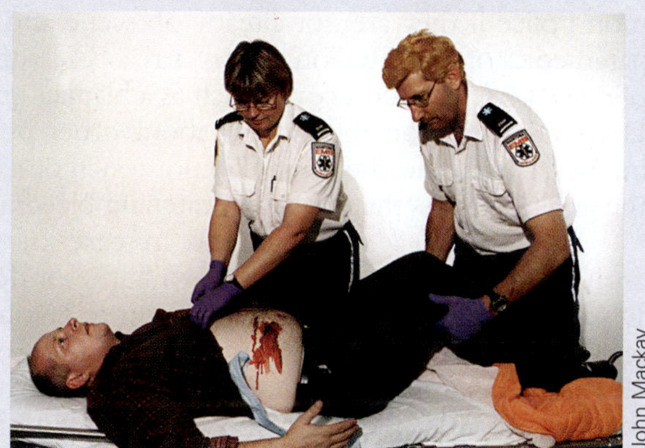

Figure 21–13a   Cut away clothing.

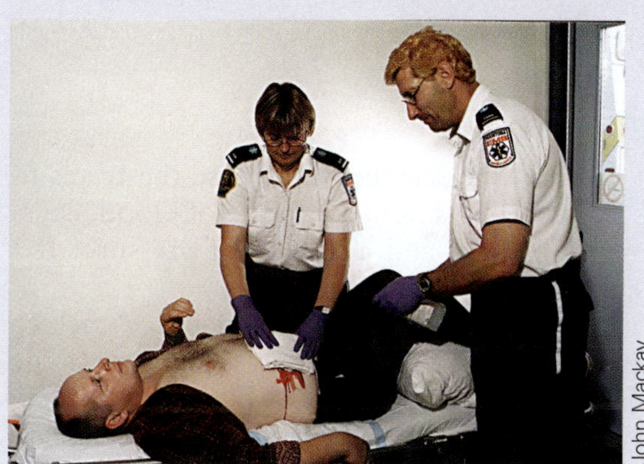

Figure 21–13b   Cover the exposed organs with a moist, bulky dressing.

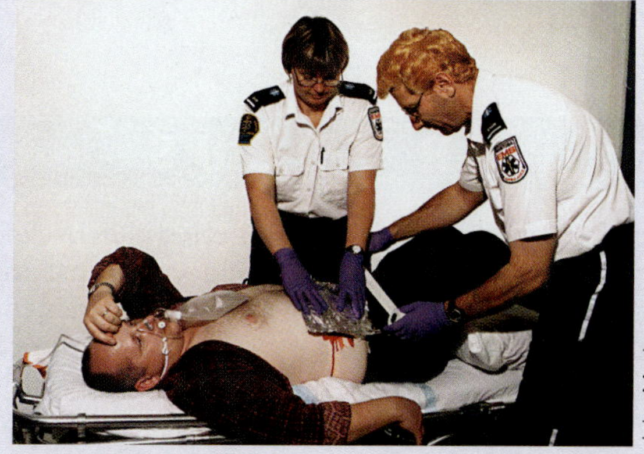

Figure 21–13c   Secure an occlusive dressing over the bulky one.

Penis

The skin of the penis can be torn or avulsed. Such injuries occur most commonly in accidents and assaults. To give emergency care, do the following:

1. Wrap the injured penis in a soft, sterile dressing that is moistened with sterile saline solution.
2. Apply a cold pack to relieve pain and reduce swelling.
3. Never remove impaled objects. Instead, stabilize them and bandage them in place.
4. If you can find avulsed skin, wrap it in sterile gauze that has been moistened with sterile saline. Send it with the patient to the hospital.

In some cases, the penis may be partially or completely amputated. Blood loss may be significant. If so, apply a sterile pressure dressing to the remaining stump to control the bleeding. Aggressive direct pressure may be needed also. If you can find the amputated penis, follow the usual procedure for preserving and transporting amputated parts with the patient.

Scrotum and Testicles

A direct blow to the scrotum can cause the testes to rupture. It can also result in a pooling of blood, causing tremendous pain and a feeling of pressure. If a testicle ruptures, it requires surgery.

To care for this emergency, apply an ice pack to the entire area to reduce swelling and pain. If the scrotal skin becomes avulsed, try to find it. Then wrap it in moist, sterile gauze. Send it with the patient to the hospital. Dress the scrotum itself in a sterile dressing moistened with sterile saline. Control the bleeding with pressure.

Female Genitalia

Injuries to the internal female organs are rare. That is because they are small and well protected, except during pregnancy when the uterus is enlarged. These injuries can result in serious blood loss and shock.

Injuries to the external female genitalia can follow straddle injuries or sexual assault. Because the area is richly supplied with blood vessels and nerves, injuries can cause severe pain and bleeding. However, they are not usually life threatening. To provide emergency care, do the following:

1. Control the bleeding with local pressure using compresses moistened with sterile saline.
2. Dress the wounds. Bandage them with a diaper-like bandage. Stabilize any impaled objects and bandage them in place.
3. Use cold packs over the dressing to relieve pain and reduce swelling. Never place anything inside the vagina.
4. Treat the patient for shock.

If you suspect sexual assault, protect the patient's privacy as you stay alert for scene safety. You should summon police if they are not already on scene and advise paramedics of the situation as they arrive. Clear the area of onlookers. Provide a cover, such as a blanket or sheet. Discreetly question the patient about other potential injuries, such as head trauma. Do not touch or examine the genitals unless there is life-threatening bleeding.

To help preserve evidence in case of sexual assault, do not allow the patient to bathe or douche. Discourage the patient from washing her hair or cleaning under her fingernails. If possible, do not clean any wounds. Handle the patient's clothing as little as possible. Bag all items of clothing and other items separately. If there is blood on any item, do not use plastic bags. Traces of evidence could be less discernible if smeared together. Follow local protocol.

EMR FOCUS

Injuries to the chest and abdomen are potentially very serious. The emergency care you give to the patient, such as applying an occlusive dressing, is vital. Another component of quality care is immediate transport to a hospital, preferably a trauma centre if one is available.

It is your responsibility to activate and update the paramedics when you have a patient with either of these serious conditions. The responding crew will begin to prepare even before they reach the scene, so your call will help expedite care. You may also be asked to help with spinal immobilization and other tasks that will help the paramedics get to the hospital faster.

Do not transport the patient in your EMR vehicle. The patient will benefit from the additional care he or she will receive from the paramedics.

Remember that the care you give is important, but prolonged scene downtimes will hurt rather than help. The care that will ultimately save the patient occurs in the hospital.

CASE STUDY FOLLOW-UP

At the beginning of this chapter, you read that EMRs were on the scene with a female patient with an open chest wound. To see how the chapter skills apply to this emergency, read the following. It describes how the call was completed.

PRIMARY ASSESSMENT *(Continued)*

Our immediate priorities were to evaluate the patient's ABCs and seal the chest wound. Fortunately, there were two of us. My partner, Meg, talked to the patient, explaining who we were and what we were doing. The patient was alert but in a lot of pain. Meg applied oxygen by non-rebreather mask. I applied an occlusive dressing.

Our general impression was that of a conscious female patient who was in a potentially serious condition. We updated the paramedics over our portable radio.

SECONDARY ASSESSMENT

The patient reported that she had been struck over the head, stabbed, and kicked by a gang of teens. We realized that this was a significant mechanism of injury, so Meg stabilized the patient's head while I began a head-to-toe exam. I got as far as the abdomen when the paramedics arrived.

PATIENT HISTORY

We didn't have time to get much of a history.

ONGOING ASSESSMENT

The paramedics arrived before we could reassess the patient.

TRANSFER OF CARE

Our hand-off report was as follows:

"This is Andrea MacPurne. She is 30 years old and was assaulted during a robbery. Multiple teens struck, kicked, and stabbed her. She is alert, with a strong pulse and adequate respirations. She has a good bump on the left side of her skull. She has a stab wound to the chest to which we have applied an occlusive dressing. We just got to her abdomen and found it reddened. It looks like she took some punches or kicks there as well. We applied oxygen. We didn't get to the history or vitals."

The paramedics understood. There were important things to do. They, too, realized the urgency and quickly immobilized the patient and prepared for transport. Meg and I later found out that the woman's wounds were mostly superficial and that she recovered well.

Always rely on the mechanism of injury, a high index of suspicion, and a careful physical examination to assess any trauma patient. Early recognition and prompt emergency treatment of injuries to the chest and abdomen can save a life.

NOCPs

4.3 e Conduct respiratory system assessment and interpret findings **S**

g Conduct gastrointestinal system assessment and interpret findings **S**

h Conduct genitourinary/reproductive system assessment and interpret findings **A**

i Conduct integumentary system assessment and interpret findings **S**

j Conduct musculoskeletal assessment and interpret findings **S**

6.1 d Provide care to patient experiencing signs and symptoms involving genitourinary/reproductive systems **S**

o Provide care to trauma patient **S**

REVIEW QUESTIONS

Page references where answers may be found or supported are provided at the end of each question.

SECTION 1

1. What are the major signs and symptoms of an injury to the chest? (pp. 314–315)
2. If a patient's chest is injured—even if the skin is not broken—what serious underlying damage should you suspect? (p. 314)
3. What are the general guidelines for emergency care of a patient with a closed chest injury? (p. 316)
4. What is the emergency medical care of a patient with blunt injuries to the chest, compression injuries to the chest, or traumatic asphyxia? (p. 316)
5. What are some of the possible complications of a rib fracture? (pp. 316–317)
6. What are the signs and symptoms of a rib fracture? (p. 317)
7. How can you recognize flail chest? In addition to following the general guidelines for emergency care of chest injuries, what must you do to help this patient? (pp. 317–318)

8. How should you dress a sucking chest wound? What can you do if the patient develops increased respiratory distress after dressing? Explain your answers. (pp. 319–320)

SECTION 2

9. What are the general signs and symptoms of an injured abdomen? (p. 322)
10. What are the general guidelines for emergency care of a patient with abdominal injuries? (pp. 322–323)

SECTION 3

11. How should you provide emergency care to a patient with an injury to his penis? (p. 324)
12. What are the emergency care guidelines for injuries to the female genitalia? (p. 324)
13. What actions and precautions should you take with a suspected sexual assault patient? (p. 324)
14. Why should plastic bags not be used to bag a patient's clothes if there is blood on them from a sexual assault? (p. 324)

22

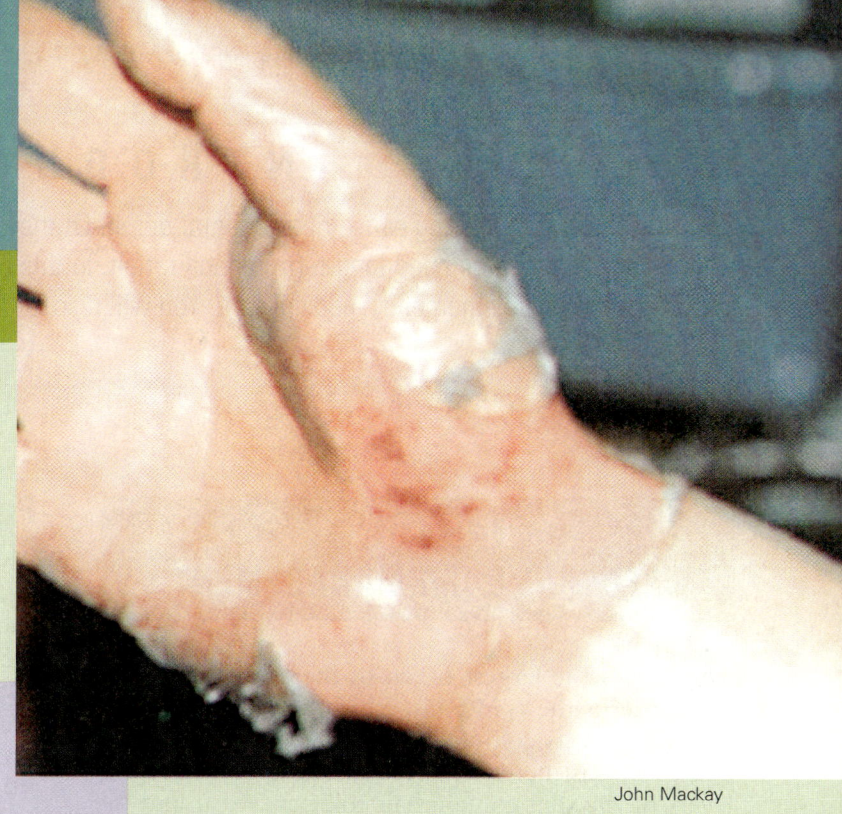
John Mackay

Burn Emergencies

OBJECTIVES

1. Describe the three severities of burns and their relationship to the depth of burn and body surface area.
2. List the areas of the body to which burns are considered more critical.
3. Outline the steps in the emergency care of burns.
4. Establish the relationship between airway management and patients with burns and describe the treatment for inhalation injuries.
5. Describe the emergency medical care for a patient with chemical burns and for one with electrical burns.
6. Demonstrate a caring attitude toward the patient and family when dealing with burns, while giving priority to the interests of the patient.

INTRODUCTION

Burns are a leading cause of accidental death. Of the people who are burned each year, many die and many more need long-term rehabilitation. In this chapter, you will learn how to assess burns and provide emergency medical care. You will also learn about the common causes of burns.

SECTION 1
GENERAL BURN MANAGEMENT

The skin is the largest organ of the body. Its outermost layer is the epidermis, which contains cells that give the skin its colour. The dermis, or second layer, contains a vast network of blood vessels. The deepest layers of the skin contain hair follicles, sweat and oil glands, and sensory nerves. Just below the skin is a layer of fat called **subcutaneous tissue**. (See Figure 4–13 in Chapter 4 for an illustration.)

The function of the skin includes protecting the deep tissues from injury, drying out, and invasion by bacteria and other foreign bodies. It helps regulate body temperature, partly by perspiration of water (and various salts). It also acts as the receptor organ for touch, pain, heat, and cold. When the skin is damaged by burns, some or all of its functions may be compromised or destroyed.

Patient Assessment

Always make sure the scene of a burn accident is safe before entering it. If the emergency involves noxious fumes, chemical spills, or electricity, call for specialized personnel to secure the scene before entering it. Never try to rescue people trapped in a fire unless you are equipped and trained to do so.

Most burn patients who die in the pre-hospital setting die from a blocked airway, inhaled toxins, or other trauma, not from the burn itself. As with all patients, perform a primary assessment. After you have assessed the ABCs and taken care of all life threats, determine the severity of your patient's burns (Table 22–1).

The severity of a burn depends on many factors, including the following:

- Depth of the burn
- Extent of body surface burned
- Which part of the body was burned
- Other complicating factors

TABLE 22–1		
DETERMINING SEVERITY OF BURNS		
Severity of Burn	**Adults**	**Infants and Children**
critical	Full-thickness burns involving the hands, feet, face, or genitals Burns associated with respiratory injury Full-thickness burns covering more than 10 percent of body surface area (BSA) Partial-thickness burns to more than 30 percent of BSA Burns complicated by painful, swollen, deformed extremity Burns encompassing any body part (for example, arm, leg, or chest)	Any full-thickness burn greater than 10 percent of BSA Any partial-thickness burn greater than 20 percent BSA Burns involving the hands, feet, face, airway, or genitals
moderate	Full-thickness burns of 2–10 percent of BSA (excluding hands, feet, face, genitals, and upper airway) Partial-thickness burns of 15–30 percent of BSA Superficial burns to more than 50 percent of BSA	Partial-thickness burns to 10–20 percent of BSA
minor	Full-thickness burns of less than 2 percent of BSA Partial-thickness burns to less than 15 percent of BSA	Partial-thickness burns of less than 10 percent of BSA

CASE STUDY

Dispatch

It was raining hard that day. As soon as we got back to the station house, my partner and I checked in and readied our truck for the next call. Before long, we were dispatched to a man hit by lightning.

Scene Assessment

Upon arrival at Costanza's Farm, we were met by a woman who told us the patient had been moved into the barn. We drove up to the building, took BSI precautions, and approached the patient.

Primary Assessment

My partner immediately stabilized the patient's head and neck. I found the patient conscious to painful stimuli only. The primary assessment revealed a patent airway, respirations that were adequate and of good quality, and no visible bleeding. We elected to place the patient on oxygen at 15 L/min by way of a non-rebreather mask. We also noted a feathery pattern of markings scattered over the patient's left arm.

Our general impression was of a middle-aged male who was conscious only to pain after being hit by lightning.

> What else should be done to assess his condition? What is the proper emergency medical care? Consider this patient as you read Chapter 22.

Depth of Burns

Burns are typically classified by depth (Figure 22–1). A **superficial burn** involves only the first layer of skin. A **partial-thickness burn** involves the epidermis and the dermis. In a **full-thickness burn**, the burn extends through all the layers of skin and may involve subcutaneous tissue, muscles, organs, and bone. Note that burns are seldom only one depth. They usually involve a combination.

You can recognize superficial, partial-thickness, and full-thickness burns as follows:

- *Superficial burns* (Figure 22–2). A superficial burn is caused by flash, flame, scald, or the sun. It is the most common of all burns and is considered minor. The patient's skin surface will be dry, and there may be some swelling. Though the skin is red and painful, the burn involves only the epidermis. A superficial burn heals in two to five days with no scarring. Peeling of the burned skin may occur. Some temporary discoloration may result.

- *Partial-thickness burns* (Figure 22–3 on p. 331). This type of burn usually results from contact with hot liquids or solids, flash or flame contact with clothing, direct flame from fire, contact with chemicals, or the sun. The skin appears moist and mottled, ranging in colour from white to red. The burn area is blistered and intensely painful. It usually requires 5 to 21 days to heal. If infection occurs, healing time can take longer.

- *Full-thickness burns* (Figure 22–4 on p. 331). A full-thickness burn results from contact with hot liquids or solids, flame, chemicals, or electricity. The skin is dry and leathery and may be a mix of colours from white to dark brown to charcoal. Often charred blood vessels are visible. While it can be very painful, the patient may feel little if nerve endings have been destroyed. Small, full-thickness burns require weeks to heal. Large ones, which may need skin grafting and other specialized burn care, can take months or years to heal. These burns often result in scarring.

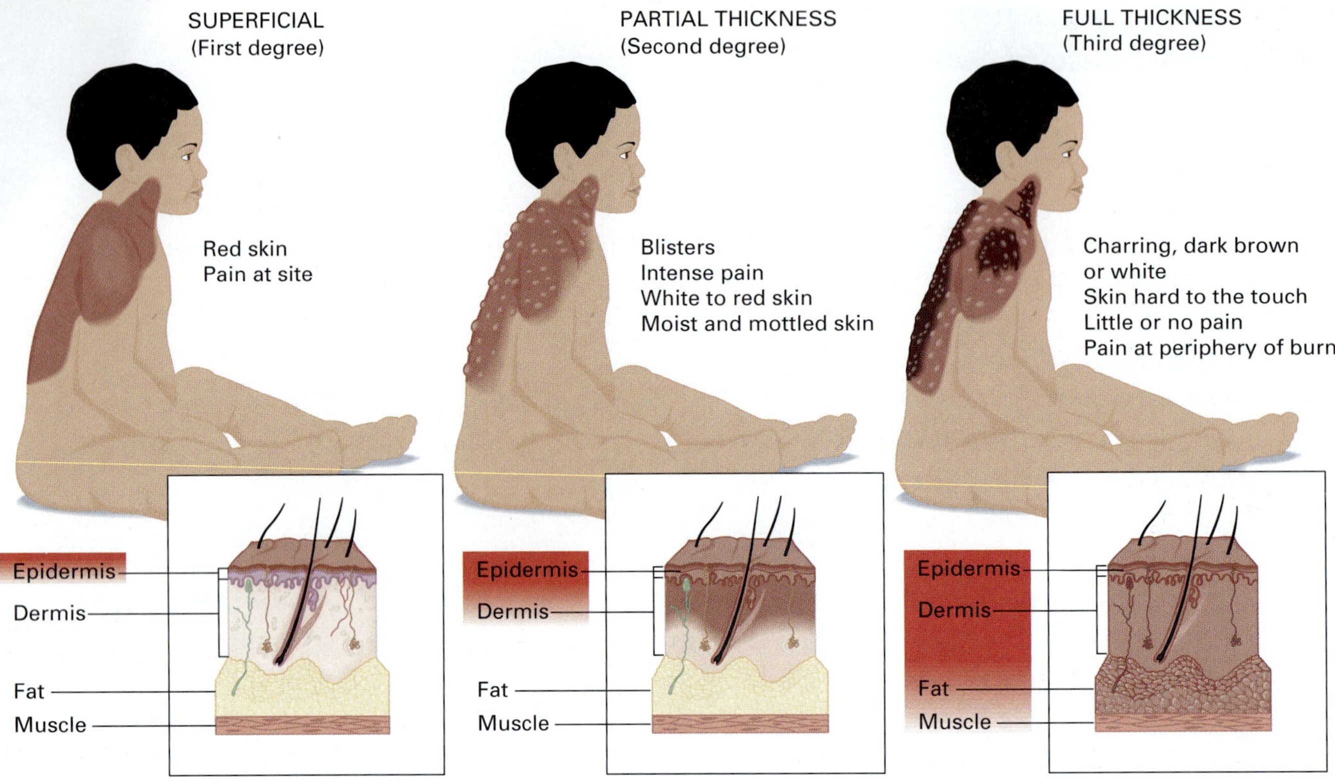

Figure 22–1 Classification of burns by depth.

Extent of Body Surface Burned

The **rule of nines** is a standardized way to estimate the amount of **body surface area (BSA)** burned. The head and neck region is considered 9 percent of the total body surface area. The posterior trunk is 18 percent. The anterior trunk is 18 percent. Each upper extremity is 9 percent, and each lower extremity is 18 percent. In an infant, the head is considered 18 percent of BSA, and each lower extremity is 14 percent of BSA. External genitalia are estimated as 1 percent of BSA in all patients (Figure 22–5 on p. 332).

An alternative method is called the **palmar surface method**. With this method, use the palm of the patient's hand—approximately 1 percent of the BSA—to estimate the size of a burn. For example, if a burn area is equal to seven palms, the burn would be estimated as 7 percent of BSA.

You will find it useful to use the rule of nines to estimate the BSA of larger burn injuries and the palmar surface method for smaller burns. Follow local protocols. However, do not spend time trying to determine a burn's exact percentage of BSA. Slight differences in percentages will not affect proper EMR care.

SUPERFICIAL BURNS

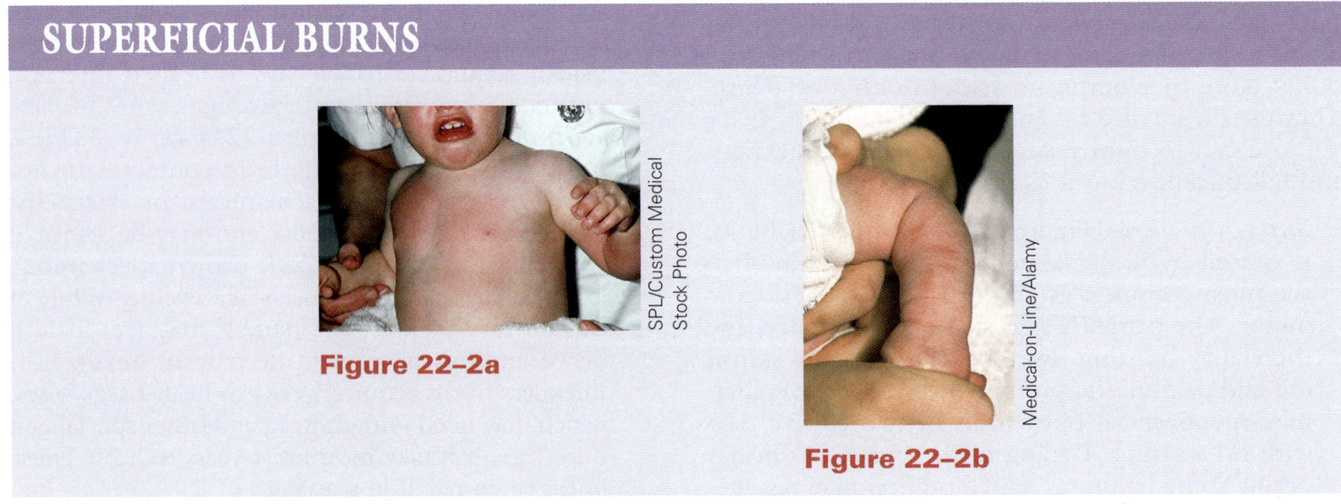

Figure 22–2a

Figure 22–2b

PARTIAL-THICKNESS BURNS

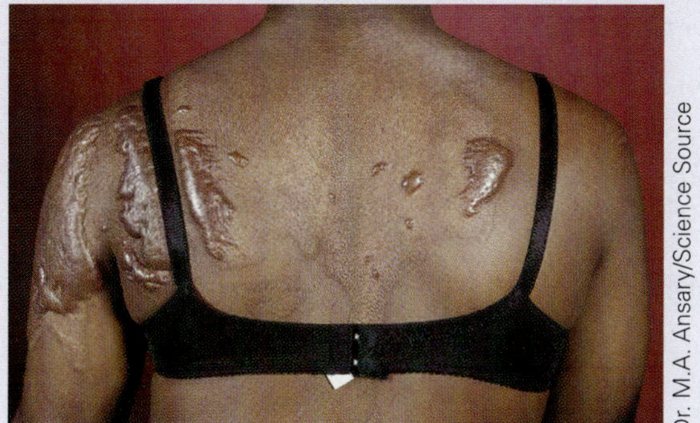

Figure 22–3a

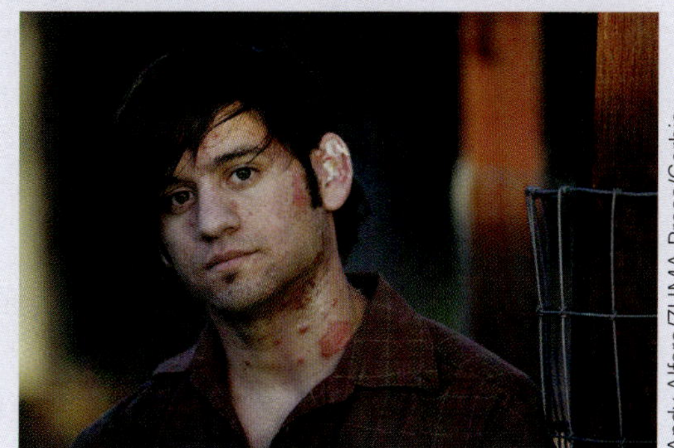

Figure 22–3b

Location of Burns

Burns to certain areas of the body are more critical than others. For example, burns to the face can compromise breathing or cause injury to the eyes. Loss of function may be the result of burns to the hands or feet. Burns to the genital area may result in loss or impairment of genitourinary function. Burns that encircle a body part, such as a joint, arm, or leg, are considered critical because of the possibility of blood vessel and nerve damage. Burns that encircle the chest can limit its ability to expand, which can result in inadequate breathing.

Arrange for patients with burns to any of these areas to be transported to a hospital or burn centre immediately.

Complicating Factors

Patients who have chronic diseases, such as heart disease or diabetes, or other injuries will always react more severely to burns, even minor ones. Therefore, try to determine the patient's medical history early in the course of care.

The age of a patient may also be a complicating factor. Children under the age of 5 years and adults over the age of 55 tolerate burns poorly. In older adults, a burn covering only 20 percent of BSA can be fatal. Because older adults and the very young generally have thin skin, they can sustain much deeper burns. Fluid loss from a burn can also affect older adults and the young more critically. Even a small fluid loss can result in serious problems. An additional problem concerns the immune system, which is immature in children and usually compromised in the older adult patient.

Please note that burns may also be the result of child abuse. Look for burn patterns that indicate a child might have been dipped in scalding water. Cigarettes are also used to burn children as a form of abuse. Follow local protocols for reporting your observations.

FULL-THICKNESS BURNS

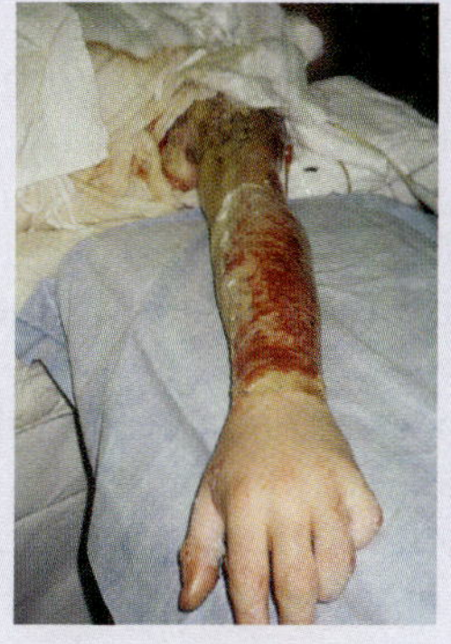

Figure 22–4a

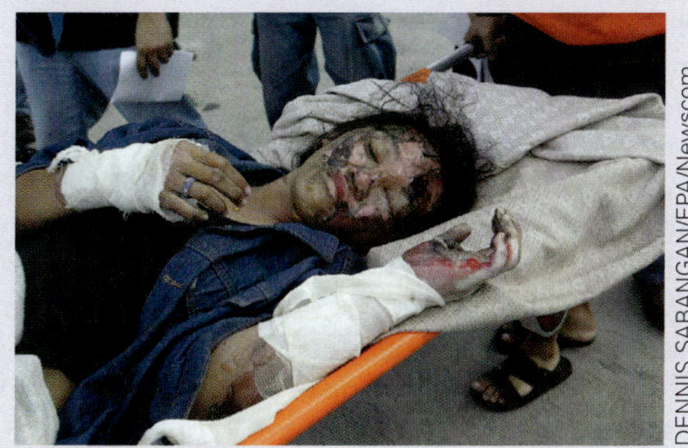

Figure 22–4b

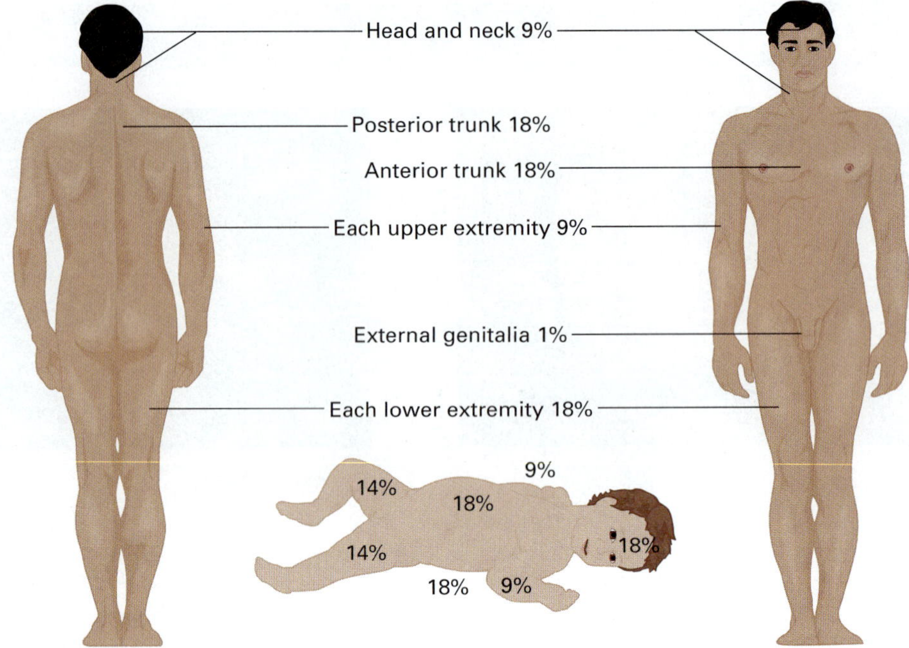

Figure 22–5 The rule of nines.

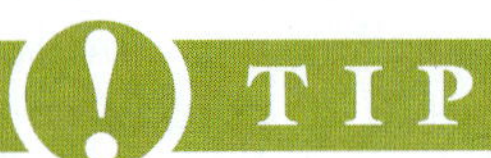

TIP

When a child anticipates or reacts to scalding burns, he or she will assume a fetal position. If you notice a burn pattern where the extremeties and chest seem strangely uninvolved, this may be indicative of abuse.

Emergency Medical Care

Once the patient has been removed from the source of the burn, provide emergency medical care. Take BSI precautions and follow these steps (Figure 22–6):

1. *Stop the burning process.* Run cold water over scald burns. Flush away chemicals with water for 20 minutes or more. Remove any smouldering clothing and jewellery. If you meet resistance, or if you see bits of foreign matter melted into the skin, cut around the area. Do not try to remove them.
2. *Perform a primary assessment.* Treat all life threats. Administer oxygen by non-rebreather mask. If your patient's breathing is inadequate, provide ventilations with supplemental oxygen.
3. *Determine the severity of the patient's burns during the secondary assessment.* Take into account the depth of burns, extent of BSA involved, location of burns, and complicating factors. Don't forget to look for other possible injuries.
4. *Cover the burns.* Use dry sterile dressings or a disposable sterile burn sheet. Do not use grease or fat, ointment, lotion, antiseptic, or ice on the burns. Do not break any blisters. If a burn involves an eye, be sure to apply dressings to both eyes (Figure 22–7).
5. *Keep the patient warm.* Treat other injuries as needed.

Proper care of burns must start as soon as possible after the injury. Loss of body fluids, pain contributing to shock, swelling, and infection may quickly follow a burn injury. Be especially alert to any sign of breathing difficulty. If the burns were caused by an electrical source, monitor the patient closely for cardiac arrest. Be prepared to administer CPR and, if you are trained and equipped, to apply an SAED. Remember that the patient's status can change suddenly, so monitor vital signs continually.

As always, do your best to calm and reassure the patient. He or she may be in a great deal of pain. The patient and family members may also be afraid of permanent scarring and disfigurement. Tell them that you are doing what is necessary to prevent further injury and contamination. Let them know that additional EMS personnel are on the way.

Also, note that patients and family members may have tried to treat the patient's burns before you arrived on the scene. Find out what they did. Include this information in your patient hand-off report. One reason why burns are so often critically damaging or even fatal is that some individuals are poorly informed about methods of care.

CARE OF BURN INJURIES

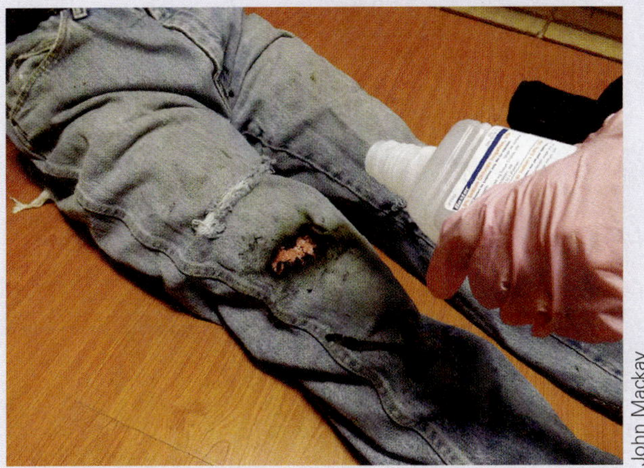

Figure 22–6a Stop the burning process.

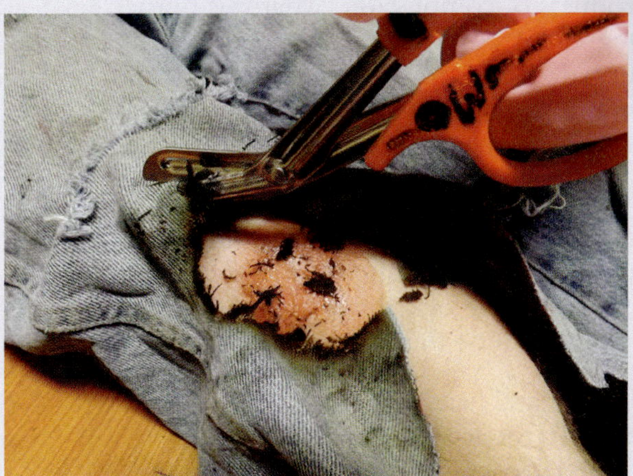

Figure 22–6b Remove all smouldering clothing.

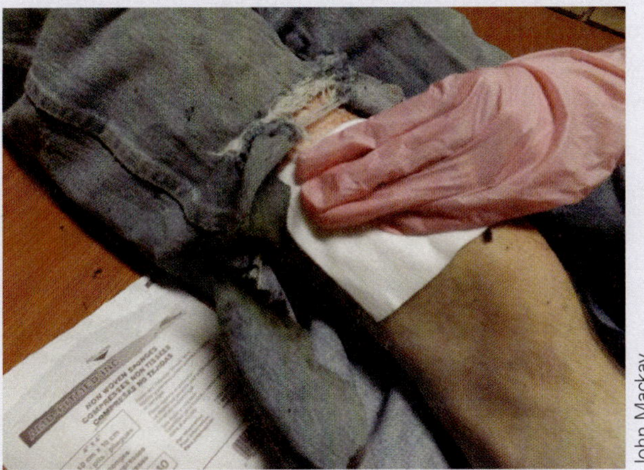

Figure 22–6c After life threats have been treated and a secondary assessment completed, cover burns with dry sterile dressings.

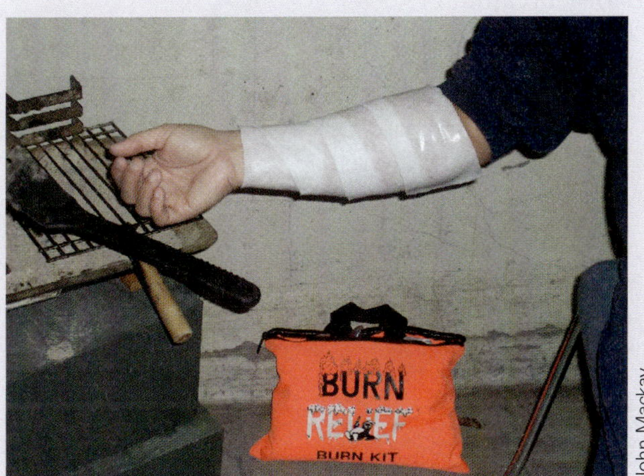

Figure 22–6d Burn dressing.

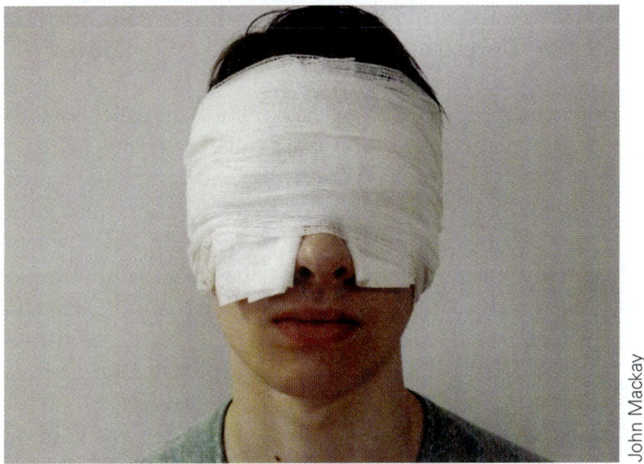

Figure 22–7 Apply dressings to both eyes, even if only one is burned.

SECTION 2
SPECIAL TYPES OF BURN INJURIES

Inhalation Injuries

More than half of all fire-related deaths are caused by smoke inhalation. About 80 percent of those who die in residential fires do so only because they inhaled heated air or smoke and other toxic gases. Smoke inhalation is the leading cause of death and a major cause of disability among firefighters. Suspect inhalation injury in any patient who was burned in a fire, especially if the patient was in an enclosed space.

The severity of an inhalation injury is determined by the following factors:

- Products of combustion (what was burned)
- Degree of combustion (how completely it was burned)
- Duration of exposure (how long the patient was exposed to the smoke or gas)
- Whether or not the patient was in a confined space

Most upper airway damage from heat inhalation consists of scorched mucous membranes and swelling, which can block the airway. Specific signs and symptoms include the following (Figure 22–8):

- Singed nasal hairs
- Burns to the face (Figure 22–9)
- Burned specks of carbon in the sputum
- Sooty or smoky smell on the breath
- Respiratory distress
- Noisy breathing
- Hoarseness, cough, difficulty speaking
- Restricted chest movement
- Cyanosis

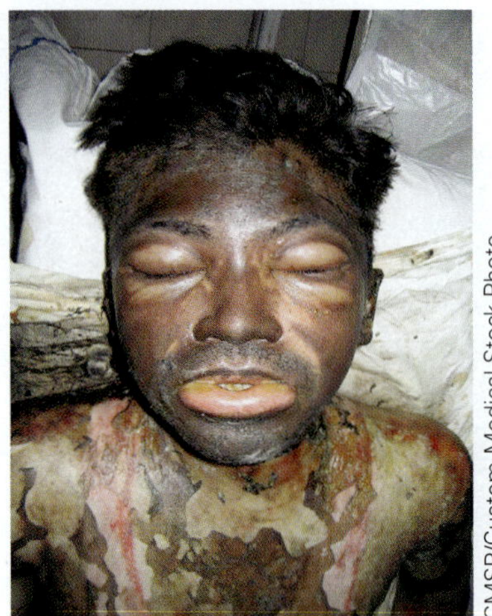

Figure 22–9 Burns to the face.

If any of these signs and symptoms are present, administer humidified oxygen if it is available. Note that this type of injury may appear to be mild at first and then become more severe. Closely monitor the patient's airway and breathing. Be prepared to assist ventilations if necessary.

> **! TIP**
>
> Carbon monoxide (CO) readily bonds with the blood's hemoglobin, and a cherry-red skin colour is a late sign of CO poisoning. Patients with acute CO poisoning require high-flow oxygenation and rapid transport to more definitive care.

Chemical Burns

It is very difficult in the field to assess the severity of chemical burns. The general guideline is to treat all chemical burns as critical. Speed is essential. The faster you stop the burning process and initiate care, the less severe the burn will be. Follow these guidelines:

- Remember scene safety. Make sure that it is safe to approach the patient. If not, wait for trained rescue personnel to arrive. When you can approach your patient, wear protective gear to avoid contamination.
- Immediately begin to flush the patient's burns vigorously with water. Do not waste time trying to find an antidote. If the patient is at home, use the shower or a garden hose. Irrigate the area continuously under a steady stream for at least 20 minutes.
- If chemical burns affect the eyes, flush them with water (Figure 22–10). Use a faucet or a hose running at low pressure. If necessary, use a pan, bucket, cup, or bottle. Have the patient remove any contact lenses.

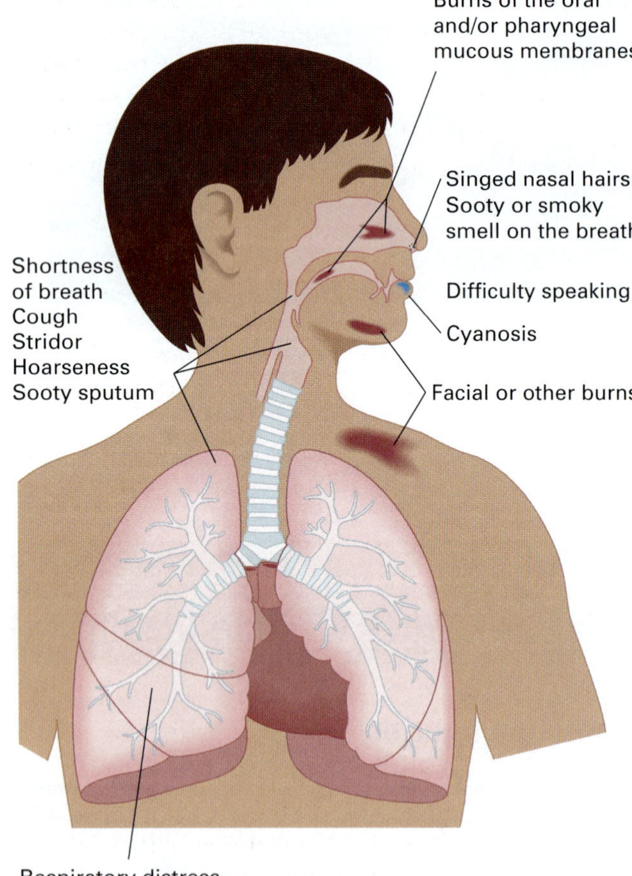

Figure 22–8 Signs and symptoms of inhalation burns.

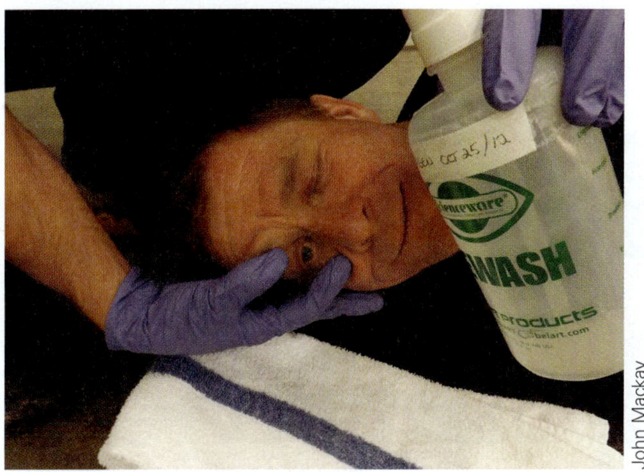

Figure 22–10 Flushing a chemical burn to the eye.

- Minimize further contamination by making sure the water runs away from the burn injury and not toward uninjured areas.

Note that you should brush off dry chemicals, such as lime powder, before flushing with water (Figure 22–11). Also, wash off phenol or carbolic acid with alcohol first and then flush the burn with water.

Electrical Burns

In any incident involving a car crash into a power pole, look for downed power lines. Sometimes they can be hidden from sight by grass or a bush. Therefore, look at the next pole down the line. Count the number of power lines at the top cross-arm. There should be the same number of lines at the top of the damaged pole. If the number is not the same, proceed as follows:

- If you suspect that lines are down, or the power pole has been weakened, notify all rescue personnel of the possible danger. Then notify the power company and request an emergency crew.
- If the soles of your feet tingle when you enter the area, go no further. You are entering an energized zone.
- Assume that a downed power line is live until the power company crew tells you otherwise. Remember that vehicles, guard rails, metal fences, and so on conduct electricity.
- If the patient's vehicle is in contact with a downed power line, tell the patient to stay inside the car. Maintain a safe distance. Never have a patient try to jump clear unless there is immediate danger of fire or explosion. Do not touch the vehicle and the ground at the same time. If you do, the current can kill you.
- Never try to remove a power line. Personnel from the power company must do it. They have the training and the proper equipment to handle the line safely.

If you approach an emergency scene involving other electrical hazards, make a visual sweep for power cords. Pull the plug before you approach or touch the patient. Remember that a power tool does not have to be on to present a shock hazard. In general, you should never try to remove a patient from an electrical source unless you are trained and equipped to do so. Never touch a patient still in contact with an electrical source.

The signs and symptoms of electric shock may include:

- Altered mental status
- Obvious severe burns
- Weak, irregular, or absent pulse
- Shallow, irregular, or absent breathing
- Multiple fractures due to intense muscle contractions

Electricity can enter one part of the body and leave from another part, so look for both entry and exit burns (Figure 22–12). Assume that there are internal injuries. Care for a patient with electrical burns (Figure 22–13) the same way you would care for any other patient with burns. However, note that an electric shock can throw a patient a significant distance. Therefore, stabilize the patient's head and neck during assessment and treatment.

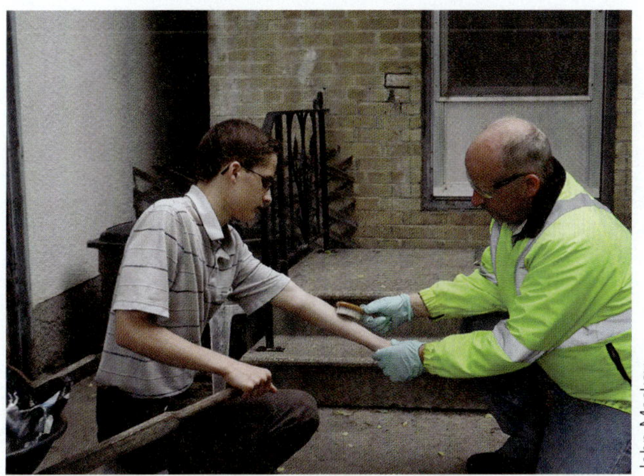

Figure 22–11 Lime powder should be brushed off the skin before flushing.

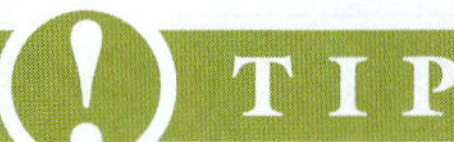

TIP

External burns do not reflect the true nature of an electrical injury. The path of the current between the entrance and exit wounds through the body can cause severe damage to organs, tissues, and other internal anatomy.

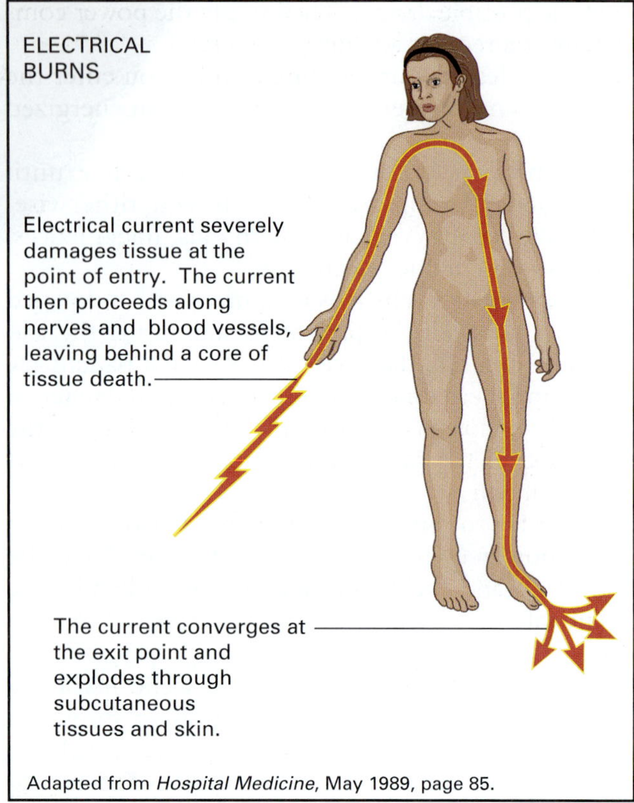

Figure 22–12   Look for an entry burn and an exit burn.

Lightning Injuries

Hundreds of electrical injuries occur each year in Canada. About 25 percent of them are lightning injuries (see Figure 22–14). A lightning bolt can pack more than a trillion watts of electricity and up to 100 million volts. Much of the electrical energy from lightning flows around, not through, a strike victim. A patient who has been struck by lightning does not hold a charge, so it is safe to approach him or her.

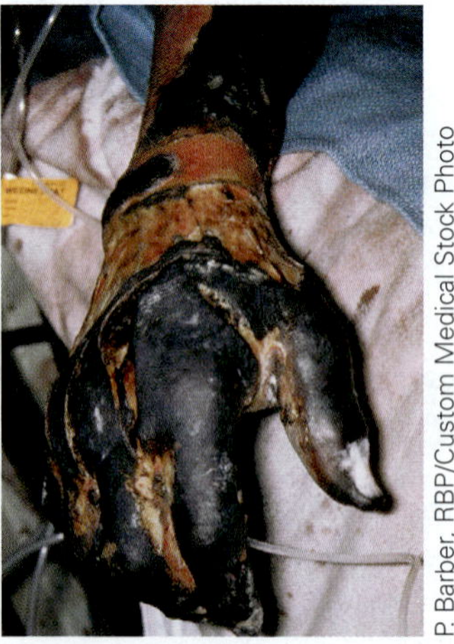

Figure 22–13   Full-thickness electrical burn.

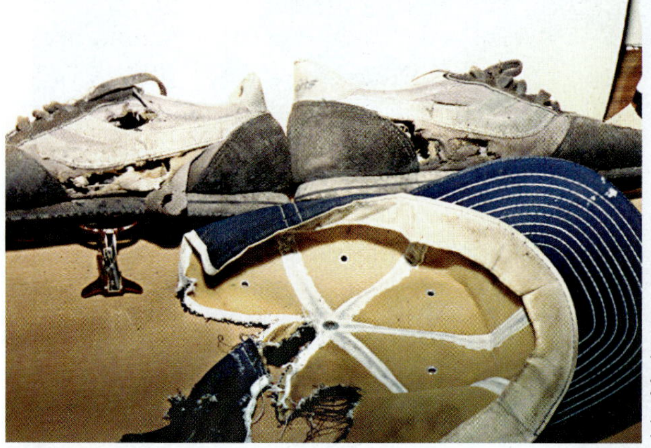

Figure 22–14   Hat and shoes from a lightning strike victim.

People are struck by lightning most often in open fields, under trees, on or near water, near tractors and heavy equipment, on golf courses, and while using landline telephones. A person may be struck directly by lightning, or lightning may splash off a nearby object. Whole groups of people can be affected by a ground strike in which lightning hits the ground and electricity ripples outward.

Most victims of lightning are knocked down or thrown, so assume possible spinal injury. Also, assume that a victim of lightning has sustained multiple injuries. Patients generally sustain the following types of injury:

- *Nervous system*. In many instances of lightning strike, the patient becomes unconscious. Few actually remember being struck. Some patients suffer partial paralysis. Occasionally, paralysis of the respiratory system causes death.
- *Senses*. Some patients experience loss of sight, hearing, and the ability to speak. Rupture of one or both eardrums (tympanic membranes) occurs in 50 percent of patients who have been struck by lightning.
- *Skin*. In a lightning burn, the skin may appear feathery, patchy, or as a scattered pattern resembling flowers. This is called ferning. The burn may be red, mottled, blue, white, swollen, or blistered. The ferning fades and disappears within days.
- *Heart*. The lightning strike itself can disrupt the heart's rhythm, but it is the complications that follow that generally lead to full cardiac arrest.
- *Vascular system*. Within seconds following the lightning strike, the patient may become unconscious, appear pale and mottled, have cool arms and legs, and lose pulses. If the injury is moderate, the conditions may correct themselves quickly. In case of severe injury, blood may coagulate, and tissues in the arms and legs may die, leading to a need for amputation. Kidney failure may also result from severe injury.

Care for lightning burns as you would any other type of burn. You should also provide manual stabilization of the patient's head and neck during emergency care and be prepared to provide basic life support. Such measures should continue even if the patient appears to be lifeless. Victims of lightning have been resuscitated as long as 30 minutes after a strike without any lasting damage.

EMR FOCUS

Burns can be painful, disfiguring injuries. The care you provide as an EMR will be vital to the patient's survival. The most critical complication of burns is the most difficult to observe. Burns to the airway can cause swelling and obstruction, which can lead to inadequate breathing or respiratory arrest. Monitor the patient very carefully for these conditions.

Safety is also a primary concern. The source of the burn (such as flames or chemicals) and a smoke- or vapour-filled environment can be a danger to EMRs. Have people who are properly trained and equipped remove the patient from a hazardous scene. Then begin emergency medical care.

CASE STUDY FOLLOW-UP

At the beginning of this chapter, you read that EMRs were on the scene with a male patient who had been hit by lightning. To see how the chapter skills apply to this emergency, read the following. It describes how the call was completed.

SECONDARY ASSESSMENT

While my partner maintained manual stabilization and monitored breathing, I conducted a head-to-toe exam. I found an entrance burn on the patient's left arm and a larger exit burn on his left foot. There appeared to be no other injuries. I covered the burns with sterile gauze. After I took a set of vital signs, which were within normal ranges, the patient moaned and tried to sit up. We encouraged him to lie still and explained what had happened.

PATIENT HISTORY

The patient was still somewhat confused, so we interviewed witnesses to the incident. They related that the man had been walking to his barn when he was struck by a lightning bolt. They knew of no medical problems or allergies. We found no medical identification tags or cards.

ONGOING ASSESSMENT

We took the patient's vital signs every five minutes or so until the paramedics arrived. There were no changes noted. His oxygen was continued without resistance. When the patient became more alert, he told us his name was Sam Costanza and gave us a brief medical history.

TRANSFER OF CARE

My hand-off report to the paramedics was as follows:

"This is Sam Costanza. He is 42. He was struck by lightning as he approached his barn some 20 minutes ago. Initially, he responded only to painful stimuli. He presented with good respirations and heart rate. During the secondary assessment, he slowly became conscious. He remembered nothing about what happened to him. The secondary assessment revealed full-thickness burns on the left arm and left foot. We covered them with sterile dressings. He says he has no significant medical history. His respirations are 20 and of good quality, pulse 90 and strong, blood pressure 140/82. His pupils are equal and reactive. His skin is warm and dry."

After the paramedics took over, we returned to our duty station and prepared our truck for the next call.

Treat all burn injuries in basically the same way: Stop the burning process, remove smouldering clothing, and dress the wounds. However, your job may not be finished there. After the primary assessment and treatment of life threats, be sure to perform a thorough secondary assessment to find and treat other injuries the patient may have. Gather a good patient history, and continue with ongoing assessment until the paramedics arrive to take over patient care.

NOCPs

3.3 a Assess scene for safety **S**
b Address potential occupational hazards **S**

4.2 f Obtain information regarding incident through accurate and complete scene assessment **S**

4.3 a Conduct Primary patient assessment and interpret findings **S**
b Conduct Secondary patient assessment and interpret findings **S**
c Conduct cardiovascular system assessment and interpret findings **S**
d Conduct neurological system assessment and interpret findings **S**
e Conduct respiratory system assessment and interpret findings **S**

i Conduct integumentary system assessment and interpret findings **S**
k Conduct assessment of the ears, eyes, nose, and throat and interpret findings **S**

5.6 b Treat burns **S**

6.1 n Provide care to patient experiencing signs and symptoms due to exposure to adverse environments **S**

6.3 a Conduct ongoing assessments based on patient presentation and interpret findings **S**
b Re-direct priorities based on assessment findings **S**

REVIEW QUESTIONS

Page references where answers may be found or supported are provided at the end of each question.

SECTION 1

1. When you estimate how severe a patient's burn may be, what four factors should you consider? (p. 328)

2. What is a superficial burn? Briefly describe its characteristics. (p. 329)

3. What is a partial-thickness burn? Briefly describe its characteristics. (p. 329)

4. What is a full-thickness burn? Briefly describe its characteristics. (p. 329)

5. What is the rule of nines? Describe how it is used. (p. 330)

6. What is the palmar surface method? (p. 330)

7. Are burns to certain areas of the body more critical than others? Explain. (p. 331)

8. Do age and chronic illness have anything to do with how severe the results of a burn may be? Explain. (p. 331)

9. What are the general guidelines for the emergency medical care of burns? (pp. 332–333)

SECTION 2

10. What special care would you provide if your patient had inhalation burns? (p. 334)

11. How would you stop the burning process if a dry chemical, such as lime powder, is involved? (p. 335)

12. What special precautions related to scene safety should you take if you are called to the scene of an electrical hazard? (pp. 335–336)

13. What other types of less obvious injuries might an electrical burn patient have sustained? (p. 335)

14. At what locations do lightning strikes most often occur? (p. 336)

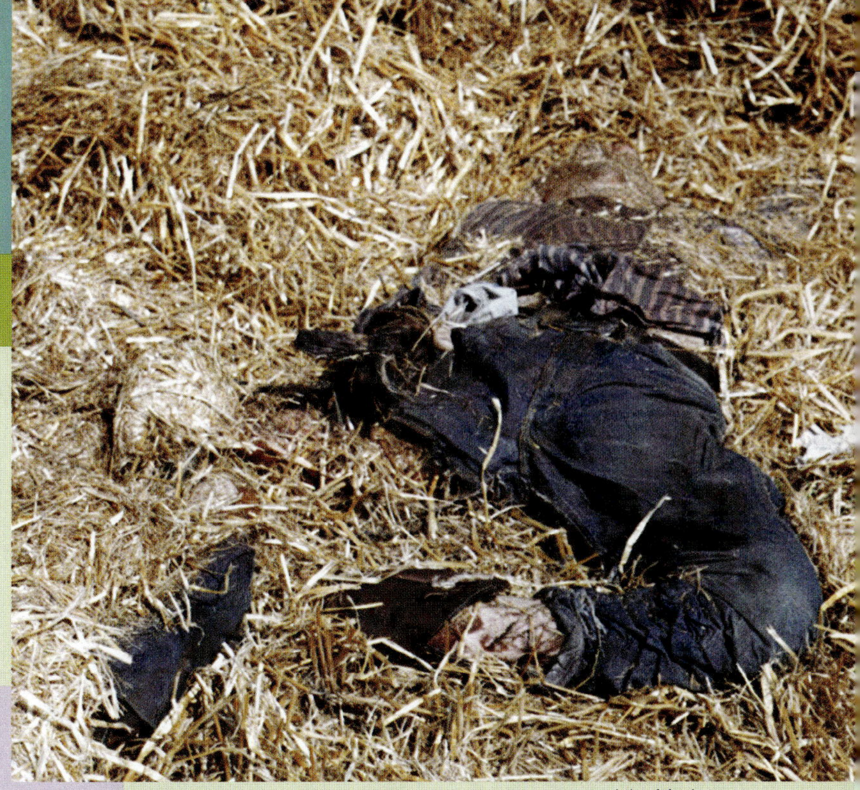
John Mackay

Agricultural and Industrial Emergencies

1. Identify seven factors involved in the high rate of injury and fatality among farmers.
2. Describe the four steps in the emergency medical care of the patient with a farm injury.
3. Identify common operational controls used on farm machinery.
4. Discuss common mechanisms of injury among agricultural workers.
5. Discuss the principles of disentanglement from farm equipment.
6. Describe how to safely approach the scene of an industrial emergency.
7. Demonstrate a caring attitude toward the patient and family when dealing with an agricultural or industrial emergency, while giving priority to the interests of the patient.

INTRODUCTION

Although more people in Canada live in cities, the death rate from accidental trauma is highest in rural areas. Agriculture involves over 300 000 people, including those in fishing and forestry. Farming is considered the nation's most hazardous occupation. The number of accidents per work hour is five times higher in agriculture than the national average for major industry. Sadly, there is little information on this topic in most EMR training, even though some form of agricultural activity exists in every province.

Farming-type injuries also occur in urban areas. For example, the pizza dough roller works on the same principles as the printing press or the agricultural combine. Workers who do snow removal, construction work, and factory work also use similar machinery and are prone to similar accidents.

SECTION 1
AGRICULTURAL EMERGENCIES

More farm workers die in work-related accidents than workers in the mining industry, construction trades, transportation, and public utilities. Why are farm accidents so serious? Consider the following:

- Most farm equipment is very complicated. As machinery becomes more sophisticated, the chances of injury increase.
- Most farmers do not use personal protective equipment.
- Farmers often use old, unsafe equipment because of the tremendous cost of replacement.
- Lengthy extrication is often needed when farmers become entangled in equipment. This can increase the severity of injuries.
- Since many farmers work alone in remote areas, they may not be missed for hours. Many farmers die from injuries that would not have been fatal if they had been discovered in time.
- There is often no phone at the scene. Many rural areas have no 9-1-1 service and no central dispatch.
- Long transport times contribute to the severity of injuries. Farms in rural areas can be long distances from hospitals.

Farmers are also under a great deal of stress. In fact, farming is rated among the top 10 percent of most stressful occupations. Farmers work long hours, often seven days a week. They rarely take breaks or vacations. They are exposed to heat, cold, and excessive noise and vibration. They also suffer the psychological stress of unstable weather conditions and financial difficulties, including unfavourable prices at harvest time.

General Guidelines for Emergency Care

Emergency care of patients with farm injuries is basically the same as for any other patient. In the case of a patient entangled in equipment and in need of rescue, follow these steps:

- Remember the priorities of airway, breathing, and circulation. Disentanglement can take up to an hour. Do not neglect the airway while the patient is being freed. If you are allowed to, administer high-flow oxygen throughout the rescue.
- If you cannot apply direct pressure to a bleeding wound, use the nearest pulse point. Sometimes the farm equipment itself helps to control bleeding by the pressure it exerts on an injury. In these cases, transport the patient while he or she is still entangled in the equipment. Most equipment can be cut to a manageable size.
- Monitor vital signs. Do it constantly so that you will not lose the patient to an undetected injury.
- Preserve amputated parts, despite their appearance. If fingers have been injured, stabilize the wrist joint. It is probably also injured.

Disentanglement requires appropriate training and assistance at the scene. Rescue should begin only when all of the following have been accomplished:

1. Farm equipment has been stabilized.
2. Engines have been shut down.
3. Other hazards, such as leaking fuel, have been controlled.
4. The patient has been stabilized.

CASE STUDY

Dispatch

When the klaxon alarm goes off, it means that an employee is caught in a baling machine. As soon as I heard it, I made sure that someone called 9-1-1. Then I went to the scene of the accident. I knew that a co-worker, Ellen, would meet me with our first-aid kit as planned.

Scene Assessment

It was quiet when I got to the scene. All equipment around the patient had been shut down. Several employees were working to set the man free. They were experts. They told me it would be a few minutes more. When I got a look at the patient, I saw he was an apprentice. He had been pulled by his sleeve into a baler. The workers who were disentangling him said it looked as if he had one or two amputated fingers.

> Consider this patient as you read Chapter 23. What may be done to assess and treat his condition?

As in any other emergency situation, attend to the feelings of the patient as best you can. Explain who you are, what you are doing, and what you plan to do. Keep the patient informed—and his or her family if they are on the scene—as you proceed with emergency care. Be the patient's liaison during extrication as well. As in any other emergency, be sure to continuously take all safety precautions. Do not let your guard down.

Common Operational Controls and Shutdown

Tractors and other farm equipment have a number of mechanisms that cause injury (Figure 23–1). They include the following:

- *Pinch points*—two objects meet to cause a pinching or pulling action
- *Wrap points*—an aggressive component moves in a circular motion
- *Shear points*—two objects move close enough together to cause a cutting action
- *Crush points*—two large objects come together to cause a crushing action
- *Stored energy*—hazards remain after machinery has been shut down

Become familiar with common operational controls. This knowledge can save you time and frustration during rescue. Some manufacturers use different symbols or colours to help the operator quickly identify controls. Colour codes include red, which indicates combined movement controls (throttle, gearshift, ground speed control). Yellow indicates auxiliary power controls (separator control, cylinder speed control, header drive control). Black indicates miscellaneous function controls.

The first step in shutting down farm machinery is to stabilize it. You can use one of several methods: block or chock the wheels, set the parking or operational brakes, or tie the machine to another vehicle. Once the machine is stabilized, shut it down as follows:

1. Enter the cab if possible. Look at the controls. Locate the ignition switch-on key and throttle lever. *If you have any doubt about how to identify the controls, do not touch them. Wait for help.*
2. Slow the engine down with the throttle. Switch off the key. If the machine is fuelled with diesel, the key may not shut off the engine. Locate a fuel or air shutoff lever. Again, if you are in doubt, do not touch the lever.
3. Pull the knob or lever to shut down the engine.
4. If you cannot shut down the engine in the cab, try the fuel tank area.
5. As a last resort, locate the fuel line or filters ahead of the fuel pump or injector pump. Interrupt the flow of fuel. Use extreme caution when cutting a fuel line. Large farm machinery can carry over 300 L of fuel.

FARM MACHINERY

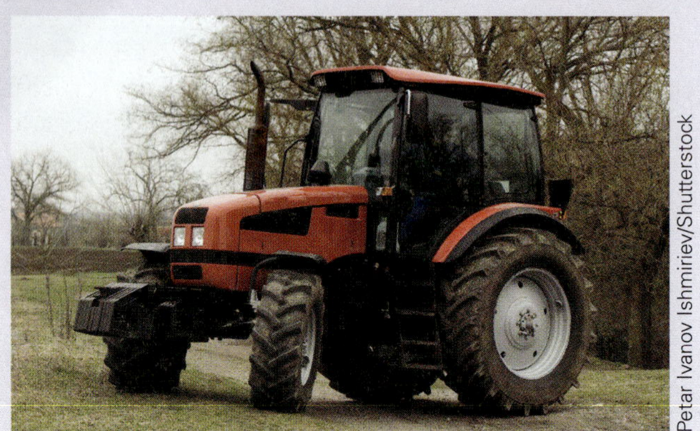

Figure 23–1a Diesel tractor.

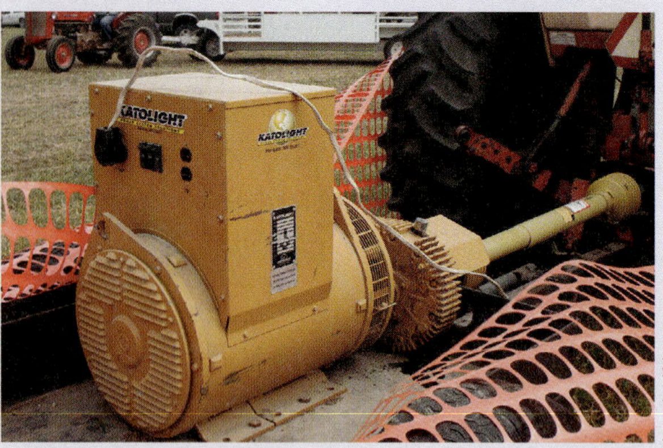

Figure 23–1b Power takeoff (PTO) shaft.

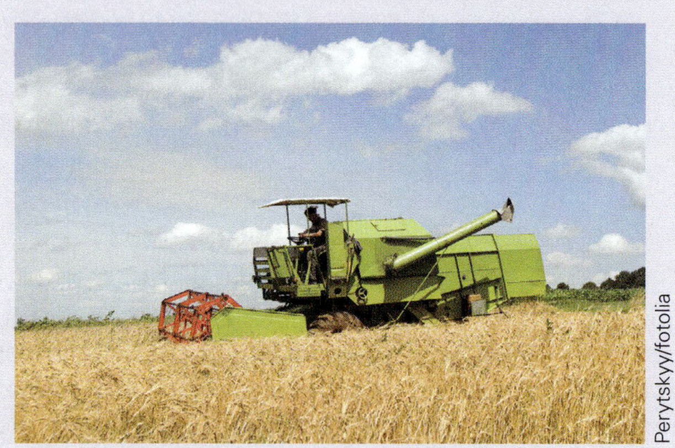

Figure 23–1c Combine with corn head.

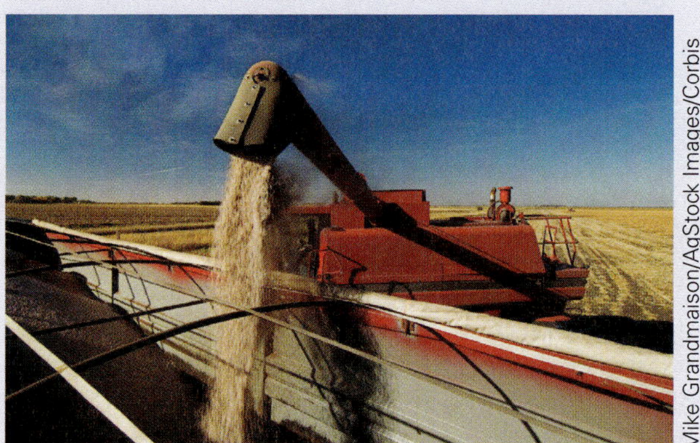

Figure 23–1d Auger and hopper with protective cage.

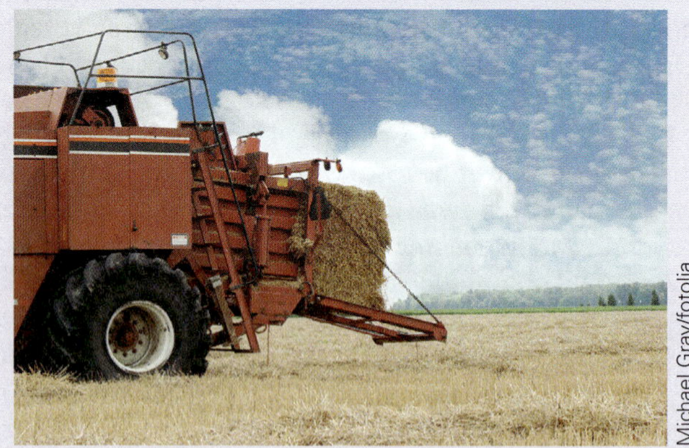

Figure 23–1e Baler for square bales.

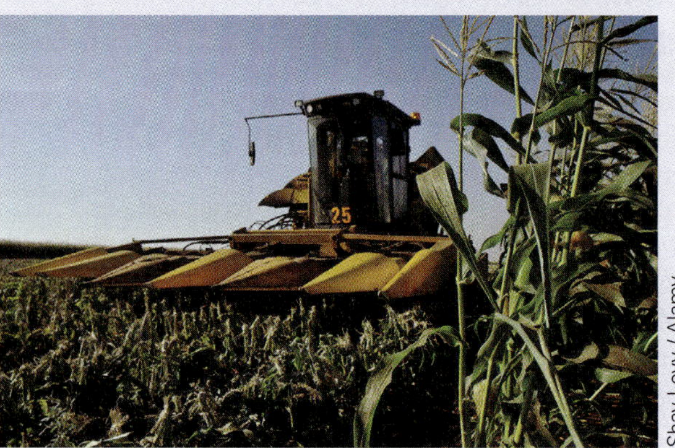

Figure 23–1f Corn picker.

6. If the engine is a diesel, loosen the fuel filter. The engine will stall.

7. If all other attempts at shutting down the machine fail, locate the air intake. Discharge a 9 kg CO_2 fire extinguisher into it. Make sure that you hold the trigger of the extinguisher until the engine comes to a complete stop. (*Warning:* This technique can cause extensive damage to the engine.)

Tractors

Tractors are the most common cause of farm-related fatalities. Most involve a tractor turning over backwards or rolling to the side. Most tractor fatalities are the result of crushing injuries.

The tractors used today fall into two categories: two-wheel drive and four-wheel drive. Engines may be fuelled by gasoline, diesel, or liquid propane. Fuel leaks, fires, and explosions can result from tractor accidents. Fire protection is critical during rescue.

Tractor Stabilization

Before rescue, a tractor engine must be shut down, the fuel controlled, and the tractor stabilized. If you are unfamiliar with the equipment, call for assistance. Local repair shops and area agriculture workers can be good resources; local farmers and neighbours may be available with expert knowledge of the machinery. Rescue teams should be capable of handling fire since there will almost certainly be spilled fuel and hot hydraulic fluid.

To stabilize the tractor, lock up the rear wheels with two one-ton or two-ton cable hoists and three chains, even if the tractor is upright:

1. Wrap one chain around the rear tire and through the high slot in the rim.

2. Wrap the second chain around the same wheel and through the low slot in the rim.

3. Attach the third chain to the front of the tractor and stretch it to a hoist.

4. Attach the other hoist to the two rear chains. If the tractor does not have slots in the rims, stretch the hoist and chains across the rear tire to a strong point on the rear of the tractor. Make sure you do not lift the secure tire off the ground during hoisting.

Patient Assessment and Emergency Care

Scene safety is a priority. Once the equipment is shut down and stabilized, reassess the area before starting patient care. When you are certain the scene is safe, assess the patient. Some points to remember follow:

- As always, determine if there is any immediate threat to life. Give aggressive management to airway, breathing, and circulation.
- Suspect possible chest injuries, including pneumothorax and sucking chest wounds. Since most tractor overturns are to the side, expect crushing injuries to the patient's head, chest, and abdomen, as well as multiple lacerations.
- Treat the patient for shock.
- Common tractor rollover injuries include burns from spilled engine coolants, transmission fluid, hydraulic fluid, and battery acid. Pay special attention to the eyes and assess for chemical burns.
- After assessment, stabilize all injuries. When there are open extremity injuries with possible broken bones, immobilize them in splints if you are trained to do so.

When possible, lift or remove the tractor from the patient once he or she is stabilized. Do not stop patient care during the lifting operations. Both efforts should continue at the same time. Be sure to call the fire crew, extrication crew, and advanced care providers as soon as possible.

Lifting Operations

During any lifting operation, a cross-crib capable of supporting the tractor must be built. This is to protect the patient and other rescuers in case the lifting devices fail or the tractor has to be let down and repositioned for another lift.

The crib should be as wide as possible. A safe rule of thumb is that the crib box should not be taller than it is wide. Also, the cribbing and lifting devices need a solid surface from which to work and function properly. This is sometimes difficult in a soft field or ditch. The rescue squad should carry several quarter-inch tread plates about 60×60 cm each. The plates will serve as a firm lifting surface on soft ground or on blacktop.

High-pressure airbags (approximately 90 to 120 psi) are the best tools available to lift a heavy, irregularly shaped machine. The bags must be placed carefully. Keep in mind the tractor's centre of gravity. It is 25 cm above and 60 cm ahead of the rear axle at the platform area where the operator places his or her feet. About 30 percent of the tractor's weight is in front of this point and 70 percent behind.

Even though airbags appear to be indestructible, they are not. Airbags are most efficient during the first 8 to 13 cm of lift. They may be stacked to get a higher lift, but they become increasingly unstable as they are inflated. Whenever possible, a cross-crib should be built to get the bag within 2 to 5 cm of the object. A steel plate should be placed between the bag and the crib to keep the crib from being knocked off during inflation.

Power spreaders or hydraulic rams also do a good job of lifting. With power hydraulic tools, the steel plate is a must for a good lifting platform. Hydraulic tools move very fast. The operator may have to wait for the crew that is building the cross-crib. The tool operator must continuously take note of the centre of gravity. He or she must also watch for unstable conditions, such as changes of angle between the lifting surface of the tool and the tractor, sinking of the tractor on the opposite side of the lift, and so on.

Hand-powered hydraulic jacks, or manual jacks, can also be used to lift a tractor. Use extreme caution if more than one jack has to be used. The cross-crib must be kept as close to the lifting device as possible. If one device becomes overloaded and fails, the other will almost certainly do the same. Cranes, wreckers, and boom trucks can also be used, if readily available, especially if you are dealing with a very large tractor. Regardless, cribs should still be built to protect the patient and rescuers from equipment failure or operator error.

When you lift or remove the overturned tractor from a patient, follow these basic rules:

- All rescuers should know exactly what their roles will be. They should also know who is responsible for hoisting commands before lifting is done. During any extrication, only one rescuer should give lifting instructions. Instructions from more than one will result in injury to rescuers and patients.
- Always try to determine the tractor's centre of gravity. Always build a crib to guard against equipment failures or operator error.
- Watch the patient during the lift to ensure that the part to be lifted is moving properly and that another part is not putting more pressure on the patient. If conditions change, the rescuer leading the lifting operation should be advised.
- Any time more than one lifting device has to be used, use extra care in coordinating the lift to keep loads from shifting.

Lifting a tractor is not like lifting an automobile. A tractor is usually heavier. (A tractor can weigh up to 15 000 kg.) It is also difficult to stabilize because of its irregular shape and because many accidents occur on soft ground. To be sure, a tractor rollover presents a difficult challenge. However, if safety precautions are taken, and if patient care and extrication are provided at the same time, this complex situation can be handled with confidence.

Power Takeoff Shafts

The power takeoff (PTO) shaft is a high-speed drive shaft that connects a tractor to farm implements, such as balers, mowers, corn pickers, forage harvesters,

and so on. It is the second most common cause of agricultural fatalities.

PTO-related accidents most often occur in fall or winter, when the farmer's heavy clothing gets caught in the shaft and pulls the farmer in. Most of these accidents involve the arms, which are usually amputated. The farmer's entire body can also get wrapped around the shaft. PTO shaft injuries are not common, but they are usually fatal.

To shut down a PTO shaft, turn off the source of power—the tractor. Some PTO shafts will freewheel in either direction when the power is shut off. Some lock up immediately. Take care, as energy can be stored in the shaft.

To disentangle the patient, do the following:

- Always assume that the patient has sustained neck and back injuries. Stabilize the patient's spine as soon as possible. Immobilize him or her before transport.
- If the patient is completely wrapped on the shaft, determine if clothing could be cut to free the patient. The PTO shaft will wrap the patient's clothing into multiple layers, making cutting difficult and time consuming. Look for the end of the wrap where clothing is only one layer thick. Cut at this point with rescue knives.
- If you must remove the PTO shaft with the patient, place a fire pry bar (over 1 m long) into the implement side of the PTO shaft to hold the stored energy. If pressure is on the coupling, the shaft will not slide apart. By reversing the shaft 2 mm, the coupling will move. Uncouple the shaft. Slide it apart. Send the section along with the patient to the hospital.
- If you cannot uncouple the shaft, cut it with a power saw, gasoline-powered circular saw, or hack saw. If nothing else will extricate the patient, cutting should be done. This procedure will release the stored energy in the shaft very quickly. Therefore, when cutting the shaft, take extreme care to prevent it from spinning. Lock the PTO shaft in place with a fire pry bar through the universal joint on both ends.
- As you remove the patient, make sure that all rescuers and bystanders stand clear to avoid further injury.
- Locate amputated parts if possible, but do not delay transport. Send the parts with the patient.

Because of the energy involved, injuries to the patient can be quite severe. The patient will need rapid treatment and transport. Aggressively control the bleeding at the site of an avulsion or amputation with trauma dressings. If advanced care is available (air transportation, ground paramedics), call for it as soon as possible.

Other Equipment

Other types of agricultural equipment include the combine, auger, corn picker, snapping rolls, and hay baler.

Combines, Snapping Rolls, and Gathering Chains

The combine is a machine used to harvest and thresh all kinds of grain. It is assembled with multiple augers, shafts, belts and pulleys, roller chains, and sprockets. Many times a farmer is injured while doing routine maintenance on the combine, such as greasing bearings or tightening belts. Combines commonly cause partial and complete amputations.

The snapping rolls and gathering chains on an older model combine (two- to four-row units) require power rescue tools and airbags, along with wooden wedges to spread the rolls. The rolls on the new models cannot be spread with conventional rescue tools. (See the "Corn Pickers and Snapping Rolls" section below.)

Just behind the combine header, and just ahead of the wheels, is a coupling device that attaches the head to the driving mechanism. This device could be a shaft with a pin in it. It could also be a set of flat gears sitting side by side with a common roller chain wrapped around them. Since it has to be released any time the head is changed, the device will be easy to get to and remove.

If you release the coupling device, you will be able to turn the header backwards slowly and keep it under control. However, because of stored energy, you may need to use a pipe wrench or large channel-lock pliers to move the shaft 2 mm forward to remove the coupling. Once the coupling has been disconnected, manual pressure on the wrench should be released with care.

Never use the self-reversing features on modern combines to remove a trapped person. The reversing feature moves too fast and for too long for you to remove a patient without causing further injury. By turning the shaft backwards, you will reverse only the head.

If the patient has been pulled into the feeder-conveyor, where the head attaches to the combine, you will have to disassemble a portion of the head and the shroud that surrounds the conveyor. This should be done by using an air chisel to cut away the sheet metal in the area.

If a torch is used, consider the fire hazards first. One spark could quickly start a fire; temporarily remove the source of supplemental medical oxygen if needed. A charged fire line should be available after the surrounding area of the field and the combine itself are washed down with water. Any remaining dust around the work area should be removed with water. Flush down the inside of the combine header and feeder house and up into the main combine.

Augers and Elevators

Combines and corn pickers are equipped with augers and elevators that move the grain through the machine. Many augers and elevators have cleanout doors and inspection covers that become traps to the unwary operator if opened while the machine is in operation.

Augers are used to move the threshed, separated, and cleaned grain from the cleaning shoe to the wagon or truck for transport. An auger is generally 10 to 30 cm in diameter with flights 8 to 28 cm apart. The elevator has a series of rubber or steel paddles attached to a drive chain that moves at over 108 m/min (metres per minute).

The power for the majority of these devices comes from the belt-and-pulley system on the combine. If a patient becomes trapped in the auger, the drive should be disconnected. Before cutting the belt or chain, place a large pipe wrench on the shaft that drives the auger. This will hold the stored energy and prevent further injuries. After the belt or chain is cut, slowly release the pressure on the shaft. Monitor the patient to be sure no further injury is being caused.

Augers can pull in victims with extreme force. They often cause complete amputation, usually of the hands and arms and sometimes of the feet and legs. Auger accidents often involve children who are not experienced enough to avoid an accident. Entanglement in augers is so severe that it often cannot be handled in the field. You may need to cut the auger free and have the patient transported with it.

If the amputation is complete, you may be able to slowly rotate the auger in its natural direction until the amputated part emerges at the end. (Never reverse an auger. It can cause increased tissue damage.) If that is not possible, you may have to dismantle the auger.

If the auger tube is held by bolts, remove them first. If not, the tube will have to be split or cut with an air chisel or a reciprocating saw. Do not use a torch. The danger of heat transfer to the patient and the threat of fire are too great. Cut a couple of metres from the patient. Look for spot welds on the flighting. Cut so that the end of the flighting nearest the patient will not spring back to cause further injury. Take care to avoid excessive vibration or movement.

Corn Pickers and Snapping Rolls

Corn pickers can be mounted on or pulled by a tractor, or they may be self-propelled. Each uses a system of rollers, chains, belts, and blades to remove corn from the stalk and then shear the corn away from the cob. Power for corn pickers is usually taken from the tractor PTO and hydraulic systems.

Corn picker accidents usually involve a hand that is crushed when a farmer tries to free trapped material in the picker. Amputation is rare, but the hand is often lost as a result of damage or infection. Extrication is extremely difficult since the machinery is in heavy metal housings and cannot be reversed.

Snapping rolls move at a normal speed of almost 4 m/s (metres per second). Generally, they can cause severe crushing injuries to the hand. Often, a weed or stalk catches between the rolls and stops them. A farmer who tries to remove the trapped material can cause the snapping rolls to start up with the slightest movement, and the rolls move more quickly than the farmer can pull back.

The majority of snapping rolls on corn pickers can be spread with the use of two wooden wedges plus a small hydraulic wedge. Use the wooden wedges for cribbing the rolls as they are separated by the hydraulic wedge. Insert one wooden wedge from the top of the rolls while the other wooden wedge is pushed in from below. Equip the bottom wedge with a rope that allows the operator to pull it through from above.

The two wedges are a must. If only one is used and the hydraulic wedge slips or is released, the one wooden wedge will be shot from the machine. If this is allowed to happen, your patient may be further injured and the rescuers jeopardized.

Snapping rolls may also be spread with the use of high-pressure airbags and two wooden wedges. The majority of power hydraulic tools may be used with the two wooden wedges. Whatever tool you use, remember some basic rules: Always use the wooden wedges for cribbing. Open the roll only as wide as necessary to remove your patient. Make sure that rescue efforts are coordinated with medical personnel.

Husking Beds

After the ears of corn pass through the snapping rollers, they enter the husking beds, one on each side of a mounted picker. The husking beds pull the leaves from the ear, exposing the kernels of corn still attached to the cob. The ear is then moved to the elevator and dropped in a wagon.

Husking beds present the greatest challenge. They are mounted on the picker with heavy-duty bearing housings (normally cast iron) and are held together with strong springs. They are also enclosed by sheet metal, which can be removed by cutting off the bolt heads with an air chisel or just by taking the machine apart with wrenches.

Once the rolls have been reached, take care to avoid uncontrolled release of the springs that hold

them together. At this point, you should release the tension-adjusting nuts or bolts. Then remove the bolts that fasten the bearing housings to the husking bed housing, again avoiding explosive release of stored energy in the springs. If you can reach the bearing housings with a power rescue tool, try to break them. However, removing the bolts by hand is the recommended and more controlled method.

Hay Baler

The hay baler compacts straw and hay into bundles. Some are small rectangular bundles. Others are massive rounded ones. The hay baler exerts forces of up to 600 kg between spring-loaded rollers. Amputations are often the result of hay baler accidents. These machines also commonly cause compression, avulsion, and wringer injuries. Because the springs can be released and the bolts cut, it is not as difficult to free a patient from a hay baler as it is from other farm equipment.

Agricultural Storage Devices

Grain Tank

Farmers who fall into the grain tanks risk death from suffocation. Always assume that a patient in a grain tank is alive, even if he or she has been trapped there for hours. Turn off electric power to the structure as soon as possible. Call the fire department and extrication teams to the scene. If advanced care providers are available, have them dispatched to the scene as soon as possible. Do not enter the structure without other rescuers to help. Any rescuer entering should be tied to a safety lifeline and be wearing a disposable mechanical filter respirator rated for dust particles.

Do not use the gravity gate or auger to release the grain. The grain flows from top to bottom, and the patient can be pulled further into the tank. Instead, cut uniform half-metre triangular holes as high as possible but still below the level of the grain. Cut in the middle of the bin sheets, avoiding the bolts, seams, and stiffeners. Open the holes simultaneously so that the grain flows out evenly. This will prevent the walls of the tank from collapsing. Once the tank begins to empty, rescuers with shovels, tractors and loads, or skid loaders may be needed to remove grain.

Once the patient is exposed, secure him or her with a lifeline. Then aggressively clear the patient's airway of grain by suctioning. After the airway has been ensured, assess for other injuries. Then a trained rescuer must fully immobilize the patient. Move the patient onto a long backboard and position a basket stretcher for extrication. A hole 60 × 60 cm can be cut at the surface of the grain to allow the stretcher to be lowered to the ground. If the grain feels cool or cold, treat the patient for hypothermia.

If the patient is only partially submerged, lower a rescuer on a harness secured with lifelines. Clear the area around the patient's head to make breathing possible and to establish an airway. Use plywood, sheets of metal, or a 250 L drum with both ends removed to keep grain away from the patient's face during extrication.

Silo

When crops are stored in silos, gas is formed by natural chemical fermentation. Fermenting crops can release high levels of carbon monoxide, methane, and nitrogen dioxide. These gases can cause serious injury or death. The presence of silo gas may be recognized by any of the following signs:

- Bleach-like odour
- Yellowish or reddish vapour hovering over the product
- Stains of red, yellow, or brown on the product or other surfaces touched by the gas
- Dead birds or insects near the silo
- Nearby livestock with signs of illness

The greatest danger of silo gas is just after harvest. However, fumes can persist and can be present when a silo is opened months later. Most silo injuries occur when a victim falls into the silo and either becomes trapped in the unloading device or is overcome by gas. Some suffer cardiac arrest in the silo.

Unfortunately, silo gas causes little immediate pain. A victim may not be aware of an injury and may die hours later because the injured lungs fill with fluid during sleep. Common reactions to silo gas include the following:

- Eye irritation
- Cough, possibly with laboured breathing
- Fatigue
- Nausea, vomiting
- Cyanosis
- Dizziness or sleepiness

Two teams are usually needed to rescue a patient from a silo. Rescuers should be lowered in and the patient lifted out through the top on a litter. Always use a self-contained breathing apparatus (SCBA) when doing rescue work at a silo.

Place an SCBA with supplementary oxygen on the patient as soon as possible. If the extrication team is delayed, or if no SCBA is available, the silo blower may be turned on to purge the air.

Be sure all patients exposed to silo gas are transported to a hospital for monitoring. Complications can develop up to 12 hours after exposure.

Manure Storage Areas

Large livestock facilities handle manure by flushing down the confinement buildings with water. The liquid is then sent to an open pond for storage. In some cases, liquid manure is stored in a structure similar to a silo. Hog farm operations are notorious for their production of methane gas as a byproduct of pig manure (Figure 23–2). Although usually well ventilated, the methane gas can accumulate in an upper airspace such as the attic. This can create both a toxic and a very combustible environment.

There are two potential injuries from liquid manure: drowning and inhaling toxic fumes. The liquid manure releases ammonia, carbon monoxide, carbon dioxide, methane, and hydrogen sulphide. Agitation of a manure pit can cause the sudden release of hydrogen sulphide. The signs and symptoms of hydrogen sulphide poisoning may include the following:

- Cough
- Irritation of mucous membranes
- Nausea
- Sudden collapse and respiratory paralysis (with high concentrations)

The primary goal of rescue is to provide ventilation to the patient. Always use backup rescuers. Always wear SCBA and lifelines. Provide aggressive airway management to the patient and, if needed, basic life support. Monitor the patient's vital signs. Treat for shock. Place the patient on high-flow oxygen. If advanced care is available (air transportation, ground paramedics), call for it as soon as possible.

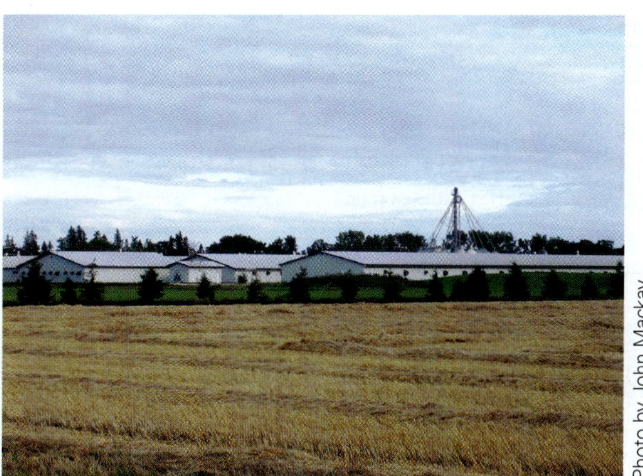

Figure 23–2 Hog farm facility.

After the patient has been pulled out from the storage area, remove all clothing from the patient and rescuers. Flush thoroughly with water and wash with green soap. All contaminated clothing must be removed before transporting the patient. If not, the clothing will give off fumes that can overcome the ambulance crew.

SECTION 2
INDUSTRIAL RESCUE

Like rural emergencies, industrial emergencies are anything but routine. Hazardous materials are often present at the scene. Heavy machinery may be involved. More than one person is usually injured, and patients may be in unusual positions, crushed beneath fallen debris, or trapped at high angles.

In any industrial rescue, follow these safety guidelines:

- If you are not familiar with the company's operations, check with staff to determine potential hazards at the scene. Make sure all hazards are controlled before you approach the patient.
- Never assume that any machine is locked and secured. Verify with company officials that all valves, switches, and levers that allow a machine to operate have been secured in the off position.
- If the patient is in a confined space or has been injured by an airborne or spilled agent, wait for specialized personnel or HazMat teams to arrive and decontaminate the scene and the patient.

Your first priority in responding to the scene of an industrial accident is to protect your own safety.

If there are hazardous materials or chemical spills at the scene, all rescuers must be protected. Call multiple response teams, including teams that can fight fire and handle hazardous materials if needed. If the site is large, designate an area where the responding units should report. Assign a rescuer to stand at the gate or site to meet incoming units and to direct them to the patients. If the patients are buried under heavy debris (such as concrete, steel reinforcements, heavy machinery, or roofing materials), call specialty teams that can hoist it away. A member of an EMS team should supervise the removal of heavy objects. Removal must be closely monitored to prevent further injury to the patient.

If a patient has been contaminated by hazardous materials, decontamination is necessary. Rescuers should not assess or treat a contaminated patient because they may become contaminated themselves. In cases of gross contamination, specially equipped rescuers may need to scrape or dissolve chemicals from the patient before assessment and treatment can take place.

If the patient is trapped at a high angle, get enough rescuers who are properly equipped for the rescue. Secondary safety belts, full-body harnesses, and rappelling harnesses can be used in high-angle rescues. Patients who are not severely injured can be lowered with full-body and rappelling harnesses. Those who are more severely injured, or who require immobilization prior to being moved, can be lowered in a basket stretcher. Regardless of which method is used, a rescuer must be lowered alongside the patient to monitor his or her condition and provide reassurance during descent.

(Specific information on how to handle hazardous materials and multiple-casualty incidents is offered in Chapters 30 and 31. Also see Chapter 34 for other special rescue situations.)

EMR FOCUS

Agricultural and industrial emergencies may be catastrophic. The machinery used in these settings is capable of causing serious injury or death with its moving parts, sharp edges, and even extreme weight. These same mechanisms of injury also work against the EMR. Therefore, unless you are trained to do so, do not attempt a rescue. You, too, may fall victim to the weight of the overturned tractor, the hazardous air and shifting materials in a silo, or the grasp of a baler.

CASE STUDY FOLLOW-UP

At the beginning of this chapter, you read that EMRs were on the scene with a male patient who was pulled into a baler. To see how the chapter skills apply to this emergency, read the following. It describes how the call was completed.

PRIMARY ASSESSMENT

Ellen and I quickly sorted out our priorities, remembering that the ABCs are always first. When the patient was free and a safe distance away from the machine, we saw that the others had been correct. There were two fingers missing, the hand was badly mangled, and the patient was going into shock. Ellen had him lie down and positioned him. I assessed his airway and breathing. Ellen applied oxygen as I worked on controlling the bleeding.

Because the plant was so large, I knew that the ambulance crew would need help to find us. Another employee volunteered to go to the main gate to meet them when they arrived.

SECONDARY ASSESSMENT

After the bleeding was under control, I performed a quick head-to-toe exam. I bandaged and splinted the patient's injured hand and wrist. A worker yelled out that he found one of the patient's amputated fingers. I wrapped it in sterile gauze and instructed him to go to the cafeteria to get some cold packs, a container with a tightly fitting lid, and at least two plastic bags. I wanted to make sure it was stored safely in case it could be reattached.

PATIENT HISTORY

The patient reported that he was allergic to penicillin but had no other problems. He answered the rest of our questions, but he was in a lot of pain.

ONGOING ASSESSMENT

Each time I took the vital signs, I wrote them down. I did that a few times. We monitored the patient closely, kept him warm, and kept checking the oxygen until the ambulance crew arrived.

TRANSFER OF CARE

When the paramedics arrived, I gave them the hand-off report:

> "This is Tom Robinson. He is 22. About 15 minutes ago, his right arm got pulled into the baler, which amputated two fingers. Tom is conscious. We had him lie down and applied oxygen. The secondary assessment did not turn up anything except the injured hand, so we bandaged and splinted it. We wrapped and bagged one of the amputated fingers. The patient had some coffee about two hours ago, nothing else today. He is allergic to penicillin. His vitals are pulse 110, respirations 18. Skin is cool and moist."

We found out later that the doctors were able to reattach the one finger. The apprentice thanked Ellen and me for saving his life when we saw him. I don't think we saved his life. He wouldn't have died from his injuries, but I'm really glad we had the training to help him.

No matter where or how your patient is found, follow the EMR's patient assessment plan from scene assessment through patient hand-off. If special rescue teams are needed to extricate the patient, ensure continued emergency medical care throughout the procedure.

NOCPs

3.3 a Assess scene for safety **S**
    b Address potential occupational hazards **S**
    c Conduct basic extrication **S**
4.3 i Conduct integumentary system assessment and interpret findings **S**
    j Conduct musculoskeletal assessment and interpret findings **S**
5.6 a Treat soft-tissue injuries **S**
5.7 a Immobilize suspected fractures involving appendicular skeleton **S**
    b Immobilize suspected fractures involving axial skeleton **S**

6.1 f Provide care to patient experiencing signs and symptoms involving integumentary system **S**
    g Provide care to patient experiencing signs and symptoms involving musculoskeletal system **S**
    n Provide care to patient experiencing signs and symptoms due to exposure to adverse environments **S**
    o Provide care to the trauma patient **S**

REVIEW QUESTIONS

Page references where answers may be found or supported are provided at the end of each question.

SECTION 1

1. What are the general procedures of emergency care for farm-related injuries? (pp. 340–341)
2. If a patient is caught in machinery, what four steps must be accomplished before disentanglement should begin? (p. 340)
3. What are some mechanisms of injury associated with farm machinery? (p. 341)
4. How many rescuers should be responsible for hoisting commands during lifting and extrication? (p. 344)
5. When a patient has debris or machinery on top of him or her, why should medical personnel monitor lifting during rescue? (p. 344)

SECTION 2

6. What are the three safety guidelines that you should follow at the scene of any industrial accident? (p. 348)
7. What are some other specialized rescue teams that you might require to assist at an industrial scene? (p. 348)

CHAPTER

24

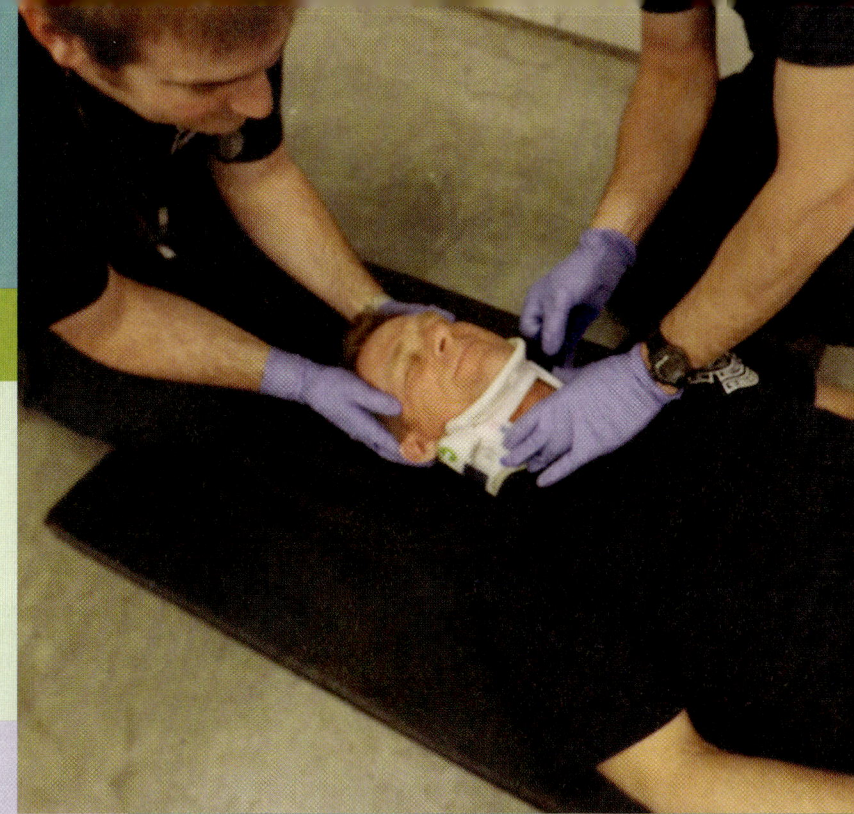

John Mackay

Injuries to the Head, Face, and Neck

OBJECTIVES

1. List 14 signs and symptoms of a head injury.
2. Describe the emergency medical care of injuries to the head.
3. Establish the relationship between facial injuries and airway management.
4. Describe the emergency care of injuries to the face, including injuries to the jaw, cheek, nose, and ear.
5. Describe the emergency care of injuries to the neck.
6. Outline the six components of the examination of an eye injury.
7. Describe the emergency care of injuries to the eye, including foreign objects; injuries to the orbits, eyelids, and globes; impaled objects; and extruded eyeball.
8. Outline the procedure for flushing chemical burns to the eye.

INTRODUCTION

Injuries to the head are among the most serious emergencies. They run a high risk of causing lifelong complications or death. Your role as the first medically trained rescuer on the scene can be critical.

While some injuries to the face and throat are minor, many can be life threatening. They can compromise the upper airway and impair the patient's ability to breathe. In addition, many injuries to the face and neck stem from impacts strong enough to cause hidden facial fractures, cervical spine damage, and skull fractures.

SECTION 1
INJURIES TO THE HEAD

A head injury may be open or closed. An open head injury is accompanied by a break in the skull, such as that caused by a fracture or an impaled object. It involves direct local damage to tissue. It can also result in brain damage.

A closed head injury does not involve a break in the skull. Even so, the brain can be seriously injured. The skull holds brain tissue, blood, and **cerebrospinal fluid**. The volume of each can vary, but the total volume cannot. Because the skull is rigid, its capacity is limited. If brain tissue swells or if bleeding occurs, pressure can build up inside the skull and cause damage to the brain.

Patient Assessment

The general signs and symptoms of a head injury include the following:

- Altered mental status, ranging from confusion to unconsciousness
- Irregular breathing
- Open wounds to the scalp
- Penetrating wounds to the head
- Softness or depression of the skull
- Blood or cerebrospinal fluid leaking from the ears or nose (Figure 24–1)
- Facial bruises
- Bruising around the eyes (raccoon eyes)
- Bruising behind the ears (Battle's sign)
- Abnormal findings in an assessment of pulses, movement, and sensation
- Headache severe enough to be disabling or that appears suddenly
- Nausea, vomiting
- Unequal pupil size with altered mental status
- Seizure activity

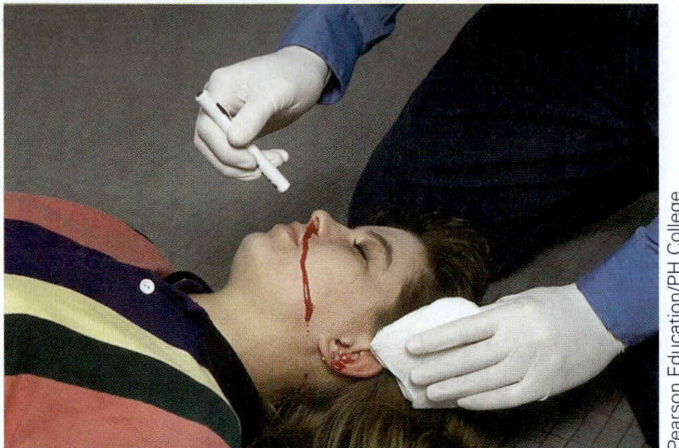

Figure 24–1 Blood or cerebrospinal fluid may come from the ears and nose of a patient with a head injury.

Suspect spinal injury in any patient with a head injury (Figure 24–2). If there is an obvious head injury, if the mechanism of injury suggests a head or spinal injury, or if a trauma patient is unconscious, immediately stabilize the patient's head and neck. Maintain manual stabilization until the patient is completely immobilized (Figure 24–3). If you are alone with an injured patient, you may be allowed to

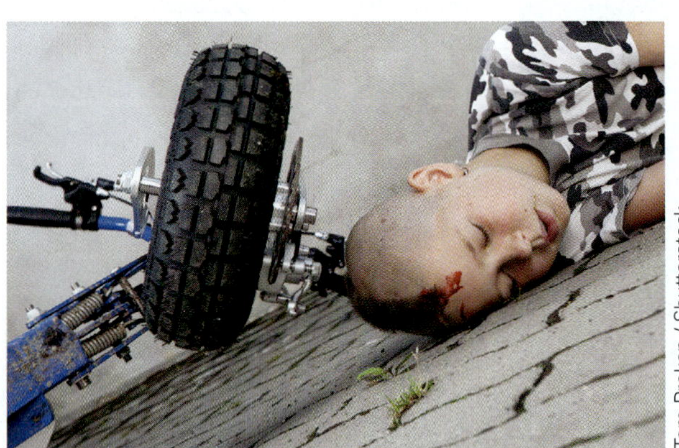

Figure 24–2 Always suspect spinal injury in a patient with a head injury.

CASE STUDY

Dispatch

Our EMR crew was preparing to go off duty when a call came in. It was 0750 hours. My partner and I jumped in the truck and headed out to the factory at 700 Mill Street. Dispatch reported that a man had fallen from the second-storey roof of the factory supply building and workers couldn't wake him up.

Scene Assessment

Although dispatch did not give us any reason to anticipate an unsafe scene, we approached with caution. The foreman met us at the gate and immediately directed us to the patient's location. The crowd that had gathered around the patient was being controlled by the company security guards. We identified ourselves and approached the patient.

Primary Assessment

My partner held the patient's head and neck while I began the assessment. The patient was not conscious to voice or painful stimuli. I opened and assessed his airway and heard gurgling sounds from his throat. Without delay, I suctioned the mouth and the gurgling sounds ceased.

The patient's respirations appeared to be adequate. We elected to place him on oxygen at 15 L/min with a non-rebreather mask. There was no visible bleeding present. Our general impression was of a male in his 30s who was unconscious after a fall.

> Consider this patient as you read Chapter 24. What would you do to assess and treat his condition?

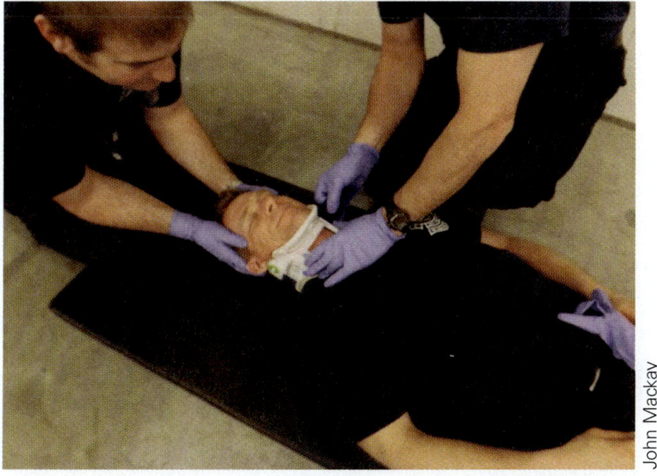

John Mackay

Figure 24–3 Maintain manual stabilization until the patient is properly immobilized.

place a rigid item on each side of the patient's head to prevent movement. Follow local protocols.

During your primary assessment, use the jaw-thrust manoeuvre to open, assess, and maintain the airway. Also, note that bleeding from the scalp may be profuse because of the large number of blood vessels there.

During your secondary assessment of the patient, look for open injuries to the head. Closed injuries may present with swelling or depression of the bones of the skull. Check for cerebrospinal fluid. This appears as a clear liquid, possibly tinged pink with blood, leaking from an open head wound or from the ears or nose.

For the head-injury patient, it is especially important for you to assess pulse, movement, and sensation in the extremities. Also, pay attention to the function of the patient's eyes and note any numbness, especially of the face, arms, or legs.

When you take the patient's history, be sure to try to find out when the injury occurred, if the patient lost consciousness, and if the patient was moved after the injury occurred. Details about what happened are crucial to medical care.

During your ongoing assessment, monitor the patient for any change in his or her level of consciousness. Keep in mind that change in a patient—not the patient's status at any one time—may be the most important sign of how a patient is doing.

General Guidelines for Emergency Care

If you suspect an injury to the head, be sure paramedics have been notified. After taking BSI precautions and establishing manual stabilization of the patient's head and neck, proceed with the following emergency care:

1. *Make the airway a top priority.* Note that oxygen deficiency in the brain is the most frequent cause of death following a head injury. Monitor the airway and breathing closely. Suction as needed. Administer oxygen in high concentrations. If ventilation is needed, use 100 percent oxygen at a rate of 22 to 25 ventilations per minute. Follow local protocol.
2. *Control the bleeding and dress open wounds.* Scalp wounds may bleed profusely, but they are usually easy to control with direct pressure. (*Note:* Never apply direct pressure to a head wound that is accompanied by an obvious or depressed skull fracture. It could drive fragments of bone into brain tissue and cause further injury.)

    Do not try to stop the flow of cerebrospinal fluid. If the fluid is leaking from the ears or a head wound, cover the opening loosely with sterile gauze dressings.

    If there is a penetrating object, do not try to remove it. Instead, stabilize it with bulky dressings.
3. *Apply a rigid cervical immobilization device if you are trained and allowed to do so* (see Chapter 25 for instructions). Maintain manual stabilization of the head and neck before, during, and after application and until the patient is immobilized on a long backboard.
4. *Monitor vital signs closely.* Watch for any sign of deterioration or change in the patient's status. If the patient has convulsions, protect him or her from injury.
5. *Calm and reassure the patient.* Continue to talk with him or her. If you can stimulate the patient, you may be able to prevent loss of consciousness.

Specific Head Injuries

Injuries to the head include skull fracture, injuries to the brain, concussion, and penetrating wounds.

Skull Fracture

The primary function of the skull is to protect the brain from injury. Because of its shape and thickness, the skull is usually broken only by extreme trauma. Suspect skull fracture with any significant trauma to the head, even if the injury is a closed one.

A skull fracture accompanied by brain injury is a serious condition that needs immediate management. The signs and symptoms of a skull fracture include the following (Figure 24–4):

- Damage to the skull, visible through lacerations in the scalp
- Deformity of the skull or face
- Pain or swelling at the injury site
- Clear or pinkish fluid dripping from nose, ears, mouth, or head wound
- Unusual size of pupils, one eye sunken
- Purplish bruising under or around the eyes (raccoon eyes)
- Purplish bruising behind the ears (Battle's sign)

Injuries to the Brain

Whether a head wound is open or closed, brain damage can be extensive. In fact, it is often more severe

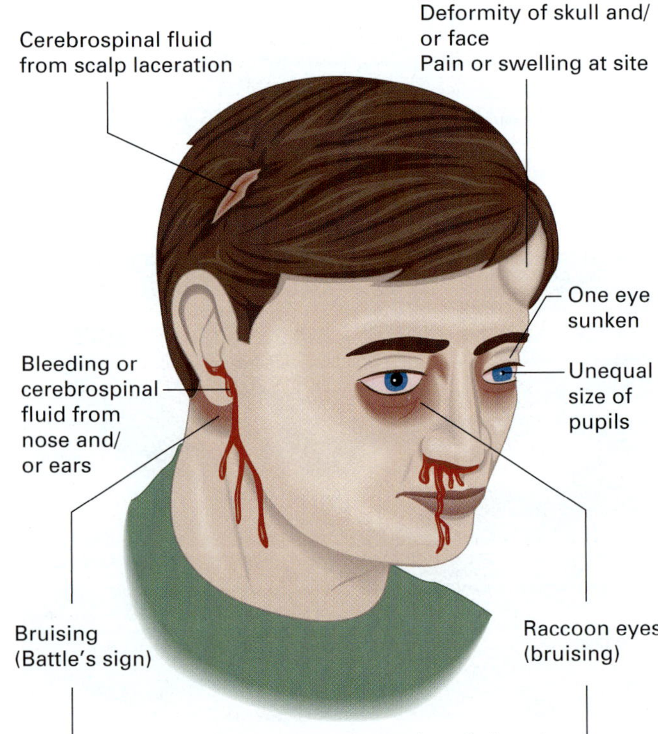

Figure 24–4 Signs and symptoms of skull fracture.

in closed injuries than in open ones. Severity depends mainly on the mechanism of injury and the force involved. However, consider all suspected head injuries to be serious. The signs and symptoms of a brain injury include the following:

- Changes in mental status, ranging from confusion to unconsciousness
- Paralysis or flaccidity, usually only on one side of the body
- Unequal facial movements, squinting, drooping, unequal or unreactive pupils, disturbances of vision in one or both eyes
- Ringing in the ears, loss of hearing in one or both ears
- Rigidity of all limbs (present with severe injury)
- Loss of balance, staggering, or stumbling gait
- Slow, strong heartbeat that gradually becomes rapid and weak (late sign)
- High blood pressure with a slow pulse
- Rapid, laboured breathing or disturbances in the pattern of breathing
- Vomiting after head injury
- Incontinence

Concussion

A concussion is a temporary loss of the brain's ability to function. There is no detectable damage to the brain. A concussion is classified as mild, moderate, or severe on the basis of the time interval before return to consciousness. The key distinguishing factor of concussion is that the signs and symptoms appear immediately or soon after impact. Then they disappear, usually within 48 hours. If symptoms develop several minutes after impact or do not subside over time, the injury is probably more serious than a concussion.

The signs and symptoms of a concussion include the following:

- Momentary confusion or confusion that lasts several minutes
- Inability to recall the period just before and after being injured
- Repeatedly asking what happened
- Mild to moderate irritability, uncooperativeness, combativeness, verbal abusiveness
- Inability to answer questions or obey commands appropriately
- Persistent vomiting
- Incontinence
- Restlessness
- Seizures
- Brief loss of consciousness

Penetrating Wounds

A penetrating wound occurs when an object passes through the skull and lodges in the brain. It often involves bullets, knives, or ice picks. A penetrating wound is an extreme emergency and almost always results in long-term damage.

If the object is impaled in the skull, do not try to remove it. Stabilize it with soft bulky dressings. Then dress the area around it with sterile gauze. If an object has penetrated the skull but you cannot see it, cover the wound lightly with sterile dressings. In both cases, permit the blood to drain. Never apply firm pressure to a head injury that might involve a skull fracture.

SECTION 2
INJURIES TO THE FACE AND NECK

General Principles of Care

While some injuries to the face and neck are minor, many can be life threatening (Figures 24–5 and 24–6). They can result from impacts strong enough to cause hidden facial fractures, cervical spine damage, and skull fractures.

For injuries of the face and neck, follow the patient assessment and general guidelines for emergency care described at the beginning of this chapter. Take spinal precautions as appropriate. Be sure the airway stays clear of fragments of teeth, broken dentures, bits of bone, pieces of flesh, and other possible obstructions.

Remember to keep the airway a priority. If bleeding into the mouth or throat threatens the airway, roll the patient onto one side to allow drainage. Be prepared to monitor the airway and breathing constantly and to suction often. Keep in mind that the patient may be very anxious about possible

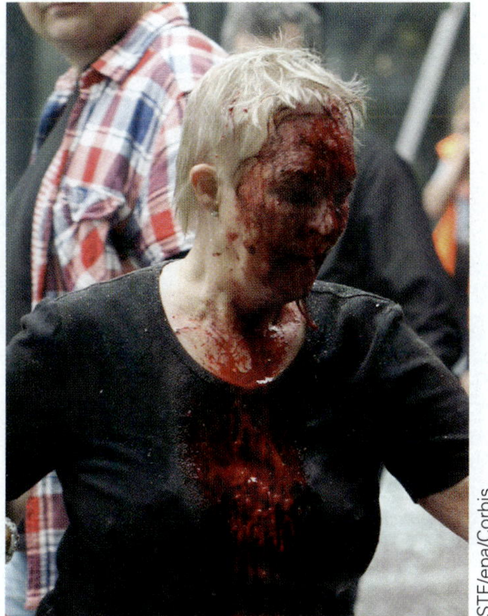

Figure 24–5 Injury to the face.

INJURIES TO THE CHEEK, MOUTH, AND JAW

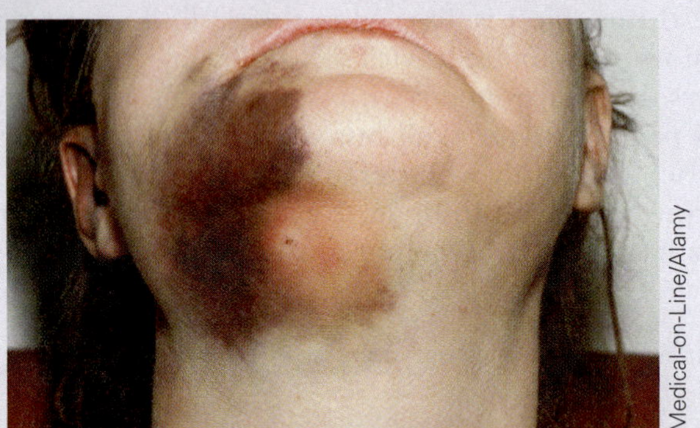

Figure 24–6a Fractured mandible.

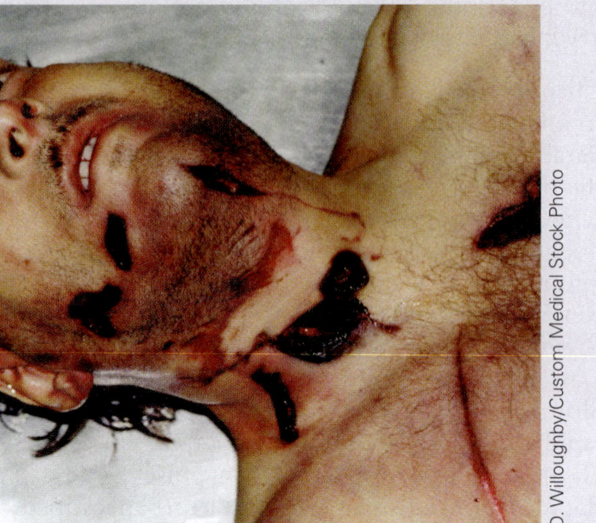

Figure 24–6b Multiple stab lacerations.

disfigurement. Reassure the patient and do your best to help him or her stay calm.

Facial Injuries

Face

Whenever there are significant soft-tissue injuries to the face, there may also be underlying fractures. The signs and symptoms of a facial fracture include the following:

- Distortion of facial features
- Numbness or pain
- Bruising and swelling
- Bleeding from the nose or mouth
- Limited jaw motion
- Teeth that do not meet normally, teeth that are missing
- Double vision (with fracture of bones around the eyes)
- Asymmetry of bones in face (before swelling)

Jaw

Patients with injuries to the face may also have a broken jaw (Figure 24–7). Such an injury can cause

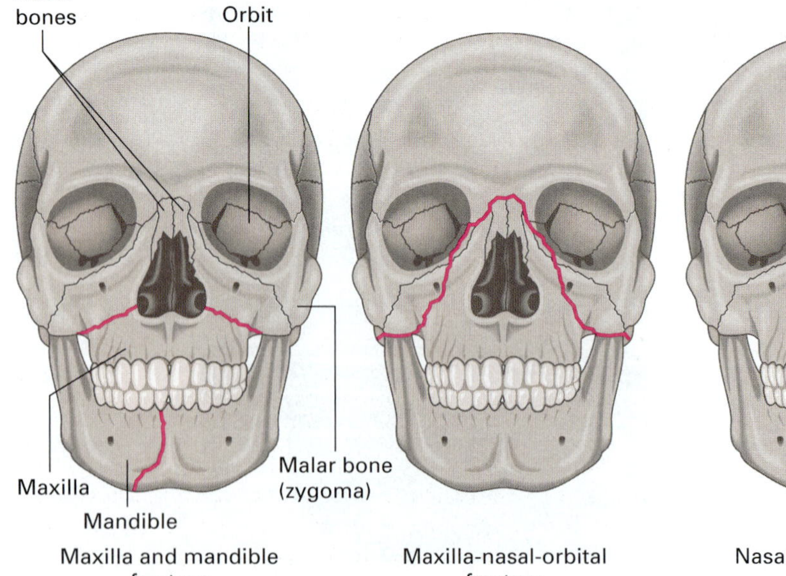

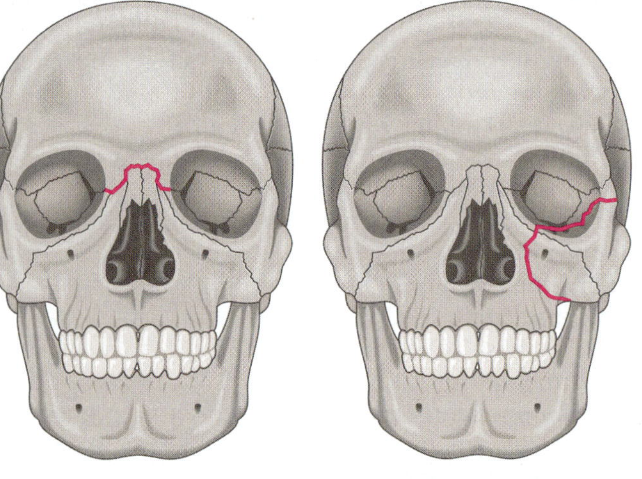

Figure 24–7 Common fractures of the face and jaw.

problems with the airway and breathing. Monitor both closely. The signs and symptoms of injuries to the jaw include the following:

- Mouth will not open or close
- Drooling of saliva mixed with blood
- Difficulty swallowing
- Pain with talking or difficulty talking
- Missing, loosened, or uneven teeth
- Teeth that do not meet normally
- Pain in area around the ears

If a tooth has been lost, try to find it. Control the bleeding from the socket with a gauze pad. If you find the missing tooth, be sure to handle it by the crown, not by the roots. Then rinse it with tap water and be careful to protect any remaining tissue. Gently pick off debris. Then put the tooth in a glass of milk. If milk is not available, wrap the tooth in moistened gauze. Do not allow the tooth to dry. Send it with the patient to the hospital. (These steps will help maximize the chances for a successful reimplantation.)

If dentures are in place and unbroken, let them stay in place. They can help support the structures of the mouth. If dentures are broken, remove them. Send them with the patient to the hospital so that the surgeon can use them to establish proper alignment of the jaw.

Cheek

If there is an impaled object in the cheek, stabilize it with bulky dressings, unless it has penetrated all the way through. If it has penetrated all the way through, it may cause enough bleeding to block the airway. So, remove it carefully. Be prepared to suction the airway.

Nose

Care for soft-tissue injuries to the nose (Figure 24–8) in the same way you would care for other such injuries. Take special care to maintain an open airway. Position the patient to prevent blood from draining into the throat.

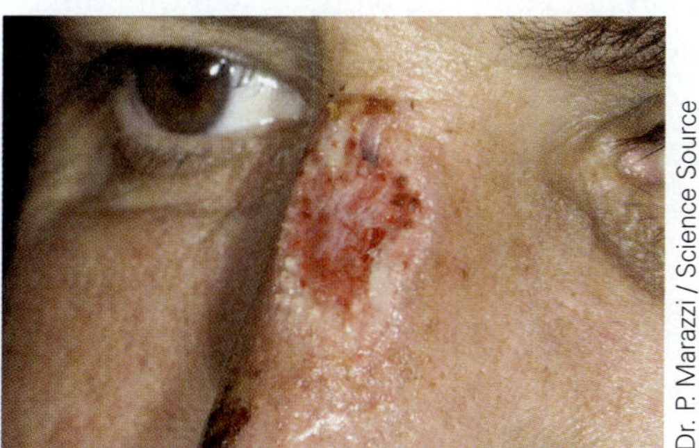
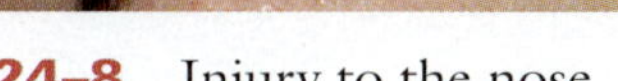
Figure 24–8   Injury to the nose.

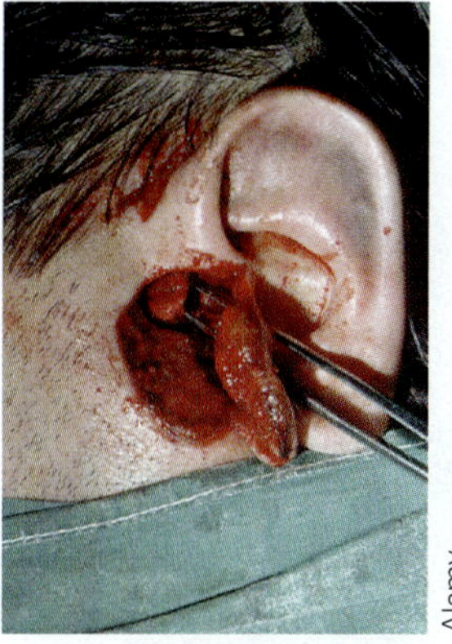
Figure 24–9   Injury to the ear.

The nose is the most commonly broken bone in the face. When it is broken, it will swell and appear to be deformed. To treat it, apply cold packs to reduce swelling. Arrange for patient transport.

Foreign objects in the nose are usually a problem among small children. Reassure the child and parents, and arrange for transport to a hospital. Do not probe or try to remove the object because special lighting and instruments are required.

Ear

Soft-tissue injuries to the ear, including avulsions, are common (Figure 24–9). Treat them as you would treat any other such injury. Keep in mind that when dressing an injured ear, you should place part of the dressing between the back of the ear and the side of the head.

Never probe the ear. Never pack it to stop bleeding from the ear canal. Blood, clear fluid, or blood-tinged fluid draining from the ear may indicate skull fracture. Place a loose, clean dressing across the opening to absorb the fluid. Do not apply pressure.

Foreign objects in the ear, such as beans or peanuts, are common among children. The patient should be transported to the hospital where good lighting and appropriate equipment are available.

Neck Injuries

Common causes of neck injury include hanging (attempted suicide), impact with a steering wheel, or running into a stretched wire or clothesline (Figure 24–10). Large wounds may involve injuries to the major vessels in the neck, which can produce massive, even fatal, bleeding. If a wound to the neck is left uncovered, air may be sucked into the vessels and cause an obstruction (air embolism).

D. Willoughby/Custom Medical Stock Photo

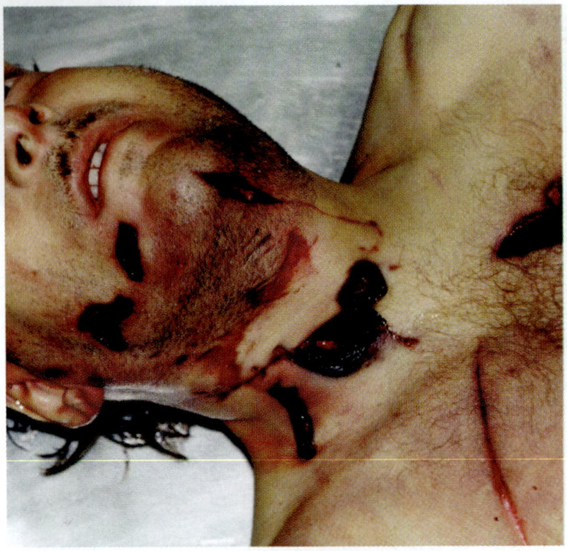

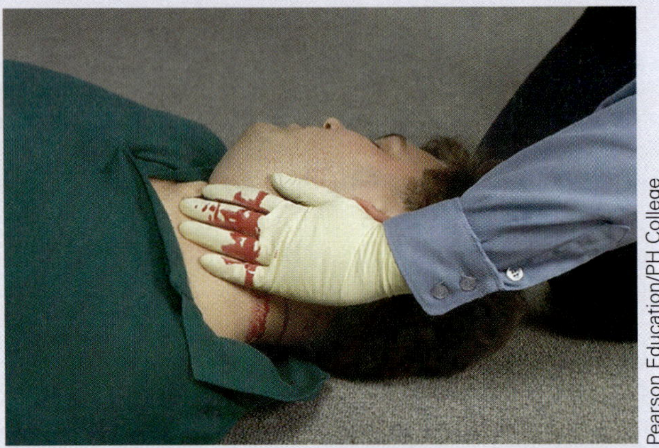

Figure 24–10 Injury to the neck.

The signs and symptoms of neck injuries include the following:

- Obvious lacerations or other wounds
- Deformities or depressions
- Obvious swelling, which sometimes occurs in the face and chest
- Difficulty speaking, loss of the voice
- Airway obstruction
- Crackling sensations under the skin due to air leaking into the soft tissues (subcutaneous emphysema)

If there is bleeding from a neck wound, apply slight to moderate pressure with an occlusive dressing. Tape down the edges of the dressing to form an airtight seal. Add a bulky dressing over the occlusive one (Figure 24–11). Never apply pressure to both sides of the neck at the same time. Never apply a pressure dressing around the neck.

SEVERED NECK VEINS

Pearson Education/PH College

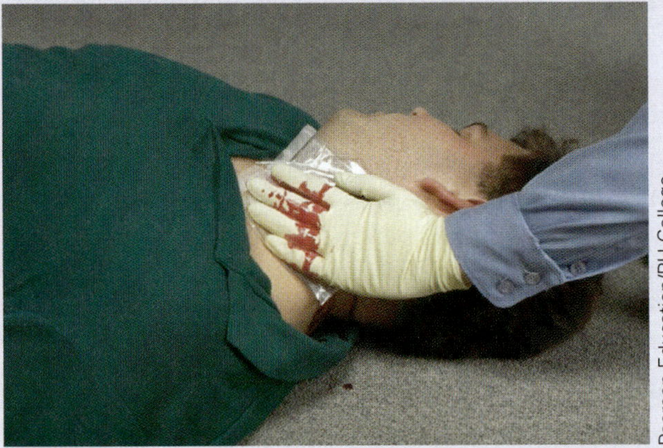

Figure 24–11a Do not delay! Place your gloved palm over the wound.

Pearson Education/PH College

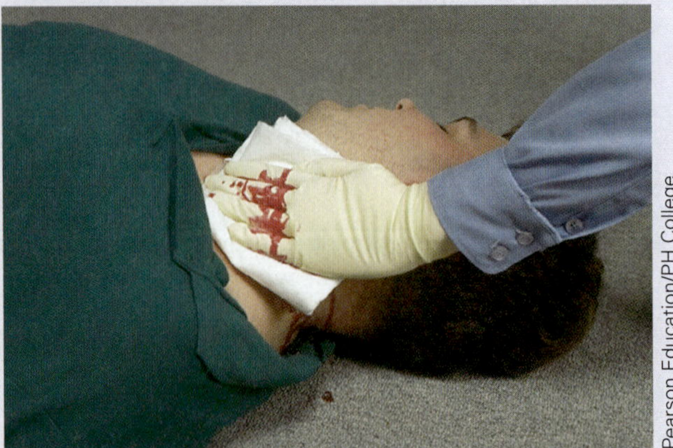

Figure 24–11b Apply moderate pressure with an occlusive dressing.

Pearson Education/PH College

Figure 24–11c Add a bulky dressing.

CAUTION: Do not compress blood vessels on both sides of the neck at once.

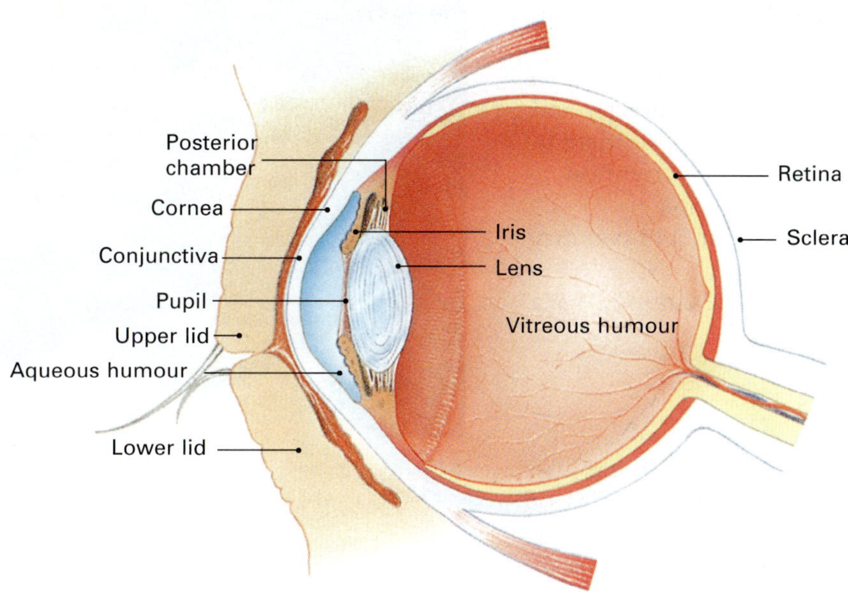

Figure 24–12　Anatomy of the eye.

If there is an impaled object in the neck, stabilize it in place with bulky dressings. Do not remove it.

Eye Injuries

For the anatomy of the eye, see Figure 24–12 above. When you assess a patient with an eye injury, find out when the injury occurred, whether or not both eyes were affected, and what symptoms the patient first noticed. Then carefully examine the eyes separately and together with a small penlight. Proceed as follows:

- *Orbits (the bones in the skull that hold the eyeballs).* Check for bruising, swelling, lacerations, tenderness, depression, and deformity.
- *Eyelids.* Check for bruising, swelling, and lacerations.
- *Mucous membranes.* Check for redness, pus, and foreign objects.
- *Globes (eyeballs).* Check for abnormal colouring, laceration, and foreign objects.
- *Pupils.* Check for size, shape, and equality (Figure 24–13). Also check for reaction to light. The pupils should be black, round, and equal in size. They should react to light by constricting.
- *Eye movement.* Check to see that the eyes can move in all directions. Check for abnormal gaze or pain upon movement.

The basic rules for emergency care of an injured eye include the following:

- Many EMS systems do not allow flushing of an injured eye unless it has a chemical injury. If the eye has been perforated, damage done during flushing will be irreversible. Follow local protocol.
- Do not put direct pressure on the eyeball. Fluids inside the eyeball are irreplaceable.
- Do not put salves or medications in the injured eye. This is a physician's responsibility.
- Do not remove blood or blood clots from the eye. But you can sponge blood from the face to help keep the patient comfortable.
- Do not try to force the eyelid open unless you have to flush out chemicals.
- Do not let a patient with an eye injury walk without help, especially up or down stairs.

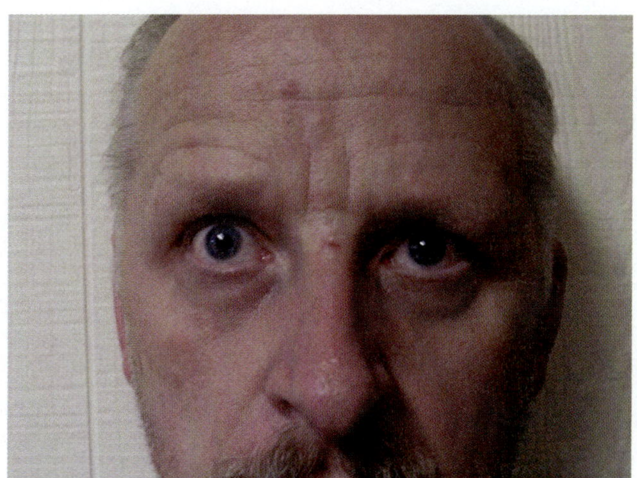

Figure 24–13　Unequal pupils.

- Patch both eyes, even if only one is injured. Eyes move together, so patching both eyes will help keep the injured eye from moving excessively. Explain everything you are doing in order to minimize the patient's anxiety. Speak directly and clearly and hold the patient's arm as appropriate to reassure him or her of your undivided attention.
- Do not allow the patient to eat or drink.
- Never panic. It will upset the patient, and you may lose his or her trust.
- An eye injury should always be examined by a physician.

Foreign Objects

Foreign objects are frequently blown or driven into the eye (Figure 24–14). They include particles of dirt, sand, cinders, coal dust, or fine pieces of metal. If not removed, they can cause inflammation, scarring, or infection. They may also scratch the cornea. The signs and symptoms of foreign objects in the eye include pain, excessive tearing, and abnormal sensitivity to light.

Do not allow the patient to rub the eyes. Rubbing can force a particle with sharp edges into the tissues, making removal difficult.

It is always safer for an EMR to allow EMS personnel with more training to remove a foreign object. However, if removal is necessary and local protocols allow it, there are several ways in which you might proceed. They are as follows:

- Hold the eyelids apart and flush the eye with clean water (Figure 24–15). Note that some EMS systems do not allow flushing except for chemical burns. Follow local protocol.
- If the object is under the upper eyelid, draw the upper lid down over the lower lid. When you let it return to its normal position, its undersurface

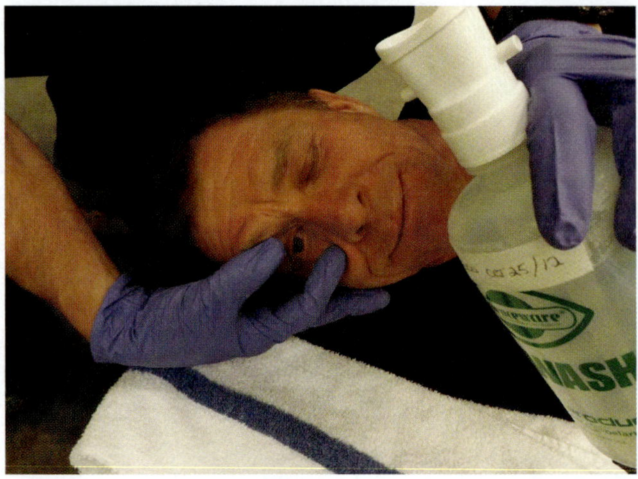

Figure 24-15 is credited:

Figure 24–15   Flushing a foreign object from the eye.

will be drawn over the lashes of the lower lid. The lashes will sweep away the foreign object.
- Grasp the eyelashes of the upper lid. Turn up the lid over a cotton swab (Figure 24–16). The foreign object may then be carefully removed with the corner of a piece of sterile gauze.

If the object is under the lower eyelid, pull down the lower lid to expose the inner surface. Then use the corner of a piece of sterile gauze to remove the object (Figure 24–16).

Should a foreign object become lodged in the eyeball, do not try to remove it. If you do, it could be forced deeper into the eye, causing further damage. In this case, place a rigid eye shield over the injured eye (Figure 24–17). Cover the opposite eye with gauze. Arrange for immediate transport to a hospital.

Orbits

Trauma to the face may result in fracture of the bones that form the orbits, or eye sockets (Figure 24–18). A patient with an orbit injury may complain of double or decreased vision, numbness above the eyebrow or over the cheek, or massive discharge from the nose.

Fractures of the lower part of the orbit are the most common. They can cause paralysis of the upward gaze; that is, the patient's eyes would not be able to follow your finger upward. Patients with an orbit fracture need hospitalization and surgery.

If there is no injury to the eyeball, place cold packs over the injured orbit to help reduce the swelling. However, if the eyeball is injured or if you are in doubt, do not apply cold packs.

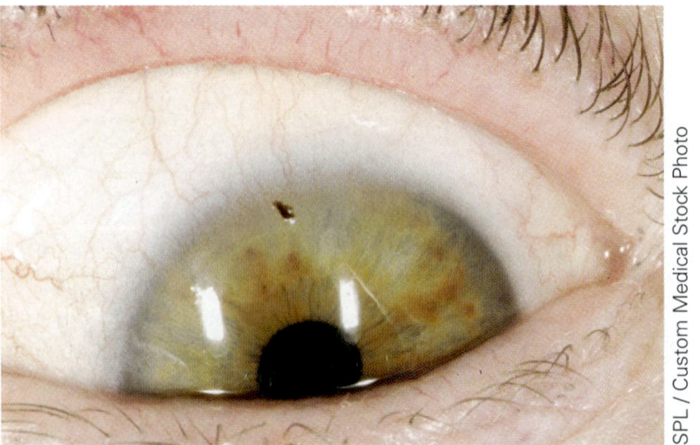

Figure 24-14 is credited:

Figure 24–14   Foreign object lodged in the eye.

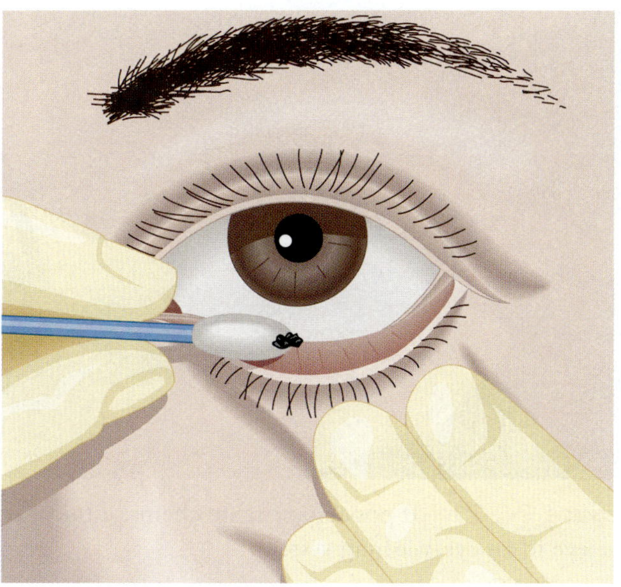

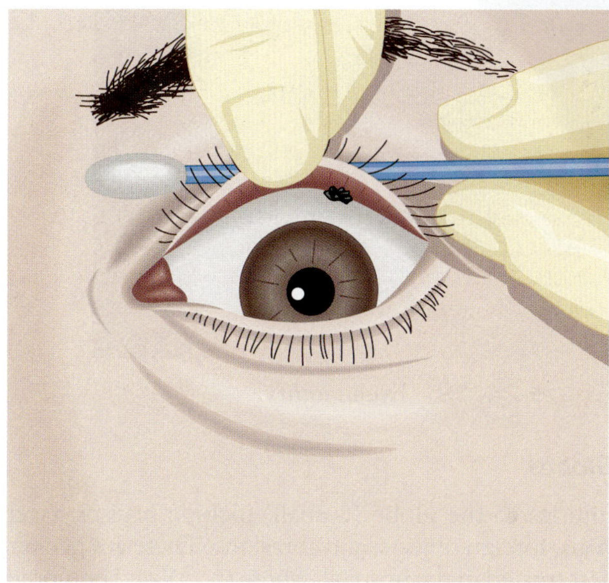

Figure 24–16   Removing foreign particles from the white of the eye.

Eyelids

Lid injuries include discoloration, burns, swelling or drooping, and laceration (Figure 24–19). Anything that damages the lid may also damage the eyeball. In general, little can be done for these injuries in the field beyond gentle patching.

To control bleeding from the eyelid, apply light pressure. No pressure should be used if the eyeball itself is injured.

Never attempt to remove embedded material, such as gravel. Use sterile gauze soaked in saline to keep the wound from drying. If the lid is avulsed, preserve it and send it with the patient for later grafting.

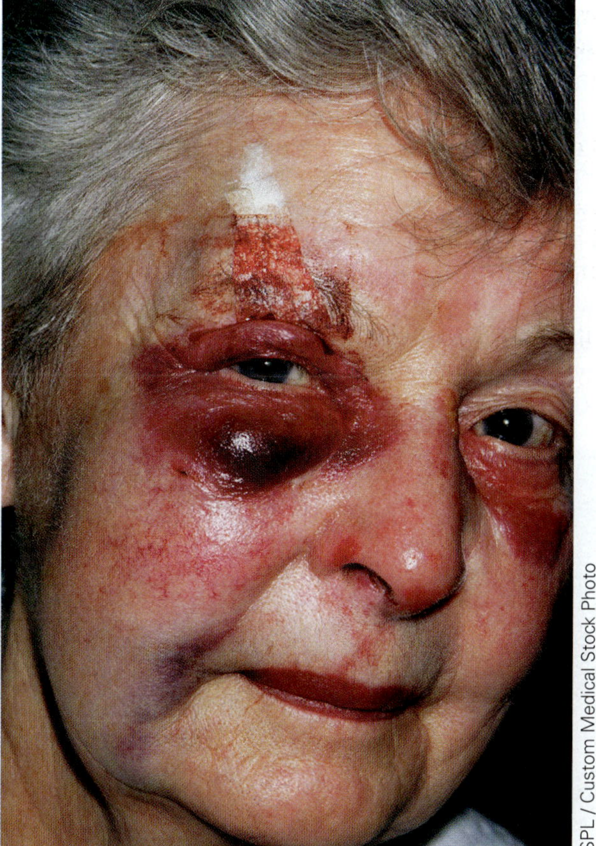

Figure 24–17   Place a rigid shield over the eye with the embedded foreign object. Cover the opposite eye with gauze.

Figure 24–18   Eye orbit injury.

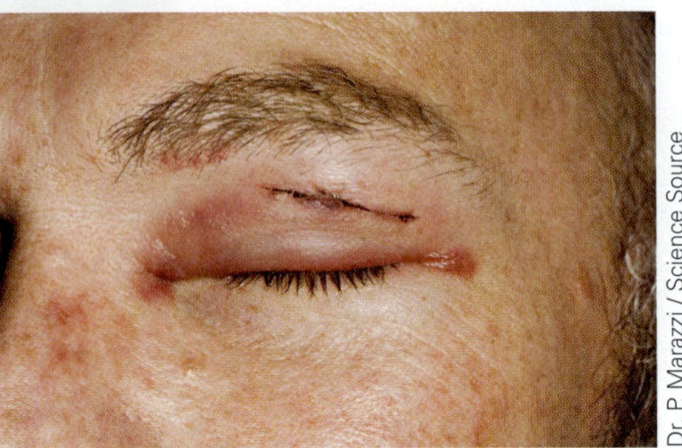

Figure 24–19 Eyelid injury.

Dr. P. Marazzi / Science Source

Globes

Injuries to the globe (eyeball) include bruises, lacerations, foreign objects, and abrasions. These are generally best treated in the hospital, where specialized equipment is available. In the field, keep the patient supine. Lightly apply patches to both eyes since eyes move together. Keep in mind that patients who have both eyes covered need a bit more patience and understanding. This is a very frightening experience for them.

Chemical Burns to the Eye

Chemical burns to the eye are quite common (Figure 24–20). They are the most urgent emergency related to the eyes. Permanent damage can occur within seconds of the injury. The first 10 minutes are crucial to the final outcome. Remember, burning and tissue damage will continue as long as the chemical remains in the eye, even if it is diluted.

To provide emergency care, begin immediate, continuous irrigation with water (Figure 24–21). Do not use anything other than water. The water does not need to be sterile, but it must be clean. Be sure to wear protective glasses. Gently hold the patient's eyelid open so that all of the chemical can be flushed away. You may have to force the eyelid open because of the patient's pain.

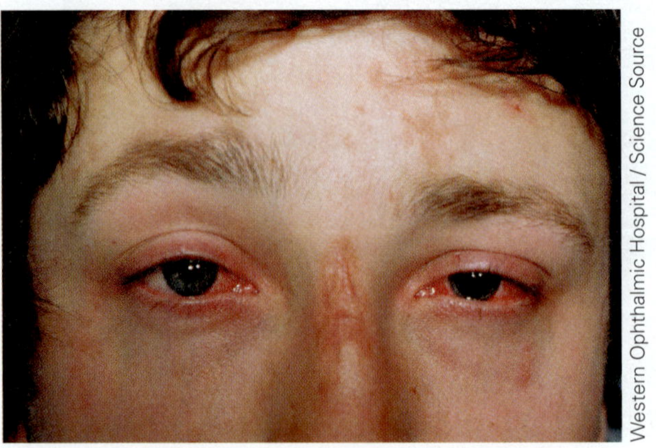

Figure 24–20 Chemical burn of the eye.

Western Ophthalmic Hospital / Science Source

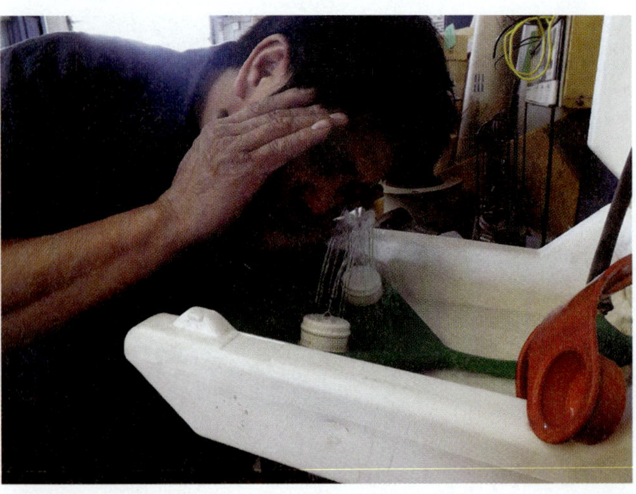

John Mackay

Figure 24–21 If possible, irrigate chemical burns to the eye in an eye-washing system.

Pour water from the inside corner across the eyeball to the outside edge. This will help avoid contaminating the uninjured eye. Irrigate continuously for 30 to 60 minutes.

Remove any solid particles from the surface of the eye with a moistened cotton swab. Contact lenses must be removed or flushed out. If not, chemicals can be trapped between the lens and the cornea. Follow local protocol.

Following irrigation, wash your hands thoroughly. Avoid contaminating your own eyes.

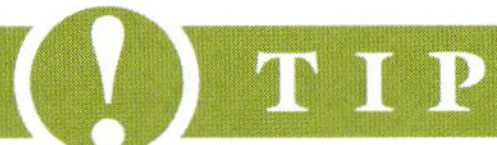

Even if you successfully flush debris from an eye, it is imperative that the patient see a physician or eye specialist who can assess the extent of injury.

Impaled Objects

Objects impaled in the eye should be removed only by a physician. You must protect the patient from further injury until he or she can reach a doctor. So, stabilize the object in place (Figure 24–22).

Begin by stabilizing the patient's head with sandbags or large pads. Keep the patient supine. Encircle the eye with a gauze dressing or soft sterile cloth. Do not apply pressure. You can then cut a hole in a single bulky dressing and slip it over the impaled object. Then place a metal shield, a Styrofoam or paper cup, or a cone over the object and the eye. The sides of the shield or cup should not touch the object at all. Hold the cup and the dressing in place with a self-adhering bandage and apply a roller bandage that covers both eyes.

IMPALED-EYE INJURY

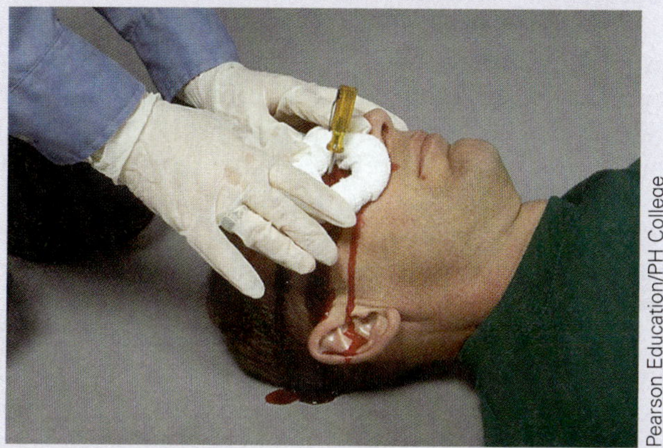

Figure 24–22a   Place padding around the object.

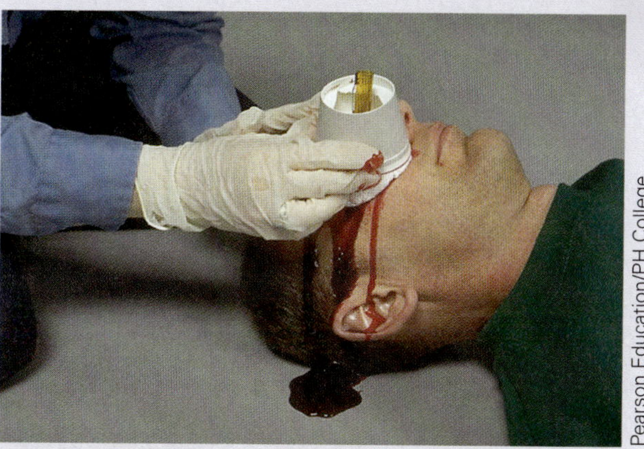

Figure 24–22b   Stabilize the object with a cup.

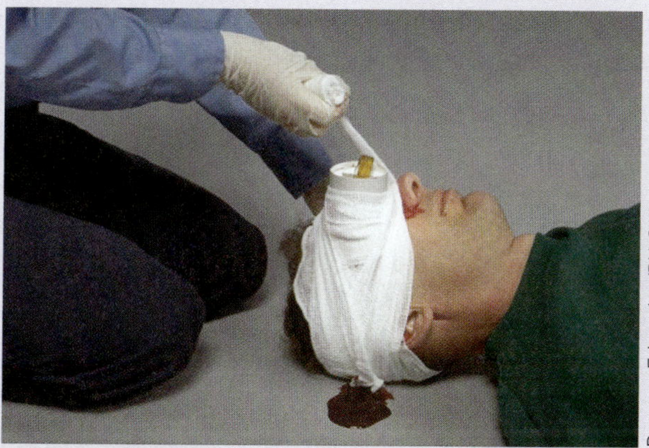

Figure 24–22c   Secure the cup in place.

After covering the patient's eyes, do not leave him or her alone. The patient could panic. Keep the patient in hand contact so that he or she knows someone is there.

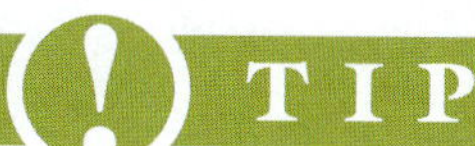

T I P

If you have access to an intravenous (IV) bag of normal saline, when required to flush both eyes you might consider running the fluid through a nasal cannula, which can straddle the bridge of the nose. You can then simultaneously flush both eyes of a supine patient in the desired direction.

Extruded Eyeball

During a serious injury, the eyeball may be knocked out of the socket, or extruded (Figure 24–23). Do not try to replace it. Instead, cover it with a moist dressing and protective cup. Do not apply any pressure. Then apply a bandage that covers both eyes.

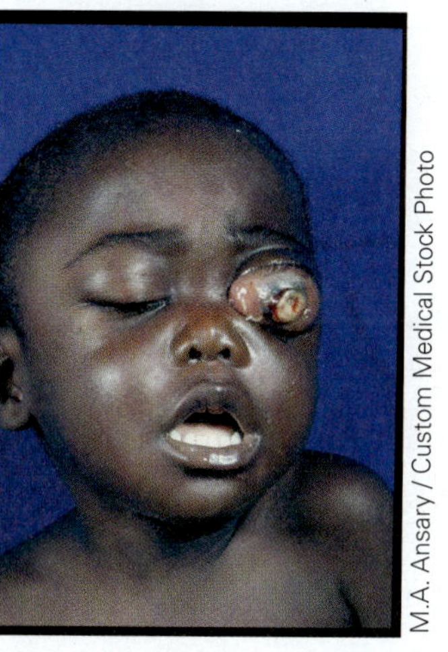

Figure 24–23   Extruded eyeball.

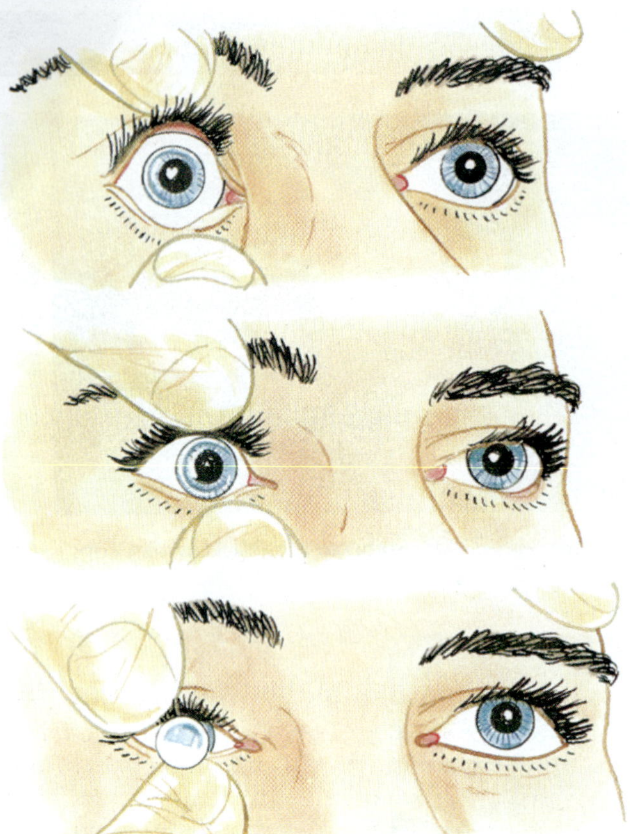

Figure 24–24 Removing hard contact lenses.

Other Eye Injuries

In all other emergencies involving the eye, patch both eyes and arrange for transport. Such emergencies include eye infections, black eye, corneal abrasions, light burns, and heat burns. Follow local protocols.

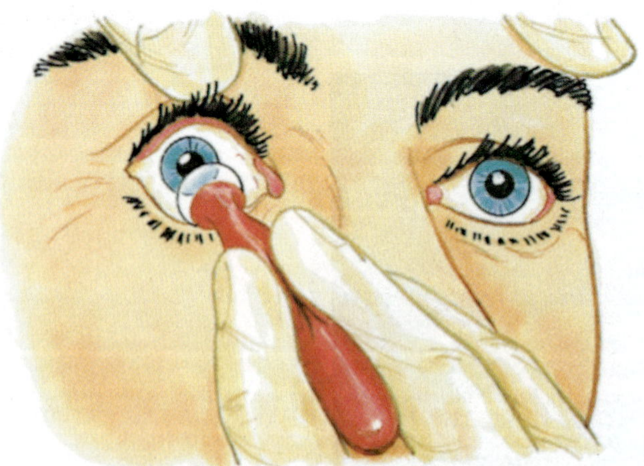

Figure 24–25 Using a moistened suction cup to remove hard contact lenses.

Removing Contact Lenses

An estimated 1.8 million people in Canada wear contact lenses. Some may wear a lens in one eye only, so be sure to examine both eyes carefully. Other patients, especially older adults, wear both contact lenses and eyeglasses. To detect lenses, shine a penlight into each eye. A soft lens will show up as a shadow on the outer portion of the eye. A hard lens will show up as a shadow over the iris. In general, remove contact lenses only when there has been a chemical burn to the eye or when it is medically necessary. Always follow local protocols.

To remove hard contact lenses (Figure 24–24), first separate the eyelids. Position the lens over the cornea by manipulating the eyelids. Place your thumbs gently on the top and bottom eyelids and open the lids wide. Gently press them down and forward to the edges of the lens. Press the lower lid slightly harder and move it under the bottom edge of the lens. Move the eyelids toward each other, allowing the lens to slide out between them. Finally, remove the lens and put it in a safe place. An alternative method is to use a moistened suction cup to remove the lenses (Figure 24–25).

To remove soft contact lenses, place several drops of saline on the lens. Then, gently lift it off by pinching it between your thumb and index finger (Figure 24–26).

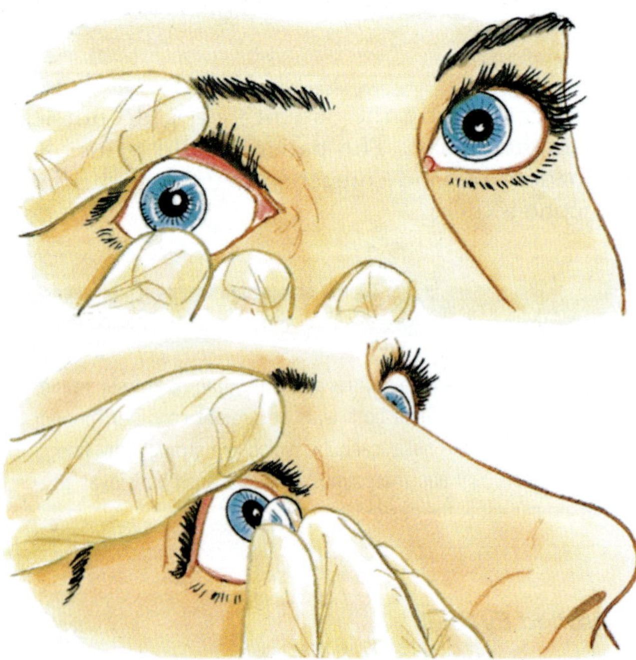

Figure 24–26 Removing soft contact lenses.

EMR FOCUS

The head, face, and neck hold very important organs and structures. The head contains the brain and a great number of blood vessels that supply the brain with oxygen. This means that injuries to the head can injure the brain and cause severe bleeding. The face and neck contain structures of the airway, which can be injured. The airway may also be compromised if severe bleeding from the head flows into it. Be alert for the possibilities. Position and suction the patient as needed.

Injuries to the head, face, and neck can also cause injuries to the spine. Take spinal precautions whenever a patient's chief complaint or mechanism of injury suggests the possibility of a spinal injury.

CASE STUDY FOLLOW-UP

At the beginning of this chapter, you read that EMRs were on the scene with an unconscious male patient. To see how the skills in this chapter apply to this emergency, read the following. It describes how the call was completed.

SECONDARY ASSESSMENT

My partner continued to monitor the airway and breathing while I conducted a head-to-toe exam. I found only a large bruise on the left side of the patient's head. His vital signs were within normal ranges.

During the assessment, the patient opened his eyes and responded to my voice. I cautioned him to be very still, told him why my partner was holding his head, and explained what I knew of what happened. Although he was somewhat drowsy, he indicated that he understood by whispering, "Okay."

PATIENT HISTORY

A company personnel officer provided the medical history that was kept on record. The patient was also able to answer some of our questions. His chief complaint was that he hurt all over. He had no known allergies and was not taking any medications. He had eaten breakfast at 0500. The patient did not remember what had happened, but his co-workers said he was performing his job when he tripped and flipped over the roof ledge. There were no eyewitnesses to the fall to the ground.

ONGOING ASSESSMENT

The patient required careful monitoring due to changes in his level of consciousness. He did not resist the oxygen mask, so we elected to continue administration. The patient was able to wiggle his toes and fingers, and he continued to respond to questions appropriately.

TRANSFER OF CARE

When the paramedics arrived, I gave them the hand-off report:

"This is Javier Gonzalez. He is 38 years old. About 15 minutes ago, he fell approximately 8 metres from the roof of this building onto the grass. No one moved him before or after we arrived on the scene. Initially, he did not respond to voice or painful stimuli. He presented with adequate respirations but needed suctioning of the airway early in the primary assessment. During the secondary assessment, he began to respond to our voices. The assessment revealed a large bruise to the left side of his head. There was no bleeding at the wound site. There is no record of previous medical problems. His vital signs are pulse 88, respirations 18, blood pressure 130/82, skin warm and dry, and pupils equal and reactive."

The paramedics took over care of the patient and told us that we had done a good job. We learned when we started our next shift that Mr. Gonzalez was diagnosed with a concussion and would be released from the hospital the next day.

As the first medically trained rescuer on the scene, you have the opportunity to make a real difference in the life of a head-injury patient. Proper assessment and treatment could save him or her from further injury, permanent disfigurement, and even death.

NOCPs

4.3 i Conduct integumentary system assessment and interpret findings **S**

k Conduct assessment of the ears, eyes, nose, and throat and interpret findings **S**

5.6 a Treat soft-tissue injuries **S**

c Treat eye injury **S**

d Treat penetration wound **S**

6.1 j Provide care to patient experiencing signs or symptoms involving the eyes, ears, nose, or throat **S**

REVIEW QUESTIONS

Page references where answers may be found or supported are provided at the end of each question.

SECTION 1

1. What are the signs and symptoms associated with a head injury? (p. 352)
2. Under what conditions should you immediately take spinal precautions in a patient who has a head injury? (p. 352)
3. What are the general guidelines for emergency care of a patient with a head injury? (p. 354)
4. Should you remove an object impaled in the skull of a patient? Describe what you should do. (p. 355)

SECTION 2

5. What are the general principles of emergency care of a face or neck wound? (pp. 355–356)
6. Why would you want to remove a penetrating object from a patient's cheek? (p. 357)
7. How would you provide emergency care to a patient with an open and bleeding neck wound? (pp. 358–359)
8. Why should you never put pressure on the eyeball? (p. 359)
9. How would you care for a patient with a chemical burn to the eye? (p. 362)
10. Even if you successfully remove debris from the eye, why is it important for a patient to visit a physician or eye specialist? (p. 362)
11. How would you care for a patient with an object impaled in the eye? (pp. 362–363)

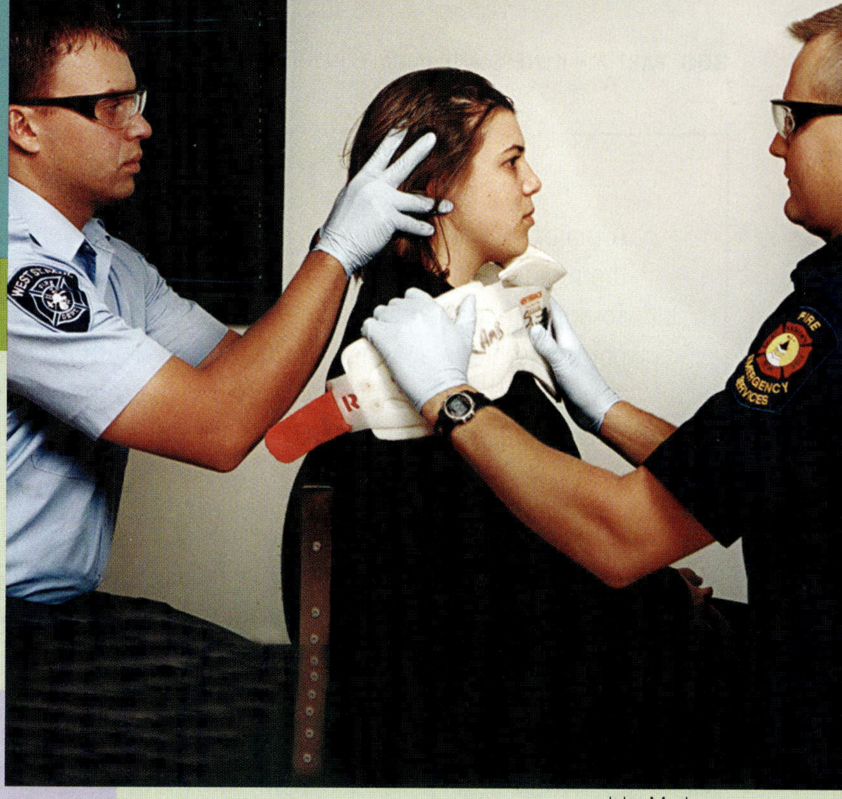

John Mackay

Injuries to the Spine

OBJECTIVES

1. Describe the implications of not properly caring for potential spinal injuries.
2. Relate the six common mechanisms of injury to the type of potential injury to the spine.
3. State 10 signs and symptoms of a spinal injury.
4. Describe the method of determining whether a conscious or an unconscious patient may have a spinal injury.
5. Relate emergency airway techniques to the patient with a suspected spine injury.
6. Discuss the sizing and application of a cervical spine immobilization device.
7. Describe how to log-roll a patient with a suspected spine injury and how to secure him or her to a long backboard.
8. Describe when and how to perform a rapid extrication.
9. Discuss the circumstances when a helmet should be removed and outline the steps for the two methods of helmet removal.
10. Demonstrate a caring attitude toward the patient and family when dealing with injuries to the spine, while giving priority to the interests of the patient.

INTRODUCTION

A major goal of EMS has always been the prevention of problems related to spinal injury. From the moment you arrive on the scene, consider the possibility of spinal injury and act accordingly. To appreciate the importance of this task, remember that failing to accomplish it can condemn a patient to life in a wheelchair or even to death. Not providing the precautionary care you are able to provide could result in civil litigation if it turns out that the patient did indeed have an injury that, left unprotected, resulted in disability or death.

SECTION 1
ANATOMY OF THE SPINE

The spinal cord lies within the spinal column. It is responsible for sending signals from the brain to the body and for receiving signals from the body and relaying them to the brain. If these signals are interrupted by injury or illness, a person could lose the ability to move, feel, or even breathe. (Review Chapter 4 for more on the musculoskeletal and nervous systems of the body.)

The spinal column is made up of 33 bones, one stacked on top of another. These vertebrae articulate, or fit and move together, so that we can bend, turn, and flex.

The spine is divided into five regions—the cervical, thoracic, lumbar, sacral, and coccygeal (Figures 25–1 and 25–2). The cervical spine starts at the base of the skull where the spinal cord begins. Its seven vertebrae not only house delicate nerve tissue, but they also support the weight of the head. This makes them especially vulnerable to injury.

The thoracic spine is supported by the rib cage. There are 12 thoracic vertebrae, one for each set of ribs. Because the ribs help protect this part of the spine, it is less frequently injured.

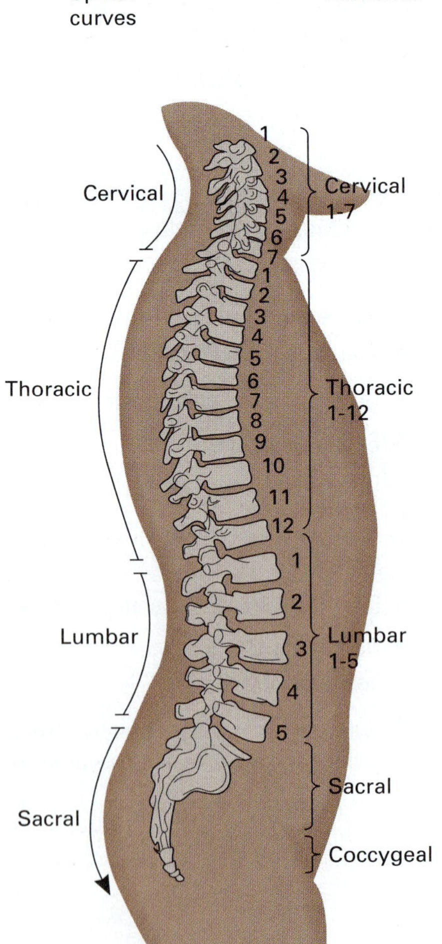

Figure 25–1 Regions of the spine.

Figure 25–2 Curves and vertebrae of the spine.

CASE STUDY

Dispatch

We were on foot patrol at the university football game. Just as the home team receiver looked as if he would score, his lone pursuer dove and hit the post head-first with full force.

Scene Assessment

The coach and team trainer ran out onto the field. Almost immediately, the trainer indicated he needed us there. We donned our gloves on the way.

When we got to the patient, we saw that the trainer was already stabilizing his head and neck. He quickly told us that the player appeared to be unconscious. We noticed the helmet was cracked along the top. We called for EMS support immediately.

Primary Assessment

My partner and I assisted the trainer, who was experienced in helmet removal. Then we used the jaw-thrust manoeuvre to open the patient's airway. It was clear of blood and secretions. Breathing was adequate but irregular. We applied 100% oxygen by non-rebreather mask, using a small portable oxygen tank. The patient's pulse was strong and bounding, and his skin was warm and dry. No bleeding was noted. We carefully applied a cervical collar.

> Consider this patient as you read Chapter 25. What else might be done to assess and treat his condition?

The next group of five vertebrae make up the lumbar spine. They carry the weight of most of the body. For this reason they are heavier and larger. The discs between the lumbar vertebrae are thicker than in other parts of the spine. Sometimes, a disc can shift, slip, or rupture. Injuries to the lumbar spine cost millions of dollars in medical expenses and lost wages every year.

The last two regions of vertebrae are the sacral and coccygeal. The sacrum has five fused vertebrae. The coccyx has four. Together they form the posterior portion of the pelvis. Because they are fused, these parts of the spine do not bend easily.

SECTION 2
SPINAL INJURIES

During scene assessment, you as an EMR must identify the mechanism that injured your patient. In doing so, you consider what occurred and what injuries may have resulted. Your index of suspicion for a spinal injury should be very high in any of the emergencies described below:

- Motor vehicle accidents (MVAs)
- Motorcycle crashes
- Pedestrian–car crashes
- Falls
- Diving accidents
- Hangings
- Blunt trauma
- Penetrating trauma to the head, neck, or torso
- Gunshot wounds
- Any speed sport accident, such as rollerblading, skateboarding, bicycling, skiing, surfing, or sledding
- Any unconscious trauma patient

Note that if the mechanism of injury suggests it (Figure 25–3 on p. 370), you should proceed as if the patient has a spinal injury—even if the patient says he or she is not injured at all. The absence of

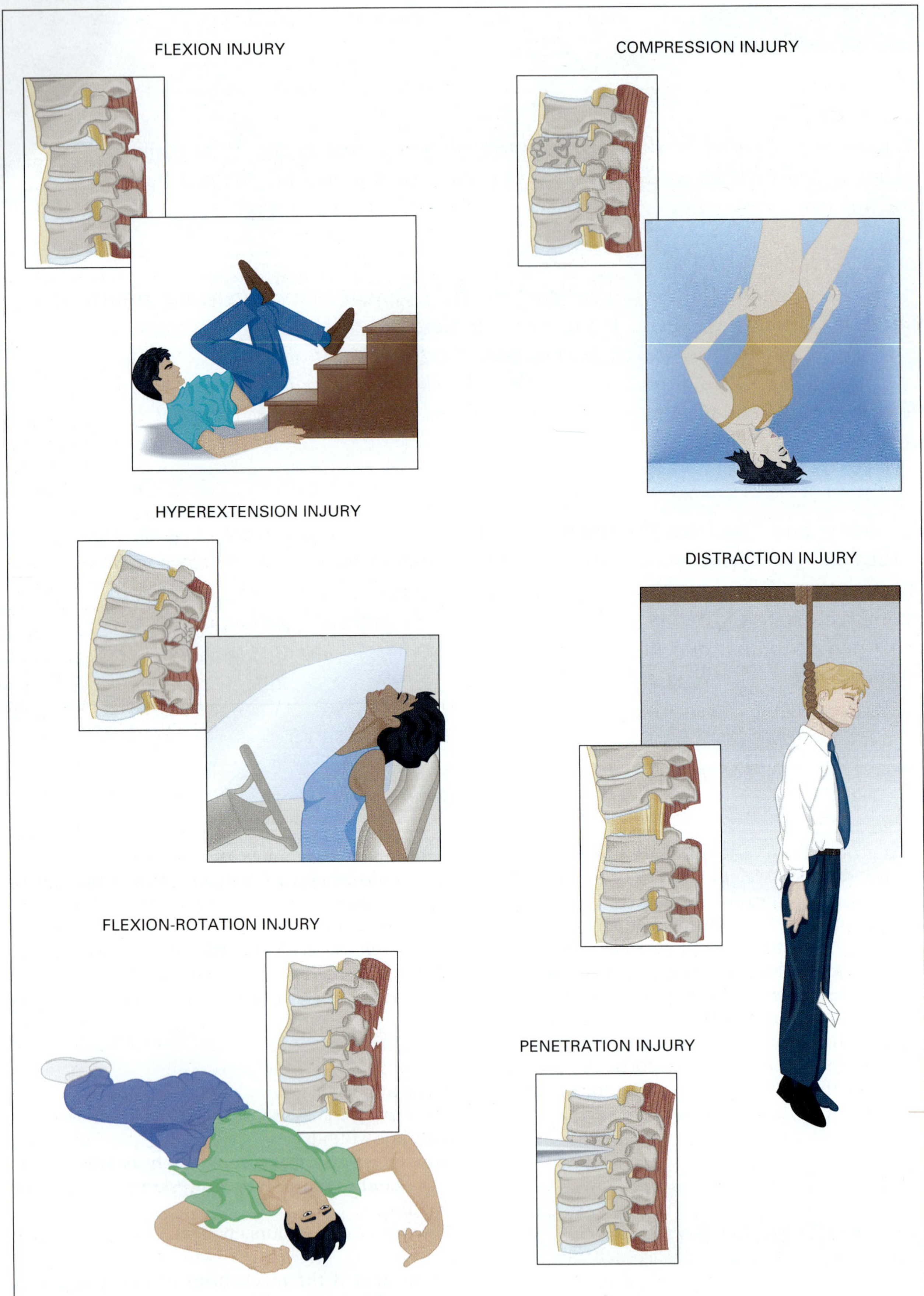

Figure 25–3 Common mechanisms of spinal injury.

back pain and having the ability to walk, move arms and legs, or feel sensation do not rule out spinal injury.

> ## (!) T I P
>
> Patients found hanging ideally require at least three rescuers to cut the rope and lower the patient to the floor if resuscitation is to be attempted without further injury. In addition to the cervical trauma, the hangman's fracture can cause severing of the spinal cord. Tracheal injury, causing airway complications, is also associated with hanging.

Patient Assessment

If you suspect spinal injury in your patient, you must protect the spine from further damage. Immediately upon completing your scene assessment, stabilize the patient's head and neck. Then assess the ABCs. Be sure to use the jaw-thrust manoeuvre to open and maintain the airway. Remember that a cervical spine injury can result in severe breathing problems, even respiratory arrest. Be sure to monitor the patient's airway and breathing continuously.

There may be no signs at all of spinal injury. However, when they do appear, they typically include one or more of the following:

- Respiratory distress
- Tenderness at the site of injury on the spinal column
- Pain along the spinal column with movement (Do not move the patient or ask the patient to move to test for this pain.)
- Constant or intermittent pain, even without movement, along the spinal column or in the lower legs
- Obvious deformity of the spine (rare)
- Soft-tissue injuries to the head, neck, shoulders, back, abdomen, or legs
- Numbness, weakness, or tingling in the arms or legs
- Loss of sensation or paralysis in the upper or lower extremities or below the injury site
- Incontinence, or loss of bowel or bladder control
- Priapism, or a constant erection of the penis (a classic sign of cervical spine injury in men)

During the secondary assessment, do not risk moving the spine by taking off the patient's shirt or coat. Cut off the patient's clothes if necessary. Be sure to ask the patient if and where the spine hurts. Stop immediately if the patient complains of pain upon palpation of the spine. Continue the assessment of other areas of the body.

Assess pulses, movement, and sensation in all four extremities (Figure 25–4 on p. 372). To assess movement, ask the patient if he or she can move the hands and feet. Then have him or her squeeze both your hands at the same time. Gauge the patient's strength and decide if it is equal on both sides. Also, have the patient push his or her feet against your hands. Again, gauge strength and equality.

To assess sensation, gently squeeze one extremity and then the other. As you do, ask questions such as these: "Can you feel me touching your fingers? Can you feel me touching your toes?"

If the patient is unconscious, or unable to follow your instructions, apply a painful stimulus to check response. Either pinch the webbing between the toes and fingers or apply pressure with a pen across the back of a fingernail. The patient should withdraw from the pain. Note the response to pain in all four extremities.

After the assessment of the front of the patient, perform a log roll so that you can assess the back. However, do so only if you are trained in its use and have enough help to do so safely. Details on how to perform a log roll are provided later in this chapter. When performing the log roll, have a backboard ready onto which to roll the patient back.

Remember that a patient may be uncomfortable, confused, and possibly afraid of paralysis or death. It is important for you to show a caring attitude. As you proceed with the secondary assessment, for example, be careful how you communicate your findings to your partner. A casual remark could terrify the patient. When you speak to the patient's family, be honest but do not alarm them unnecessarily.

General Guidelines for Emergency Care

If the mechanism of injury suggests a possible spinal injury, stabilize the patient's cervical spine immediately. This means placing your gloved hands just behind the patient's ears. Then hold the patient's head firm and steady in a neutral, in-line position. *Neutral* means the head is not flexed forward or extended back. *In-line* means the patient's nose is in line with the navel.

If you find that the patient's head is not in line, you must gently put it there. Stop at once if the conscious patient complains of pain or if you feel resistance in the unconscious patient. In this case, stabilize the head and neck in the position in which they were found.

Manual stabilization may be released only when the patient is immobilized from head to toe on a long backboard. When possible, have another rescuer maintain manual stabilization so that you can be free to care for the patient.

In general, emergency care for a suspected spinal injury patient proceeds as follows:

1. Take BSI precautions. Observe the mechanism of injury.

ASSESSING PULSE, MOVEMENT, AND SENSATION

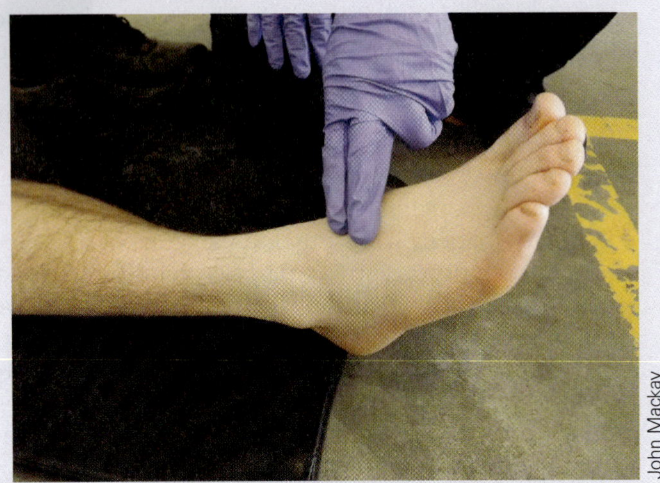

Figure 25–4a   Feel for a pulse in all the extremities.

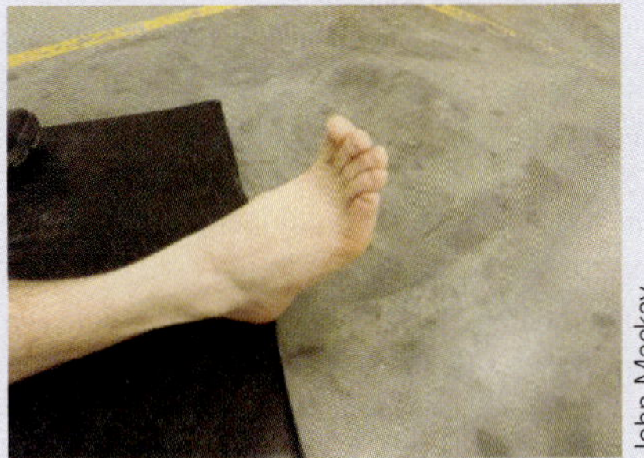

Figure 25–4b   See if the feet and toes can move.

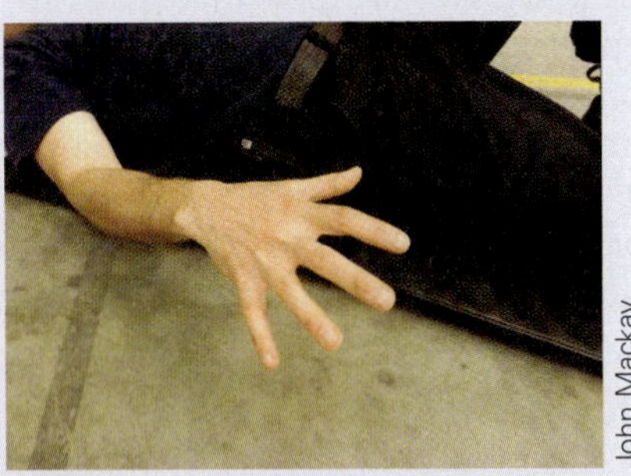

Figure 25–4c   See if the hands and fingers can move.

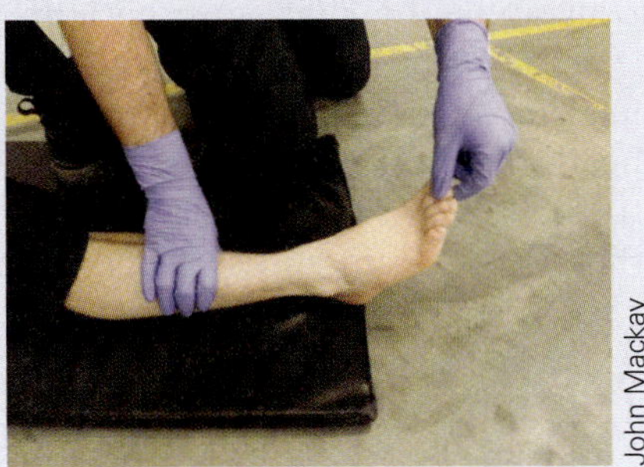

Figure 25–4d   Touch the toes to assess for sensation.

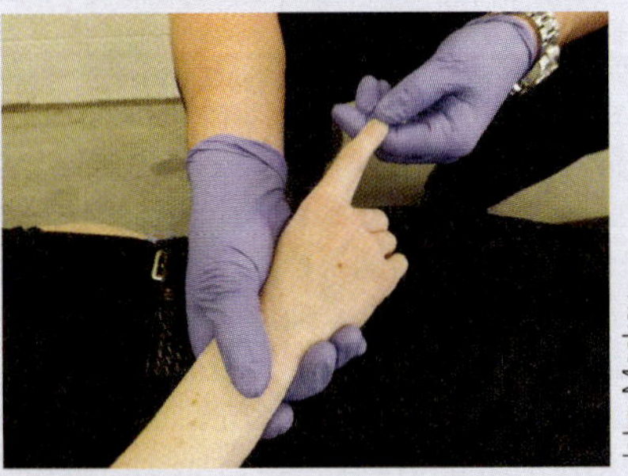

Figure 25–4e   Touch the fingers to assess for sensation.

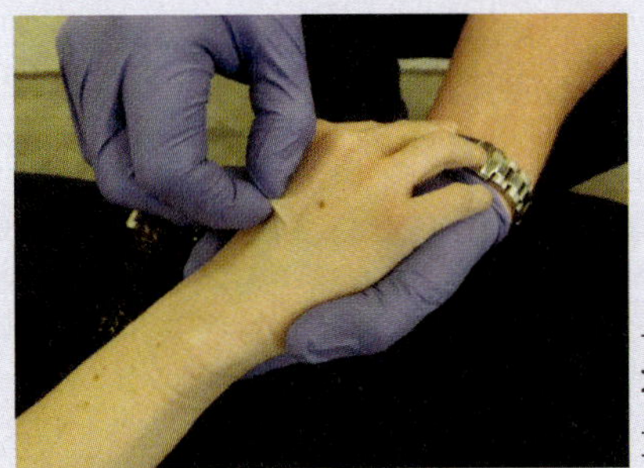

Figure 25–4f   If the patient is unconscious, see if he or she responds to painful stimuli.

2. Stabilize the patient's head and neck immediately (Figure 25–5). Keep the patient from moving.

3. Then perform a primary assessment and provide treatment. Be sure to open and maintain the airway with the jaw-thrust manoeuvre. Insert an oropharyngeal or nasopharyngeal airway if needed. Suction without turning the patient's head.

4. Provide high-flow oxygen via a non-rebreather mask. If the patient stops breathing or if breathing is inadequate, assist with artificial ventilation. Maintain neutral, in-line stabilization throughout.

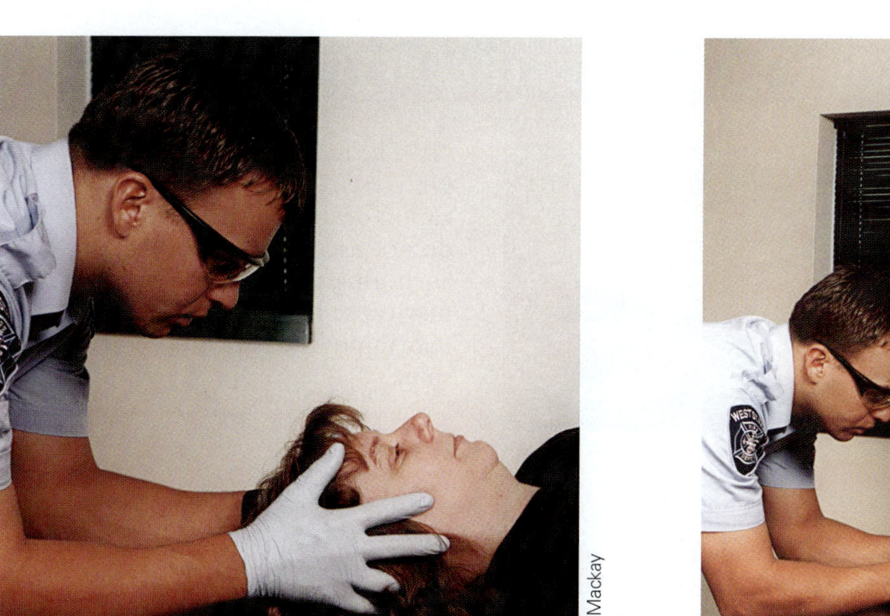

Figure 25–5 Manual stabilization means holding the patient's head firmly and steadily in a neutral, in-line position.

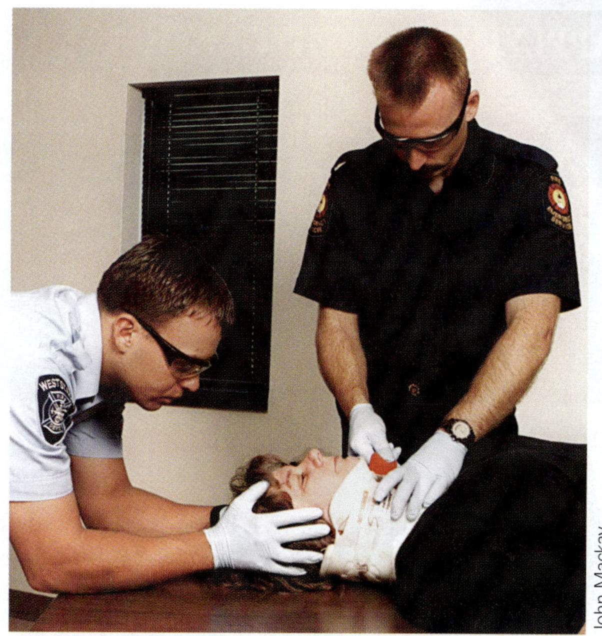

Figure 25–6 If you are allowed, apply a rigid cervical immobilization device to the patient.

5. Perform a secondary assessment and provide treatment. Be sure to monitor the patient's airway and breathing continuously.
6. Maintain manual stabilization until the patient is completely immobilized.

Immobilization Techniques

Many EMS systems allow EMRs to immobilize a suspected spinal injury patient. Even if your system does not, you may be called to assist the paramedics. Become familiar with the techniques. They include cervical immobilization, long backboard immobilization, rapid extrication, and helmet removal.

Remember: Never attempt to treat or move a spinal injury patient unless you have the proper equipment, training, and personnel.

Cervical Immobilization

After a primary assessment, a rigid cervical immobilization device, or extrication collar, should be applied to the patient (Figure 25–6). Various types are available. However, never use a soft collar in the field. They are nothing more than cotton-covered foam rings, which do not prevent movement of the head and neck.

Use rigid or hard collars in the field. They are designed to prevent the patient from turning, flexing, and extending the head. They can restrict movement by up to 70 percent. The remaining 30 percent must be accomplished by manual stabilization.

Follow the manufacturer's instructions for applying a cervical collar, or C-collar. Though instructions will vary, all collars are supported at the same points: the maxilla (jaw), shoulders, and clavicles. Note that failure to fit a patient properly can aggravate the injury.

Before application, be sure that jewellery and long hair have been moved away from the area. In addition, examine and palpate the patient's neck before the collar is applied.

In general, to apply a rigid cervical collar to a supine patient, follow these steps (Figure 25–7):

1. Slide the posterior portion of the collar into the gap under the patient's neck.
2. Then flip the anterior portion under the chin.
3. Secure the collar with the Velcro strap. Be careful not to pull too hard on one end. It can twist the patient's head.

> ## ⓘ T I P
>
> EMS professionals appreciate having their equipment as ready as possible for use. One idea that has dual benefits is to open your packaged cravats or triangular bandages, fold and wrap them in a ready-to-use fashion, and secure them with an elastic band. This band can also be used later to tie up a patient's long hair into a bun, which will enable you to have better access for assessment and treatment—including C-collar application—of a trauma patient.

APPLYING A RIGID CERVICAL IMMOBILIZATION DEVICE

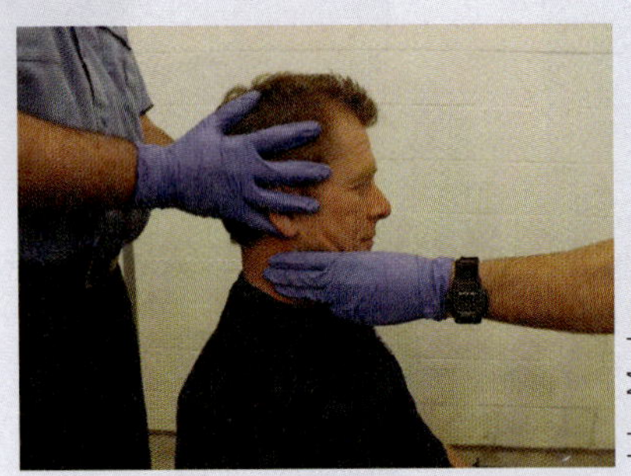

Figure 25–7a

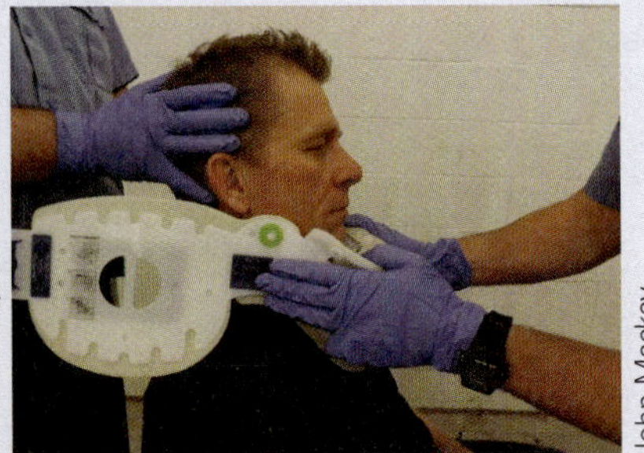

Figure 25–7b

NOTE: Do not use soft collars. Only use rigid cervical immobilization devices in the field. Also, do not use the chin piece as an anchoring point for the collar. This may cause hyperextension, which may injure the patient's cervical spine.

SIZING

It is critical to select a collar that is the correct size. Too tall can over-extend the neck, force the jaw closed, and limit access to the airway. Too short can lead to inadequate immobilization. Too tight can impede blood flow. One way to measure collar size is to use your fingers to compare the neck size to the corresponding area of the collar.

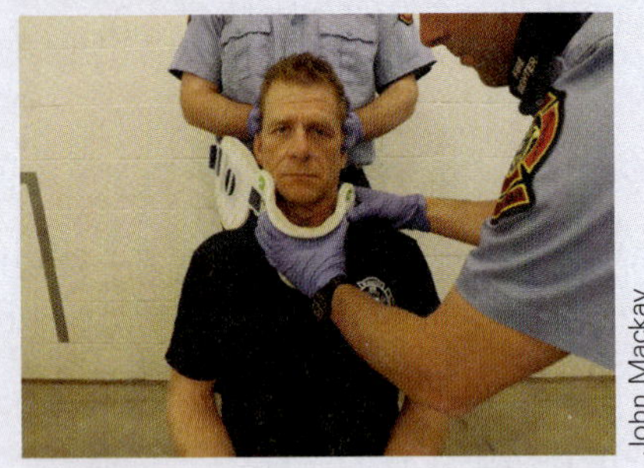

Figure 25–7c

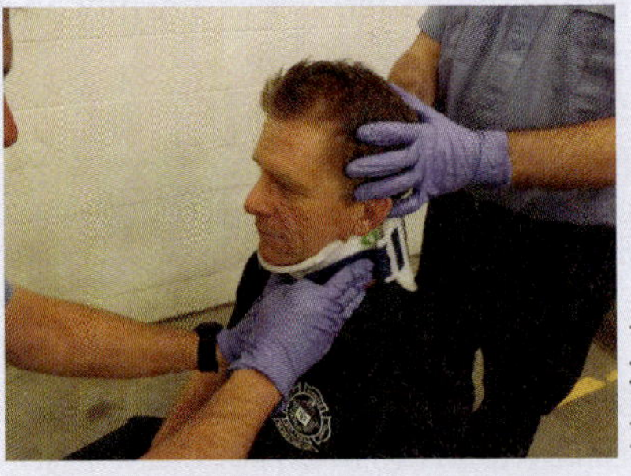

Figure 25–7d

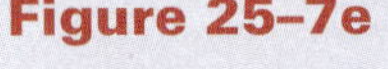

Figure 25–7e

SEATED APPLICATION

The patient's chin must be well supported by the chin piece. To accomplish this, slide the collar up the patient's chest wall. If the collar is pushed directly inward, it may be difficult to position the chin piece and, therefore, to apply the collar tightly enough.

TIGHTENING

Grip the "trache" hole as you tighten the collar. Then check to see that the collar fits according to the manufacturer's instructions.

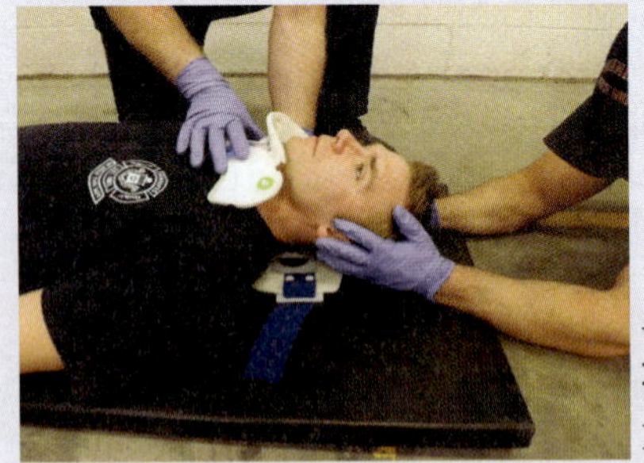

Figure 25–7f

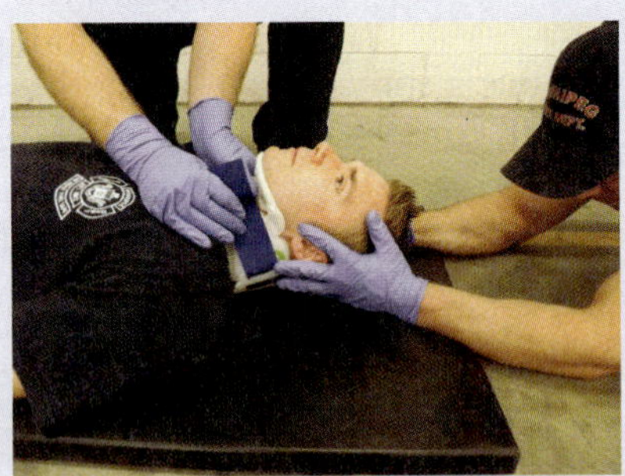

Figure 25–7g

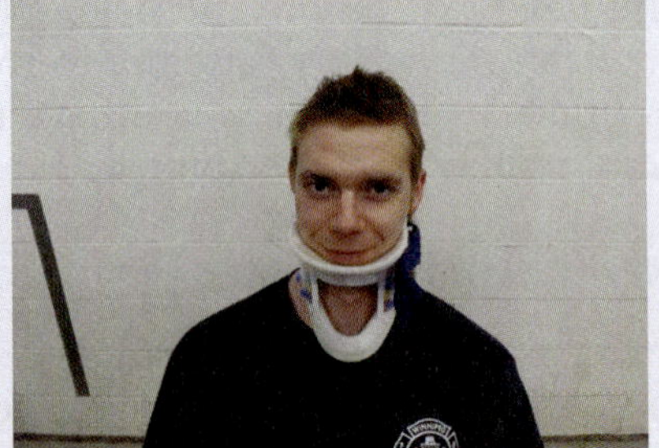

Figure 25–7h

SUPINE APPLICATION

Slip the collar underneath the patient's neck. Then rotate the collar up along the chest until the chin piece is properly positioned.

WARNING

Always check for neutral alignment and proper fit. Improper sizing or application may allow the patient's chin to slip inside the collar. This must be prevented.

If your patient is sitting, move the collar up the chest until the chin is trapped. Then slide the posterior portion around the back of the neck and fasten it. Whatever position your patient is in, you must maintain manual stabilization of the head and neck.

Release it only when the patient is completely immobilized on a long backboard.

Long Backboard Immobilization

All patients with suspected spinal injury must be immobilized onto a long backboard. To immobilize a supine or prone patient, you must first roll the patient onto the side, slip the board under him or her, and roll the patient back. This procedure is called a log roll.

To perform a log roll safely, you need at least three rescuers, preferably four, who are trained in the procedure. One should stay at the head to maintain manual stabilization and to coordinate the move. The other two should position themselves along one side of the patient's body. Proceed as follows (Figure 25–8):

1. Maintain manual stabilization of the patient's head and neck. Continue to do so until the patient is completely immobilized.
2. Apply a rigid cervical immobilization device.
3. Assess pulses, movement, and sensation in all four extremities.
4. Position the patient. Place the patient's arms straight down by the sides if possible.
5. Position the rescuers. At the signal of the rescuer at the head, the other two should reach to the far

THREE-RESCUER LOG ROLL

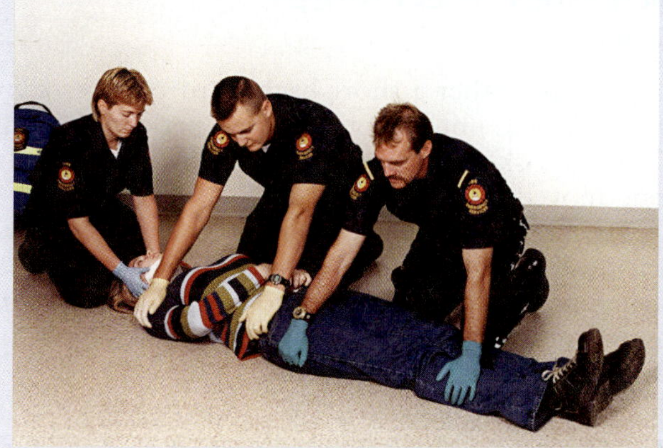

Figure 25–8a   Maintain the patient's head and neck in a neutral, in-line position.

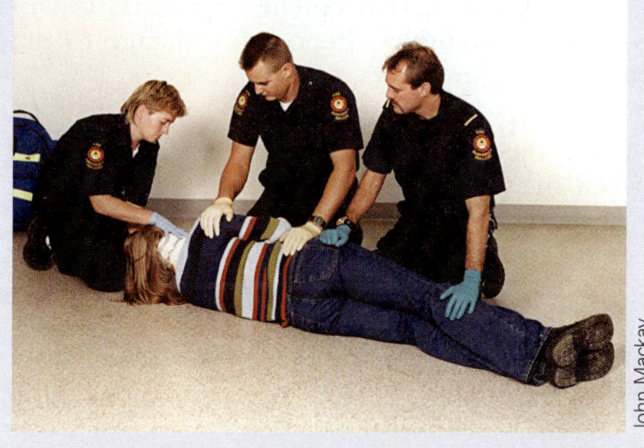

Figure 25–8b   Roll the patient onto the side.

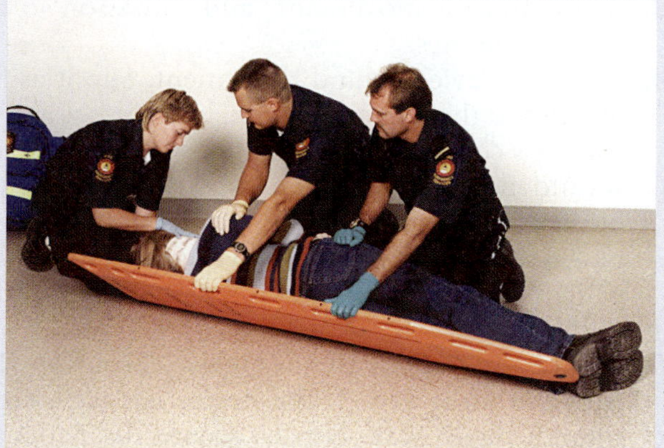

Figure 25–8c   A bystander or one of the three rescuers should move the long backboard into place.

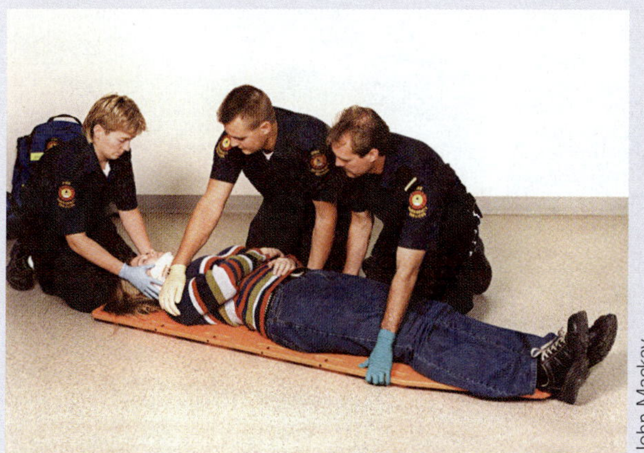

Figure 25–8d   Lower the patient onto the long backboard.

side of the patient. One rescuer should position his or her hands on the shoulder and the hip. The second rescuer should position the hands at the thigh and lower leg.

6. On signal, the rescuers should simultaneously roll the patient onto the side. Note that this is a good time to assess the patient's posterior if it has not been done already.

7. Position the board. A fourth person—another rescuer, a family member, or bystander—should push the board under the patient. If no one else is available, one of the rescuers at the side may lean over the patient, grab the backboard, and pull it under the patient.

8. On signal, the rescuers should simultaneously roll the patient back down and onto the board. If the patient is not in the middle of the board, gently pull the patient down and then up again until he or she is straight on the board. This is done at the shoulders and hips and by pulling in alignment with the long axis of the spine. Never push a patient over to the middle of the backboard.

9. Reassess pulses, movement, and sensation in all four extremities. Report any change to the incoming paramedics.

Once the patient is in place, pad the spaces between the patient and the board (Figure 25–9). For an adult, pad anywhere along the length of the body to maintain neutral alignment and provide comfort. For an infant or child, also pad under the shoulders. This is to keep the relatively larger head from flexing forward. Take care to avoid extra movement.

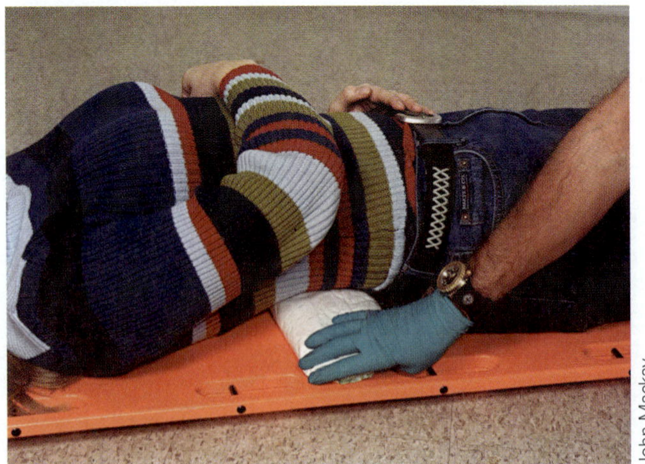

Figure 25–9 Pad the gaps between the patient and the board.

Your next step is to secure the patient to the long backboard. It should always be done in this order (Figure 25–10 on p. 377):

1. Immobilize the torso first. If you have to turn the patient laterally in order to facilitate vomiting during immobilization, a secured thorax better enables you to maintain alignment of the head and spine. If you turn a patient with only the head secured to the board, the thorax may compromise proper cervical alignment.

2. Immobilize the head next. The head must always be immobilized after the torso. Take a great deal of care not to lock the jaw in place. If the patient needs to vomit, the patient must be able to open his or her mouth.

3. Immobilize the legs last.

4. Withdraw manual stabilization of the head and neck.

5. Reassess pulses, movement, and sensation. Report any change to the incoming paramedics.

Short Backboard or Vest-Type Immobilization

You can use either a short backboard or a vest-type device to help immobilize a seated patient. It minimizes the risk of further injury while the patient is being moved to a long backboard.

To apply a short backboard or vest to a seated patient, follow the steps outlined below. Remember to maintain manual stabilization throughout, until the patient is completely immobilized. Proceed as follows (Figure 25–11 on p. 378):

1. Maintain manual stabilization of the patient's head and neck. If possible, hold the patient's head and neck from behind.

2. Apply a rigid cervical immobilization device.

3. Assess pulses, movement, and sensation in all four extremities.

4. Slide the device behind the patient. Slip it as far down into the seat as possible, but not below the patient's coccyx. The top of the short backboard should be level with the top of the patient's head. The body flaps of the vest should fit snugly under the patient's armpits. Try not to jostle the patient or the rescuer who is maintaining manual stabilization.

5. Secure the patient to the device. Strap up the patient's torso first. If the device has leg straps, tighten those next. Finally, secure the patient's head. To make sure the head and neck remain in neutral alignment with the rest of the spine, you may need to pad behind them.

SECURING A PATIENT TO A LONG BACKBOARD

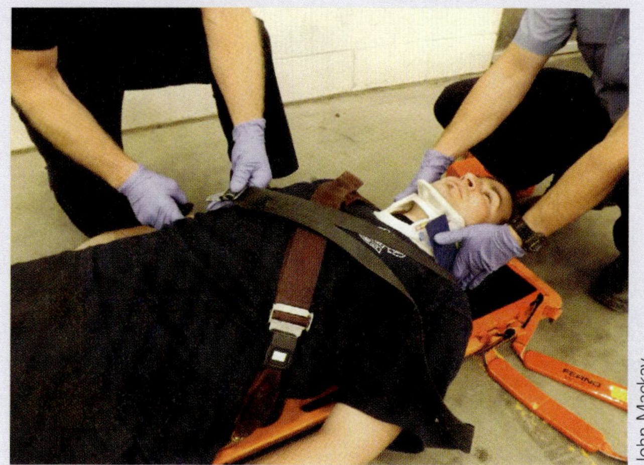

Figure 25–10a Immobilize the patient's torso first.

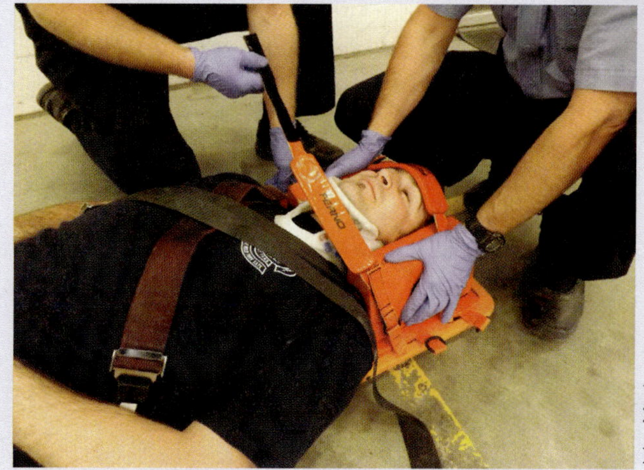

Figure 25–10b Immobilize the head next.

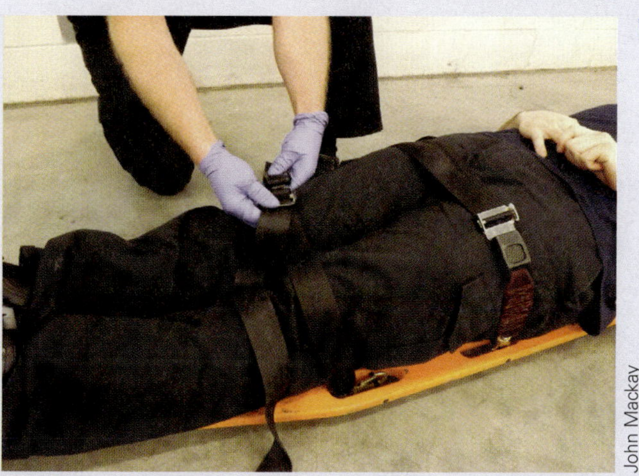

Figure 25–10c Finally, immobilize the patient's legs and feet.

To move the patient to a long backboard, position it under or next to the patient's buttocks. Rotate the patient until his or her back is in line with it. Then lower the patient onto the long backboard. If you utilized a vest type of device, then you must release the leg straps before you secure the patient to the board.

Follow the instructions outlined above for securing the patient. Release manual stabilization when the patient is completely immobilized.

Rapid Extrication

In general, rescuers should move a sitting spinal-injury patient only after short backboard immobilization.

However, in certain emergencies, there is not enough time. A rapid extrication may need to be performed in the following circumstances:

- The scene is not safe. For example, there is a threat of fire or explosion, a hostile crowd, or extreme weather conditions.
- Life-saving care cannot be given because of the patient's location or position.
- There is an inability to gain access to other patients who need life-saving care.

In general, a rapid extrication must be performed by a team of three or more rescuers.

SECURING A PATIENT WITH AN EXTRICATION VEST

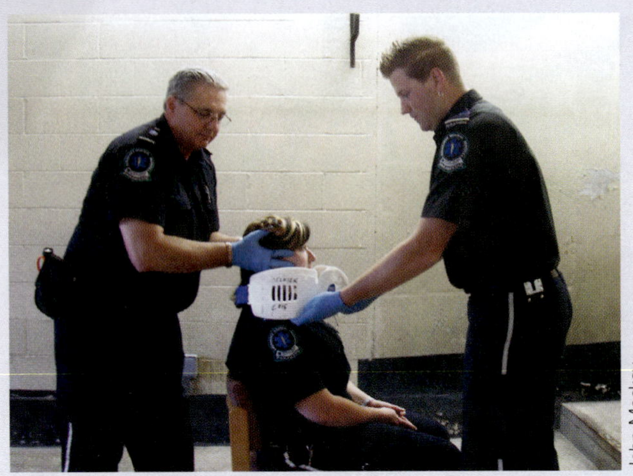

Figure 25–11a   Manually stabilize the head and neck. Then, apply a rigid cervical collar.

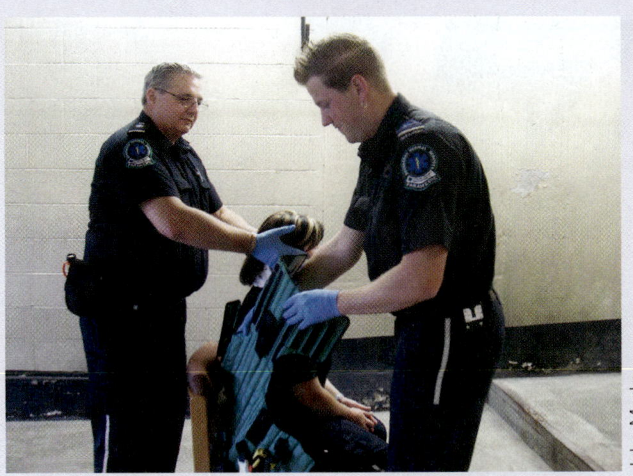

Figure 25–11b   Position the extrication vest behind the patient.

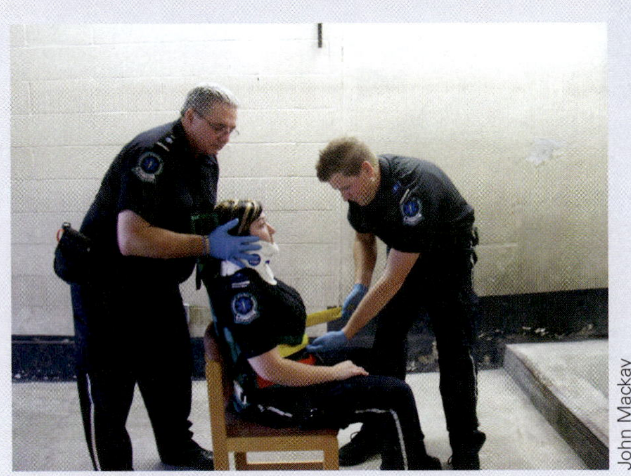

Figure 25–11c   Secure the torso and leg straps.

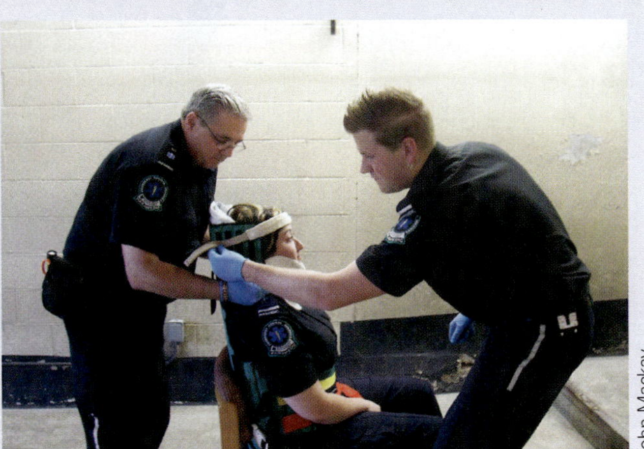

Figure 25–11d   Pad behind the head if necessary and secure the head straps.

The objective is to move a sitting patient to a long backboard with only manual stabilization of the spine. To do so, proceed as follows (Figure 25–12):

1. Bring the patient's head into a neutral, in-line position. This is best done from behind or to the side of the patient.
2. Apply a rigid cervical immobilization device.
3. Rotate the patient into position. Do so in several short, coordinated moves until the patient's back is in the vehicle's open doorway and his or her feet are on the adjoining seat.
4. Bring the long backboard in line with the patient. It should rest against the patient's buttocks.

5. Lower the patient onto the long backboard and slide him or her into position in short, coordinated moves.
6. Secure the patient to the backboard. Release manual stabilization only when the patient is completely immobilized on a long backboard.

It may be necessary to hand off manual stabilization to someone else during the procedure. Be sure it is maintained continuously until the patient is completely immobilized. If the level of danger does not afford you even the time to apply a C-collar, remove the patient by using the shirt drag technique (see Figure 6–7 on p. 69), using your forearms to provide as much cervical stability as possible.

RAPID EXTRICATION

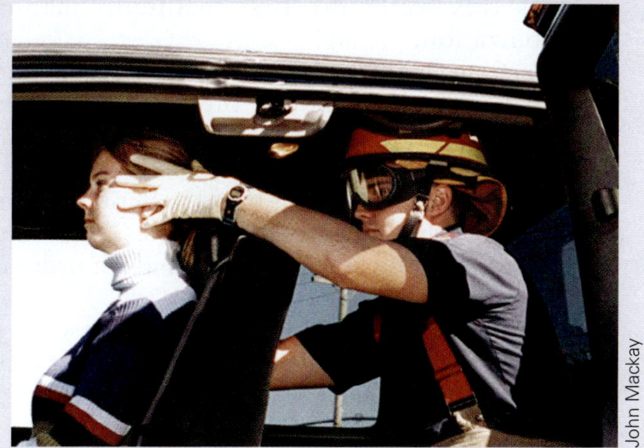

Figure 25–12a Bring the patient's head into a neutral, in-line position.

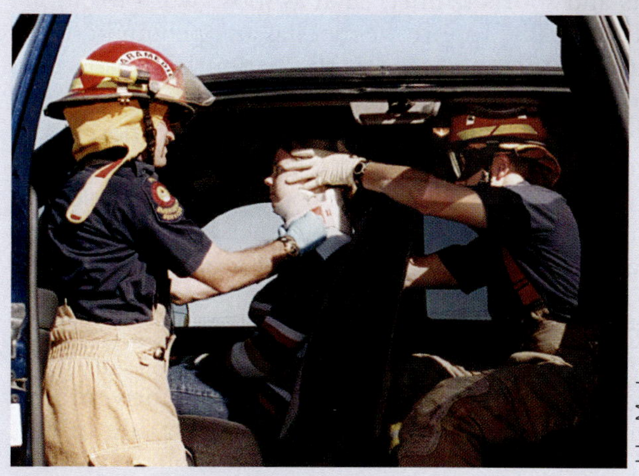

Figure 25–12b Apply a rigid cervical immobilization device.

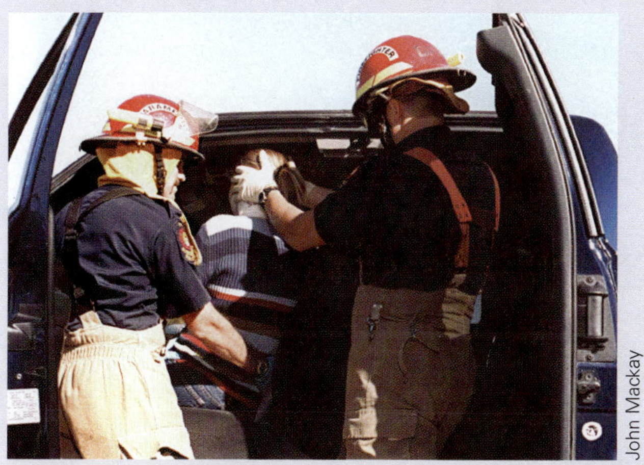

Figure 25–12c Rotate the patient into position.

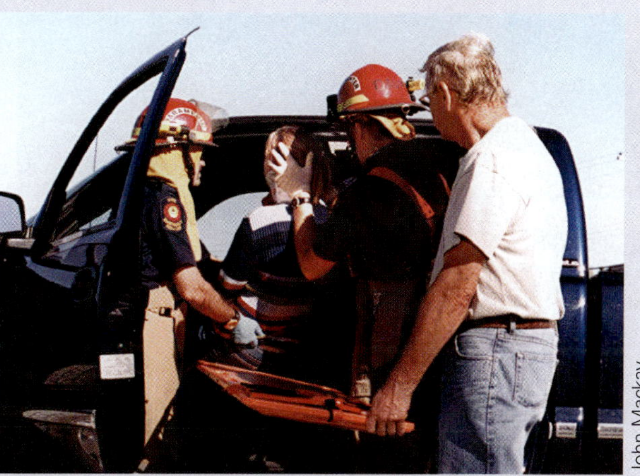

Figure 25–12d Bring the long backboard in line with the patient.

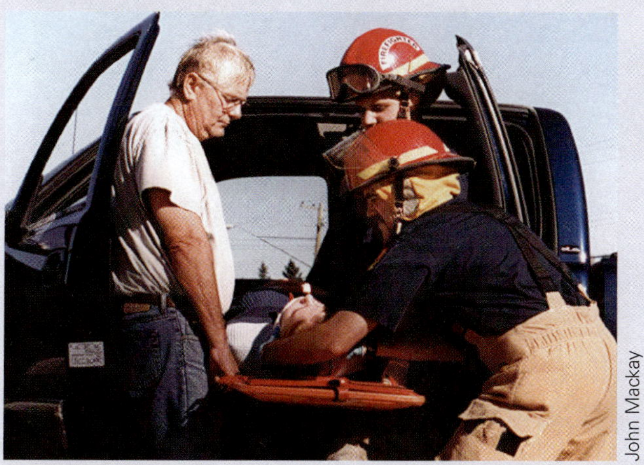

Figure 25–12e Lower the patient onto the long backboard.

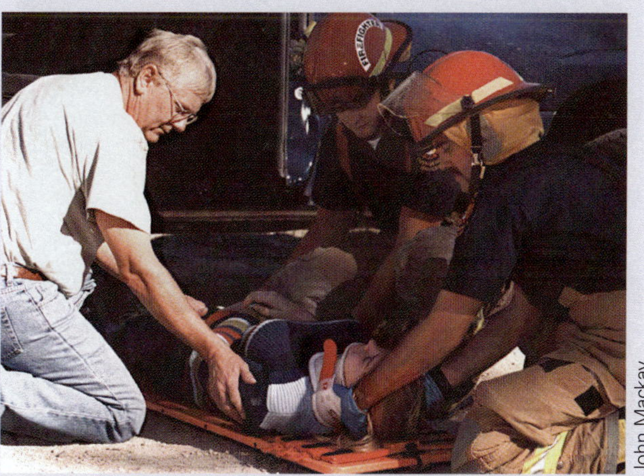

Figure 25–12f Slide the patient into position in small steps and secure the patient to the backboard.

Helmet Removal

There are two basic types of helmets: motorcycle helmets and sports helmets such as those worn for football. Typically, a sports helmet has an opening in front that allows easy access to the patient's airway. For many, the face shield can be unclipped or snapped off for easy removal. A full-face motorcycle helmet, however, will prevent access to the patient's airway.

In general, if your patient can be properly assessed and the airway maintained, a helmet should be left in place. Do not attempt to remove a helmet by yourself. Wait for help. If it must be removed, follow these steps (Figures 25–13 and 25–14):

1. Stabilize the helmet to prevent movement. The rescuer at the head holds each side of the helmet and places his or her fingers on the lower jaw.
2. Loosen the chin strap. The second rescuer does this while the first maintains manual stabilization.
3. Transfer stabilization. To do so, the second rescuer places one hand on the mandible at the angle of the jaw. He or she then places the other hand at the back of the head.
4. Slip off the helmet about halfway. Be sure to pull it wide so that it can clear the ears. The second rescuer then adjusts his or her hands in order to maintain alignment of the head.
5. Remove the helmet completely. The rescuer at the head then takes over manual stabilization until the patient is completely immobilized.

HELMET REMOVAL

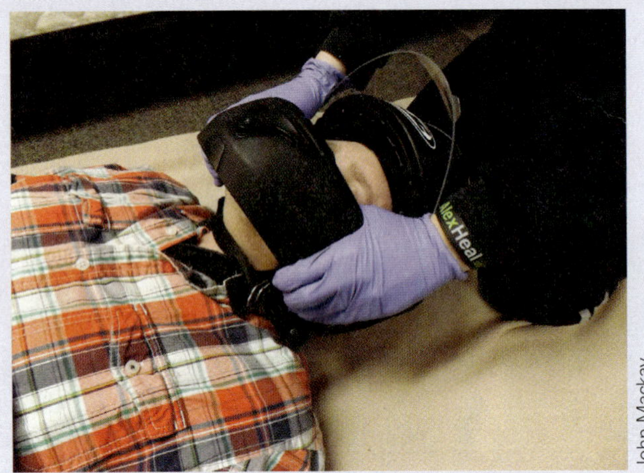

Figure 25–13a Stabilize the helmet, head, and neck to prevent movement.

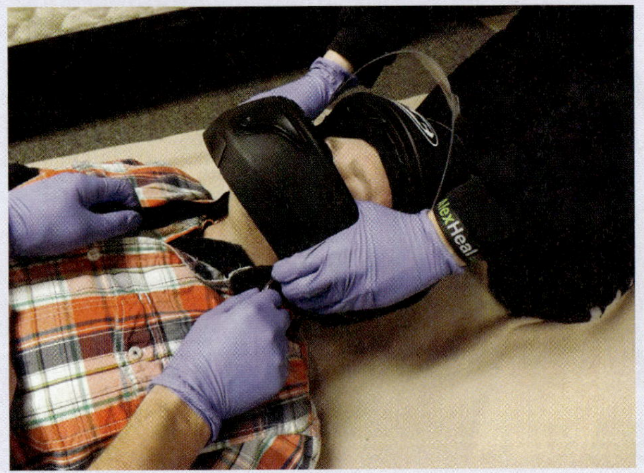

Figure 25–13b The second rescuer loosens the chin strap while the first maintains manual stabilization.

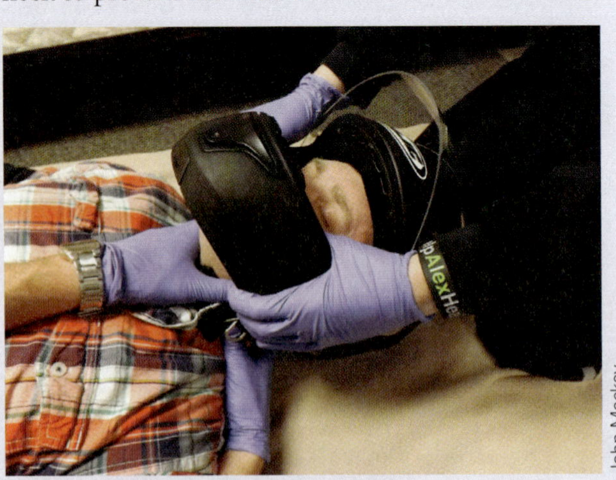

Figure 25–13c Transfer stabilization to the second rescuer.

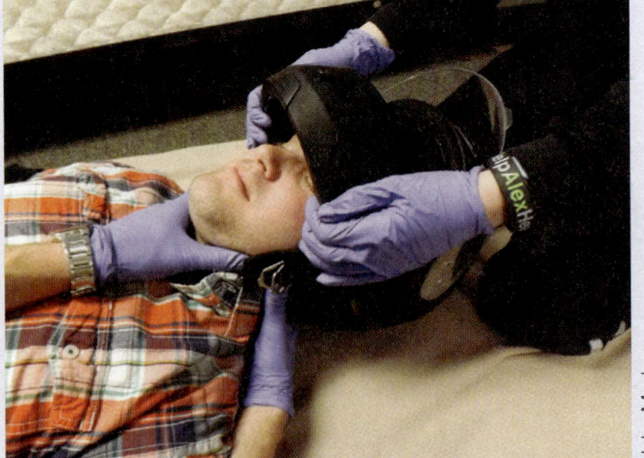

Figure 25–13d Slip off the helmet about halfway while the second rescuer maintains an in-line position of the head.

HELMET REMOVAL *(continued)*

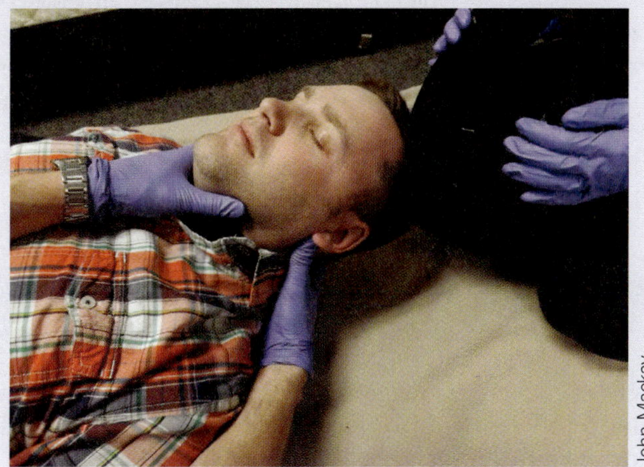

Figure 25–13e The second rescuer adjusts his or her hands to maintain manual stabilization.

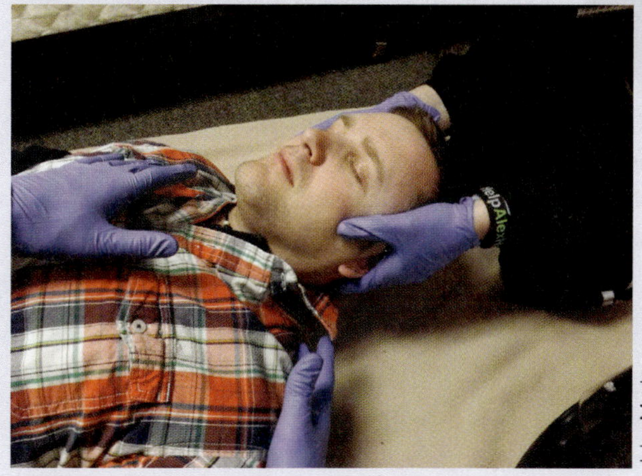

Figure 25–13f When the helmet is completely removed, transfer manual stabilization to the rescuer at the head.

HELMET REMOVAL—ALTERNATIVE METHOD

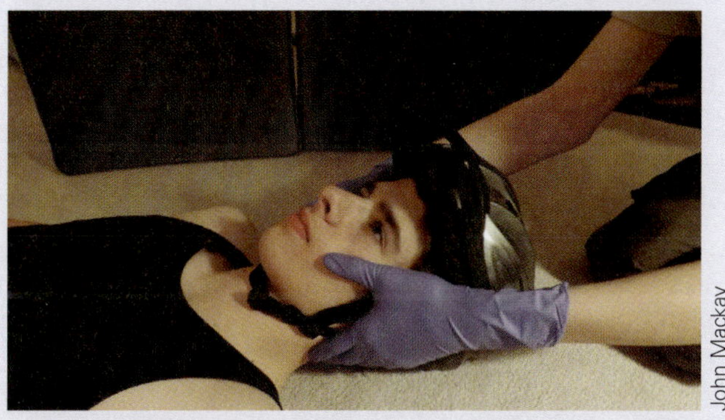

Figure 25–14a Stabilize the helmet, head, and neck to prevent movement.

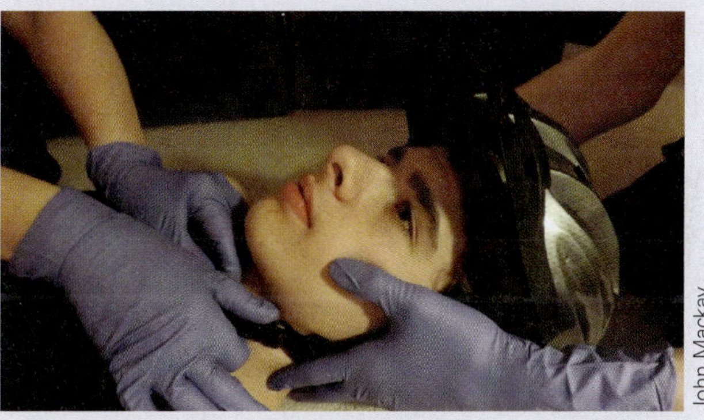

Figure 25–14b The second rescuer removes the chin strap while the first maintains manual stabilization.

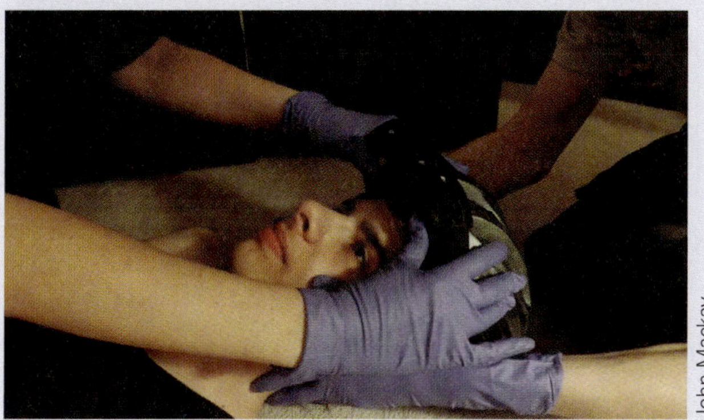

Figure 25–14c The second rescuer removes the helmet. Full-face helmets will have to be tilted back to clear the nose.

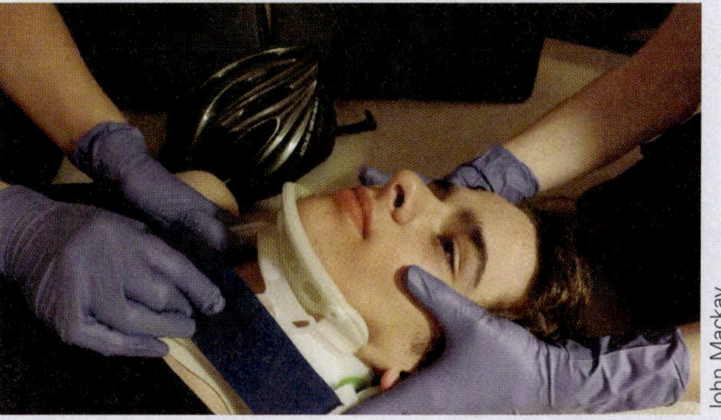

Figure 25–14d Apply a rigid cervical collar, and maintain manual stabilization until the patient is completely immobilized.

EMR FOCUS

Even after a collision with heavy damage to the crash vehicles, there may be patients with a complaint of only minor pain or no pain at all. It is just as important to take spinal precautions with these patients as with patients who complain of pain. Never assume a patient is uninjured if the mechanism suggests injury. That is for the hospital physicians to decide.

An EMS instructor wrote this simple but powerful message on the chalkboard during an EMR class: "Quadriplegia is forever." (Quadriplegia is the inability to use any of the extremities because of a spinal cord injury.) Use caution with every patient who has a possible spinal injury. The consequences of not doing so are extremely serious!

CASE STUDY FOLLOW-UP

At the beginning of this chapter, you read that EMRs were caring for a male patient with possible head and spinal injuries. To see how the chapter skills apply to this emergency, read the following. It describes how the call was completed.

SECONDARY ASSESSMENT

The ETA of the ambulance was about three minutes. I began a secondary assessment as the team trainer carefully removed the patient's pads. My partner maintained manual stabilization and asked the coach about the patient's history.

My first obvious finding was a deformity and swelling on the top of the patient's head. Clear fluid and blood seeped out of his ears. His facial bones all appeared to be intact.

PATIENT HISTORY

The coach got the patient's medical history card from his pack at the sideline. It indicated that the player had no known allergies and that he did not take any prescribed medication. His last physical by the team doctor was unremarkable. He had no other significant past medical history.

The coach told my partner that the team players had eaten lunch about an hour before the game.

ONGOING ASSESSMENT

We maintained manual stabilization. Since the patient was unconscious and his respirations were somewhat irregular, we watched his breathing carefully. We also checked his pulse again. We radioed for the ambulance to bring immobilization equipment and to drive right onto the field.

TRANSFER OF CARE

When the paramedics arrived, I told them what we knew:

"This is Henry Jones, 21 years old. He struck a steel goal post, shattering his helmet and sustaining a head injury. He was unconscious upon our arrival, and that hasn't changed. His respirations have been irregular but deep. We'll have to assist his breathing soon. Pulse has dropped from 80 to 56. We removed the helmet and pads with the assistance of the trainer. We manually stabilized his head and neck the whole time. The coach has his history—nothing of note."

We helped to log-roll the patient onto a long backboard. The paramedics radioed the trauma centre to report a possible neurosurgical emergency.

Head and spinal injuries are among the most devastating injuries a patient can suffer. Always be alert to the possibility that an injury to the spine may have occurred. Do everything you can to protect it from further harm. Remember, if the mechanism of injury suggests it, treat for it.

NOCPs

3.2 b Transfer patient from various positions using applicable equipment and/or techniques **S**

c Transfer patient using emergency evacuation techniques **S**

d Secure patient to applicable equipment **S**

5.7 a Immobilize suspected fractures involving axial skeleton **S**

6.1 o Provide care to trauma patient **S**

REVIEW QUESTIONS

Page references where answers may be found or supported are provided at the end of each question.

SECTION 1

1. Which of the five regions of the spine is most vulnerable to injury? Why? (p. 368)

SECTION 2

2. What are five emergencies in which your index of suspicion for spinal injury should be high? (p. 369)

3. When should you begin manual stabilization of the cervical spine? When may you release it? (p. 371)

4. What is the basic emergency care for a suspected spinal injury patient? (pp. 371–373)

5. Under what circumstances would rapid extrication be appropriate? (p. 377)

6. When should a helmet be left in place? (p. 380)

7. How many rescuers are required to properly perform helmet removal? (p. 380)

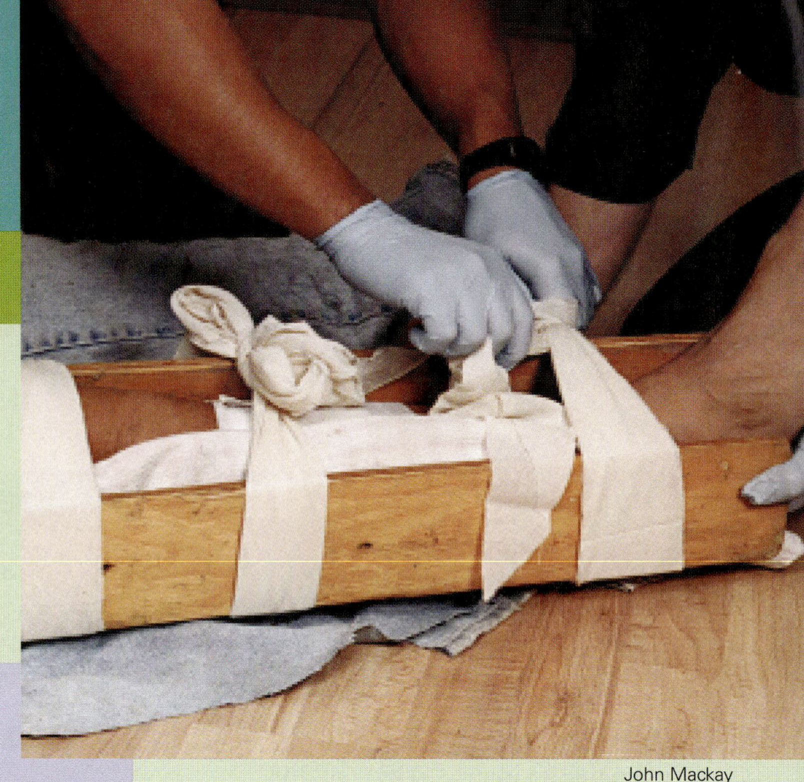

John Mackay

Musculoskeletal Injuries

OBJECTIVES

1. Differentiate between an open and a closed musculoskeletal injury and outline the emergency medical care of each.

2. State five clear reasons for splinting a musculoskeletal injury.

3. Compare the following splints: rigid, traction, circumferential, improvised, and sling and swath.

4. List 10 general rules for splinting a musculoskeletal injury.

5. List four complications of improper splinting.

6. Describe the type of splint and the method used to splint the following parts of the upper extremities: clavicle, shoulder, shoulder and humerus, elbow, forearm and wrist, hand and fingers.

7. Describe the type of splint and the method used to splint the following parts of the lower extremities: pelvis, hip, femur, knee, tibia and fibula, ankle and foot.

8. Demonstrate a caring attitude toward the patient and family when dealing with musculoskeletal injuries, while giving priority to the interests of the patient.

INTRODUCTION

Injuries to muscles, joints, and bones are some of the most common emergencies you will encounter in the field. They can range from a pulled muscle or twisted ankle to life-threatening breaks in a femur. Regardless of whether the injury is mild or severe, your ability to assess your patient and provide the appropriate emergency care can help prevent permanent disability and disfigurement.

SECTION 1
INJURIES TO BONES AND JOINTS

The musculoskeletal system is made up of more than 200 bones and over 600 muscles. Together, they give the body its shape, protect internal organs, and provide for movement. Any time bones and muscles are injured, one of those functions is either temporarily or permanently impaired. Turn to Chapter 4 to review the structures of the musculoskeletal system.

Bones and muscles may be injured in four basic ways:

- A bone is broken (fracture).
- A muscle or a muscle and tendon are overextended (strain).
- A joint and ligament are injured (sprain).
- A bone is moved out of its normal position in a joint and remains that way (dislocation).

Mechanisms of Musculoskeletal Injury

As you conduct your scene assessment, consider the mechanism of injury. A mechanism of musculoskeletal injury may involve direct, indirect, or twisting forces (Figure 26–1). The mechanism can give you a good idea of how extensive an injury may be.

With a direct force, an injury occurs at the point of impact. For example, imagine that a patient is in an MVA. When he or she is thrust forward, one of the knees strikes the dashboard. The resulting broken kneecap is caused by that direct force or direct blow.

With an indirect force, the energy of a blow travels along a path away from the point of impact. For

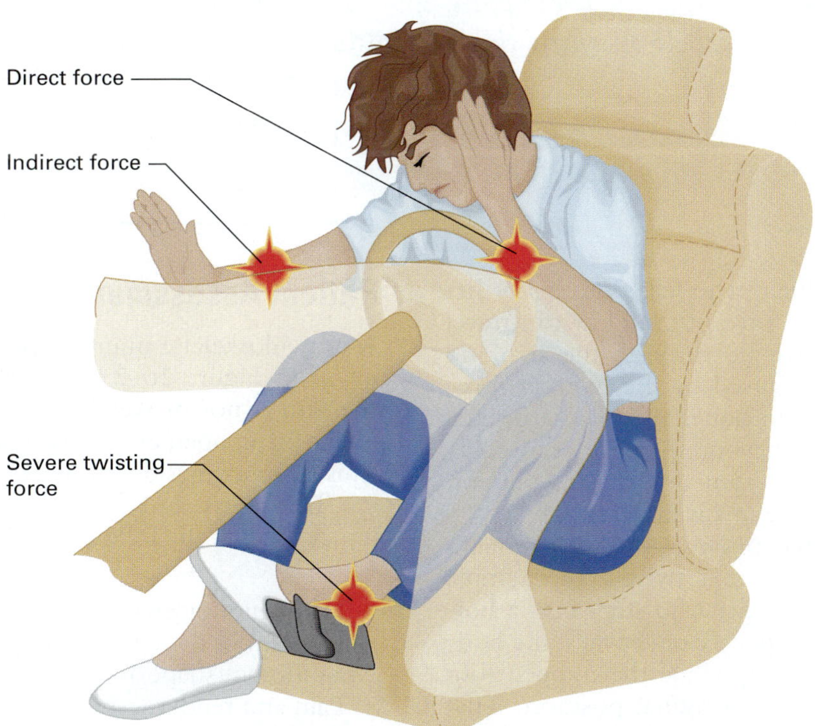

Figure 26–1 Different types of force can cause different types of injury.

CASE STUDY

Dispatch

The temperature outside was dropping rapidly, and snow flurries had already started. I was just sitting down for an evening of television when the tones went out: "Portage Fire/Rescue and Ambulance Unit 2: MVA on the overpass at east junction of Hwy 1 and 1A."

Scene Assessment

As my partner and I approached the scene, we could see several cars on the bridge. Most of them were off the road and against the guardrails. We were just stopping when we saw a police cruiser slide into a slow spin and glide past us.

We exited our unit when the road was flared off and the scene was safe. The police then directed us to vehicle #3. It had been struck by another vehicle and had skidded into the guardrail.

Primary Assessment

Our patient was a 19-year-old woman who was in the driver's seat. Her left thigh was bulging so much that we could see the deformity through her jeans. She was holding her leg tightly and appeared to be in a great deal of pain. My partner stabilized her head and neck while I began the primary assessment.

The patient was alert and cooperative. Her speech was clear. Her pulse was strong and fast, and her skin was cold and dry. There was no gross external bleeding. She had no trouble breathing, no chest pain, and no apparent injuries to her head. She did not have her seatbelt on when the car crashed into the guardrail.

> Consider this patient as you read Chapter 26. What may be done to assess and treat her condition?

example, think of a patient who falls onto his or her outstretched hand. The force of the blow can travel from the hand and wrist up through the arm and shoulder. The injuries caused by the indirect force could include broken arm bones and even a broken clavicle. Therefore, look beyond the injury caused by a direct force when you examine a trauma patient. Additional injuries may be involved.

With a twisting force, one part of a limb remains stationary while the rest of it twists. An example would be the case of a jogger who steps into a hole and gets a foot caught. When he or she falls, the body would pull the leg one way while the trapped foot would hold it firmly in its original position. That could twist the limb, causing any of its bones or joints to break. Suspect injuries beyond the most obvious one when you examine your patient.

Patient Assessment

A musculoskeletal injury is classified as either closed or open (Figure 26–2). In a closed extremity injury, the skin is not broken at the injury site. It remains intact. In an open extremity injury, the skin is broken. This is sometimes due to protruding bone ends.

The signs and symptoms of musculoskeletal injury include the following (Figure 26–3):

- Deformity or angulation (Compared to the uninjured limb, the injured one is a different size or has a different shape.)
- Pain and tenderness
- Grating, or crepitus (This is the sound or sensation of broken bones grinding against each other.)
- Swelling

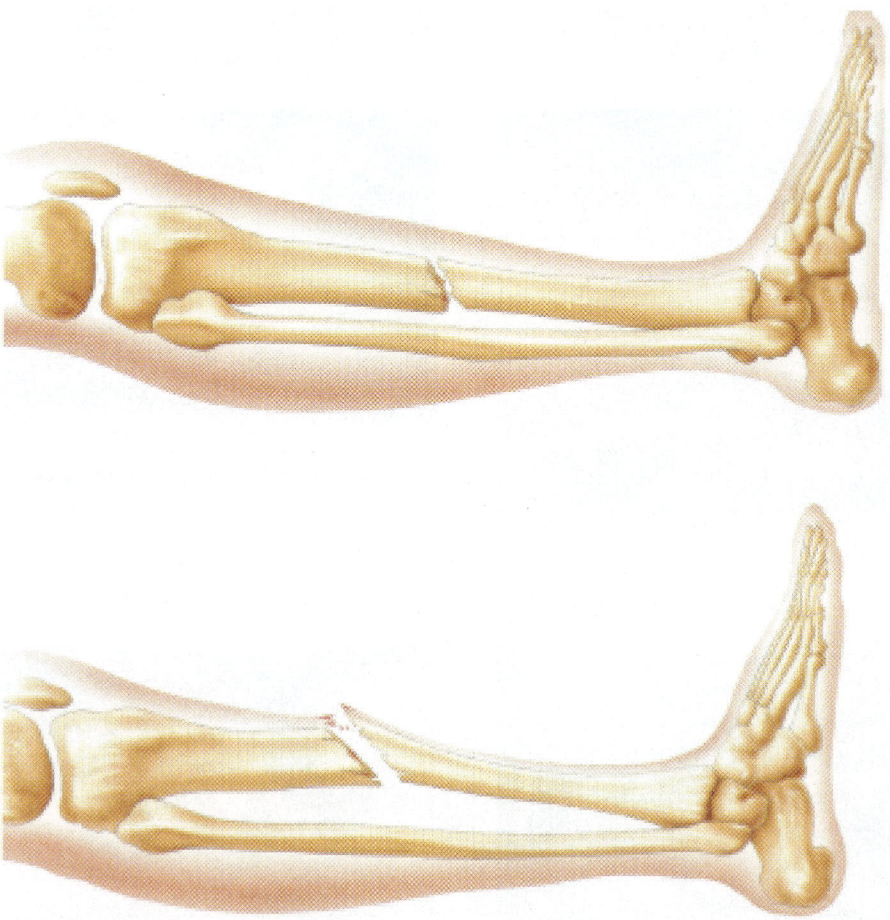

Figure 26–2 A closed injury vs. an open one.

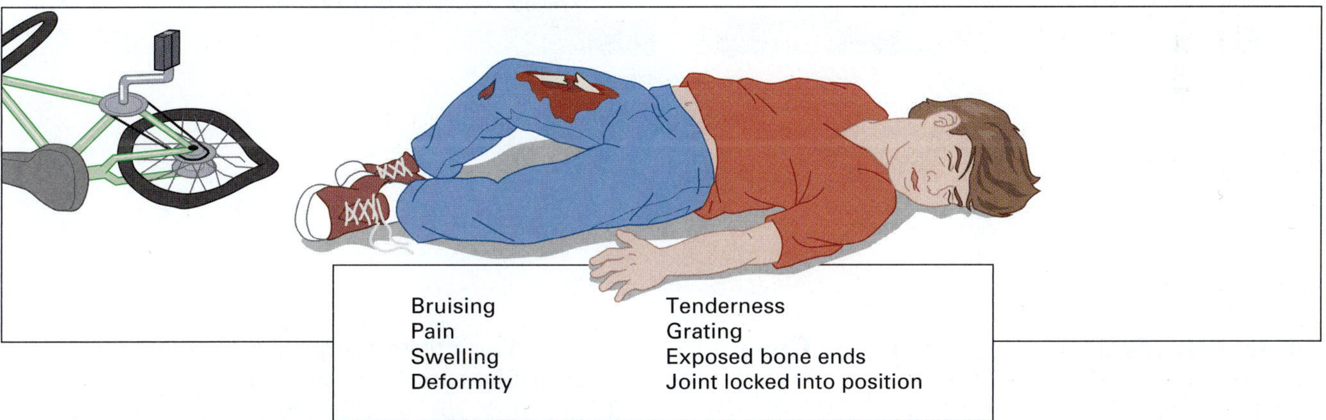

Figure 26–3 Signs and symptoms of bone or joint injuries.

- Bruising or discoloration
- Exposed bone ends (Figure 26–4)
- Joint locked in position
- A snap or crack heard by the patient at the time of the incident

An injury that causes pain, swelling, or deformity in an extremity may be the result of a fracture, sprain, strain, or dislocation. Because these injuries look so much alike in the field, you do not need to figure out which is which. Instead, always treat a painful, swollen, or deformed extremity as if it involved a broken bone.

When examining a patient with a musculoskeletal injury, remember that he or she may be in a great deal of pain. Be careful not to move the injured limb or jar the body. Be gentle and reassuring to the patient and his or her family.

OPEN MUSCULOSKELETAL INJURIES

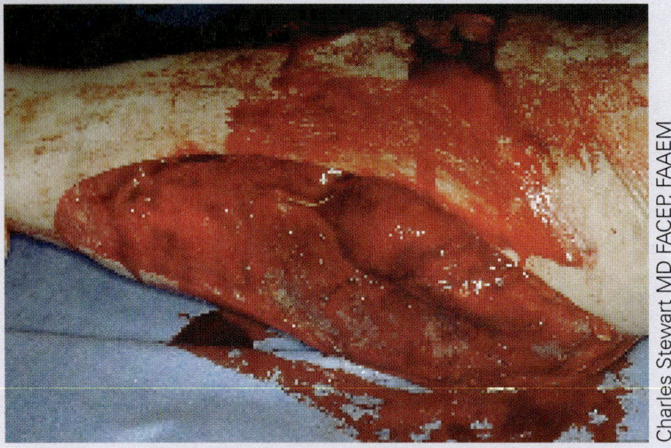

Figure 26–4a

Charles Stewart MD FACEP, FAAEM

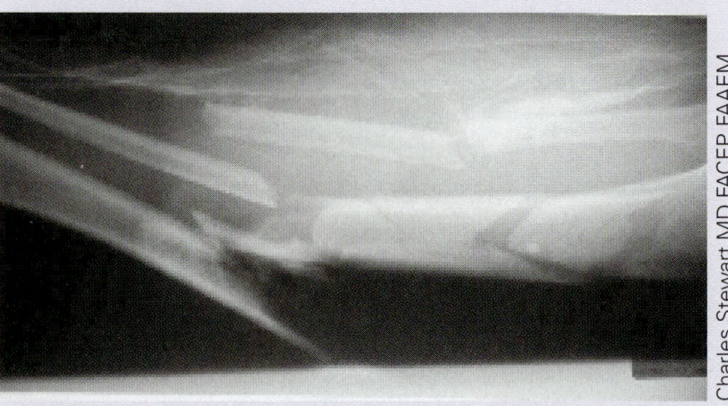

Figure 26–4b Radiograph of the limb in Figure 26–4a, showing broken bones both above and below the surface.

Charles Stewart MD FACEP, FAAEM

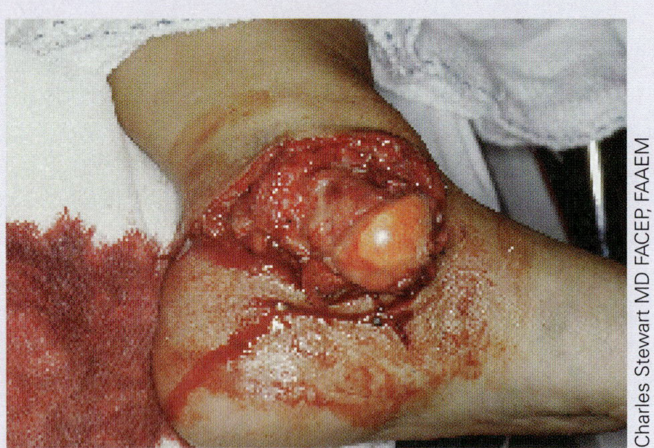

Figure 26–4c

Charles Stewart MD FACEP, FAAEM

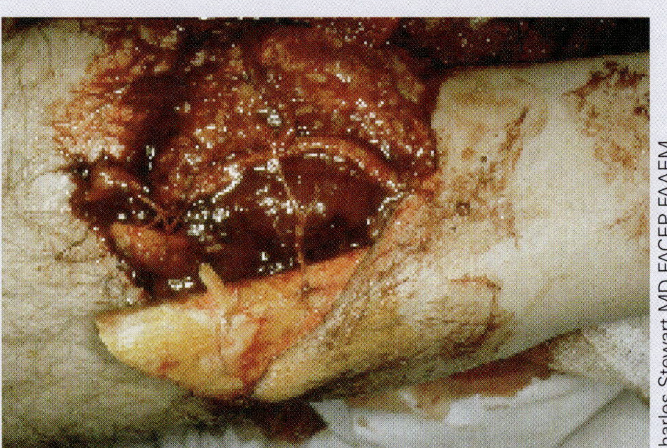

Figure 26–4d

Charles Stewart MD FACEP, FAAEM

General Guidelines for Emergency Care

As an EMR, you must not be distracted by gruesome-looking injuries, especially when treating a patient with multiple trauma. Simply put, your priority is life before limb. Remain focused on treating the life threats you identify in the primary assessment. Once that is done, you can turn to limb-threatening injuries.

Generally, emergency care proceeds in the following manner:

1. *Take BSI precautions.*
2. *Identify and treat life threats.* If indicated, maintain manual stabilization of the patient's spine as you complete the primary assessment. If it is available, administer oxygen.
3. *Stabilize the injured extremity* after you have completed a secondary assessment. Hold it manually above and below the injury site. Maintain manual stabilization until the limb is completely immobilized in a splint.
4. *Expose the injury site.* To avoid jarring the limb, you may need to cut away clothing. If possible, also remove jewellery.
5. *Treat any open wounds.* Control the bleeding. If necessary, apply pressure to the appropriate pressure point. Be careful to avoid applying any pressure to broken bone ends. Then dress any open wounds with sterile dressings.

6. *Allow the patient to rest in a position of comfort* while you wait for the arrival of the paramedics. Apply a cold pack to the injured area. It can help reduce pain and swelling. You may also wish to pad under the patient's injured limb to prevent discomfort. Continue to assess for pulse, movement, and sensation below the injury site. Record any changes.

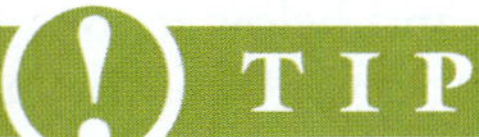

! TIP

Assess and reassess CWCM distal to a fracture:

C — Colour

W— Warmth

C — Circulation

M— Movement

Manual stabilization of the injured limb is maintained to help prevent further injury. Without it, a simple closed injury could become an open one. Another important reason for manual stabilization is to prevent and reduce pain.

While you are stabilizing an injured limb, do not intentionally replace any protruding bones. Do not apply manual traction (pull the limb) in an attempt to straighten a limb or realign the bones, except when you are authorized to do so. Only trained medical personnel should attempt traction in the field. Be sure to follow all local protocols.

Maintain manual stabilization of an injured extremity until it is completely immobilized with a splint. Even if you find that you have to stay in an uncomfortable position for some time, maintain stabilization. The patient's best interests must be your foremost consideration. If you are trained and allowed to do so, splint the injured extremity after you have performed the steps described above.

SECTION 2
SPLINTING MUSCULOSKELETAL INJURIES

Any device used to immobilize a body part is called a splint. A splint may be soft or rigid. It can be commercially manufactured, or it can be improvised from virtually any object that can immobilize the limb (Figure 26–5).

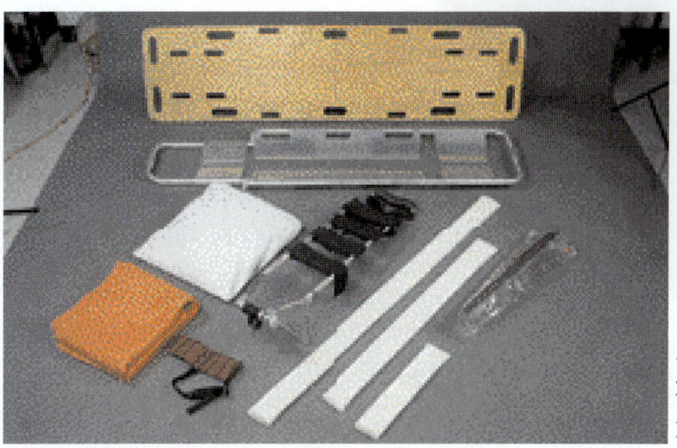

Figure 26–5 Examples of splints.

There are five good reasons for splinting a musculoskeletal injury:

- To prevent motion of bone fragments or dislocated joints
- To minimize damage to surrounding tissues, nerves, blood vessels, and the injured bone itself
- To help control the bleeding and swelling
- To help prevent shock
- To reduce pain and suffering

The EMRs in your system may have limited authority in the use of the various types of splints to immobilize musculoskeletal injuries. Make sure you follow all local protocols.

Types of Splints

Some common types of splints are rigid splints, traction splints, circumferential splints, improvised splints, and the sling and swath. All are designed to accomplish the same task: they must immobilize an injured extremity.

Rigid Splints

Rigid, padded boards are the most common type of splint. They may be made of wood, aluminum, wire, plastic, cardboard, or compressed fibres. Some are shaped specifically for arms or legs. Others are pliable enough to be moulded to fit any appendage. Some come with washable pads. Others must be padded before being applied.

A rigid splint must be applied in line with the bone. Then it must be anchored to the limb with cravats that are secured with square knots (or straps or Velcro closures). Remember, never place a cravat across the injury site. It could cause further injury and pain.

Traction Splints

A traction splint is a mechanical device that provides a counter pull to alleviate pain, reduce blood loss, and minimize further injury. It holds a limb in alignment but does not realign broken bones. Several types of traction splints are available, and application procedures vary according to manufacturer. As an EMR, you should use a traction splint only if you are specifically trained and allowed to do so. Follow local protocols.

Circumferential Splints

This type of splint completely surrounds, or envelops, the injured limb. An example is an air splint. It can be inflated, either mechanically or manually, until it forms a semi-rigid sleeve around the injured limb. An advantage of an air splint is that the compression it provides helps reduce the swelling. Air splints need to be checked and rechecked if transport of the patient includes temperature or elevation changes.

Improvised Splints

An improvised splint can be made from a cardboard box, cane or walking stick, ironing board, rolled-up magazine, umbrella, broom handle, catcher's shin guard, or any similar object. It must be long enough to extend past the joints and prevent movement on both sides of the injury. It should also be as wide as the thickest part of the injured area.

A self-splint may also be effective. In fact, in some cases, a patient will not permit any other type of splint to be applied. In a self-splint, the injured limb is secured against the patient's body with a cravat or roller bandage. Gaps between the limb and body are then padded with bulky dressings or similar material as appropriate.

Sling and Swath

An injured limb can be supported by the sling, while a swath keeps the limb protected and immobile against the body. When applying a sling, be sure to keep the knot off the back of the patient's neck. It can be very uncomfortable there.

General Rules of Splinting

Keep these general rules of splinting in mind (Figure 26–6):

- Be sure you have taken BSI precautions before splinting.
- Do not release manual stabilization of an injured extremity until it is properly and completely immobilized.
- Never intentionally replace protruding bones or push them back below the skin.
- You can't assess what you can't see. Therefore, cut away all clothing around the injury site before applying a splint. In addition, remove all jewellery from the injury site and below it. Bag the jewellery and give it to the patient, a family member, or the police.
- Control the bleeding and dress all open wounds before applying a splint.
- If a long bone is injured, immobilize it and the joints above and below it.
- If a joint is injured, immobilize it and the bones above and below it.
- If a limb is severely deformed by the injury, or if the limb has no pulse or is cyanotic below the injury site, align it with gentle manual traction (pulling). If there is pain or grating (crepitus), stop pulling immediately. Perform this procedure *only if you are specifically trained and allowed to do so.* Follow all local protocols.
- Pad a splint before applying it to help keep the patient as comfortable as possible.
- Before and after applying a splint, assess pulse, movement, and sensation below the injury site. Try to keep pulse sites exposed so you can reassess. You should reassess every 15 minutes after applying a splint, and record your findings.

For all the obvious benefits that splints provide, they can also cause complications if they are applied incorrectly. *Improper* splinting can do the following:

- Compress nerves, tissues, and blood vessels under the splint, which can aggravate the injury and cause further damage
- Move displaced or broken bones, causing even further injury to nerves, tissues, and blood vessels
- Reduce blood flow below the injury site, endangering the life of the limb
- Delay transport of a patient who has a life-threatening problem

Remember that patients who have a painful, swollen, deformed extremity may be in considerable pain. They may also be concerned about regaining full use of the limb. Therefore, as you provide emergency care, consider their feelings. Be gentle and reassuring.

GENERAL RULES OF SPLINTING

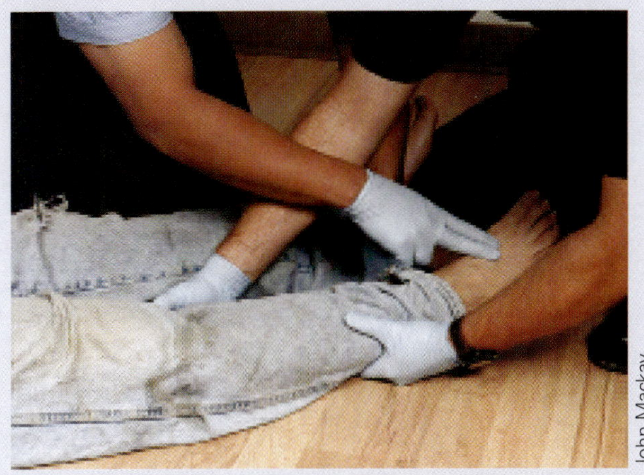

Figure 26–6a   Stabilize the limb and assess pulse, movement, and sensation below the injury site.

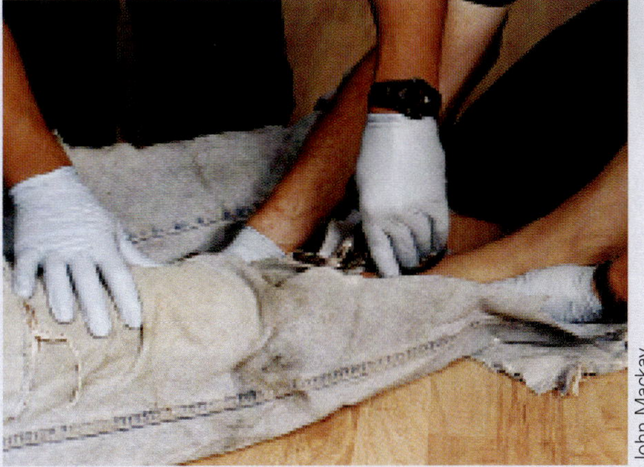

Figure 26–6b   Cut away clothing to expose the injury.

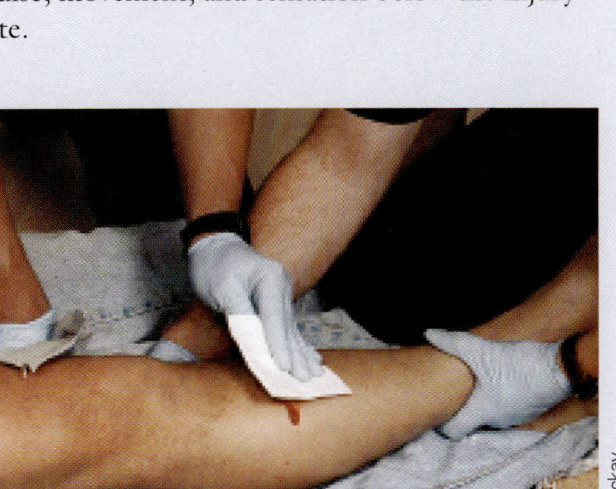

Figure 26–6c   After controlling bleeding, place a sterile dressing over any open wounds.

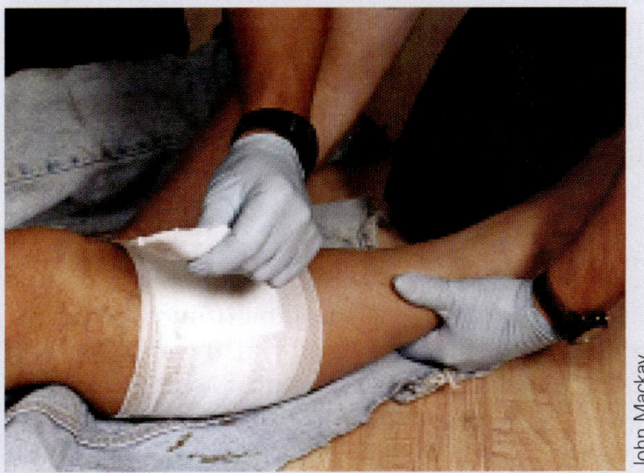

Figure 26–6d   If there is severe deformity, absence of pulse, or cyanosis in the extremity, align it with gentle traction if you are allowed to do so. Maintain it until the limb is completely immobilized.

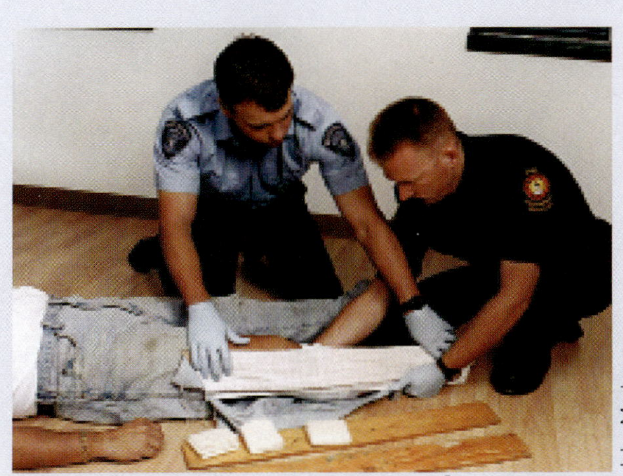

Figure 26–6e   Pad the splint.

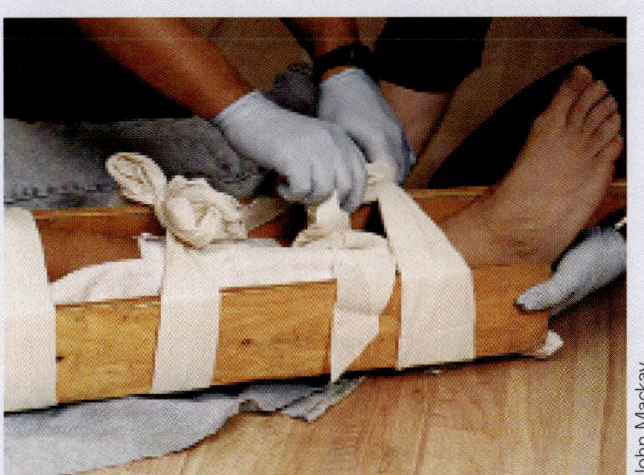

Figure 26–6f   Secure the limb to the splint and reassess pulse, movement, and sensation.

APPLYING A SLING AND SWATH

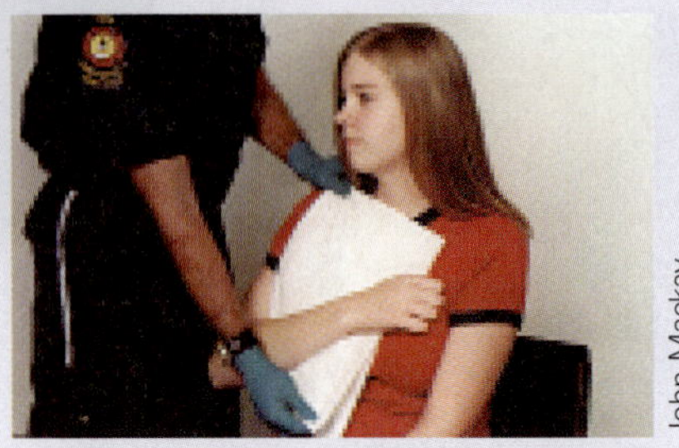

Figure 26–7a Place a pad between the injured arm and the chest.

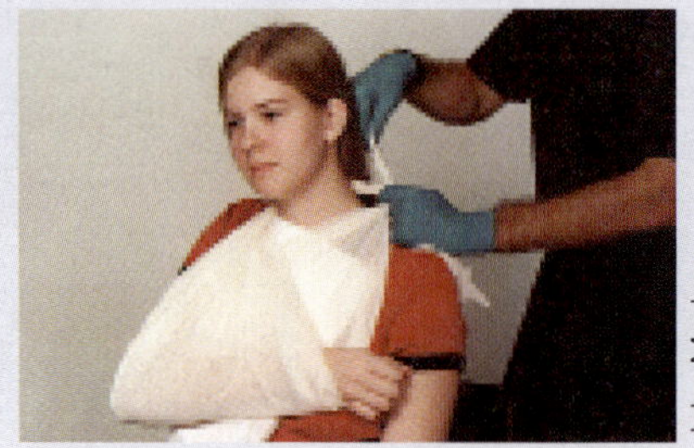

Figure 26–7b Support the injured arm with a sling.

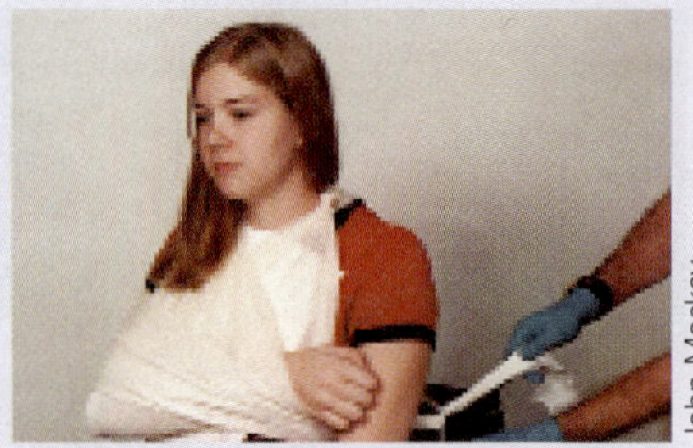

Figure 26–7c Immobilize the arm with a swath.

Splinting the Upper Extremities

Clavicle

An injury to a shoulder will often result in the fracture of a clavicle. When a clavicle is broken, the patient's shoulder may appear to have dropped. The clavicle itself may look crooked and deformed. The best way to splint it is to apply a sling and swath (Figure 26–7).

Shoulder

A dislocated shoulder is a common injury. Patients have often had the same injury many times before. The dislocated shoulder will appear to be deformed. You may also see a hollow in the upper arm below the clavicle. The patient frequently complains of severe pain and may refuse to let anyone touch the arm.

Attempt to apply a sling and swath to the arm. Padding the void between the body and the arm may be helpful. Use a small pillow, towels, or even trauma dressings for padding.

In a shoulder dislocation, there is a danger of injuring nerves and arteries. A great deal of care must be taken when applying the sling and swath.

Shoulder and Humerus

The humerus may break at mid-shaft or at the shoulder. It is thick and fairly strong. If it is injured, suspect other injuries nearby.

Manually stabilize the arm as soon as possible. Then check for pulse, movement, and sensation below the injury site. Apply a rigid splint to the outside of the arm and pad the voids. Then apply a sling and swath (Figure 26–8). Do not forget to reassess pulse, movement, and sensation. See Figure 26–9 for an alternative method of splinting the humerus.

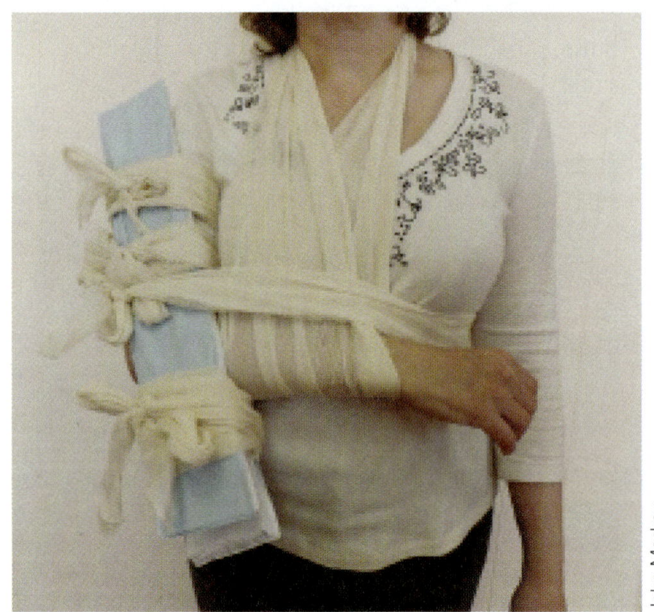

Figure 26–8 Fixation, or rigid, splint with a sling and swath.

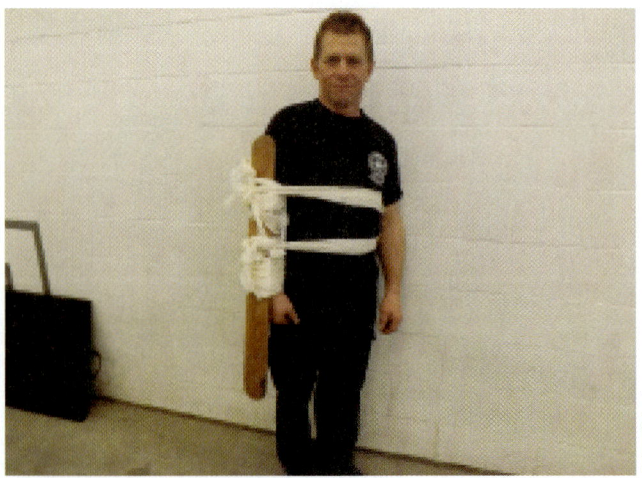

Figure 26–9 Fixed splint for a humerus injury.

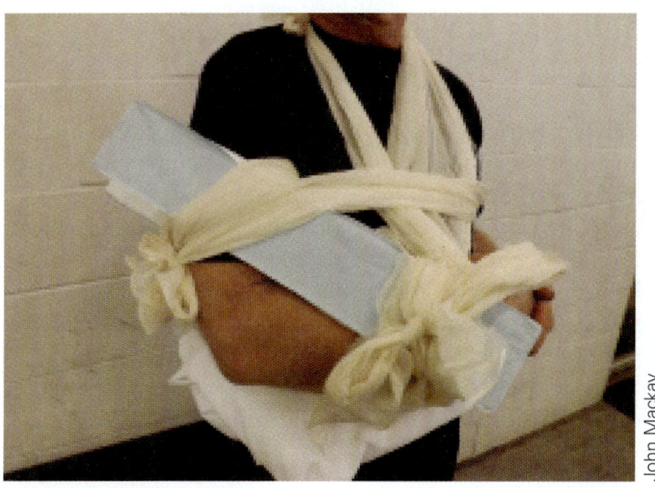

Figure 26–10   Injured elbow immobilized in a bent position.

Elbow

The elbow should be splinted in the position in which it was found. Do not attempt to straighten it. If the arm is bent at the elbow, splint the injury with a sling and swath (Figure 26–10). However, if the deformity is severe, you may elect to use a large, flat pillow or even a blanket wrapped around the limb and secured to the chest with a strap.

If the elbow is straight, then the entire arm should be splinted from the armpit to the fingertips on two sides (Figure 26–11).

Forearm and Wrist

Forearm and wrist injuries are very common. They must be supported from the elbow to the finger-tips. First, splint the injured area with a short arm

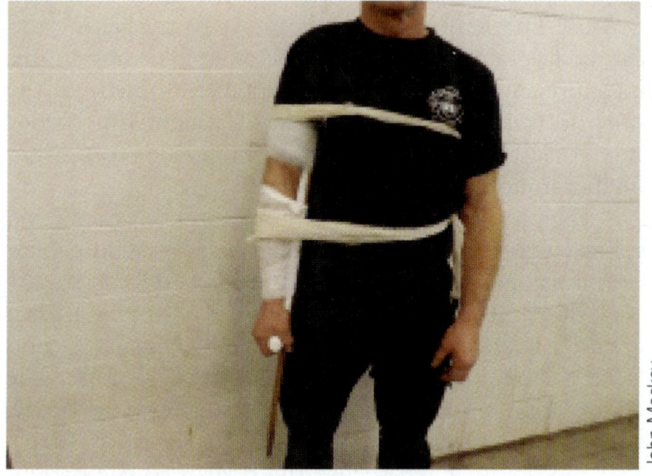

Figure 26–11   Injured elbow immobilized in a straight position.

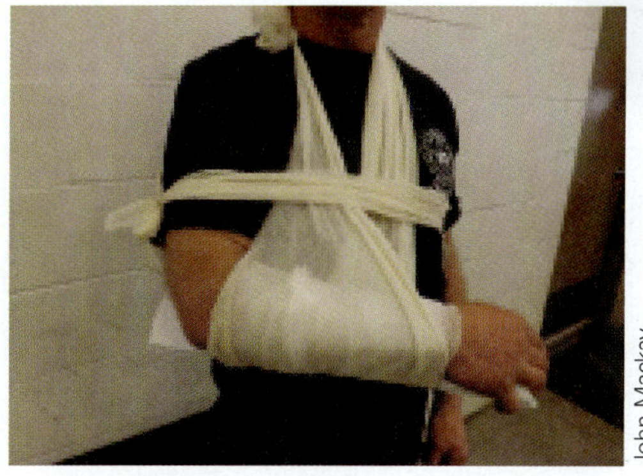

Figure 26–12   Immobilization of an injury to the forearm, wrist, or hand.

board. Then a sling and swath should be applied (Figure 26–12).

If the injury is a closed one, a circumferential splint may be used instead. Be sure the splint extends from the elbow to beyond the hand (Figure 26–13).

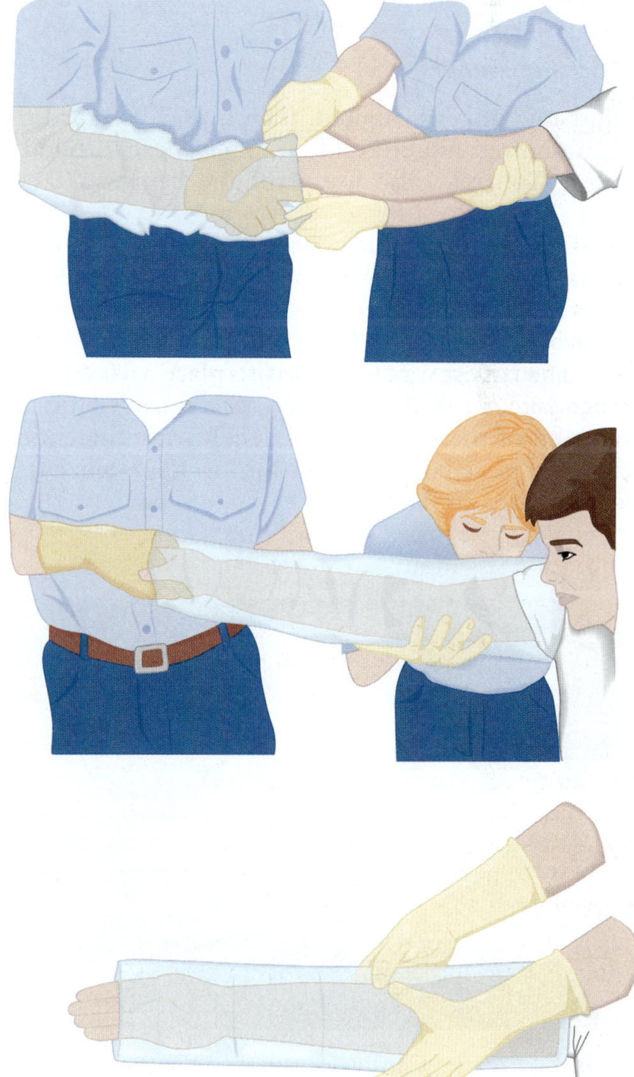

Figure 26–13   Applying an air splint.

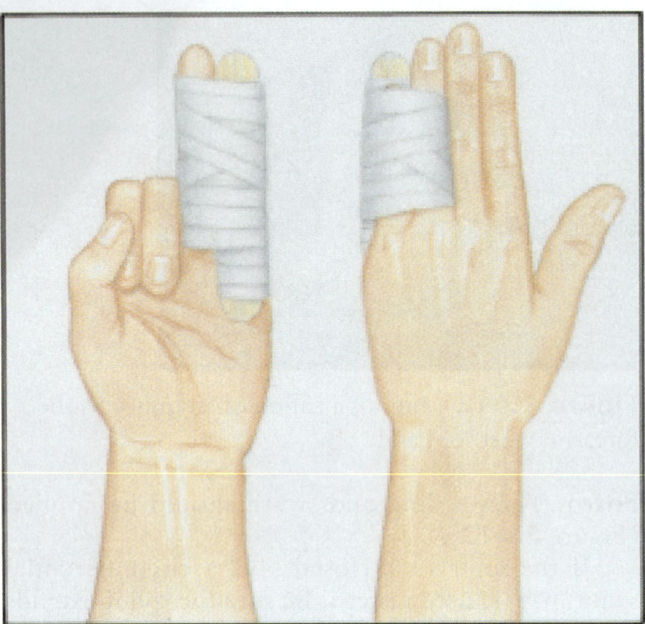

Figure 26–14   A tongue depressor used as a splint.

Hand and Fingers

If just one finger is injured, then it may be taped to the uninjured finger beside it. This is called buddy taping. You may also use a tongue depressor as a splint (Figure 26–14).

If there is more than one finger involved, or if the hand injury is the result of a fight, the entire hand needs to be immobilized.

A hand must be splinted in the position of function. The easiest way to do it is to place a 10 cm roll of bandage, a rolled hand towel, or a small ball inside the palm of the injured hand. Then wrap the entire hand and place it on an arm board to immobilize the wrist (Figure 26–15).

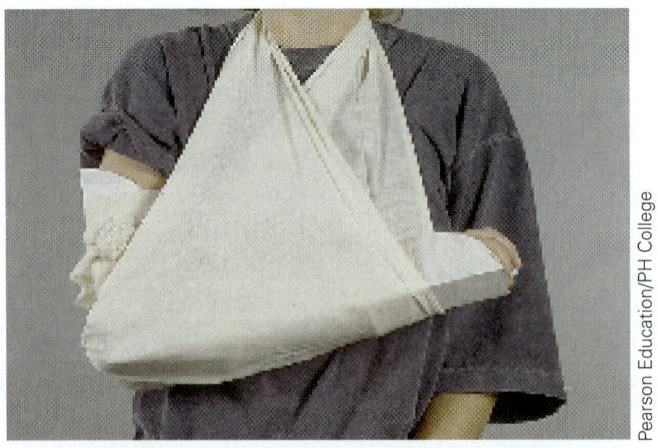

Pearson Education/PH College

Figure 26–15   Cardboard splint of the forearm, wrist, or hand.

Splinting the Lower Extremities

Pelvis

Pelvic injuries can be life threatening because a large amount of blood can quickly be lost into the lower abdomen. Suspect shock with any pelvic injury.

The patient must be placed on a long backboard. Pad between the legs and consider putting a blanket on each side of the patient's hips. Then, secure the patient's whole body to the backboard. Keep the patient warm. If you suspect shock, the foot end of the backboard may be elevated slightly, provided it does not compromise the splinting.

Hip

The hip is actually the proximal end of the femur, where the femur fits into the pelvis. Fractures of the hip are common in severe frontal car crashes. They are also common in older adults as the result of a fall.

With a broken hip, the leg on the injured side may be shorter than the other leg and externally rotated. The patient will complain of pain when the leg is moved or when the hips are gently compressed.

When you perform a primary assessment of a patient with a possible hip injury, be sure to assess and treat life-threatening problems first, including shock. Then stabilize the patient's hip. The best method is to immobilize the patient's whole body on a long backboard.

Femur

With such mechanisms of injury, consider the need for spinal immobilization in addition to the femur. Older adults, however, may more readily suffer lower extremity fractures from simple falls or twisting as a result of their decreased bone density. The result of a break is usually a marked deformity of the thigh, as well as a great deal of pain and swelling. Any femur fracture can be dangerous. The femoral artery lies next to the femur and can be lacerated by broken bone ends. Bleeding in this location can be very difficult to detect. Sometimes the only outward sign is swelling in the thigh. Emergency care consists of immobilizing the bone ends to prevent further injury.

The preferred method of immobilization is a traction splint (Figure 26–16). Remember, use a traction splint only if you are specially trained and allowed to do so.

Alternative care involves using two long boards to create a fixation splint. The inner board must extend from the groin to below the bottom of the foot. The outer board must extend from the armpit to below the bottom of the foot (Figure 26–17 on p. 396). Pad the voids. Then secure the boards to the patient with cravats at the shoulders, hips, knees, and ankles.

APPLYING A TRACTION SPLINT

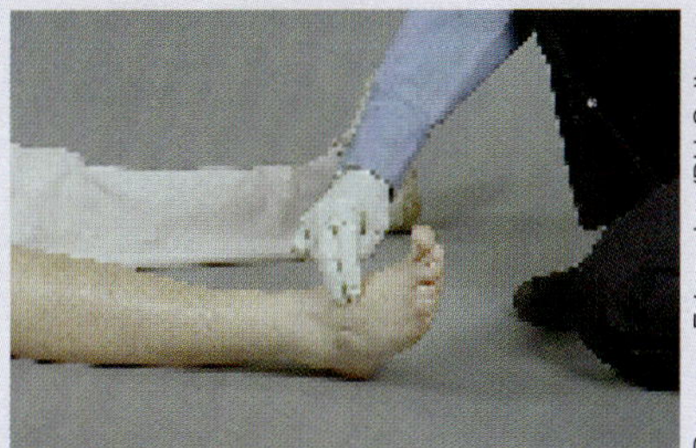

Figure 26–16a Assess pulse, movement, and sensation below the injury site.

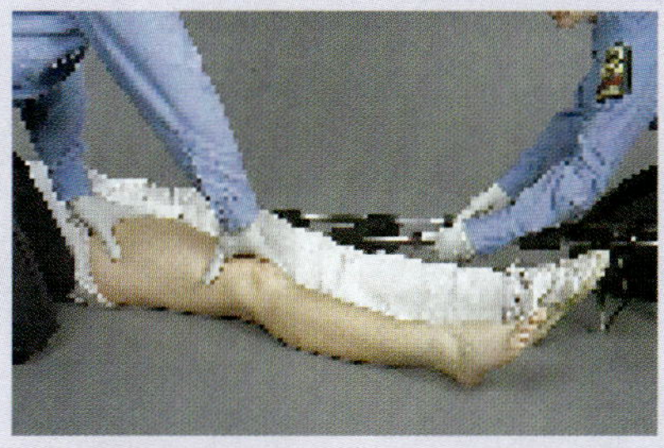

Figure 26–16b Manually stabilize the limb.

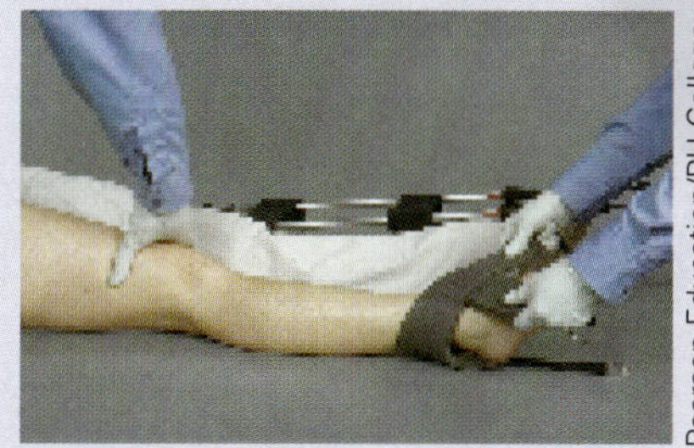

Figure 26–16c Apply the ankle hitch.

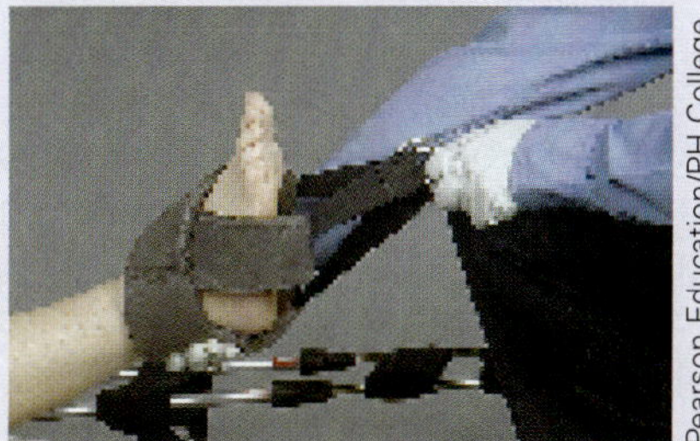

Figure 26–16d Apply and maintain manual traction. Position the splint.

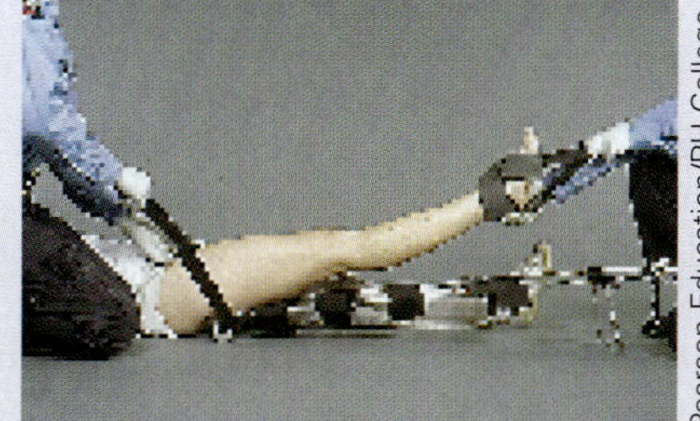

Figure 26–16e Attach the ischial strap.

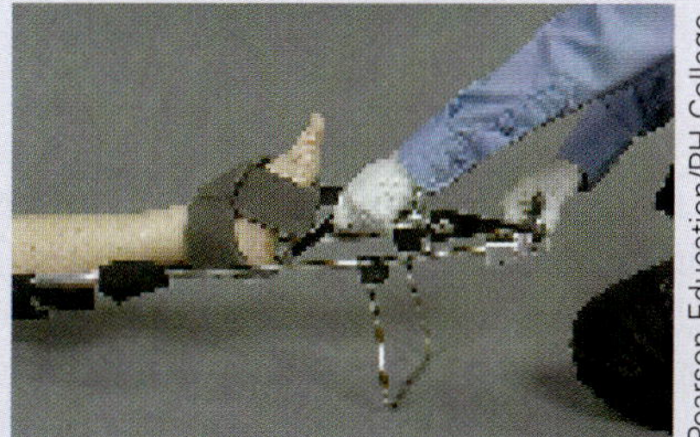

Figure 26–16f Fasten the splint to the ankle hitch. Apply mechanical traction.

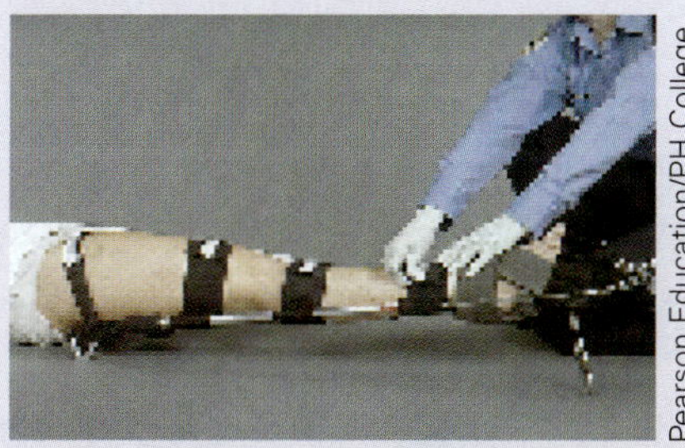

Figure 26–16g Fasten leg support straps in place.

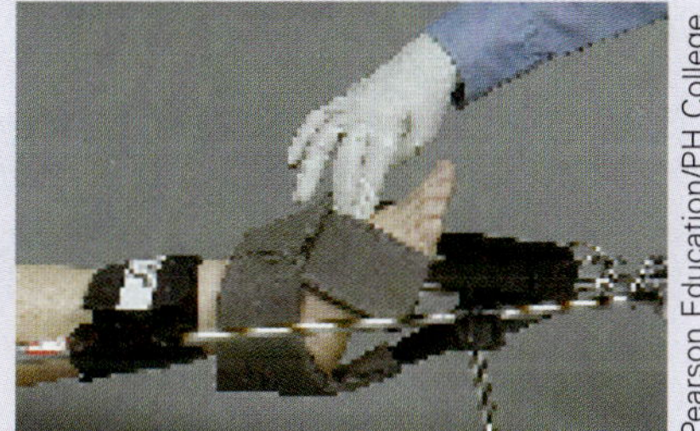

Figure 26–16h Reassess pulse, movement, and sensation below the injury site.

Knee

There are many types of knee injuries. Emergency treatment is basically the same. If you find the injured leg in a straight position, use two padded long boards to splint it in the position found. Place the first on the inner thigh so that it extends from the groin to beyond the foot. Place the second on the outer thigh so that it extends from the hip to beyond the foot. Then secure the boards to the patient with cravats.

If you find the knee in a bent position, immobilize it in the position found. The bones above and below it should be splinted with two padded short boards (Figure 26–18).

Tibia and Fibula

Open fractures of the tibia are common because only thin layers of skin protect it. Usually, fractures of the fibula are not so readily apparent since it is not a weight-bearing bone. Whichever one of the two bones is injured, the procedure for splinting remains the same.

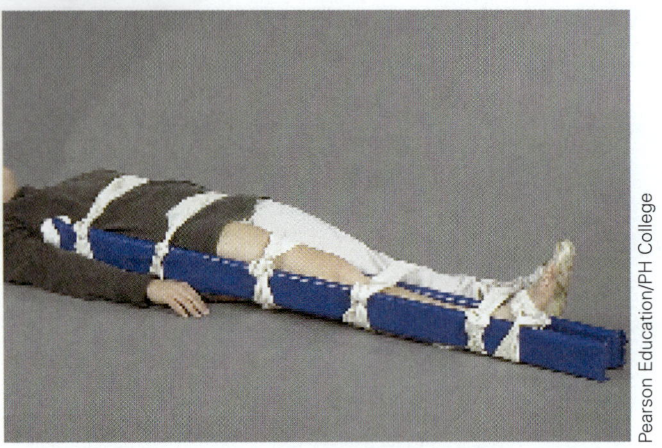

Figure 26–17 A high femur fracture immobilized in a fixation splint.

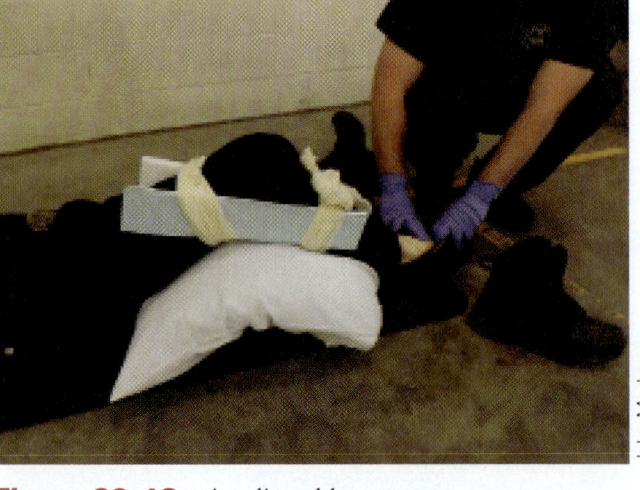

Figure 26–18 A splinted knee.

Use two padded long boards (Figure 26–19). Place the first on the inner thigh so that it extends from the groin to below the foot. Place the second on the outer thigh so that it extends from the hip bone to below the foot. Then secure the boards to the patient with cravats.

An alternative method for a closed injury to the tibia or fibula is to use a circumferential splint. Make sure it extends beyond the knee and covers the entire foot. One drawback of an air splint is that you will not be able to assess colour, warmth, circulation, or movement (CWCM) distal to the fracture, as suggested in the TIP box on page 389.

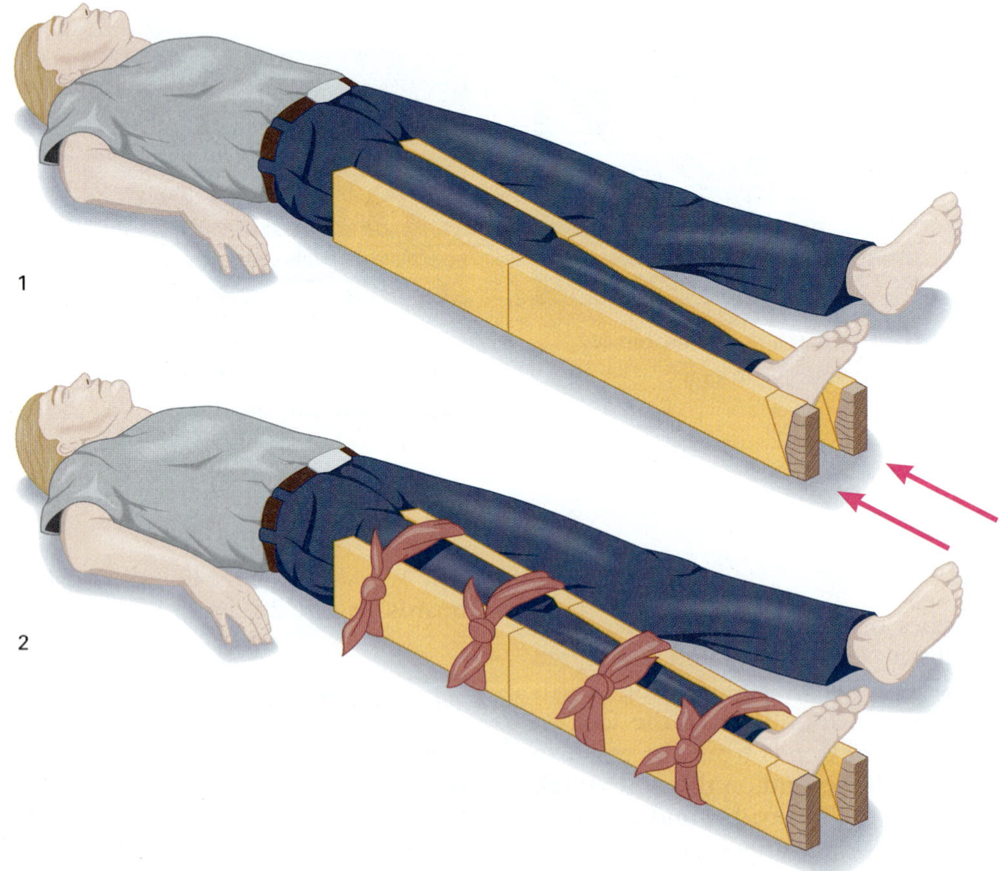

Figure 26–19 Fixation splint of the tibia/fibula using padded boards.

Ankle and Foot

The foot is commonly injured by heavy objects falling onto it or by twisting forces during a fall. The ankle bears so much weight that it does not take much movement in the wrong direction to make it unstable. Whether the injury is to the ankle or to the foot, it is splinted in the same way.

Circumferential splints work well in these cases. However, the easiest splint may be a pillow. Simply wrap the pillow, or a blanket, around the foot. Then secure it with cravats at the toes and the shin. The more cravats applied, the better (Figure 26–20).

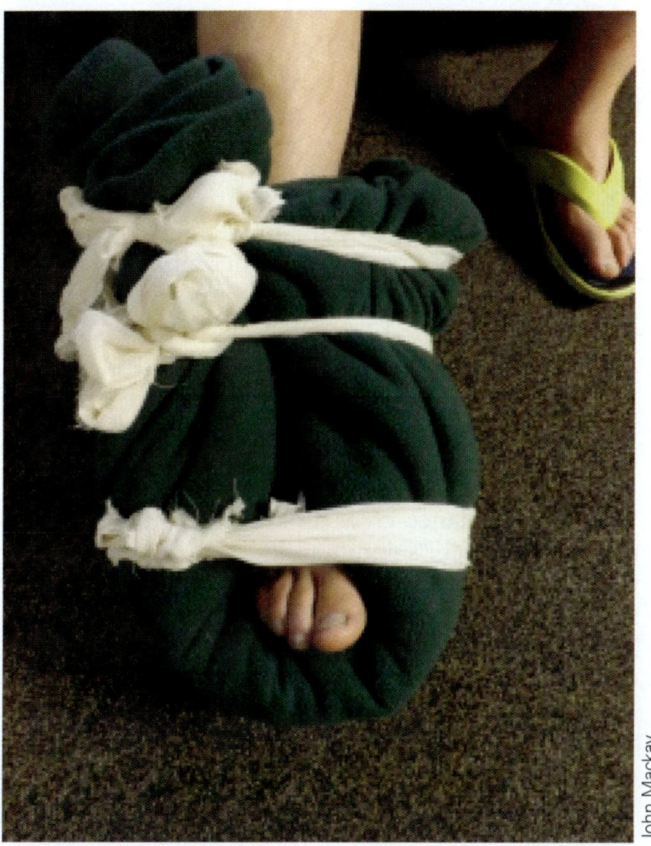

Figure 26–20 Blanket-roll splint of the ankle and foot.

EMR FOCUS

Patients may be aware of only one obvious injury, but it is your responsibility to perform a thorough patient assessment. Do not let an injury that is gruesome, but relatively minor, make you miss a life-threatening injury or condition, such as an open chest wound or shock. As you assess a patient with musculoskeletal injuries, keep the following tips in mind:

- The mechanism of injury can alert you to hidden injuries.
- Broken bones can be serious. They bleed and they cause shock. If there is a possibility that your patient has more than one broken bone, the potential for shock and other hidden injuries is very high.
- Examine the extremities last. The more important areas—the head, neck, chest, and abdomen—must be examined first because they contain the vital organs.

In the first 10 minutes, it is important to make accurate decisions based on your assessment findings. Treat injuries and conditions that are a threat to life first.

CASE STUDY FOLLOW-UP

At the beginning of this chapter, you read that EMRs were caring for a patient with a painful, swollen, deformed thigh. To see how the chapter skills apply to this emergency, read the following. It describes how the call was completed.

SECONDARY ASSESSMENT

A quick secondary assessment revealed no other deformities, open injuries, tenderness, or swelling. At this point, an RCMP officer took over manual stabilization of the femur above and below the injury site. I cut open the patient's jeans and saw that there was no obvious bleeding. The skin was unbroken.

PATIENT HISTORY

During the interview, I asked the patient if she had heard a popping or snapping sound. She said yes. Then I asked her to describe the pain on a scale of 1 to 10, with 10 being the worst. She said 10. She also said that she had consumed two or three beers but had not taken any type of medication.

ONGOING ASSESSMENT

We monitored the patient carefully. We were especially concerned about shock because of the possible femur fracture. We continued to check her pulse and respirations every five minutes. Her airway remained clear. Her respirations remained at 24 and adequate. Her pulse was 106 and strong.

TRANSFER OF CARE

When Ambulance Unit 2 arrived, I gave a quick hand-off report:

> "This is Lynn Solomon. She is 19 and was involved in a low-speed auto collision. Her chief complaint is pain in her left mid-thigh. She is awake and alert, and her airway is patent. Her breathing is rapid. She is not having trouble breathing. We put her on oxygen via non-rebreather mask. She is not bleeding externally. Her vital signs are respirations 24, pulse 100, blood pressure 120/90, and skin is cold and dry. She said that she had two or three beers."

The ambulance crew took over manual stabilization of the patient's femur and further medical care. It wasn't long before the patient was extricated, packaged, and on the way to Portage Hospital. We proceeded to keep our promise to contact her parents and tell them where she and her wrecked car were being taken.

> Musculoskeletal injuries are usually painful and obvious. Even so, you should always assess for and treat life-threatening problems first. Remember—life before limb!

NOCPs

4.3 j Conduct musculoskeletal assessment and interpret findings **S**

5.7 a Immobilize suspected fractures involving the appendicular skeleton **S**

b Immobilize suspected fractures involving the axial skeleton **S**

6.1 g Provide care to a patient experiencing signs and symptoms involving musculoskeletal system **S**

o Provide care to trauma patient **S**

REVIEW QUESTIONS

Page references where answers may be found or supported are provided at the end of each question.

SECTION 1

1. What is the function of the musculoskeletal system? (p. 385)
2. What is the difference between an open and a closed extremity injury? (p. 386)
3. Is the emergency care you give to a patient with a fracture any different from the care you give to a patient with a strain, a sprain, or a dislocation? Why or why not? (p. 387)

4. What are the general emergency care guidelines for a painful, swollen, deformed extremity? (pp. 388–389)

SECTION 2

5. What are the reasons for splinting a painful, swollen, deformed extremity? (p. 389)
6. What kind of material can an improvised splint be made of? (p. 390)
7. What are five general rules of splinting? (p. 390)
8. What are some of the possible complications of improper splinting? (p. 390)
9. What are two of the classic signs of a broken hip? (p. 394)

27

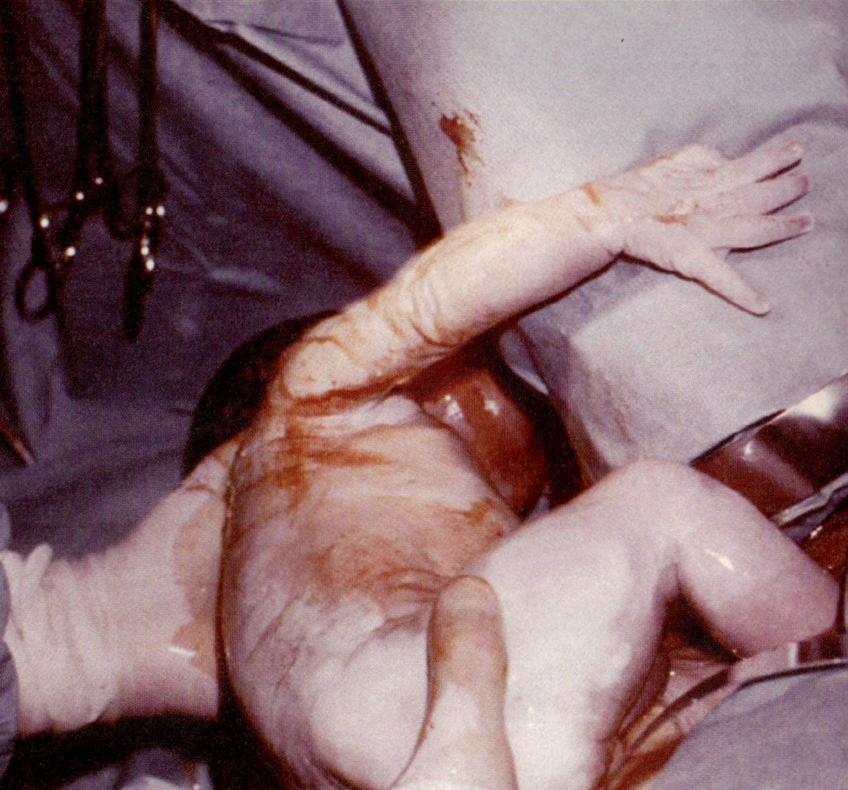

Educational Images Ltd./Custom Medical Stock Photo

Childbirth

O B J E C T I V E S

1. Identify the following structures: birth canal, placenta, umbilical cord, amniotic sac.
2. Define the following terms: crowning, bloody show, labour, spontaneous abortion.
3. State the indications of an imminent delivery.
4. Establish the relationship between BSI precautions and childbirth.
5. Outline the steps in the pre-delivery preparation of the mother.
6. Describe the steps to assist in a delivery, including the care of the baby as the head appears, the suctioning of the baby, and the cutting of the umbilical cord.
7. Describe the steps in the delivery of the placenta and the steps in the emergency medical care of the mother after delivery.
8. Outline the steps in caring for the newborn.
9. Describe emergency medical care of a patient who is suffering from the complications of pregnancy, including toxemia, spontaneous abortion, ectopic pregnancy, placenta previa, and abruptio placentae.
10. Describe emergency medical care of a patient who is suffering from the complications of childbirth, including prolapsed umbilical cord, breech birth, limb presentation, multiple births, and premature birth.
11. Demonstrate a caring attitude toward the patient and family when dealing with pregnancy and childbirth, while giving priority to the interests of the patient.

INTRODUCTION

A pregnant woman is too often rushed to a hospital, usually because the EMR is afraid that the baby will be born before the mother can get there. In most cases, there is no need for haste. Childbirth is a normal, natural process. Only a few situations will require that the mother reach the hospital quickly.

EMRs are often called to help pregnant patients. Become familiar with the nature of childbirth and the emergency medical care of both the mother and the newborn.

SECTION 1
THE PROCESS OF CHILDBIRTH

Anatomy of Pregnancy

The uterus is the organ that contains the developing fetus, or unborn baby (Figure 27–1). A special arrangement of smooth muscles and blood vessels in the uterus allows for great expansion during pregnancy and forcible contractions during labour and delivery. It also allows for rapid contractions after delivery, which help to constrict blood vessels and prevent excessive bleeding.

During pregnancy, the wall of the uterus becomes thin. The cervix (neck of the uterus) contains a mucous plug that is discharged during labour. The expulsion of this plug is known as the bloody show and appears as pink-tinged mucus in the vaginal discharge.

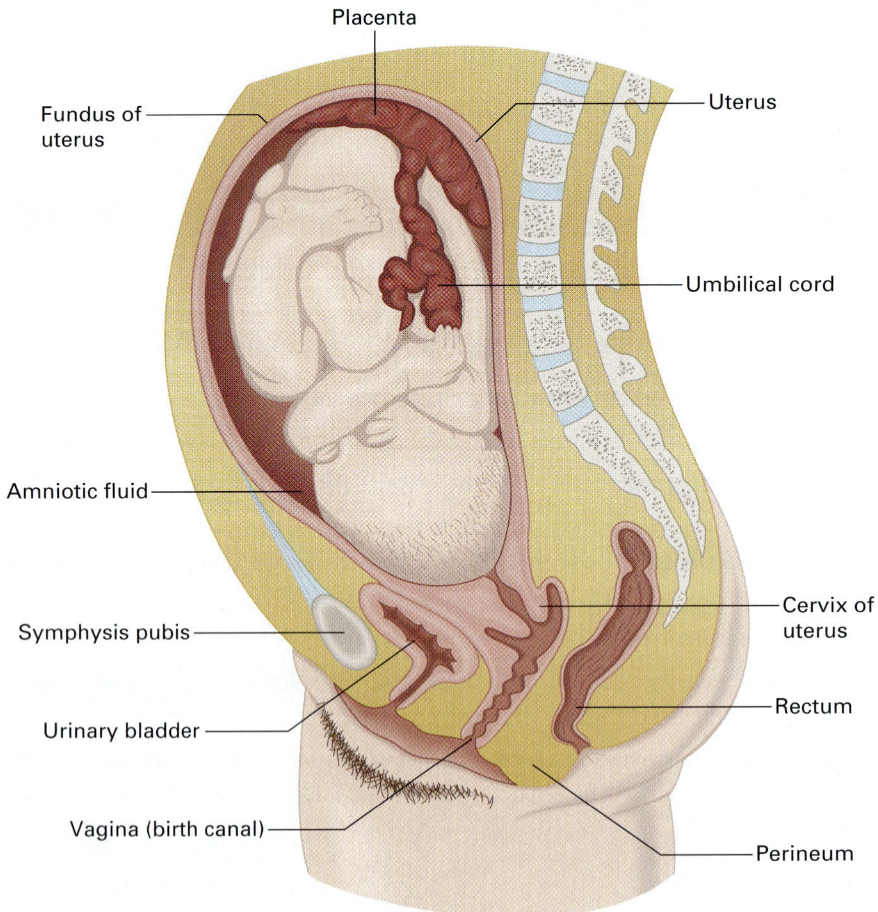

Figure 27–1 Anatomy of pregnancy.

CASE STUDY

Dispatch

My radio sounded the alert tones for an ambulance to respond to a call for a 28-year-old woman in labour. Before I was able to acknowledge the dispatcher, I heard, "Be advised a heavy snowfall advisory has been posted and all roads are considered hazardous for travel." A snowplow was being asked to respond to the ambulance station. As the municipal bylaw enforcement officer, I had access to a four-wheel drive, and knew I could get to the scene.

I informed dispatch that my ETA would be 5 to 10 minutes. She reported back that the ambulance could be 20 to 30 minutes. I found the OB kit, got my jacket on, and went out the door.

Scene Assessment

I arrived at a farmhouse residence and did a quick safety check of the area. I then advised the dispatcher of the road conditions and best access for the ambulance. Once inside the house, I was met by the husband who informed me that his wife was due to deliver in a few weeks, but her water had broken and she was now in labour. I was led to the bedroom where the wife was lying on the bed.

Primary Assessment

The patient looked up at me and said, "The baby is coming—now."

> Consider this patient as you read Chapter 27. How would you proceed?

The placenta is a disc-shaped organ on the inner lining of the uterus. Rich in blood vessels, it provides nourishment and oxygen to the fetus from the mother's blood. It also absorbs waste from the fetus and takes it into the mother's bloodstream. The mother's blood and the baby's blood do not mix. The placenta also produces hormones, such as estrogen and progesterone, that sustain the pregnancy.

After the baby is delivered, the placenta separates from the uterine wall and delivers as the afterbirth. It usually weighs about 500 g (grams) or about one-sixth of the baby's weight.

The umbilical cord is the unborn baby's lifeline. It is an extension of the placenta through which the fetus receives nourishment. The umbilical cord contains one vein and two arteries. The vein carries oxygenated blood to the fetus. The arteries carry deoxygenated blood back to the placenta. When the baby is born, the cord resembles a sturdy rope about 55 cm long and 2.5 cm in diameter.

The amniotic sac, or bag of waters, is filled with a fluid in which the fetus floats. The amount of fluid varies. It is usually from 500 to 1000 mL. The sac of fluid insulates and protects the fetus during pregnancy. During labour, part of the sac is usually forced ahead of the baby, serving as a resilient wedge to help dilate (expand) the cervix.

The birth canal is made up of the cervix and the vagina. The vagina is about 8 to 12 cm long. It originates at the cervix and extends to the outside of the body. Its smooth muscle layer stretches gently during childbirth to allow the passage of the baby.

A full-term pregnancy lasts approximately 280 days. Toward the end, the baby is usually in a head-down position, which brings the uterus down and forward. Mothers can often feel the difference and say that the baby has dropped. This position is most favourable for the baby's passage through the birth canal.

Stages of Labour

Labour is the term used to describe the process of childbirth. It consists of contractions of the uterine wall that force the baby and, later, the placenta into the outside world. Normal labour is divided into three stages: *dilation, expulsion,* and *placental* (Figure 27–2). The length of each stage varies greatly for each woman and under different circumstances.

First Stage: Dilation

During this first and longest stage, the cervix becomes fully dilated. This allows the baby's head to progress from the uterus into the birth canal. Through uterine contractions, the cervix gradually stretches and thins until the opening is large enough to allow the baby to pass through.

The contractions may begin as an aching sensation in the small of the back. Within a short time, the contractions become cramp-like pains in the lower abdomen. These recur at regular intervals, each one lasting about 30 to 60 seconds. At first, the contractions usually occur 10 to 20 minutes apart and are not very severe. They may even stop completely for a while and then start again. Appearance of the mucous plug, or bloody show, may occur before or during this stage of labour. Also before or during this stage, the amniotic sac may rupture, resulting in a gush of fluid from the vagina. When this occurs, the patient may tell you that her water has broken.

Stage one may continue for up to or beyond 18 hours for a woman having her first baby. Women who have had a child before may experience only two or three hours of labour. By the end of the first stage of labour, contractions occur at regular three- to four-minute intervals, last at least 60 seconds each, and feel very strong. The patient may indicate that she is having a considerable amount of discomfort.

Second Stage: Expulsion

During this stage, the baby moves through the birth canal and is born. Contractions are closer together and last longer: 45 to 90 seconds each. As the baby moves downward, the mother experiences considerable pressure in her rectum, much like the feeling of a bowel movement.

When the mother has this sensation, she should lie down and get ready for the birth of her child. The tightening and bearing-down sensations will become stronger and more frequent. The mother will have an uncontrollable urge to push down. This she may do. There will probably be more bloody discharge from the vagina at this point and possibly some anal excretion as well.

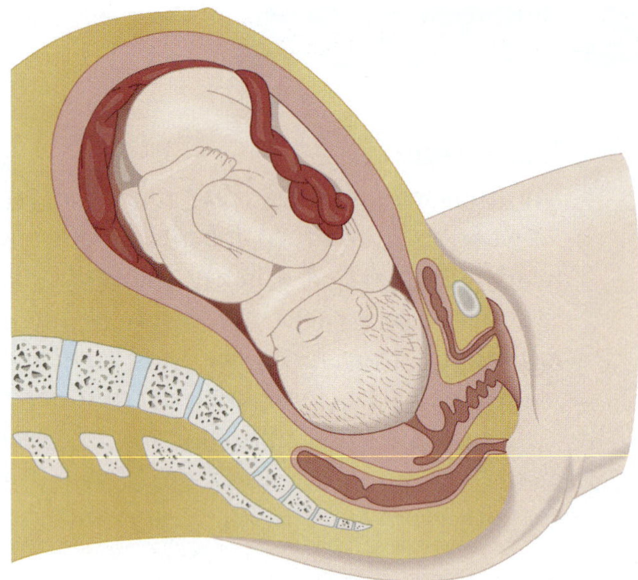

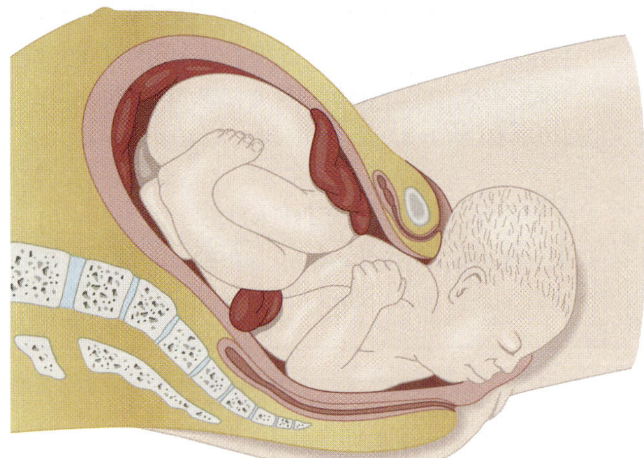

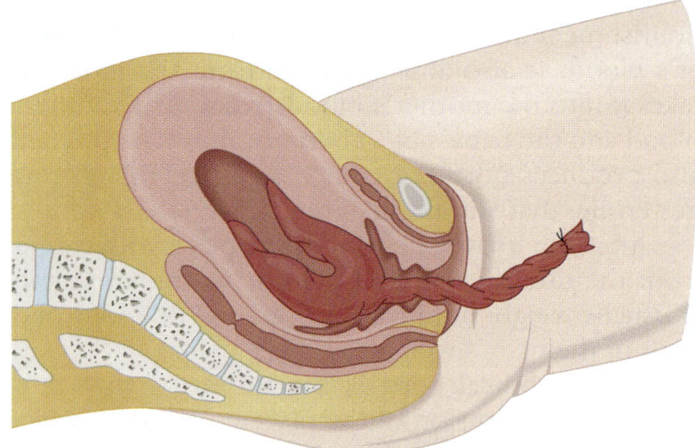

Figure 27–2   Three stages of labour.

Soon after, the baby's head appears at the opening of the birth canal. This is called crowning. The shoulders and the rest of the body follow.

Third Stage: Placental

During this stage, the placenta separates from the uterine wall. In most instances, it is then spontaneously expelled from the uterus.

Patient Assessment

Childbirth is a natural, normal process. It is not an illness or disease. It is, however, physically traumatic. Complications can be life threatening to both the mother and the baby. During history taking, confirm which medications or street drugs or other substances the mother has been taking during pregnancy.

If you are called to the scene of a birth, perform scene and primary assessments and provide treatment as you would for any patient. Give the mother calming reassurance. Then assess her condition to see if there will be time for transport to the nearest medical facility or if she will have the baby on the scene. Update the EMS.

Generally, you should expect to assist in the delivery of the baby on the scene in the following circumstances:

- You have no suitable transportation.
- The delivery of the baby can be expected within five minutes.
- The hospital or physician cannot be reached due to a natural disaster, bad weather, or some kind of catastrophe.

To determine if you should have the patient transported, time the contractions. Follow these steps:

1. Place your gloved hand on the mother's abdomen, just above her navel. Feel the involuntary tightening and relaxing of the uterine muscles.
2. Time these involuntary movements in seconds. Start from the moment the uterus first tightens until it is completely relaxed.
3. Time the intervals between contractions in minutes from the start of one contraction to the start of the next.

If the contractions are more than five minutes apart and traffic and weather conditions are not a problem, the mother usually has time to be transported safely to a hospital. If the contractions are two minutes apart, she probably does not have time. Prepare to help deliver the baby where you are.

If the contractions are between two and five minutes apart, you must make a decision based on a number of factors. Ask the mother a few questions and conduct a simple assessment. The mother is usually nervous and apprehensive, so be gentle and kind. Show confidence and support. Ask these questions:

- Have you had a baby before? (The birth may take longer in a first pregnancy.) Are you having contractions? How far apart are they? Has the amniotic sac ruptured? (or Did your water break?) If so, when?
- Do you feel the sensation of a bowel movement? (If yes, the baby's head is pressing against the rectum and the baby will soon be born. Do not let the mother sit on the toilet.)
- Do you feel like the baby is ready to be born?

Examine the mother. She should be on her back with knees bent and legs spread. Inspect the vaginal area, but do not touch it except during delivery and when your partner is present.

Determine if there is crowning. If you can see bulging in the vaginal area, and either the head or another part of the baby is visible, prepare to deliver the baby where you are. Report your findings to the paramedics.

Never ask the mother to cross her legs or ankles. Never tie or hold her legs together to try to delay delivery. Never delay or restrain delivery in any way. The pressure could result in death or permanent injury to the baby.

Also, be alert to the possibility of a condition known as supine hypotensive syndrome. This condition may occur when the pregnant patient lies on her back. The combined weight of the uterus and the fetus presses on the great vein that collects blood from the lower body and delivers it to the heart. This vein is called the inferior vena cava. That pressure can impede the blood that returns to the heart, causing the amount of blood that circulates through the body to decrease. You may observe signs of shock in your patient, including reduced blood pressure, increased pulse, and pale skin colour. Also, be alert for fainting.

To avoid supine hypotensive syndrome, the patient should be in a sitting position, if appropriate, or lying on her left side. If you suspect the condition, position the patient on her left side and treat for shock.

Preparation for Delivery

Always act in a professional manner. Be calm. Reassure the mother. Tell her that you are there to help with the delivery. Provide as much quiet and privacy for her as you can. Get rid of distractions. Hold her hand and speak encouragingly to her. Help the mother concentrate on breathing regularly with the contractions. Wipe the mother's face. Give her ice chips only if allowed by local protocol. (The mother should not eat or drink anything once labour starts.) The woman's partner, a family member, or another rescuer can help.

At the very least, the following materials and equipment should be included in your obstetrical (OB) kit:

- Sheets and towels (sterile, if possible)
- One dozen 10 × 10 cm gauze pads
- Two or three sanitary napkins
- Rubber suction syringe
- Baby receiving blanket
- Surgical scissors for cutting the umbilical cord
- Cord clamps or ties
- Foil-wrapped germicidal wipes
- Wide tape or sterile cord
- Large plastic bags

All materials used during delivery should be sterile or at least as clean as possible. This is to protect both the baby and the mother from contamination and infection.

In addition, because delivery results in exposure to a great deal of blood and other body fluids, you must wear personal protective equipment. Put on eyewear, a face mask, protective gloves, a disposable gown, and shoe coverings, if possible. Handle soaked dressings, pads, and linens carefully. Place them in separate bags that will not leak. Then seal and label the bags. Scrub your arms, hands, and nails thoroughly *before and after* the delivery, even if you were wearing gloves.

In addition, do the following:

- Be prepared to provide basic life support to both the mother and the newborn, including treatment for shock.
- Help the mother relax with each contraction. Inhaling causes muscles to tighten; therefore, have her exhale with each contraction. Encourage her to keep breathing slowly but comfortably. Tell her not to strain or push during the first stage of labour.
- The amniotic sac may rupture if it has not already done so. There may also be some blood-tinged mucus. These fluids increase as labour progresses. If you have a clean towel, place it under the mother's buttocks to absorb the fluids. Always wipe in a down-and-away direction to minimize contamination. Discard soiled towels or sheets used for this purpose. Replace them frequently with clean ones.
- If the patient feels more comfortable sitting, reclining, or in some other position during the first stages of labour, let her do so.

- As the contractions become longer and closer together, the patient should lie down on a flat, firm surface that she can push against. It is easiest for you if the mother is on an elevated surface. However, if the floor is the only firm surface available, use it. Pad it with folded sheets, towels, or blankets. Elevate the mother's buttocks about 5 cm with an additional pad of folded sheets or towels. The pad, which should extend about 60 cm in front of her, will help support the slippery baby when it is born.
- When the mother is in position, her feet should be flat on the surface beneath her. Her legs will naturally spread apart because of the size of her abdomen. Do not pull them apart any further. Remove any constricting clothing or push it above the mother's waist.
- Create a sterile field around the opening of the vagina. Place a sterile or clean sheet under the mother's hips. Touching only the corners of the sheet, have the mother lift her hips while you place one fold well under her hips. Unfold it toward her feet. If you have time, place another sheet or towel over the mother's abdomen and legs, leaving the vaginal area uncovered. Direct the best possible light toward the mother's genitals. Do not touch the vagina at any time.
- During the second stage of labour, when the mother bears down, remind her not to arch her back. She should curve forward and bring her chin to her chest to avoid excessive straining. Have her hold her breath for 7 to 10 seconds as she bears down. Holding the breath longer will cause too much straining, broken blood vessels, and tearing of the area around the vagina.

Delivery of the Baby

See Figure 27–3 for photographs of the delivery of a baby and the placenta.

1. *Place the palm of your hand on top of the baby's head.* When it crowns, apply very gentle pressure to prevent an explosive delivery.
2. *Break open the amniotic sac if it has not already broken.* Tear it or pinch it open with your fingers, and push it away from the newborn's head and mouth. Note that the baby can safely inhale clear amniotic fluid. However, if there is **meconium staining** (greenish or brownish fluid), the baby has had a bowel movement; if the excretion is inhaled, it could cause pneumonia.

   In the case of meconium staining, clean the area around the mouth and nose of the baby

CHILDBIRTH

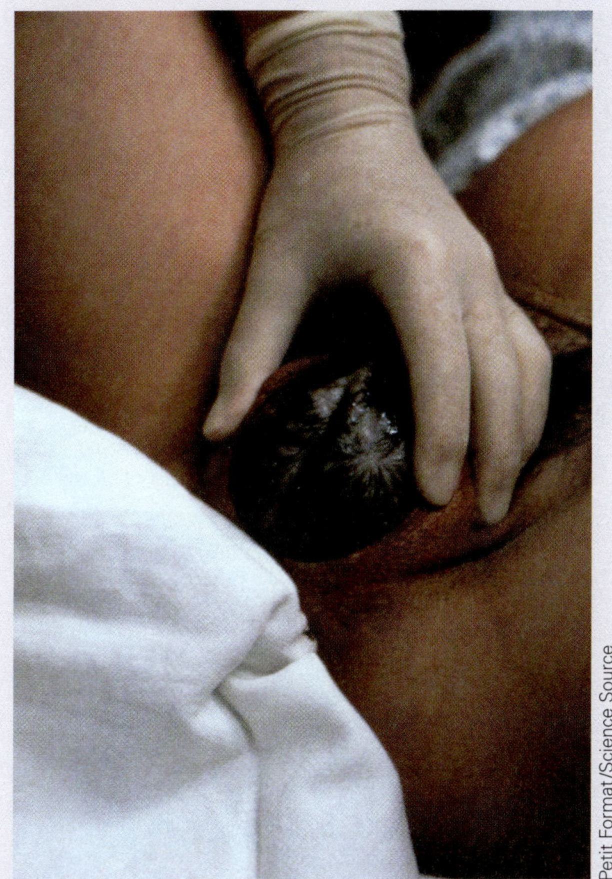

Figure 27–3a   Crowning.

Petit Format/Science Source

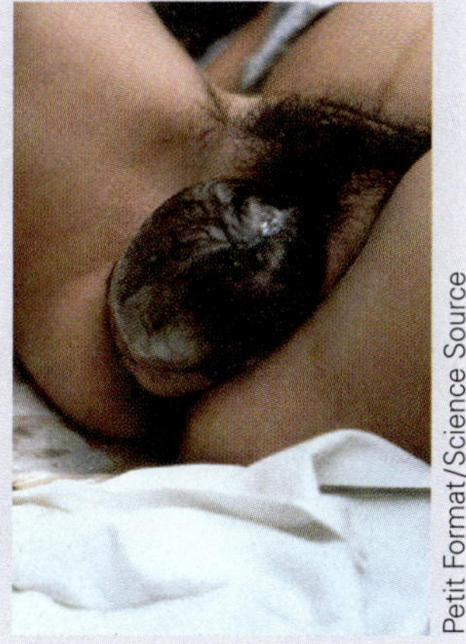

Petit Format/Science Source

Figure 27–3b   Head delivers and turns.

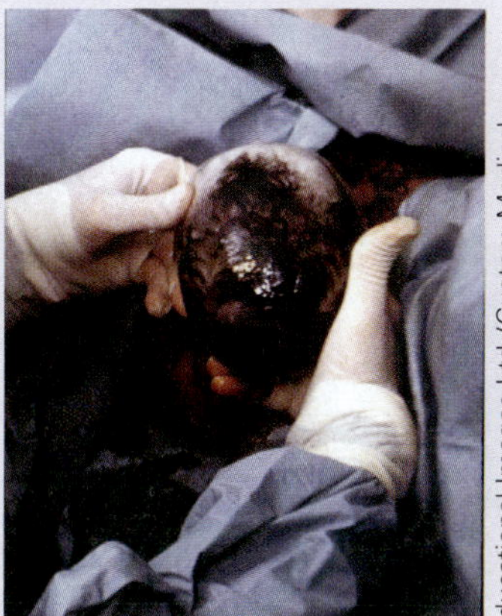

Educational Images Ltd./Custom Medical Stock Photo

Figure 27–3c   Shoulders deliver.

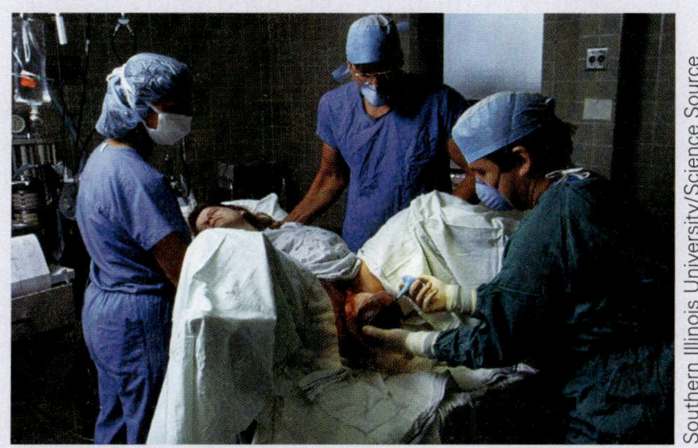

Southern Illinois University/Science Source

Figure 27–3d   Chest delivers.

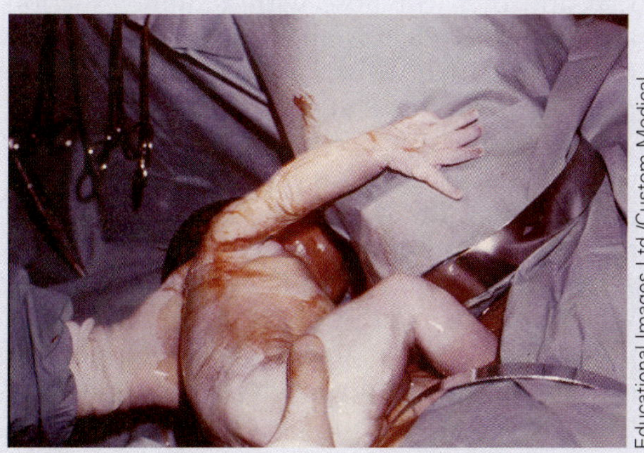

Educational Images Ltd./Custom Medical Stock Photo

Figure 27–3e   Legs and feet deliver.

CHILDBIRTH *(continued)*

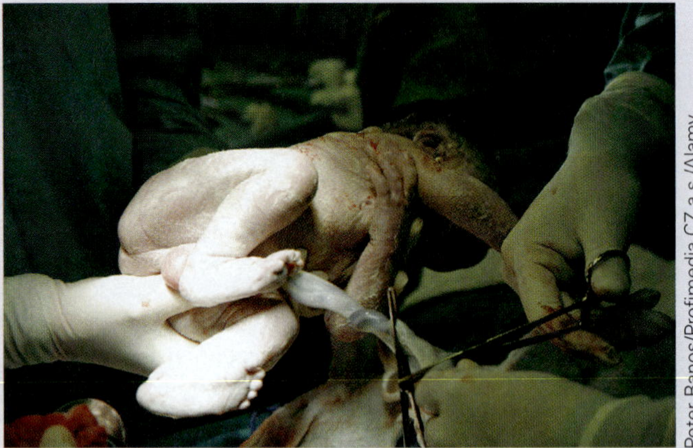

Figure 27–3f Cutting of the cord.

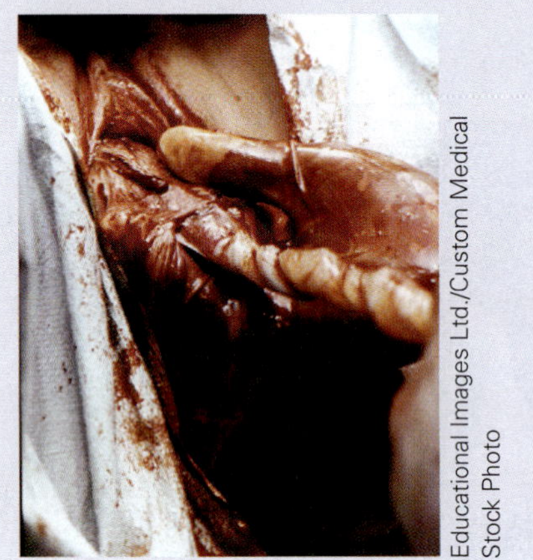

Figure 27–3g Placenta begins to deliver.

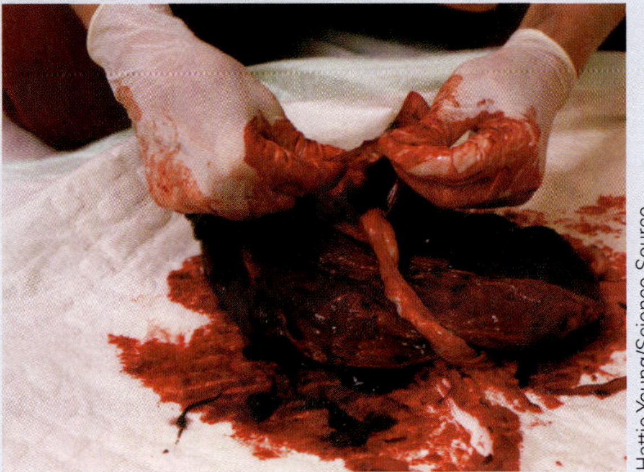

Figure 27–3h Placenta delivers.

once the head is delivered. Suction the mouth first and then the nose with a rubber suction syringe. Expel all air from the suction bulb prior to placing it in the baby's mouth or nose. Release the bulb to create suction.

Suctioning may need to be repeated in order to clear the airway. Note that meconium staining can be a life-threatening event. Consider requesting an advanced life support unit to assist.

3. *Determine the position of the umbilical cord.* When the baby's head delivers, check to see if the umbilical cord is around the baby's neck. If it is, use two gloved fingers to slip the cord over the baby's shoulder. If you cannot dislodge it, attach two clamps a few centimetres apart. Then cut between the clamps.

4. *Support the baby's head.* As soon as the baby's head is born, place one hand below it. Spread the fingers of your other hand gently around it. Avoid touching the fontanelles (the soft spots at the top of the head). In most normal presentations, the baby's head will be face down. Then it turns so that the nose is toward the mother's thigh.

5. *Remove fluids from the baby's airway.* Use a rubber bulb syringe to suction mucus from the baby's mouth first and then the nose. Make sure you fully compress the syringe before you bring it to the baby's face. Avoid contact with the back of the mouth. Insert the tip no more than 2.5 cm into the mouth. Slowly release the bulb to allow fluid to be drawn into the syringe.

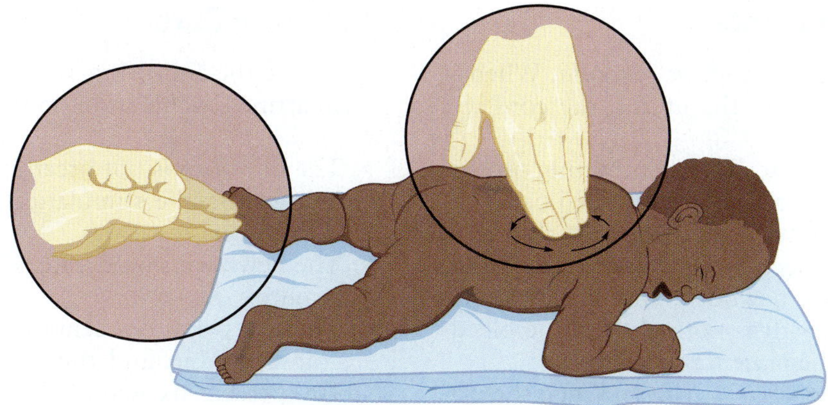

Figure 27–4 Stimulate breathing by rubbing the back or flicking the feet.

If a syringe is not available, wipe the baby's mouth and then the nose with gauze.

6. *Support the baby with both hands as the rest of the body is born.* Once the shoulders are delivered, the rest of the body will appear quickly. Note that you should never pull the baby from the vagina. Never touch the mother's vagina or anus. Handle the baby's slippery body carefully. Do not put your fingers in the baby's armpits. Pressure on the nerve centres there can cause paralysis.

7. *Grasp the feet as they are delivered.* Do not pull on the umbilical cord. Position the baby level with the mother's vagina until the umbilical cord is cut. The neck should be in a neutral position. Note the time of delivery.

8. *Dry, wrap, and position the newborn.* Gently dry the newborn with towels. Then wrap him or her in a clean, warm blanket. Place the baby on his or her side, head slightly lower than the trunk. Turn the baby's head slightly to one side to allow mucus and fluid to drain from the nose and mouth. Only the face should be exposed.

9. *Clean the newborn's mouth and nose.* Wipe blood and mucus from the baby's mouth and nose with sterile gauze. Suction the mouth first and then the nose. The reverse order may cause a newborn's gasp reflex to cause aspiration of mucus or meconium. The newborn should cry almost immediately.

10. *If the baby is not breathing, provide tactile stimulation.* Rub the back gently or slap the soles of the feet (Figure 27–4). Administer oxygen as soon as possible. Usually, placing an oxygen mask near the baby's face and allowing the oxygen to blow by is effective. Do not use oxygen tubing without a mask. The force of the oxygen coming out of the tube can be harmful. If you still get no response, start artificial ventilation. (See "Newborn Care" on p. 408 for details.)

11. *Clamp or tie and cut the umbilical cord when it stops pulsating,* provided that your EMS system allows you to do so (Figure 27–5). Place two clamps or ties on the cord about 8 cm apart. Position the first clamp about four finger-widths (15 cm) from the baby. Use sterile surgical scissors to cut the cord between the two clamps or ties. Check the end of the cord periodically for bleeding and control any that occurs.

12. *Record the time of delivery.*

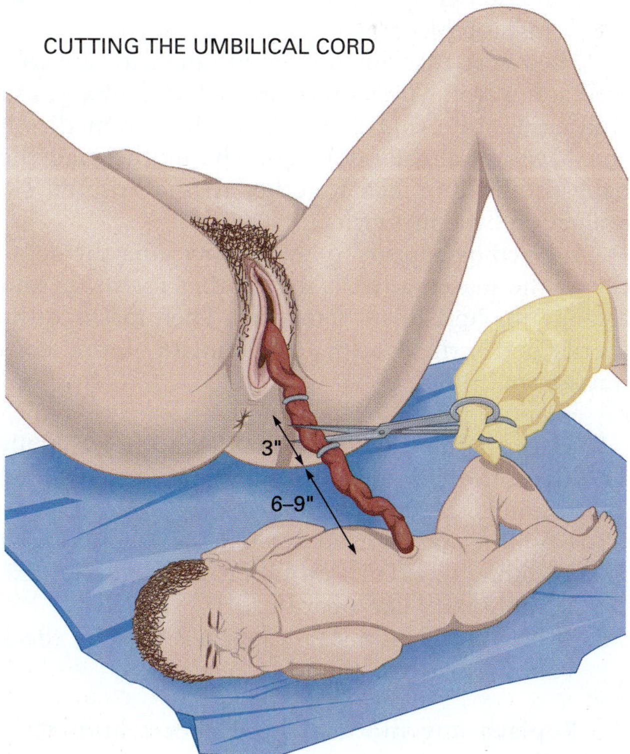

Figure 27–5 Cutting the umbilical cord.

Delivery of the Placenta

1. *Observe for the delivery of the placenta.* When it starts to separate from the uterus, the cord will appear to be longer.
2. *Feel for contractions.* The contracting uterus should feel like a hard, grapefruit-sized ball.
3. *Encourage the mother to bear down as the uterus contracts.* The placenta usually delivers within 10 minutes of the newborn, and almost always within 30 minutes. It is normal for some bleeding to occur as the placenta separates.
4. *Wrap the placenta when it delivers.* When the placenta appears, slowly and gently guide it from the vagina. Never pull. If you have not cut the cord, wrap the placenta in a sterile towel and place it next to the baby. Wrap the baby and the placenta in a third sheet or blanket. If the cord is cut, place the placenta in a plastic bag to be taken to the hospital where a physician can confirm the delivery is complete.

After the placenta delivers, check the mother's vaginal bleeding. Up to 500 mL of blood loss is normal and usually well tolerated by the mother. Place two sanitary napkins over the opening of the vagina. Touch only the outer surfaces of the pads. Do not touch the mother's vagina. At this time, ask the mother if she plans to breastfeed the baby. If so, now is a good time to encourage her to start. Breastfeeding helps the uterus to contract, which decreases its size and helps stop bleeding.

Make sure that the mother and the baby are covered and warm. The mother, as well as the baby, can chill easily following birth. Alert the paramedics if you have not already done so. The mother and the baby should be taken together to the hospital for evaluation by a physician.

If bleeding appears to be excessive after the delivery of the placenta, treat the mother for shock and arrange for immediate transport. Then massage the uterus as described below to stimulate uterine contractions:

1. Place the medial edge of one hand horizontally across the abdomen, just superior to the symphysis pubis. Extend your fingers.
2. Cup your other hand around the uterus. Use a kneading or circular motion to massage the area. It should feel like a hard ball.
3. If bleeding continues to appear excessive, check your massage technique.

Replace any blood-soaked sheets and blankets while waiting for transportation. Place all soiled items in a marked infection-control bag and seal it.

Newborn Care

If any of the following three conditions exist, perform artificial ventilation on the newborn:

- The newborn is not breathing after drying, warming, and tactile stimulation, or there are gasping respirations.
- The newborn's pulse rate is less than 100 beats per minute.
- There is persistent central cyanosis, or bluish discoloration, around the chest and abdomen after 100 percent oxygen has been administered.

The recommended rate for assisting a newborn's ventilations is between 40 and 60 breaths per minute. Keep in mind that a baby's lungs are very small and require very small puffs of air. Never use mechanical ventilation on a newborn. A BVM device may be used, but it must be the appropriate size for a newborn. Remember to observe for chest rise. Reassess after 30 seconds. For proper positioning of the head, a towel may be placed under the baby's shoulders.

If breathing and pulse are absent, or if the pulse rate is less than 60 beats per minute, start CPR. The target rate for compressions is at least 120 per minute. The ratio of compressions to ventilations for the newborn is 3:1, so you should be delivering one breath every two seconds, or about 30 rescue breaths per minute. Recheck the heart rate every 30 seconds and continue as necessary.

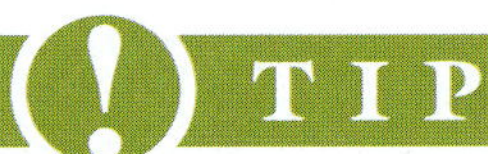

Whether or not you expect complications, you should notify the incoming crew if delivery is imminent. As soon as the baby is born, there are now two patients who each require individual attention. A second ambulance should be dispatched since one is not usually adequate for attending to two patients.

SECTION 2
COMPLICATIONS OF PREGNANCY AND CHILDBIRTH

Complications of Pregnancy

Toxemia of Pregnancy

About 5 percent of women develop toxemia (or poisoning of the blood) during pregnancy. It occurs most frequently in the last trimester (last three months). It most often affects women in their 20s who are pregnant for the first time. Women with a history of diabetes, heart disease, kidney problems, or high blood pressure are at greatest risk.

The signs and symptoms of toxemia include the following:

- High blood pressure (very common)
- Swelling in the extremities (very common)
- Sudden weight gain (1 kg or more per week)
- Blurred vision or spots before the eyes
- Pronounced swelling of the face
- Decreased urinary output
- Severe and persistent headache
- Persistent vomiting
- Pain in the upper abdomen
- Sudden seizures

To provide emergency medical care for toxemia of pregnancy, arrange for immediate transport of the patient. Position the patient on her left side to avoid compressing the inferior vena cava. Keep the patient calm. If you are allowed to do so, administer oxygen.

If the mother suffers a seizure, monitor her breathing closely. When the seizure stops, elevate her head and shoulders and administer high-flow oxygen.

Gestational Diabetes

During the weight gain of pregnancy, an expectant mother is at greater risk of developing problems with controlling her blood sugar. Gestational diabetes is a concern for both mother and baby, so be sure to include this information in your history taking and your patient hand-off report.

Spontaneous Abortion

Often called a miscarriage, a spontaneous abortion is the loss of pregnancy before the 20th week. It occurs naturally, unlike abortions that are deliberately performed in either legal or illegal settings. The signs and symptoms include the following:

- Vaginal bleeding, often heavy
- Pain in the lower abdomen that is similar to menstrual cramps or labour contractions
- Passage of tissue from the vagina

To provide emergency care, arrange for immediate transport. Treat the patient for shock. Save any passed tissue by packaging it in a sealed bag. The bag should be transported with the patient for evaluation by a physician.

Ectopic Pregnancy

A woman has two fallopian tubes. Each one extends up from the uterus to a position near an ovary. Each month an egg is released from an ovary into a fallopian tube. The fallopian tube conveys the egg toward the uterus, and the sperm from the uterus toward the ovary.

In a normal pregnancy, a fertilized ovum (egg) is implanted in the uterus. In an ectopic pregnancy, a fertilized ovum is implanted outside the uterus. It could be in the abdominal cavity, on the outside wall of the uterus, on the ovary, or on the outside of the cervix, but in 95 percent of cases, the ovum is implanted in the fallopian tube.

An ectopic pregnancy is a severe medical emergency. The expanding fertilized ovum eventually causes rupture of a blood vessel and severe abdominal bleeding. It is the leading cause of death among pregnant women in their first trimester (first three months).

The signs and symptoms of ectopic pregnancy include the following:

- Sudden, sharp abdominal pain on one side (If the bleeding is extensive, the pain will become more diffuse.)
- Pain under the diaphragm or pain radiating to one or both shoulders
- Tender bloated abdomen
- Vaginal spotting or bleeding
- Missed menstrual periods
- Weakness when sitting
- Signs of shock

Suspect ectopic pregnancy in any woman of childbearing age when the above signs and symptoms are present. To provide emergency care, arrange for immediate transport. Place the patient on her back with knees elevated. Keep the patient warm. If you are allowed and able to, administer oxygen.

Placenta Previa

Placenta previa occurs when the placenta is positioned in the uterus in an abnormally low position. When the cervix dilates, the fetus moves, or labour begins, the placenta separates from the uterus. This puts both the mother and the baby in danger.

The signs and symptoms include the following:

- Severe, usually painless bleeding from the vagina
- Signs of shock

To provide emergency care, arrange for immediate transport. Elevate the patient's legs. Maintain body temperature. If possible, administer 100 percent oxygen by mask.

Abruptio Placentae

Another major cause of bleeding during pregnancy is abruptio placentae. It is the leading cause of fetal death after blunt trauma. Life threatening for both the mother and the baby, it needs to be quickly recognized and treated.

There are several causes of abruptio placentae, including toxemia and trauma. Whatever the cause, the normally implanted placenta begins separating from the uterus sometime during the last three months of pregnancy. Bleeding begins, but it is often behind the placenta and the mother is unaware of it. Shock then develops in the mother, and the baby does not get enough oxygen.

The signs and symptoms include the following:

- Bleeding from the vagina, generally not in great quantities
- Severe abdominal pain
- Rigid abdomen
- Signs of shock

To provide emergency care, arrange for immediate transport. Monitor vital signs carefully, and treat for shock. Administer 100 percent oxygen via a mask.

Complications of Childbirth

Prolapsed Umbilical Cord

In some situations, the umbilical cord comes out of the birth canal before the baby. When this happens, the baby is in great danger of suffocating.

The cord is compressed against the birth canal by the baby's head, which cuts off the baby's supply of oxygenated blood from the placenta. Emergency care is extremely urgent. Arrange for immediate transport. Follow these steps:

1. If possible, have the mother lie down on her left side. The knees should be drawn up to her chest, or her hips and legs should be elevated on a pillow.
2. If possible, administer high-flow oxygen to the mother.
3. With your gloved hand, gently push the baby up the vagina far enough so that the baby's head is off the umbilical cord. Maintain pressure on the baby's head and keep the cord free until medical help arrives. This is controversial in some areas. Follow local protocol.
4. Do not try to push the cord back into the vagina. Cover the cord with a sterile towel moistened with clean, preferably sterile, water.

Breech Birth

In a breech birth, the baby's feet or buttocks are delivered first (Figure 27–6). Whenever possible, the mother should be taken to the hospital for the birth. If that is not possible, follow these guidelines:

1. Position and prepare the mother for a normal delivery.

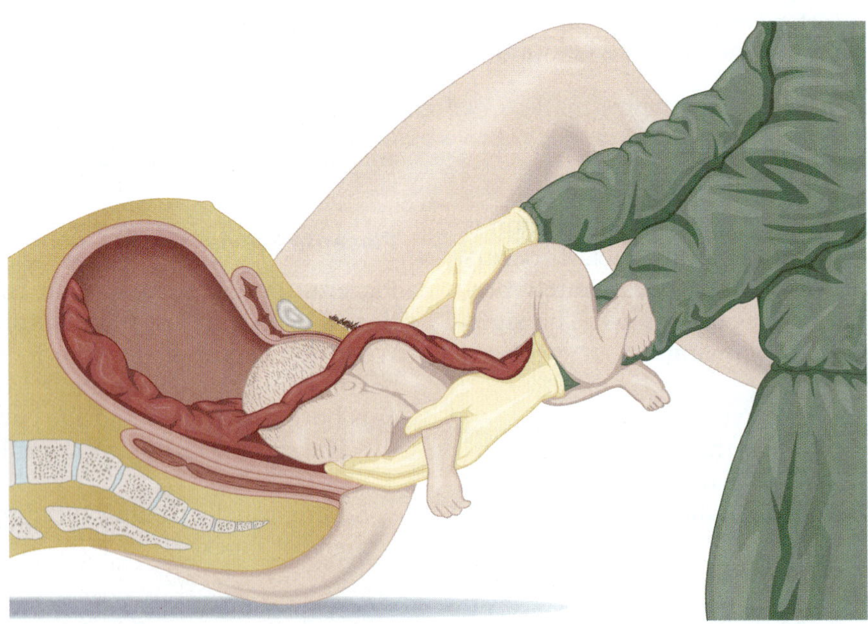

Figure 27–6 In breech birth, the baby's feet or buttocks deliver first.

2. Let the baby's buttocks and trunk deliver on their own. Never try to pull the baby from the vagina by the legs or trunk.
3. Place your arm between the baby's legs. Let the legs dangle astride your arm. Support the baby's back with the palm of your other hand.
4. The head should follow on its own within three minutes. If it does not, you need to prevent the baby from suffocating because the baby's head will compress the umbilical cord, preventing the flow of oxygenated blood from the placenta.
5. Place the middle and index fingers of your gloved hand alongside the baby's face. Your palm should be turned toward the face. Form an airway by pushing the vagina away from the baby's face until the head is delivered. Once the head is delivered, hold the baby's mouth slightly open with your finger so that the baby can breathe.

Umbilical Cord Around the Neck

If the umbilical cord is wrapped around the baby's neck in the birth canal, do the following:

1. Try to gently slip the cord over the baby's shoulders or head.
2. If you cannot, and the cord is wrapped tightly around the neck, place clamps or ties 8 cm apart on the cord. Quickly, but carefully, cut between the two clamps or ties. Unwrap the cord from around the neck.
3. Deliver the shoulders and body, supporting the head at all times.

Limb Presentation

If the baby's arms or legs come out of the birth canal first, it means that the baby has shifted so much in the uterus that a normal delivery is not possible. The baby will have to be delivered by a physician. Delay can be fatal. Never pull on the baby by the arms or legs. The mother must be taken immediately to a hospital. Transport without delay.

Multiple Births

Twins are delivered the same way as single babies, one after the other. In fact, since twins are smaller, delivery is often easier. Identical twins have two umbilical cords coming out of a single placenta. If the twins are fraternal, rather than identical, there will be two placentas.

The mother may not be aware that she is carrying twins. You should suspect that twins are present if one or more of the following conditions exists:

- The abdomen is still very large after one baby is delivered.
- The baby's size is out of proportion to the size of the mother's abdomen.
- Strong contractions begin again about 10 minutes after the baby is born.

The second baby is usually born within minutes and almost always within 45 minutes. About one-third of second twins are breech. To manage a multiple birth, follow these guidelines:

- After the first baby is born, clamp and cut the cord to prevent bleeding in the second baby.
- If the second baby has not delivered within 10 minutes, the mother should be transported to a hospital for the birth.
- After the babies are born, the placenta or placentas will be delivered normally. You can expect bleeding after the second birth.
- Keep the babies warm. Twins are often born early and may be small enough to be considered premature. Guard against heat loss until they can be taken to a hospital.

Premature Birth

If a woman gives birth before the 36th week of pregnancy, or if the baby weighs less than 2.5 kg, the baby is considered to be premature. Premature babies are smaller and redder. They have heads that are proportionately larger than in full-term babies. Because they are very vulnerable to infection, special care must be taken.

- Keep the baby warm with a blanket or swaddle. If you lack other supplies, use aluminum foil as an outer wrap.
- Keep the baby's mouth and nose clear of fluid by gentle suctioning with a bulb syringe.
- Prevent bleeding from the umbilical cord. A premature baby cannot tolerate losing even a little blood without being at risk for shock.
- Administer passive oxygen, if you are permitted to, by blowing it gently across the baby's face. Never blast oxygen directly into the face.
- Since premature babies are so vulnerable to infection, do not let anyone breathe into the baby's face. Do everything you can to prevent contamination.

EMR FOCUS

Calls for emergency childbirth are rare compared with other types of calls. Unlike other calls, childbirth is not an injury or illness. Families have delivered babies outside hospitals for centuries. In modern times, hospital deliveries are usually preferred.

If you are called to the scene where the delivery of a baby is imminent, remain calm. Remember what you have learned and keep in mind that you are assisting in a natural process.

Become familiar with the procedures and protocols in your area. In the event of complications, you will need to care for the newborn and the mother until they are turned over to the paramedics for transport to a hospital.

Boiling water, as seen in the movies, is not one of the duties of an EMR: however, warming up blankets can be a duty for a bystander if enough people are on scene.

CASE STUDY FOLLOW-UP

At the beginning of this chapter, you read that an EMR was on the scene with a patient who was preparing to give birth in her home. To see how the chapter skills apply to this emergency, read the following. It describes how the call was completed.

PRIMARY ASSESSMENT *(Continued)*

I introduced myself to the patient and assured her that I had been trained to handle childbirth situations. As we talked, I determined that she was alert and oriented with a good airway and adequate respirations. Her pulse was strong and regular and her skin warm and slightly sweaty. There was no evidence of bleeding.

I moved next to the patient and explained that the ambulance was on the way. At this point, I told both parents what needed to be done until the paramedics arrived and how they could help. Then I updated dispatch.

PATIENT HISTORY

The patient, Mrs. Sahar Hakimi, told me that it was her second pregnancy and that there had been no problems with the delivery of the first baby. The doctor had told her that the pregnancy was normal. She reported that her water had broken 45 minutes before and contractions were two minutes apart with a 50-second duration. She said she felt pressure on her rectum, as if she had to move her bowels.

I asked where her other child was, and she said that her daughter was at a neighbour's.

SECONDARY ASSESSMENT

I asked Mrs. Hakimi for permission to examine her for crowning and to prepare her for delivery. She agreed. Acting quickly, I made sure I had on all appropriate personal protective equipment. Her husband was next to her, holding her hand and trying to reassure her.

The baby's head had crowned. I placed my hands gently on the head. The shoulders and the rest of the baby followed rapidly. Using the bulb syringe from the OB kit, I suctioned the baby's mouth first and then the nose. The baby cried loudly. It was a girl. I wrapped her in a warm towel and placed her on her mother's belly. I then clamped the umbilical cord.

ONGOING ASSESSMENT

Not long after the birth, Mrs. Hakimi delivered the placenta. I placed it in a container for the paramedics to transport with the patient. Although the mother was tired, she was in good spirits and had no unusual complaints or distress. Her mental status was normal, and her vitals were stable.

After the baby was cleaned up a bit, her colour appeared to be normal. Her respirations were 48. Pulse was 146 and regular. She was actively moving around and had a good strong cry.

TRANSFER OF CARE

When the paramedics arrived, I gave them the hand-off report. They quickly packaged the patient and the baby and moved them to the ambulance. They had reached the residence quickly, considering the weather. The snowplow driver was my new hero. Even though there were no complications, and you could say it had been a textbook delivery, my heart was still racing as I watched them drive away.

Childbirth is a rare and exciting event for an EMR. Remember that birth is a natural process. You are there to assist the mother and then care for her and the baby after delivery. Your top priorities are the same as for any call. They are scene safety and the ABCs of your patients—both mother and child.

NOCPs

4.3 f Conduct obstetrical assessment and interpret findings **A**

l Conduct neonatal assessment and interpret findings **A**

6.1 q Provide care to obstetrical patient **S**

6.2 a Provide care for the neonatal patient **S**

REVIEW QUESTIONS

Page references where answers may be found or supported are provided at the end of each question.

SECTION 1

1. What is the function of each of the following: placenta, umbilical cord, amniotic sac? (p. 401)

2. What happens during the first stage of labour? The second stage? The third stage? (pp. 402–403)

3. How can you determine how fast and how close together the contractions are? (p. 403)

4. What information must you have to decide if a birth is imminent? (p. 403)

5. What is supine hypotensive syndrome? How can you avoid it? (p. 403)

6. What part of the baby usually presents first in a normal delivery? (p. 402)

7. What can you do to assist a mother in the delivery of the baby? Briefly describe the process. (pp. 404–407)

8. When does the placenta usually deliver? What should you do with it when it does? (p. 408)

9. What are the normal respiratory and heart rates for a newborn? (p. 408)

SECTION 2

10. What would you observe with a prolapsed cord? (p. 410)

11. What would you observe in a breech birth? (pp. 410–411)

12. What is the emergency medical care for a delivery with limb presentation? (p. 411)

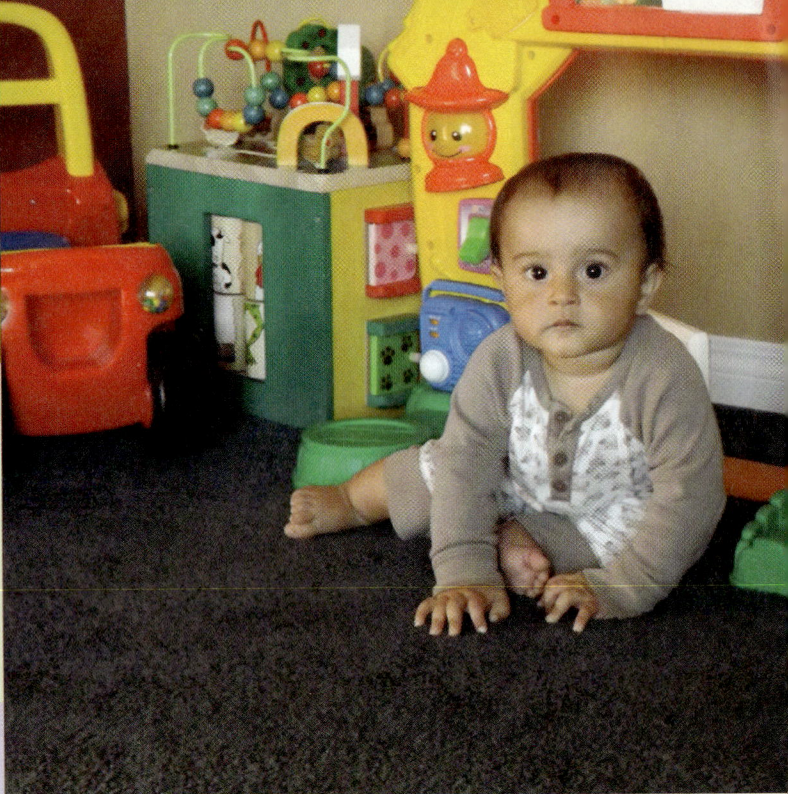

John Mackay

Infants and Children

OBJECTIVES

1. Describe characteristics associated with the five stages of infant and child development.
2. Outline the differences between the anatomy and physiology of the infant, child, and adult patient.
3. Describe and demonstrate primary assessment of the infant or child, including the seven common signs and symptoms of early respiratory distress in infants and children.
4. Describe and demonstrate secondary assessment of the infant or child, including special considerations for assessing pulse, respiration, blood pressure, temperature, skin condition, and capillary refill.
5. Discuss emergency medical care of the infant and child trauma patient.
6. Identify the signs and symptoms of shock in cases of trauma or dehydration in infants and children.
7. Discuss common respiratory emergencies in infants and children, including croup, epiglottitis, and asthma, and describe their emergency medical care.
8. List common causes and describe the management of seizures in infants and children.
9. Discuss management of cases of suspected sudden infant death syndrome (SIDS).
10. Summarize the signs and symptoms and describe the medical-legal responsibilities of the EMR in cases of possible child abuse and neglect.
11. Understand the EMR's own emotional response to a difficult infant or child call and recognize the need for EMR debriefing.
12. Demonstrate a caring attitude toward the patient and family when dealing with illness or injury in infants and children, while giving priority to the interests of the patient.

INTRODUCTION

Over 4000 children die in Canada each year. Approximately one in four children will sustain an injury that will require medical care. Most children are injured as a result of MVAs. Burns and drowning are the next most frequent types of injury. Respiratory problems are the most serious of medical emergencies.

While your assessment approach to the ill or injured child is somewhat different from your approach to an adult, your patient care plan is the same. This chapter focuses only on the particular needs of infants and children and how you can address those needs in emergency situations. It is intended to supplement the emergency care information found in the rest of the book.

SECTION 1
THE PEDIATRIC PATIENT

There are times when determining the age of a young patient may be difficult. Even though age is a common benchmark for certain types of treatment, not all young patients physically mature at the same pace. For example, some 12-year-olds may be smaller than average. Some eight-year-olds may look older. Use your best judgment when the exact age of a patient is unknown.

Developmental Characteristics

Knowing the characteristics of children at each age can help you in an emergency. You will have a good idea of what to expect from them and how best to communicate. See Table 28–1 on page 417 for a summary of childhood development by age.

As an EMR, your encounters with **pediatric patients** (infants and children) will be when they are ill or injured. They are apt to be frightened before you arrive. When you do get on-scene, the presence of an unfamiliar person will add to what the patient already perceives as a frightening situation. Children pick up on anxiety easily. Therefore, it is very important to stay calm. Children at any age often take their cue from what they observe. If the adults on the scene stay calm, a pediatric patient is also more likely to stay calm.

When dealing with younger children, it helps to get down to their eye level. Do not stare. Include them in your conversation. Do not make sudden movements when performing an assessment or providing emergency care. If the child is old enough to understand, ask his or her permission to remove

a piece of clothing or to touch the body. If a child holds out a hand, or allows you to examine some part of his or her body, seize the moment. The rule in pediatric care is to examine and palpate what you can when the opportunity presents itself.

With adolescents, it is important to be sensitive to their feelings of modesty. In many ways, they are young adults. Permanent disfigurement may be a major concern. They are also very sensitive to peer pressure and may need to be reassured that what they tell you will be held in confidence. Of course, you would still be free to include relevant information in your pre-hospital care report or in any report to emergency medical providers who have a need to know.

Dealing with Caregivers

With pediatric patients, it is important to understand that caregivers, especially parents, may be very upset and concerned. In fact, when a child is ill or injured, the EMR should view the situation as one that involves a family, not just a child. Anticipate a variety of responses from caregivers. A few of the more common are crying, emotional outbursts, anger, guilt, and confusion. Some of this emotion may be directed at EMS personnel. Keep your own safety in mind but do not take it personally. Caregivers need support and understanding.

As the assessment of the patient progresses, explain to the caregivers what is being done, and, if time permits, tell them why. If appropriate, ask them to assist with emergency care. For example, a parent can hold an oxygen mask near the infant's face (Figure 28–1 on p. 417).

On occasion, you may encounter a parent who will not let you help an ill or injured child. That parent may insist on remaining in control. Avoid becoming defensive. The parent's behaviour has nothing at

CASE STUDY

Dispatch

My partner and I had just finished lunch when tones came over the speaker in the squad room. The dispatcher's voice followed: "Fire 413, respond to a third-party call of a child struck by a car in the 400 block of Broadway Ave. Be advised that an ambulance is being dispatched. Time of call is 14:23 hours."

En route to the call, we were informed that the child's condition was unknown and that the ambulance would be delayed.

Scene Assessment

Police led us through the crowd to the scene of the incident. We saw that the child was out of the roadway on the grass. A very upset father was beside the child. While my partner tried to introduce herself to the father and calm him down, I questioned a witness. She told me that the car had been travelling at about 25 km/h (kilometres per hour) when it hit the child. She said that the child appeared to glance off the left front of the vehicle, fall to the ground, and roll onto the grass.

By that time, my partner had calmed the father down and gotten consent to provide emergency medical care.

Primary Assessment

The patient was on her side and not moving. She responded only to pain and had snoring respirations. She was little. Her father said she was six years old.

> Consider this patient as you read Chapter 28. Will assessment of the six-year-old be any different from the assessment of an adult? How about treatment? Will it be different or about the same?

all to do with you. Remember, even though they may be coping in the only way they know how, ultimately the child is the patient. If you are called, you must make sure the patient is not in need of emergency medical care.

The following techniques may help in situations where parents are especially anxious:

- Your first priority is to protect the health and safety of the patient. If parents are making unsafe demands, try an approach of reserved confrontation. Explain that your opinion and procedures are based on sound medical knowledge and that their demands are obstructing what is considered appropriate and in the child's best interests.

- Realize that the parents may be correct. They usually know their children extremely well. The parent of a chronically ill child probably has a good grasp of what is going on.

- Regardless of how the parents behave, treat them with courtesy, respect, and understanding. Avoid raising your voice. Tell them that you know they want to help.

- Let the parents stay as close to the patient as possible as long as they are not interfering with care. If medically appropriate, the child can be held by a parent. Consider letting the parents do something for the child in order to help focus their attention away from you.

- Whatever you do, do not react with anger.

TABLE 28–1
CHILDHOOD DEVELOPMENT BY AGE

Common Term	Age	Characteristics and Behaviours
Infant	Birth to 1 year	Knows the voices and faces of parents May cry to indicate hunger, discomfort, or pain Will want to be held by a parent or caregiver Has difficulty identifying the precise location of an injury or source of pain
Toddler	1–3 years old	Very curious at this age, so possibility of poison ingestion May be distrustful and uncooperative Usually does not understand what is happening, which raises level of fear May be very concerned about being separated from parents or caregivers May be helpful to use a stuffed toy in gaining trust
Preschooler	3–5 years old	Able to talk, but still may not understand what is being said to him or her; use simple words May be scared and believe what is happening is his or her fault Sight of blood may intensify response; sometimes a bandage helps
School age	6–12 years old	Should cooperate and be willing to follow the lead of parents and EMS provider Have active imaginations and thoughts about death Continual reassurance is important
Adolescent	13–18 years old	Acts like adult Able to provide accurate information Modesty is important Has fears of permanent scarring or deformity May become involved in mass hysteria; be tolerant and do not get caught up in it

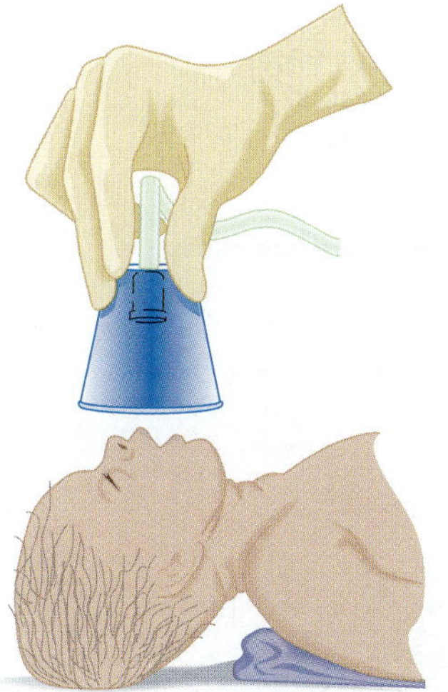

Figure 28–1   Blow-by oxygen using tubing and a paper cup. Never use a Styrofoam cup.

Using Appropriate Equipment

The correct equipment in the correct size for the pediatric patient is extremely important for quality care. The following list of EMS equipment is appropriate for the different needs of infants and children:

- Airway adjuncts in pediatric sizes
- Face masks, oxygen masks, and nasal cannulas in pediatric sizes
- BVM resuscitator with oxygen enrichment attachment (If the BVM device has a pop-off valve, it must be possible to close it.)
- Bulb syringe for suctioning
- Blood pressure cuffs in pediatric sizes
- Pediatric stethoscope
- Cervical immobilization devices in various pediatric sizes

- Backboards made especially for infants and children
- New, clean stuffed animal toys to be used to comfort or distract the patient

Patient Assessment

Scene Assessment

When entering a scene where there is an emergency involving a child, many EMS rescuers say, "Ninety percent of the assessment is done from the doorway."

That is not really true. However, you can take a second or two to try to get the big picture. Observations you can make from the doorway in addition to your usual scene assessment include the interaction between the patient and parents, general appearance of the environment, and signs of possible **non-accidental trauma** (child abuse).

During scene assessment, see how the caregivers are reacting, and, if appropriate, consider how best to involve them in the assessment and treatment of the patient. You may be called to treat infant or child patients at a location other than where they were injured or became ill. It is not uncommon for adults to pick up a child in order to provide comfort or assistance. Understand they meant no harm. Ask the caregivers the following specific questions:

- Why was EMS called?
- What is the chief complaint?
- Has the child been moved? If so, where did the incident occur?

Be alert to the possibility of poison ingestion or a fall.

Primary Assessment

To assess an infant's or child's level of consciousness, determine from the caregiver what is normal. If a patient appears to be conscious but is unable to recognize his or her own parents, consider this a serious medical emergency.

Remember that an infant's or child's anatomy is not the same as an adult's (Figure 28–2). However,

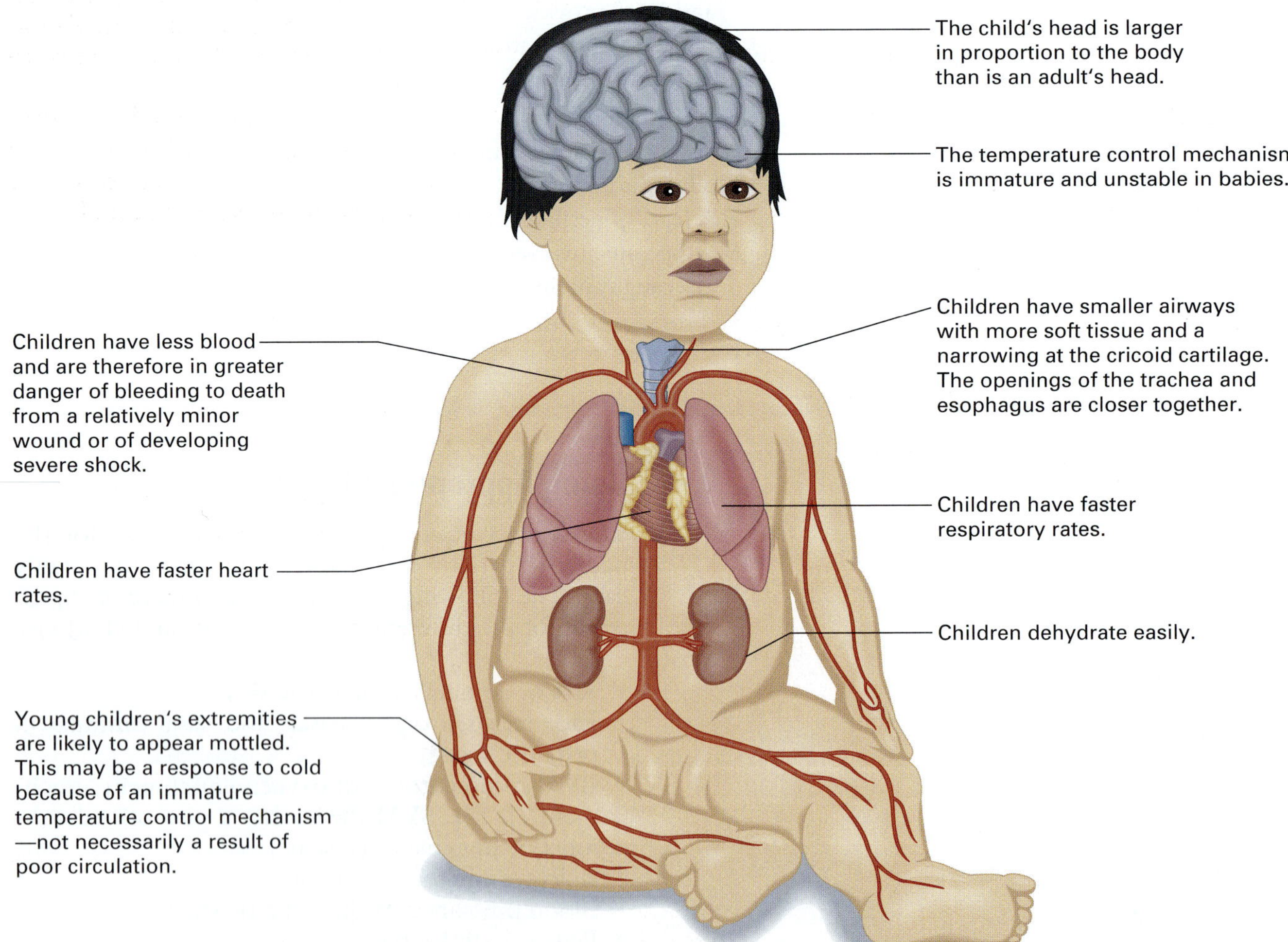

Figure 28–2   The anatomy of an infant or child is not the same as an adult's.

assessment and treatment of the ABCs are as critical to the pediatric patient as to any other. The single most important manoeuvre is to ensure an open airway. When trauma is suspected, always use the jaw-thrust manoeuvre to open the airway. Never hyperextend the head and neck. The head of an infant or young child is large in proportion to the rest of the body. One way to properly position the head in a neutral position is to place a towel with a fold or two under the patient's shoulders.

> ## (!) T I P
>
> A crying child, although difficult to communicate with, is a welcome sight and sound.
>
> Screaming = Breathing
>
> Silence or lethargy may be a result of respiratory distress.

Common signs in infants and children that indicate early respiratory distress are as follows (Figure 28–3):

- Noisy breathing, such as stridor, crowing, or grunting
- Cyanosis
- Flaring nostrils
- Retractions (drawing back) between the ribs or around the shoulders
- Use of accessory muscles to breathe
- Breathing with obvious effort
- Altered mental status

Immediately provide oxygen if any of these signs are evident. Continually monitor for signs of respiratory distress. If an infant's respirations are fewer than 20 per minute or a child's are fewer than 10, assist ventilations.

Assess circulation by palpating the infant's brachial pulse. Palpate the unconscious child's carotid or femoral pulse. Palpate the conscious child's radial or brachial pulse.

When you assess the pediatric patient's circulation, remember that inadequate oxygen can slow the heart. Provide oxygen as soon as you detect a slow pulse. Use a mask that is the correct size for the patient. When the patient is not breathing and has no gag reflex, an oropharyngeal airway should be inserted to assist in maintaining an open airway. (See Chapter 7 for a review of how to insert airway adjuncts.)

Control any external bleeding immediately. Children have the ability to compensate for blood loss longer than an adult can. However, decompensation (failure of the heart to maintain sufficient circulation of blood) is a very rapid process. It is imperative to monitor pediatric patients constantly.

After primary assessment and treatment, update the paramedics. For those patients with significant airway problems, respiratory or cardiac arrest, or the possibility of shock, rapid transport is indicated.

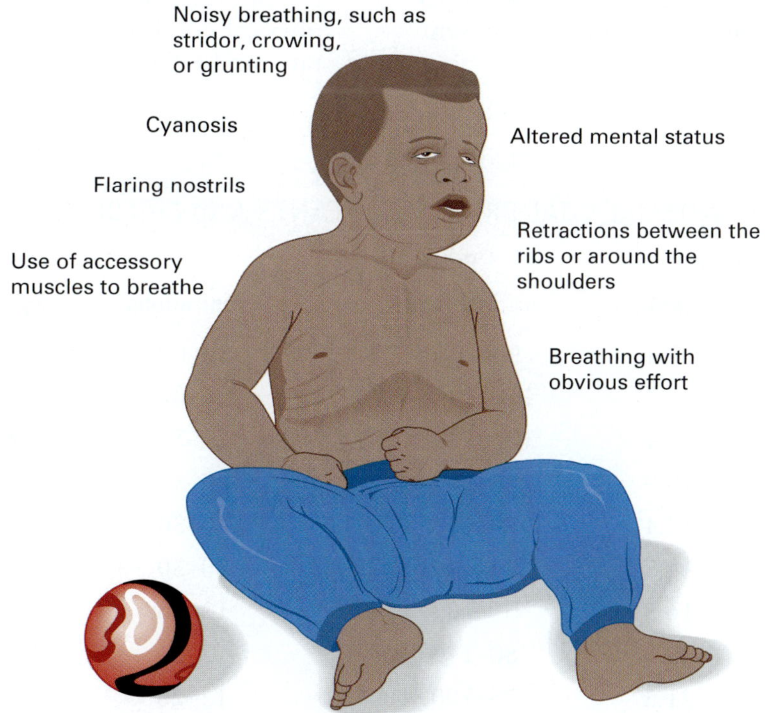

Figure 28–3 Signs of early respiratory problems.

Note: The most important care you can give a pediatric patient is done in the primary assessment. Never stop required airway care to perform a secondary assessment or gather a patient history.

Patient History

If time permits, gather a medical history. Keep in mind that anxious, upset parents and a screaming child can be unnerving. If possible, talk to the child and involve the caregivers. Interview witnesses. Avoid asking questions that require only a yes or no answer. If responses to questions seem inconsistent or if they do not correspond to your primary assessment, try rephrasing the questions.

When you take a SAMPLE history for a medical patient, include questions such as these: When did the signs and symptoms develop? How have they progressed? Is the problem a recurring one? If so, has the child been seen by a physician? If so, is the specific diagnosis known? What treatment was received?

When you take a SAMPLE history for a trauma patient, ask for the details of the accident, such as the time it occurred, mechanism of injury, and emergency care already given.

Secondary Assessment

It is difficult to assess pain in children. They may lack the body awareness and the vocabulary necessary to describe it. Children may not be able to separate the fear they feel from their physical condition. Ask the parents, if possible, how the child usually responds to pain. This may give you some idea of how the present condition compares.

The bodies of infants and children can hide injury for some time. Only after their compensatory abilities fail will you see changes in vital signs. The changes may occur very quickly, and the patient's condition may deteriorate very fast. Take the vital signs of infants and children more frequently than you would in adults. Table 28–2 summarizes normal vital signs for infants and children. Pay attention to your overall impression of how the patient looks and acts. Your observations may tell you more about the status of the child than any one vital sign.

When you do assess a pediatric patient's vital signs, keep the following in mind:

- *Pulse*—Use the brachial pulse in an infant and the radial pulse in a child. If the radial pulse is not clear, check the brachial pulse. If the pulse is too rapid or too slow, immediately examine the patient for problems such as signs of respiratory distress, shock, or head injury.

  Rapid pulse may indicate oxygen deficiency, shock, or fever. It may also be faster than normal in scared or overly excited children. A slow pulse in a child must first be presumed to be a sign of hypoxia (inadequate oxygen in the blood). Other causes of slow pulse may include pressure in the skull, depressant drugs, or a rare medical condition.
- *Respiration*—Children sometimes breathe irregularly. Monitor respirations for a full minute to determine rate. Do it frequently. (You may also need to place your hand on a belly breather's abdomen to get an accurate breathing rate.) Rates in children change easily due to emotional and physical conditions. An increase from a previous rate can be significant.

TABLE 28–2
NORMAL VITAL SIGNS FOR INFANTS AND CHILDREN

Age	Weight (lbs.)	(kg)	Pulse (average)	Respirations	Average Blood Pressure Systolic	Diastolic
1–28 days	7.4	3.4	94–145 (125)	30–60	80	46
3 months	12.5	5.7	110–140 (120)	24–35	89	50
6 months	16.5	7.4	100–140 (120)	24–35	89	55
1 year	22.0	10.0	98–160 (120)	20–30	89	60
2 years	27.0	12.4	90–140 (110)	20–30	96	62
3 years	31.0	14.5	80–120 (100)	20–30	96	64
4 years	33.6	16.5	65–132 (100)	12–26	96	65
5 years	41.0	19.0	80–110 (100)	12–26	96–98	66
6 years	47.0	21.5	75–100 (100)	12–25	96–98	70
10 years	71.0	32.3	70–110 (90)	12–21	110	74

The quality of breathing is also important. Determine if it is adequate. Observe to see if the child is working to breathe and using accessory muscles. Look for retractions. Note if breathing is noisy. Shortness of breath may indicate the need for you to assist ventilations.

- *Blood pressure*—Falling or low blood pressure in a pediatric patient can be a late indicator of shock. Be sure to use a blood pressure cuff that is the correct size for your patient. Use a pediatric stethoscope if available. Do not take a blood pressure reading in children under three years of age.
- *Temperature*—Feel the arms and legs of infants and children to see if they are cold. The torso may be warm in comparison. If your patient is not in a cold environment, cold hands and feet may indicate shock. Taking a rectal temperature and using a glass thermometer are not recommended for field use by EMRs.
- *Skin condition and capillary refill*—Always look at the pediatric patient's skin for signs of injury.
- Note skin colour. Though a newborn may have a mottled colour on the hands and feet, a child should not have a bluish discolouration. Be alert. Be sure to assess capillary refill (Figure 28–4). If it takes more than two seconds, the patient may be in shock. A delayed capillary refill should be considered an emergency in the pediatric patient.

Many children with head or spinal injuries suffer nervous system damage as well. Damage to the nervous system is the cause of traumatic death at least two-thirds of the time. If the patient's history suggests trauma, or if there is a significant mechanism of injury, manually stabilize the infant's or child's head and neck immediately. Remember that children do not have the same verbal skills as adults and their response to stimuli may be different. The parents may be able to describe a normal response. Assess for damage to the nervous system as follows:

- Determine the level of consciousness. If the patient appears to have an altered mental status, ask the parents to describe the normal level.
- Check the pupils. Find out if they are of equal size and, if practical, how they respond to light.
- Examine the head, neck, and spine for signs of injury.
- Check to see if the patient responds to verbal and painful stimuli. Pinch the skin between the thumb and forefinger.
- Check the patient's ability to recognize familiar objects and people.
- Check the patient's ability to move the arms and legs purposefully.
- Check to see if there is clear or bloody fluid draining from the ears.

If you suspect damage to the nervous system, keep your patient as still and calm as possible. Provide in-line stabilization of the patient's head and neck. Apply a cervical collar. Do not allow untrained people to move the patient. If it has not already been done, update the paramedics and continue to assess vital signs.

When you care for an infant or child, be aware of the following special conditions and situations (Table 28–3):

- Monitor an infant's breathing continually. Infants have proportionally larger tongues that can easily block the airway if relaxed.
- Head injuries are more likely in infants and children. When you suspect an injury above the clavicles, or when the mechanism of injury is unknown, provide in-line stabilization. Apply a C-collar.
- Always support the head when you lift an infant. Before the age of nine months, an infant cannot fully support his or her own head.
- During the secondary assessment, check the anterior fontanelle (soft spot) on the top of an infant's skull. If you see a bulge, there may be pressure inside the skull. If you see a depression, the infant may be dehydrated and in shock. (The fontanelle stays open for up to two years after birth.)
- Injuries to the extremities can damage the growth plates, with long-term effects. Carefully assess the extremities, including pulses, capillary refill, and skin condition. Be careful not to cause additional pain. Follow local protocols for splinting.
- Stop the bleeding as quickly as possible. Even though children can compensate for blood loss longer than an adult can, a minor amount of blood loss in an adult would be more significant for a child. Be alert to open fractures, which tend to bleed profusely.

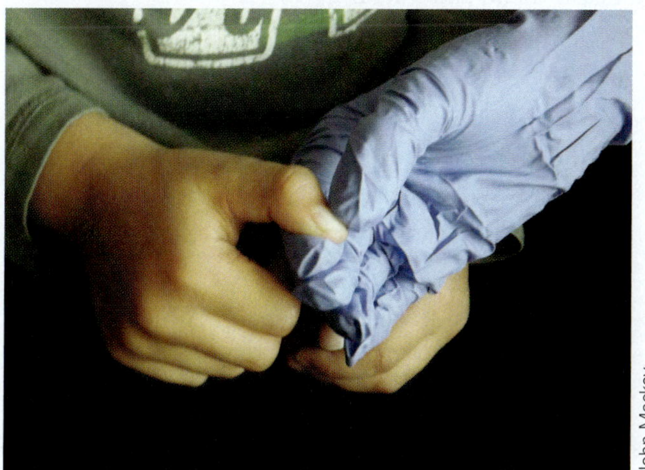

John Mackay

Figure 28–4 Assess capillary refill in infants and children under six years of age.

TABLE 28–3
ANATOMICAL DIFFERENCES BETWEEN INFANTS OR CHILDREN AND ADULTS

Anatomical Differences	Impact on Assessment and Treatment
Larger tongue	Can block airway
Reduced size of airway	Can become easily blocked
Abundant secretions	Can block airway
Baby teeth	Can easily dislodge and block airway
Flat nose and face	Difficult to obtain good airway seal with face mask
Proportionally large head	Must maintain neutral position to keep airway open and in-line stabilization of head and neck Greater potential for heat loss and for head injuries in trauma cases.
Soft spots on head	Bulging soft spots may indicate intracranial pressure; sunken ones may indicate dehydration
Thinner and softer brain tissue	Consider head injury more serious than in adults
Short neck	Difficult to stabilize and immobilize
Shorter and narrower trachea, with more flexible cartilage	Can close off trachea with overextension of the neck
Faster respiratory rate	Muscles fatigue easily, which can lead to respiratory distress
Primarily nose breathers (newborns)	Airway more easily blocked
Abdominal muscles used to breathe	Difficult to evaluate breathing
More flexible ribs	Lungs more easily damaged May be significant injuries without external signs
Heart can sustain faster rate for longer period of time	Can compensate longer before showing signs of shock and usually decompensates more quickly than an adult
More exposed spleen and liver	Significant abdominal injury more likely Abdomen more often a source of hidden injury
Larger body surface	Prone to hypothermia
Softer bones	Can easily bend and fracture
Thinner skin	Consider burns to be more serious than in an adult

- A child's skin surface is large compared to the body mass. This makes children more susceptible to dehydration and hypothermia. Response to burns can also be more severe. Watch for signs of shock.
- Make sure that a cervical collar fits correctly. Note that some children have a very short neck. Such a device may not work on them. Use a rolled towel instead.
- Children often get their arms, legs, hands, feet, or heads trapped under or in rigid structures. The injured child is sometimes in pain and is almost always in a panic. Calm the child first. Then see if he or she can move independently. Lubricate the skin surface with baby oil or a water-soluble lubricant. Make sure it is not applied near the patient's mouth, nose, or eyes. If sawing or cutting is needed, make sure the child is protected with a heavy, fire-resistant cover. Someone can keep talking to the child to provide encouragement. After the child is freed, perform a complete patient assessment.

The following are helpful hints for conducting a secondary assessment:

- If possible, assess the child while he or she is on the parent's lap (Figure 28–5).

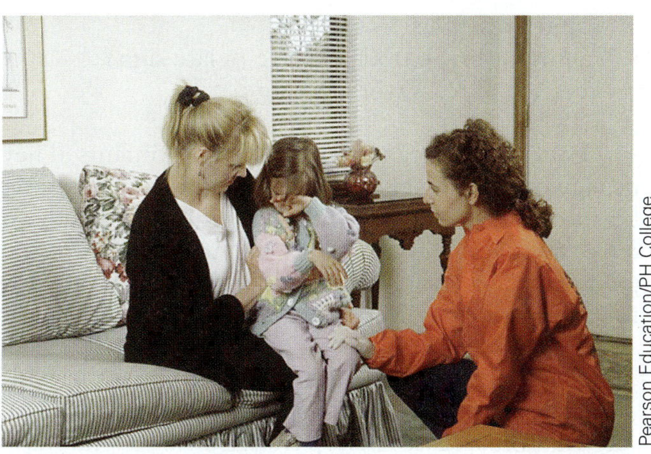

Figure 28–5   Having the child sit on a parent's lap can have a calming influence.

- Prepare yourself so that you can radiate confidence, competence, and friendliness. Remember that children between one and six years of age seldom like strangers.
- Get as close as you can to the child's eye level. Sit next to the child if possible. When it comes time for a hands-on assessment, do it in the least threatening way. Consider starting at the toes and working your way up to the head.
- Explain what you are doing in terms a child can understand. Follow up on the child's questions. Maintain eye contact but do not stare. Speak in a calm, quiet voice. Even infants will respond to a calm voice, and an apparently unconscious child may absorb much of what you say.
- Younger children tend to take any statement literally. For example, if you say you want to take a pulse, they may think you intend to take something away from them. Watch your phrasing. Older children do not like being talked about. Talk with them directly.
- Be gentle. Do everything you can to reduce the amount of pain that a child must endure. However, when there will be pain, be honest.

  "It will hurt when I touch you here, but it will last only a second. If you feel like crying, it's okay." Children can tolerate pain if they are prepared for it and are given adequate support. With children under school age, keep the most painful parts of the assessment for the end. It will help if the child is kept on a parent's lap.

- Do not lie to a child. Always be honest. This does not mean you need to explain everything that is going on, but when you do answer questions or perform a procedure that could be uncomfortable, be candid.
- If a child is not calm enough to be treated, you must restrain the patient. But be sure it is absolutely necessary. Only when care is compromised should the child be separated from a parent.

- A stuffed animal toy may help win the confidence of a young child. It may also help to distract the child during assessment and treatment. Very shy children sometimes talk through a stuffed animal. For example, they may not tell you where they hurt but might tell where the animal hurts, thereby giving you information about themselves.

Ongoing Assessment

The ongoing assessment is the same for infants and children as it is for adults. It never ends as long as you are caring for the patient.

Patient Hand-Off

Just as you would for adult patients, include the following in your infant or child hand-off report:

- Age and sex of the patient
- Chief complaint
- Level of consciousness (AVPU)
- Airway and breathing status
- Circulation status
- Secondary assessment findings
- SAMPLE history
- Treatment, interventions, and the patient's response to them

SECTION 2
COMMON PEDIATRIC EMERGENCIES

Trauma

Injuries are the leading cause of death in infants and children. Blunt injury is the most common. Basic life support and trauma management in infants and children are similar to those provided to adults. Remember to treat as you go; that is, as you assess the patient's ABCs, take care of any problem you find. Remember that children may take longer to go into shock, but when they do, it usually develops more rapidly than in adults.

Always suspect trauma when infants and children are passengers in an MVA. Suspect unrestrained passengers of having head and neck injuries. Suspect blunt trauma to the abdomen if the child was wearing a lap belt but not a shoulder belt. Fully restrained passengers often have abdominal and lower spinal injuries. The car seats in which infants ride are often fastened improperly, so suspect head and neck injuries in these patients.

It may be beneficial, for both you and the transporting crew, to immobilize a child right in the car seat. This is done by applying a cervical immobilization device to the patient and placing padding between the child and the seat to prevent movement. This procedure should not be used if the child has serious injuries or the potential for serious injuries since the car seat may prohibit airway maintenance and other important emergency medical care.

If a child is immobilized in a car seat, never tip the seat back. The position may impair breathing by putting pressure on the child's diaphragm. Always make sure that the seat remains upright.

If a child riding a bicycle has been struck by a car, suspect head, spinal, and abdominal injuries. If the child was walking when struck, suspect head, abdominal, and pelvic or femur injuries.

Shock

A major cause of shock in children is dehydration due to vomiting and diarrhea related to infection. Another cause is blood loss due to trauma.

Children tend to compensate for shock more efficiently than adults. When they decompensate, it is a rapid process that can be devastating. Blood pressure may drop so far and so fast that the patient may go into cardiac arrest. You must, therefore, constantly monitor the injured patient for signs and symptoms of shock. Continually monitor the vital signs, including capillary refill.

The signs and symptoms of shock in the pediatric patient include the following (Figure 28–6):

- Altered mental status, from anxiety to unconsciousness
- Apathy or lack of vitality (This may present as the inability of the child to identify a parent—an ominous sign.)
- Delayed capillary refill
- Rapid or weak and thready pulse
- Pale, cool, clammy skin
- Rapid breathing
- Falling or low blood pressure (a late sign)
- Absence of tears when crying

Hypothermia can intensify shock in infants. They usually cannot shiver to warm themselves. Therefore, be sure to keep them warm. Remember especially to cover an infant's head. While you are waiting for the paramedics to arrive on the scene, follow these steps for emergency medical care of an infant in shock:

1. Have the patient lie flat. Make sure that the position does not interfere with breathing.
2. Be prepared to assist ventilations. Provide oxygen as appropriate.
3. Keep the patient warm and as calm as possible.
4. Monitor vital signs continuously.

Remember that a relatively small blood loss in a pediatric patient can be very dangerous. For example, a newborn usually has less blood than the contents of a soda can. When there is significant visible blood loss, or suspected internal bleeding, constant monitoring and rapid transport are essential.

Respiratory Emergencies

There is nothing more important than controlling the airway and ensuring adequate breathing in a pediatric patient. The equation "no airway = no patient" is as true with children as it is with adults. The American Heart Association reports that more than 90 percent of pediatric deaths from foreign body airway obstruction occur in children under five years of age. Of those, 65 percent are infants. It is estimated that most could be saved by early detection.

Note that there are some differences in the way you manage a child's airway due to their different anatomy (Figure 28–7). They are as follows:

- Children are more susceptible than adults to respiratory problems. They have smaller air passages

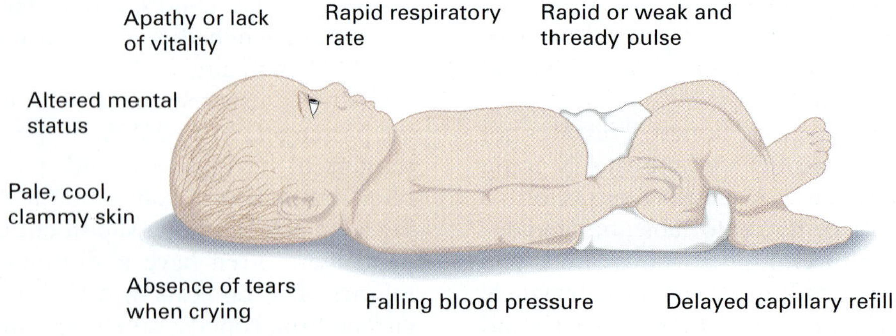

Figure 28–6 Signs of shock in an infant or child.

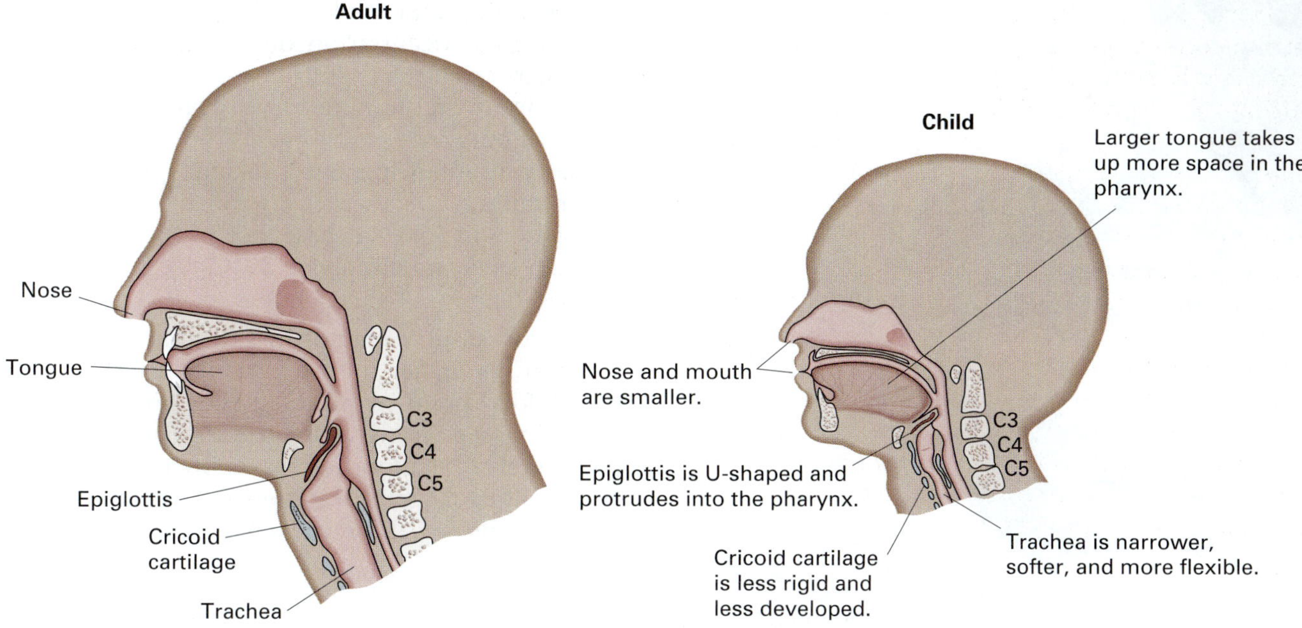

Figure 28–7 Comparison of the airways of an adult and an infant or child.

and less reserve air capacity. A child's airway can be compromised by minor trauma or infection. Be especially attentive to ensuring a clear and open airway.

- A child's airway structure is not as long or as large as an adult's. A child's airway can close off if the neck is flexed or extended too far. The best position is a neutral or a slightly extended position. If the child is flat on his or her back, place a thin pad or towel under the shoulders to keep the head and neck properly aligned. Monitor signs of breathing.
- Because of immature accessory muscles, children use their diaphragms to breathe. If there are no reasons to prevent you from doing so, place a child in a position of comfort. That is usually a sitting position.
- Children have a large tongue that can block the airway. Make sure the tongue lies forward. If the jaw-thrust manoeuvre is used, make sure your hand stays on the bony part of the chin (Figure 28–8). Positioning your fingers too low can cause the tongue to be pushed back to block the airway.
- Infants and children tend to breathe mostly through their noses. They also have abundant secretions. Be prepared to suction often to make sure the nose stays clear (Figure 28–9).
- Apply oxygen by way of a mask. Humidified oxygen is preferred, but never withhold or delay oxygen in order to have it humidified. If a child will not tolerate a mask, hold it slightly away from his or her face.

- If an infant or child is having a respiratory emergency, notify the incoming paramedic unit and be sure an advanced life support (ALS) team is en route if available.
- Even if the signs and symptoms of a respiratory emergency subside, it is still important for the child to be transported to a hospital and inspected by a doctor.

For emergency care of infants and children with respiratory emergencies, see Chapter 7. For more information about respiratory problems in all patients, see Chapter 13.

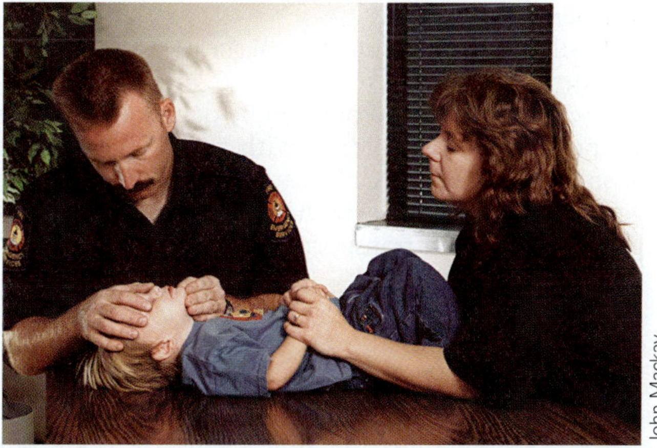

Figure 28–8 Airway obstruction may be relieved in an infant or child by keeping the head in a neutral or slightly extended position.

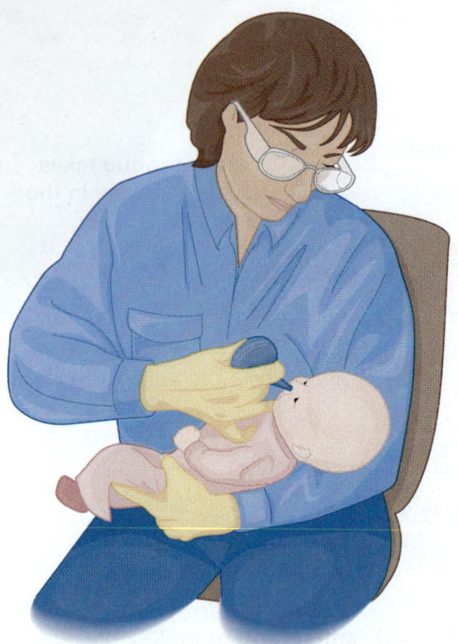

Figure 28–9 Use a bulb syringe for suctioning.

Croup

Croup is a common viral infection of the upper airway. It is most common in children between the ages of one and five years. With croup, swelling progressively narrows the airway. As the child breathes, he or she may produce strange whooping sounds or high-pitched squeaking. There may be hoarseness. The child's cough is typically described as a seal's bark. Episodes of croup occur more commonly at night.

As the child gets worse, he or she may experience the following signs of respiratory distress:

- Breathing with effort, including nasal flaring and retractions
- Rapid breathing
- Rising pulse
- Paleness or cyanosis
- Restlessness or altered mental status

Severe attacks of croup can be dangerous. About 10 percent of all children with croup need to be hospitalized. Treat a child with croup the same way you would treat one with any respiratory emergency. Arrange for transport to the nearest hospital as quickly as possible.

Epiglottitis

Epiglottitis is caused by a bacterial infection that inflames the epiglottis. It often resembles croup but is more serious. Left untreated, epiglottitis can be life threatening. The signs and symptoms may include the following:

- Occasional noise while inhaling
- Anxious concentration on breathing (The child may try to stay very still.)
- Sitting up and leaning forward, usually with chin thrust outward
- Pain on swallowing and speaking
- Drooling
- Changes in voice quality
- High fever (usually above 39°C)

If you suspect epiglottitis, do not ask the child to open his or her mouth. Do not try to examine the child's throat or place anything in the mouth. Touching the larynx can cause the airway to close completely. In all other ways, treat the child as you would for any respiratory emergency. Arrange for transport to the nearest hospital as quickly as possible.

Asthma

Asthma is common among children, especially those with allergies. However, it should always be considered a serious medical emergency. Parents are usually aware of the child's history and can recognize an asthma attack. Determine if the child is on medication.

An acute asthma attack occurs when the bronchioles go into spasm and constrict. This causes the bronchial membranes to swell and become congested with mucus, which interferes with the ability to exhale. As a result, air gets trapped in the lungs, the chest gets inflated, breathing becomes impaired, and oxygen deficiency occurs.

Especially critical signs and symptoms include the following:

- Rapid, irregular breathing, especially in younger children
- Exhaustion
- Sleepiness and changes in level of consciousness
- Cyanosis
- Rapid pulse and dropping blood pressure
- Signs of dehydration
- Wheezing (high-pitched breathing sounds)
- Quiet or silent chest (In the late stages of respiratory distress, respirations may become so shallow that they no longer make any noise. Do not be fooled into believing that the child has gotten better. The condition has, in fact, worsened.)

Emergency care is the same as for any respiratory emergency. Be sure to monitor the airway and breathing constantly. Arrange for transport to the nearest hospital as quickly as possible.

Cardiac Arrest

Most cardiac arrests in infants and children result from airway obstruction and respiratory arrest. It is therefore extremely important to ensure an open airway and adequate breathing in your pediatric patients.

The signs and symptoms of circulatory failure in the pediatric patient are as follows:

- Increased or decreased heart rate
- Unequal central (femoral) and distal pulse rates
- Poor skin colour and delayed capillary refill
- Altered mental status

In cases of cardiac arrest in infants and children, perform five cycles of CPR before phoning for help, unless there is someone available to make the call for you. In cases of drowning, cold water drowning, and hypothermia, an extensive resuscitation effort may be needed. Children have remarkable recuperative capacity. The sooner ALS is initiated, the better the outcome will be. CPR techniques vary for infants, children, and adults. See Chapter 8 for details of emergency care.

Seizures

Febrile seizures are those caused by high fever. They are the most common type of seizure in children. Seizures in children may be caused by infection, poisoning, trauma, decreased levels of oxygen, epilepsy, hypoglycemia, inflammation of the brain, or meningitis. They may also have unknown causes. All seizures, including febrile seizures, should be considered potentially life threatening.

During most seizures, a child's body may exhibit any of the following:

- Arms and legs become rigid.
- The back arches.
- Muscles may twitch or jerk in spasm.
- Eyes roll up and become fixed, with dilated pupils.
- Breathing is often irregular or ineffective.
- The bladder and bowels lose control.

The child may be completely unconscious. If the seizure lasts long enough, the child will show signs of cyanosis. The spasms will prevent the child from swallowing. He or she will push the saliva out of the mouth, which will appear to be frothing. If the saliva is trapped in the throat, the child will make bubbling or gurgling sounds. This may mean that the airway needs suctioning when the seizure has ended. After the seizure, the child often appears extremely sleepy.

To obtain a patient history, ask the parents the following questions:

- Has the child had seizures before? How often? Is this the child's normal seizure pattern? Have the seizures always been associated with fever, or do they occur when the child is well? Did others in the family have seizures when they were children?
- How many seizures has the child had in the last 24 hours? What was done for them?
- Has the child had a head injury, a stiff neck, or a recent headache? Does he or she have diabetes?
- Is the child taking seizure medication? Could the child have ingested any other medicines?
- What did the seizure look like? Did it start in one part of the body and progress? Did the eyes move in different directions?

The emergency care of childhood seizures includes the following:

1. During the seizure, the tongue may relax and shift backwards, decreasing the size of the air passage. To prevent this, as well as to encourage draining of mucus and frothing saliva, place the patient in the recovery position. Do so only if there is no possibility of spinal injury. Do not put anything in the patient's mouth.
2. Do not restrain the child during the seizure. Place the child where he or she cannot fall or strike something. An open space on the floor, with furniture and other objects moved away, is fine. If the child is on a bed that does not have sides, it may be necessary to move the child to prevent a fall.
3. Loosen any clothing that is tight and restricting, especially around the neck or face.
4. After the seizure, make sure that the airway is open. Be prepared to suction.
5. Administer high-concentration oxygen. Hold the mask slightly away from the patient's face until the seizure is completely over. If breathing is diminished or absent and the airway is clear, assist ventilations with a BVM device or a pocket face mask with an oxygen enrichment attachment. Follow local protocols.
6. Assess for injuries that may have occurred during the seizure.

If the seizure lasts longer than a few minutes, and recurs without a recovery period, then the seizure may be status epilepticus. This condition is a true medical emergency. Notify the incoming paramedic unit immediately. (See Chapter 14 for more information on seizures.)

Sudden Infant Death Syndrome (SIDS)

Sudden infant death syndrome (SIDS) is defined as the sudden death of infants in the first year of life. It used to be more commonly known as crib death or cot death.

SIDS cannot be predicted or prevented. In fact, it is still not completely understood. It almost always occurs while the infant is sleeping. The infant is typically healthy, born prematurely, and between the ages of four weeks and seven months when he or she suddenly dies. No illness has been present, though there may have been recent cold symptoms. There is usually no indication of a struggle.

Managing the SIDS Call

Always initiate the emergency medical care immediately when you discover an unconscious patient. Unless the infant has rigor mortis (stiffness), immediately initiate basic life support, even if other signs make the effort appear futile. Begin CPR and have someone update the EMS crew en route.

The extreme emotional condition of the parents makes them victims as well. They will be in agony from emotional distress, remorse, and feelings of guilt. Avoid any comments that might suggest blame. Help them feel that everything possible is being done, but do not offer false hope. Follow local protocols.

When you can, obtain a brief medical history of the infant. This should not delay life-support efforts. If necessary, have other medical personnel find out the following: When was the child put in the crib? What was the last time the parents looked in on the baby? What were the circumstances concerning the discovery of the infant's condition? What was the position of the baby in the crib? What was the physical appearance of the infant and the crib? What else was in the crib? What was the appearance of the room and home? Are there medicines present, even if it is for the adults? What is the behaviour of the people present? What has been the general health of the infant? Have there been any recent illnesses? Does the infant take medication or have any allergies?

After the ambulance personnel take over, encourage the parents to accompany their baby. Offer to stay with their other children until other caregivers arrive. Support the parents in any way possible.

Note that it is very common for EMRs to experience such emotions as anxiety, guilt, or anger after a SIDS call. Ignoring these feelings will not cause them to go away. They may even have a serious negative impact on your mental health. After a SIDS case, a critical incident debriefing session is very helpful. Talk out your feelings with colleagues and family members. Do not hold them inside.

Child Abuse and Neglect

The definition of **abuse** is improper or excessive action so as to injure or cause harm. The term **neglect** refers to giving insufficient attention or respect to someone who has a claim to that attention and respect. Child abuse, or non-accidental trauma, occurs in all parts of our society. The frequency of child abuse or neglect in Canada is increasing, with hundreds of abused children dying every year. Child abuse has been a leading cause of infant and child deaths over the last three decades.

During an emergency call, the adult (usually a parent) who abuses a child often behaves in an evasive manner. He or she may volunteer little information or give contradictory information about what happened. However, a call for child abuse may be a cry for help. Do not be judgmental. Focus on the child.

Some forms of abuse are difficult to recognize on the scene. For example, broken bones at various stages of healing can be identified only at the hospital. However, you may be able to recognize some forms of physical abuse and neglect (Figure 28–10). The signs and symptoms may include the following:

- Multiple bruises in various stages of healing
- Injury that is not consistent with the mechanism of injury described by the caregivers
- Patterns of injury that suggest abuse, such as cigarette burns, whip marks, or hand prints
- Fresh burns, such as scalding in a glove or dip pattern
- Burns not consistent with the history presented by the caregivers
- Untreated burns

Also suspect possible abuse when there are repeated calls to the same address, when the caregivers seem inappropriately unconcerned or give conflicting stories, and when the child seems afraid to discuss how the injury occurred. If an infant or child presents with unconsciousness or seizures, or signs of severe internal injuries but no external signs, suspect central nervous system injuries or shaken baby syndrome.

The signs and symptoms of neglect include the following:

- Lack of adult supervision
- An appearance of malnourishment
- Unsafe living conditions
- Untreated chronic illness, such as asthma
- Delay in reporting injuries

If you suspect abuse or neglect, first and foremost make sure that the environment is safe for the patient. Provide all necessary emergency care.

CHILD ABUSE AND NEGLECT

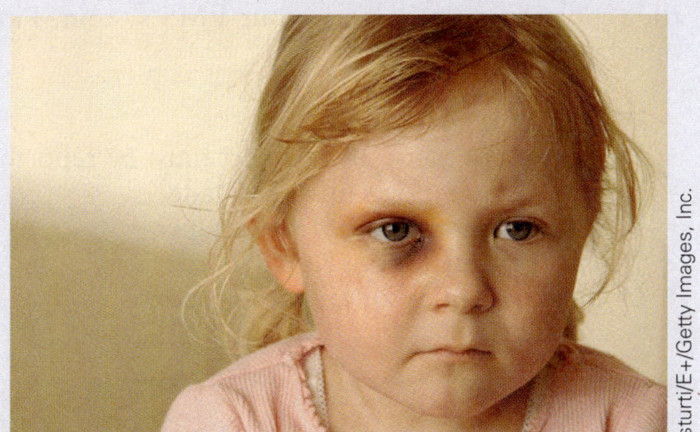

Figure 28–10a Physical child abuse.

sturti/E+/Getty Images, Inc.

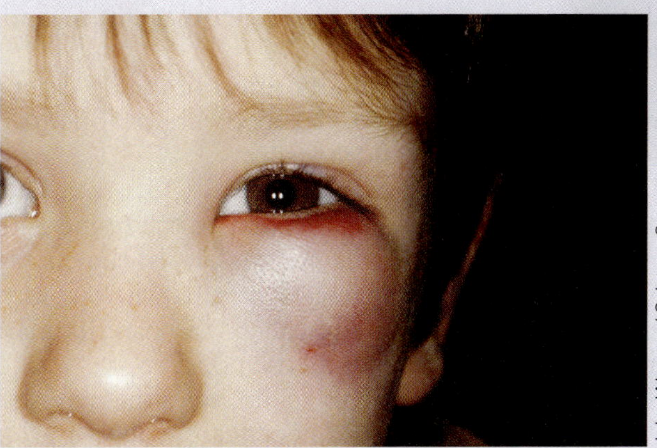

Figure 28–10b Physical child abuse.

John Watney / Science Source

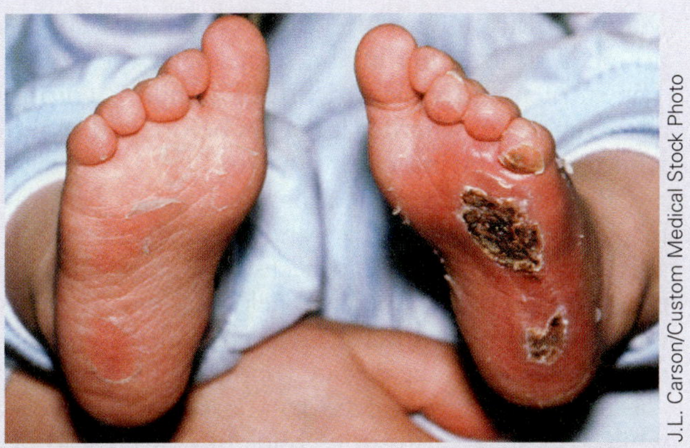

Figure 28–10c Child neglect: lack of appropriate medical care.

J.L. Carson/Custom Medical Stock Photo

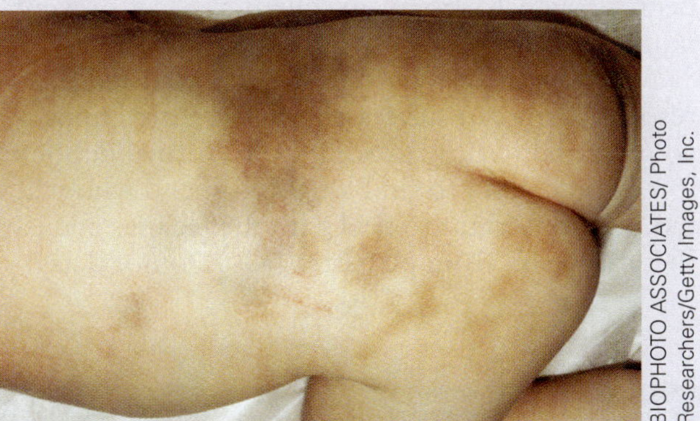

Figure 28–10d Child abuse: death from multiple injuries.

BIOPHOTO ASSOCIATES/ Photo Researchers/Getty Images, Inc.

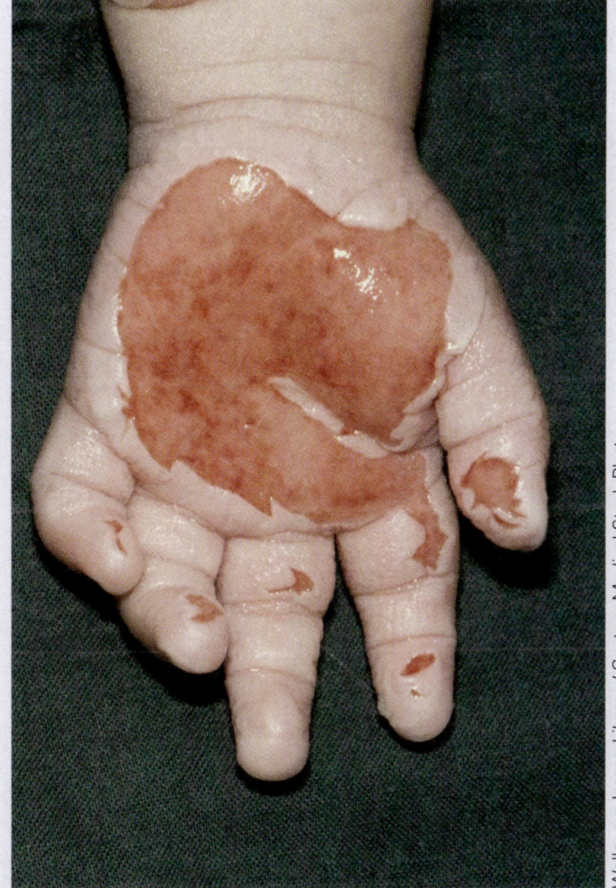

Figure 28–10e Physical abuse: burns from hand being held on an electric stove burner.

Wellcome Image Library / Custom Medical Stock Photo

As time permits, observe the child and the caregivers. Look for objects that might have been used to hurt the child. Look for signs of neglect in the general appearance of the child. Sometimes abuse and neglect are well hidden.

If you find yourself in a position of giving emergency care to a possible victim of child abuse or neglect, follow these guidelines:

- If it can be done safely, gain entry to the home and access to the child. If the parents placed the emergency call, you will probably get in without any difficulty. If someone else called, the parents may resist. You may need to call the police.
- If you are asked to help the child, calm the parents. Tell them that if the child needs care, you will provide it. Tell them that that is the only reason you are there. Speak in a low, firm voice.
- Focus attention on the child while you administer emergency care. Speak softly. Use the child's first name. Do not ask the child to recreate the situation while the parents are present.
- Do a full patient assessment. Treat as you go. Note any suspicious abrasions, bruises, lacerations, and evidence of internal injury. Also look for signs of head injury. Remember that you are there to provide emergency care, not to determine child abuse.
- Update the paramedics in the same way you would for any other child in need of care and transport.
- You are not expected to deal with child abuse issues on the spot unless the child is in danger. In all suspected cases, the child should be transported from the scene.
- Never confront the parents with a charge of child abuse. Being supportive and non-judgmental with the parents will help them be more receptive to others providing emergency care.
- Accusations can delay transport. Instead, report objective information to the transporting unit's crew. Report only what you see and what you hear. Do not comment on what you think.
- Maintain total confidentiality regarding the incident. Do not discuss it with your family or friends.

You must always report your suspicions of child abuse to the proper authorities. It is critical for you to learn the reporting laws in your own province and the reporting protocols for your EMS system. Find out the following:

- Who must report the abuse
- What types of abuse and neglect must be reported
- To whom the reports must be made
- What information an EMR must give
- What immunity an EMR is granted
- Criminal penalties for failing to report

SECTION 3
TAKING CARE OF YOURSELF

Many children who die from accidents are pronounced dead either at the scene or at the hospital. The sudden and violent death of a child is emotionally wrenching, whether it occurs before you arrive or while you are giving care.

Recognize your reactions. Feelings of fear, rage, helplessness, anxiety, sorrow, and grief are common. It is also common for rescuers to feel shame and guilt, even if they did everything possible to help the child. These feelings are particularly intense if the child dies. Remember, some children will die despite your best efforts.

As an EMR, you need to control your emotions while you are treating the child. In this way, you can render the best assistance possible. After the case is over, however, you need to deal with your feelings. Talk them out. Use any critical incident stress debriefing (CISD) team that you have access to. CISD has been proven to be an excellent way to prevent or minimize long-term problems.

Not finding a way to talk about your feelings and resolve them can have a serious negative impact on your mental health. In addition to formal debriefing, it may be helpful to find a trusted friend who will listen. It is important to deal with the feelings and issues that can result from pediatric calls. Do not delay!

EMR FOCUS

Some points to remember about the assessment and emergency care of pediatric patients follow. One EMS rescuer calls them words for the wise:

- Maintaining a good airway and ensuring quality breathing are the two most important concerns for an EMR when dealing with a pediatric emergency.

- When assisting ventilations, be sure to watch for chest rise. This is a good indicator of whether or not your breaths are effective.
- If you do not have an airway, you will not have a patient.
- With pediatric patients, all roads lead to the ABCs.

- Children tend to compensate longer before going into shock. Be alert! They decompensate rapidly.
- Children are prone to hypothermia. Keep them warm.
- When performing a patient assessment, take what you can when you can get it. For example, if a child holds out a hand, it is a good time to check the pulse or capillary refill.

- When the age of a child is unknown, use your best judgment based on the size of the child.
- In cases of abuse or neglect, EMS personnel may be the only advocates a child has.
- When you treat a traumatized child, you are treating a family.
- The interests of the infant or child must always be placed as the foremost consideration when making any and all patient care decisions.

CASE STUDY FOLLOW-UP

At the beginning of this chapter, you read that EMRs were on the scene with an unconscious six-year-old patient who had been hit by a car. To see how the chapter skills apply to this emergency, read the following. It describes how the call was completed.

PRIMARY ASSESSMENT *(Continued)*

We found the patient unconscious with snoring respirations. My partner and I knew what we had to do in one word: airway. We got into position, applied manual stabilization, and turned her for better airway assessment and control. While my partner held her head and neck in line, I applied a cervical collar. A jaw-thrust manoeuvre stopped the snoring. Further examination of the mouth showed that two baby teeth had been knocked out and there was blood in the mouth. Suction took care of it. Breathing appeared to be adequate. I applied oxygen by way of a pediatric non-rebreather at 10 L/min.

Just then, dispatch informed us that the ambulance would be on the scene in about four to five minutes. We reported our general impression of the patient. "A six-year-old female was struck by a vehicle. The airway is open, and she is breathing on her own. The patient is conscious to pain only." We advised that the ambulance should continue to respond with lights and sirens—code 4.

SECONDARY ASSESSMENT

We covered the patient with a blanket to maintain body heat and decided to proceed with a head-to-toe exam. Our findings included swelling with discolouration on the left forehead above the eye. Pupils were reactive but sluggish. The lower left arm was observed to be deformed and swollen. We found her respirations were 12 and shallow, which was slower than our last assessment, so we assisted ventilations.

PATIENT HISTORY

The father reported that the child was in good health and had no allergies.

ONGOING ASSESSMENT

We continued to assist ventilations until the ambulance crew arrived.

TRANSFER OF CARE

When the paramedics got on the scene, we gave them the hand-off report:

> "This is Tisa Kotto, six years old. She was hit by a car travelling approximately 25 km/h about 20 minutes ago. We log-rolled her onto her back, applied a C-collar, and administered oxygen. She has an injury to the left forehead, two teeth knocked out, and a swollen, deformed left arm. Her vitals are pulse 60, strong, regular; respirations 12 and shallow. We assisted ventilations. There is no medical history of allergies."

A few days later, we went to the trauma centre and asked about this patient. We were told that her head injury had required surgery, but she was doing well and was expected to make a full recovery. One of the doctors asked what had happened and we gave him all the details. He listened intently. When we were done, he said that opening the airway and alerting the paramedics to the slowing respirations may have made the difference in the patient's outcome.

Learn the unique aspects of providing emergency medical care to pediatric patients. One of the most important is that you are not treating just the patient. A calm, professional, reassuring approach can help minimize the impact of the emergency on both the patient and the family.

NOCPs

6.2 b Provide care for pediatric patient **A**

REVIEW QUESTIONS

Page references where answers may be found or supported are provided at the end of each question.

SECTION 1

1. How is scene assessment for an emergency involving an infant or child different from that involving an adult? (p. 418)

2. How is the primary assessment different? (pp. 418–420)

3. How is taking vital signs in an infant or child different from taking them in an adult? (pp. 420–421)

4. What can an infant's fontanelle tell you about his or her physical condition? (p. 421)

5. Why must you be more concerned about a small amount of blood loss in an infant or child than you would be in an adult? (pp. 421, 424)

6. What are some techniques you can use to help make the secondary assessment less threatening to the pediatric patient? (pp. 422–423)

SECTION 2

7. What is the leading cause of death in infants and children? (p. 423)

8. What are the signs and symptoms of shock in the pediatric patient? What is the emergency medical care? (p. 424)

9. What are some of the differences in the way you manage the airway of a pediatric patient? (pp. 424–425)

10. What is croup and in what age group is it most common? (p. 426)

11. What are some of the common causes of seizures in infant and child patients? Which ones are considered life threatening? (p. 427)

12. How would you manage a sudden infant death syndrome (SIDS) call? (p. 428)

13. What are the signs and symptoms of possible child abuse and neglect? (pp. 428–430)

CHAPTER

29

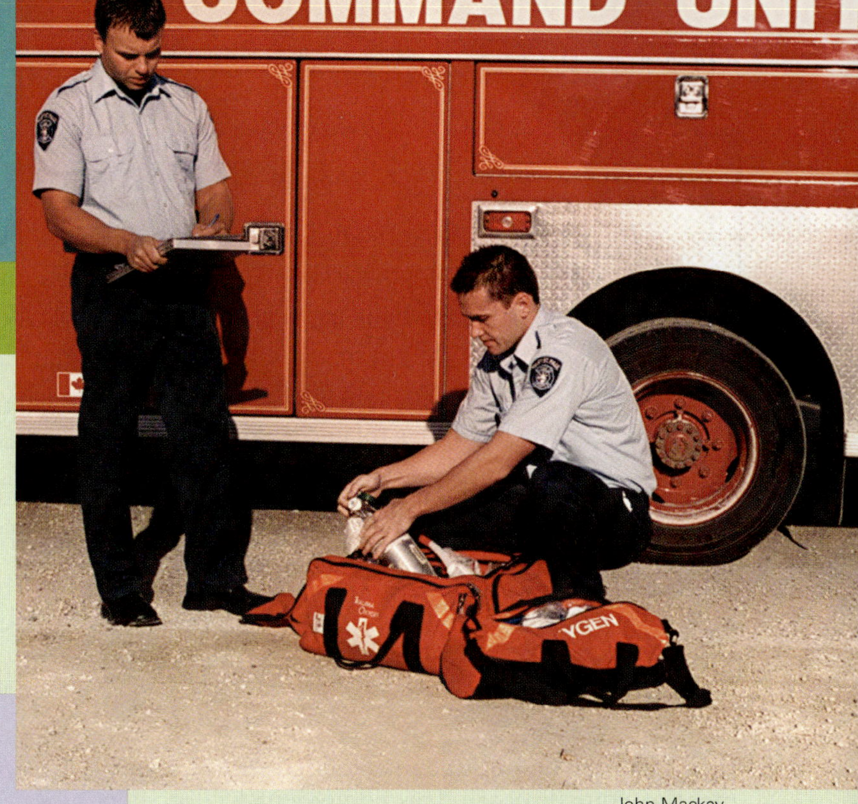
John Mackay

EMS Operations

OBJECTIVES

1. Discuss the medical and non-medical equipment needed to respond to a call.
2. List the phases of an EMS response.
3. Discuss ways of driving an emergency vehicle safely, including how to use seat belts, lights, and sirens properly.
4. Describe how to stay safe in traffic while on foot, including wearing protective equipment, parking and exiting a vehicle, and channelling traffic away from a scene.
5. Discuss safety tips for travelling in the patient compartment of an ambulance, including how to brace oneself, secure a patient, secure equipment, and perform CPR.
6. Explain the rationale for having the unit prepared to respond.

INTRODUCTION

This chapter is meant to provide you with a brief overview of some of the operational aspects of out-of-hospital emergency care. You will learn the six basic phases of an emergency response and become familiar with the medical and non-medical equipment used on the scene.

Even if you are not required to drive an emergency vehicle, become familiar with emergency vehicle safety. Since there may be a situation in which you are asked to travel in an ambulance, this chapter also provides related basic safety precautions.

SECTION 1
RECOMMENDED EMS EQUIPMENT

When you are on duty, you should have EMS equipment at your disposal. This equipment will include the following items (Figure 29–1):

- Equipment for airway and breathing
  - Adjunct airways
  - Suction devices
  - Pocket masks or other artificial ventilation devices
- Equipment for bleeding control and bandaging
  - Dressings of various types and sizes
  - Bandages of various types and sizes
  - Materials to stabilize impaled objects
  - Sterile saline
  - Scissors
  - Adhesive tape
- Equipment for patient assessment
  - Stethoscope
  - Wristwatch
  - Penlight
  - Sphygmomanometer
  - Pre-hospital care report forms
  - Pen and notebook
- Miscellaneous equipment
  - OB (obstetrical) kit
  - Blankets
  - Triage tags
  - Chemical cold and heat packs
  - Personal protective equipment for BSI precautions, such as disposable gloves, masks, eyewear, and gowns
  - Antiseptic liquid or wipes, waterless hand-washing solution, and bags or containers for contaminated materials
  - Turnout gear, heavy-duty and puncture-proof gloves, shatter-resistant eye protection and hearing protection, and other clothing, such as waterproof and reflective clothing, that will protect you from environmental hazards
  - Flares, cones, or reflective triangles for protection against traffic
  - Fire extinguisher
  - Flashlight and spare batteries
  - Local street maps
  - Latest edition of the *Emergency Response Guidebook* for hazardous material incidents
  - Personal flotation device
- Optional equipment (Depending on the equipment utilized and taught in your service, you may be trained to use some or all of the following items.)
  - Oxygen administration equipment
  - Splints
  - Backboards
  - AED (or SAED)
  - Body armour

Even when an EMR is off duty, he or she may come upon the scene of an injury or illness. That is why so many EMRs have their own personal protective equipment in their vehicles and in their homes. Be sure you carry only the equipment you are authorized to use.

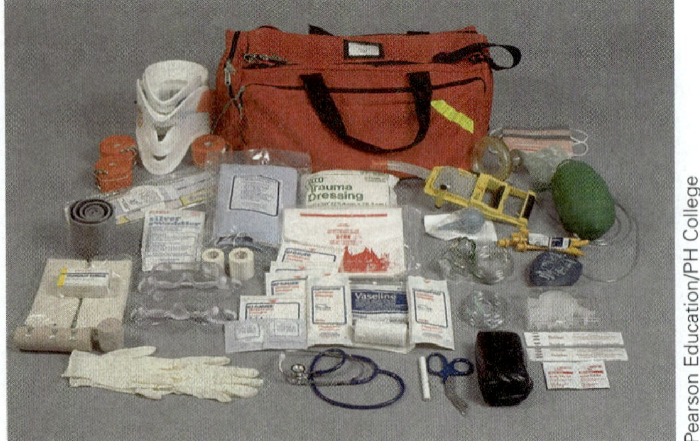

Figure 29–1 A basic EMR jump kit.

Pearson Education/PH College

CASE STUDY

Dispatch

Our EMS unit was dispatched to PTH 401 for an MVA. That stretch of highway had the reputation for some really bad collisions.

Scene Assessment

We knew from experience that most crashes at this location were caused by lack of visibility. There was a light grade that prevented drivers from seeing the road ahead. Cars would go too fast and then couldn't stop for something on the road. This meant that one crash usually turned into five or six.

Consider the scene as you read Chapter 29. What can the EMRs do to keep it safe for themselves, for other rescuers, and for the patient?

Always use extra caution when off duty. You may not have radio contact or all the protective clothing you are used to having. You may also not be wearing clothing that identifies you as an EMS responder. Take extra time to explain to the patient who you are and that you are trained to help.

SECTION 2
PHASES OF A RESPONSE

There are six general phases of an EMS response. They are preparation, dispatch, en route to the scene, arrival on the scene, transfer of care, and post-run activities.

Preparation

It is in the preparation phase of an EMS response that you report for duty and remain available for calls. Obviously, this phase is not the most exciting part of your job, but it may be the most important. That is because it's also the time when you must check and ready your equipment for service. Supplies should be checked each day. They should also be restocked, cleaned, or maintained after each run.

If you drive an EMS vehicle while on duty, inspect it daily (Figure 29–2). Your employer or volunteer organization should have a clear protocol for performing regular service and maintenance, reporting vehicle

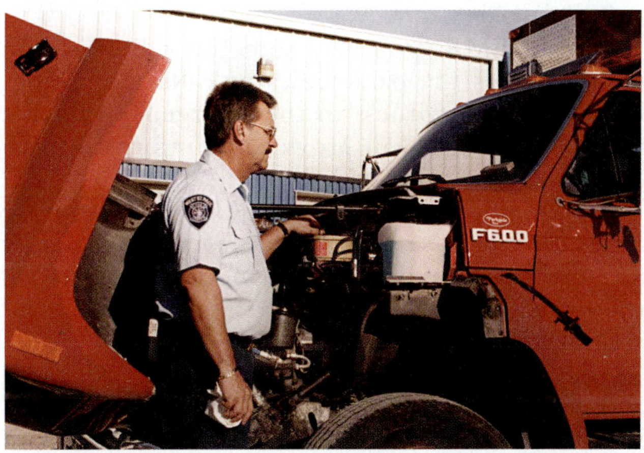

Figure 29–2 Check and ready your EMS vehicle.

problems, and taking vehicles out of service when they are unsafe. Legally, you may be liable for damage caused by a malfunctioning vehicle if you were aware of the problem. You may also be within your rights to refuse to use a vehicle you have reason to believe is unsafe.

Dispatch

Dispatch is the formal beginning of an EMS response (Figure 29–3). Dispatchers get important information from callers who report an emergency. That information includes the following:

- Nature of the call
- Name, exact location, and call-back number of the caller

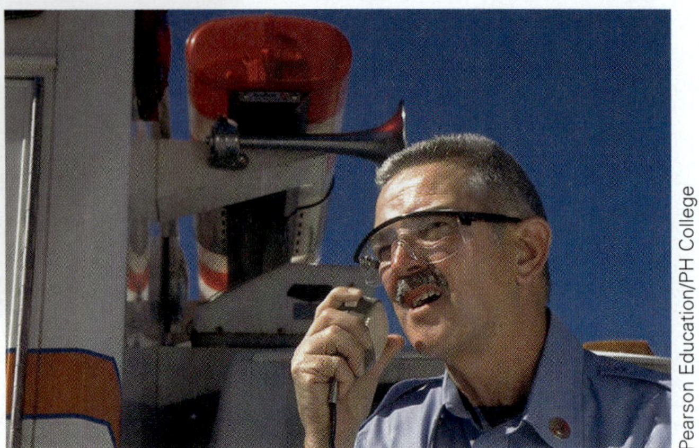

Figure 29–3 Dispatch is the formal beginning of an EMS response.

- Location of the patient
- Number of patients and the severity of the patient's problem
- Any other special problems or considerations that may be pertinent

As an EMR, you may sometimes be the one who activates the paramedics by calling dispatch. Other times, a witness to the emergency will dial 9-1-1. He or she will provide the information to the dispatcher who will, in turn, give it to you. Write the information down so that you can refer to it en route. Use it to prepare yourself physically and mentally for the call. Do not hesitate to ask the dispatcher to repeat or restate information if anything is unclear.

Note that while you are en route to the scene, an emergency medical dispatcher may give specific, life-saving instructions to the caller to perform until you arrive.

En Route to the Scene

Travelling to the scene involves much more than speed. Responses must also be safe. Excessive speed or carelessness will result in a crash, which will prevent you from helping the people who need it.

When responding, be sure to know the exact location of the emergency. Have a route planned for your response. Using a few extra seconds to confirm your route on a map may actually save you more time and embarrassment. Wear your seat belts at all times in moving vehicles. Notify the dispatcher when you have begun your response so that other emergency teams will be aware that you are responding and so that the time may be logged.

Arrival on the Scene

Notify dispatch when you arrive on the scene. Approach cautiously. If you have driven to the scene, park your vehicle in a safe place. Then complete your scene assessment in a rapid, organized, and efficient manner. If it is not safe, leave immediately and call for appropriate backup. Always remember to leave yourself an exit. Once you have determined that the scene is safe to enter, proceed with your patient assessment plan.

You can't help anyone at a scene if you don't get there safely yourself!

Transfer of Care

By the time the responding paramedics arrive on the scene, you may already be performing an ongoing assessment and beginning to package your patient. (The term **package** refers to getting the patient ready to be moved and includes such procedures as stabilizing impaled objects and immobilizing injured limbs.)

Be prepared to give a concise and accurate patient hand-off report. Be ready to assist the paramedics with packaging or lifting and moving the patient if they request your help (Figure 29–4).

Post-Run Activities

Advise dispatch when you are ready to return to your station. Then, after you turn in your pre-hospital care report, prepare for your next call. This means cleaning and disinfecting any equipment that may have

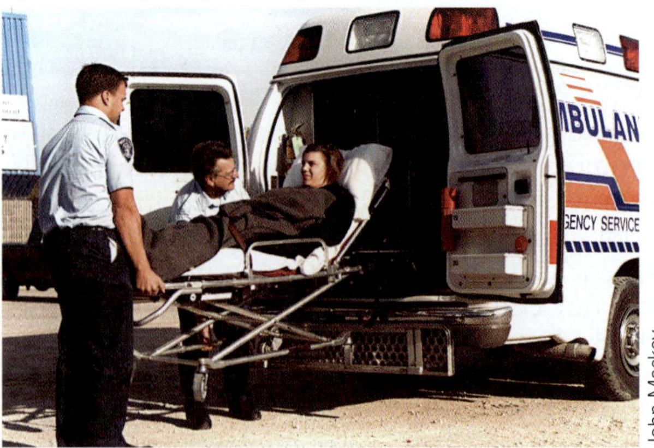

Figure 29–4 After hand-off, be prepared to assist the paramedics if you are asked to do so.

become soiled, as per your local protocols. Replace any disposable supplies. Change any soiled clothing. If necessary, fuel your vehicle. Finally, notify dispatch that you are in service and ready for another call.

SECTION 3
EMERGENCY VEHICLE SAFETY

Many rescuers spend a lot of time in traffic, both while driving and while moving around on foot at emergency scenes. If you have not had a basic safety course, check into the possibility of enrolling in one. It is a good idea to take advantage of refresher courses too.

Driving Safely

Basic Safety Tips

Statistics show that haste is unnecessary in about 95 percent of all emergency runs. Only about 3 to 5 percent of all runs are true life-or-death situations. Yet, 1 in 10 ambulances is involved in a collision every year. Unless the situation is critical, travel at the posted speed limit. Excess speed makes an emergency vehicle less stable and poses a greater risk to you and others.

Safe driving depends on common sense and good judgment. The following basic tips can improve driver safety:

- Learn all local and provincial guidelines related to driving emergency vehicles before you drive one. By law you must always exercise due regard for the safety of others. That includes yourself.
- When you can, travel in pairs. For example, the rescuer who is not driving can help the driver find the route, clear right-hand intersections, watch the road, and, in case of litigation, act as a witness who can substantiate the record.
- If you need to back up your vehicle, do so slowly and carefully. Use all available mirrors and have your window open. Have your partner take a position near the rear of the vehicle and act as a spotter (Figure 29–5).
- Know your territory. Take alternative routes whenever possible to avoid potential problems, such as tunnels, bridges, and railroad crossings. Besides the obvious advantage of arriving on the scene more quickly when you know your territory, you can also avoid collisions caused by trying to read a map while you drive.
- Exercise extra caution when travelling in congested or rush-hour traffic in urban areas or in areas around industrial centres at shift change.

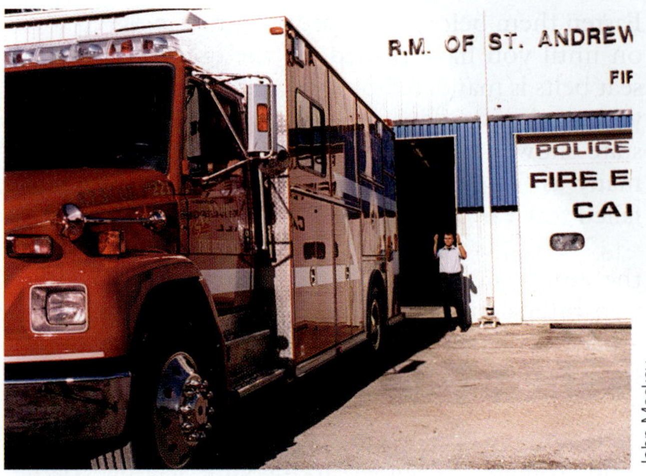

Figure 29–5   When backing up, have your partner act as a spotter.

- Sudden braking is especially dangerous at high speeds. Remember that stopping time increases dramatically as speed increases. Plan for sudden stops.
- If the nature of the emergency requires you to drive at increased speeds, exercise particular caution on curves and hills. Brake to a safe and comfortable speed before you enter a curve. Then stay on the outside of the curve (Figure 29–6). As you leave the curve, speed up carefully, gradually, and steadily. When travelling downhill, use a lower gear instead of the brakes to maintain control of the vehicle.

Seat Belts

When in an emergency vehicle, always wear proper safety restraints, including lap and shoulder belts.

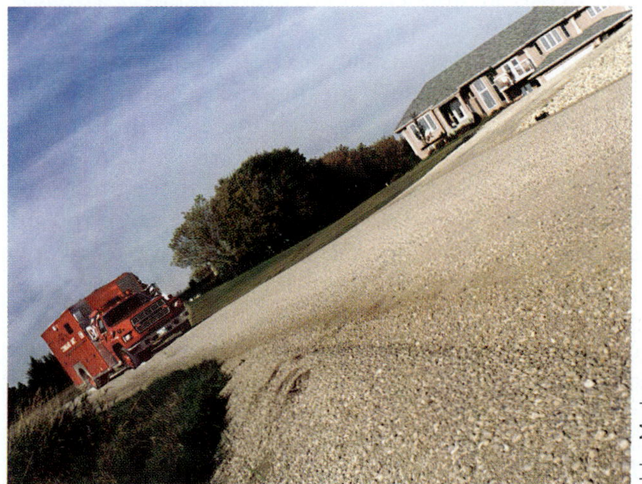

Figure 29–6   Use extra caution when driving on curves and hills.

Fasten them before you start the ignition. Keep them on until you have turned off the ignition. Wearing seat belts is mandated by law in all provinces. A three-year study of ambulance collisions in one American state showed a shocking rate of non-compliance. As many as 50 percent of those driving an ambulance failed to wear their seat belts.

Never take off safety restraints as you approach the emergency scene. Research shows that the last two intersections before arriving on the scene are especially dangerous for rescue drivers who try to save time by disengaging restraints. Generally, unless you are responding to an emergency or attending to a patient in the back, yours is just another vehicle on the road. You are also subject to the same seat belt laws.

Lights and Sirens

Whenever you respond to an emergency in a vehicle, be it during the day or night, use headlights and emergency lighting. Headlights can help alert other drivers in case emergency lights blend in with traffic lights, the tail lights of cars travelling in opposite directions, the colour of buildings, or holiday decorations. Use minimal lighting in heavy fog. Turn off the headlights when you park. If you need to alert oncoming traffic while parked, leave the emergency lights on.

Always use emergency lights and sirens as required by your local protocols. Note, however, that a siren can have a bizarre effect on the driver of an emergency vehicle. Some drivers are easily hypnotized by a siren and lose the ability to negotiate curves and turns. A siren can also disorient or cause panic in other drivers. (Never pull up behind another driver and blast the siren.) Finally, a siren may not be effective because it is often not heard. Insulation in newer vehicles can mask the sound of an approaching siren, as can a loud radio, conversation, pelting rain, thunder, dense shrubbery, trees, and buildings. To clear traffic quickly, use your vehicle's horn in conjunction with emergency lights and siren.

A significant safety advantage is to turn off your lights and siren as you approach the scene of an injury or illness. Lights and sirens attract crowds and can add to the chaos that may already exist. If there are hostile people on the scene, you can take the first step toward calming and controlling the scene by arriving discreetly.

Remember that once you turn off your lights and siren, you are no longer driving an authorized or right-of-way emergency vehicle. You are subject to all the laws meant to govern regular traffic.

Hearing Protection

Chronic exposure to loud noises poses a danger to hearing. The trauma associated with repeated loud noise can cause permanent hearing loss. If your EMS system allows EMRs to drive or ride in emergency vehicles, take the following precautions to protect your hearing:

- Keep the windows closed while the siren is in use.
- Wear ear plugs or ear muffs to protect your ears. Be aware that these devices may prevent you from hearing other emergency vehicles as they approach. Use caution and always follow local protocols.
- If you can, move the siren speakers from the top of the cab to the front grille. This move can reduce the decibel level by about 5 percent.

Avoid prolonged or repeated loud noise off the job, too. Protect yourself against loud music, high-volume radios and televisions, loud chainsaws, lawn mowers, hydraulic tools, generators, and other loud noises.

Driving an Ambulance

As soon as a patient is loaded into an ambulance, the driver is responsible for at least three lives: his or her own, the partner's, and the patient's. In many cases, there may be multiple patients, family members, other helpers, or student riders. Most ambulances accommodate as many as six.

If your EMS system allows EMRs to drive ambulances, follow these guidelines to help ensure a safe trip:

- Except in the most critical situations, do not exceed the posted speed limit. Excessive speed is unsafe for everyone in the ambulance, especially for the patient. Speed poses special hazards at intersections and on curves.
- Start and stop smoothly. Make the transition from one speed to another gradually to avoid aggravating the patient's illness or injury and to avoid disrupting patient care in the back.
- Drive at a steady but safe speed. If you keep your speed even, you can often time your approach to intersections and travel through with the green light. Also, avoid weaving through traffic. It can compromise the patient.
- Whenever you can, avoid rough dirt roads, potholes, and other hazards that can jostle the patient. The inner two lanes of a four-lane highway are the smoothest. The lane closest to the gutter on city streets is the roughest. If you see that you are going to drive over a bump, railroad tracks, or a stretch of rough road, warn those in the back so that they can protect themselves.

As part of a driver training program, many drivers are required to lie on the stretcher while the instructor drives the ambulance. Even at low to moderate speeds, the experience from the point of view of the patient is often enlightening. (Do not use the lights, sirens, or drive at increased speeds for training purposes unless you are at an approved training facility.)

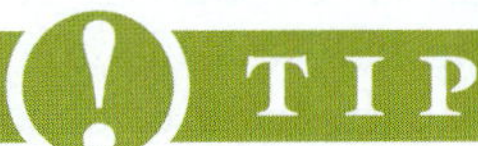

> **TIP**
>
> If you can drive your unit for about 10 minutes with a 1 L carton of milk standing in your cab without overturning it, you will not only serve your passengers well, you may also avoid a lot of spills!

Staying Safe in Traffic on Foot

As soon as you get out of your vehicle at the scene, you are at risk from oncoming traffic. Even while your focus is on the patient or the scene itself, you must never compromise your own safety.

Park for Maximum Safety

Turn off your headlights as soon as you park to prevent blinding oncoming drivers. If necessary, leave the parking lights on or leave the ambulance warning lights flashing to alert oncoming traffic.

Whenever you can, park on the shoulder of the road or in a driveway, in front of or behind the crash scene. Never park alongside a crash. If you are on a one- or two-lane road with no accessible parking areas, position your vehicle so that it blocks the entire roadway. This should prevent other vehicles from squeezing by. When the police are at the scene, follow their directions for vehicle placement.

An important part of ensuring your safety is to visually scan the scene as you approach. Note areas of vulnerability or potential danger. Pinpoint places where you could seek concealment or protection. If you are with a partner, plan how you will approach the scene before doing so. You may decide that your partner will go to the passenger who is still in the green car, for example, and you will go to the driver who is lying on the gravel.

Protect yourself from environmental hazards at the scene by parking at a safe distance. Park at least 50 m away from a burning vehicle and at least 600 m from an accident involving hazardous materials. Whenever possible, park uphill and upwind of any hazardous material or fire. Avoid parking on or driving over spilled liquids and broken glass.

Exiting a Vehicle Safely

A specific transition takes place as soon as you leave your vehicle. You move from your sanctuary to someone

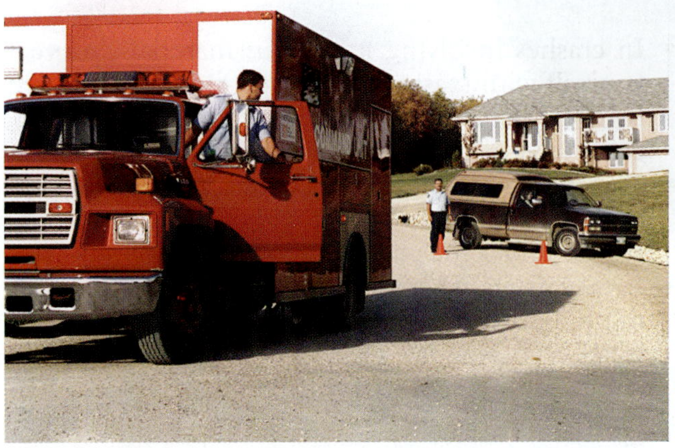

Figure 29–7 Slowly and cautiously open the door when exiting your vehicle.

else's turf, and that makes you vulnerable. Follow these tips for the greatest protection:

- Before you open the door, check the rear-view mirror to determine how much traffic is approaching from behind. If you can, wait a minute or two until traffic passes.
- Open your door slowly to alert passing motorists that you are getting out (Figure 29–7). Move carefully but quickly away from passing or oncoming traffic.
- If you have passengers in the rear compartment, have them get out through the rear doors instead of a side door, which might open into passing traffic.
- Be especially cautious about hazards at the scene, such as broken glass, twisted metal, or spilled gasoline. In any crash involving trucks, immediately assess for hazardous materials.
- If the scene is safe to enter, walk purposefully to the patient. Running is a signal to others that you are out of control, and it causes your heart to race. The unwelcome boost to your pulse and adrenaline level can hinder your ability to effectively treat the patient.

Wear Protective Equipment

Plenty of rescues take place outdoors in the dark and in bad weather. An essential for every rescuer is reflective clothing. That includes reflective tape, a reflective vest, or other gear if you have access to it. If you are channelling traffic away from the crash scene while waiting for the police, it is essential that you wear as much reflective gear as possible. It will help you be visible to drivers who may have pitted windshields, frayed windshield wipers, or drug or alcohol impairment.

Depending on the situation, consider the following protective gear:

- In crashes involving hazardous materials, protect yourself with masks, gowns, and gloves as dictated by local protocols. In accidents involving grain, cement, or similar materials, wear a dust respirator.
- If there is any risk of falling debris, wear an impact-resistant protective helmet with reflective tape and a strap under the chin.
- In situations where splashing may occur (including splashing of blood and other body fluids), wear safety goggles specified for work with power equipment. If you usually wear eyeglasses, get clip-on side shields.
- To protect yourself against the cold, wear gloves, a warm hat, long underwear, and several layers of medium-weight clothing.
- Depending on the rescue situation, you may need rubber or waterproof boots and slip-resistant waterproof gloves.

Channelling Traffic Away from the Scene

While waiting for the arrival of law enforcement, you need to channel traffic away from the scene. This is not only for the safety of the patients and bystanders but also for your own safety and that of the other rescuers. Your goals should be as follows:

- To channel the regular flow of traffic around the scene, preventing additional collisions and injuries
- To monitor traffic so that there is minimum disruption
- To clear the scene so that other emergency vehicles can reach the patients quickly

Unless there is a distinct hazard that dictates otherwise, keep traffic moving even if the roadway is blocked. Rather than bringing traffic to a standstill, try to reroute traffic to an alternative road. To effectively channel traffic, you need additional rescue personnel and attention-getting devices such as flares, chemical lights, or reflective cones. Follow these general guidelines:

- Make sure all those who are channelling traffic are wearing adequate reflective clothing or tape so that they can be seen clearly by approaching drivers.
- Visual signals given by rescuers must be clear. The approaching drivers need to understand quickly and exactly what you want them to do.
- Place flares, chemical lights, or reflective cones 3 to 5 m apart for approximately 30 m toward the oncoming traffic.

If the collision is on a two-lane highway, the flares or cones should be placed in both directions. On a curve or hill, place them at the beginning of the curve or at the crest of the hill. They should direct other motorists around the crash scene, at least 15 m from the wrecked vehicles. Use this general rule: The flares or cones should begin far enough from the scene so that a car can safely stop before it hits the scene, even if the driver did not notice the flares or cones from a distance.

Many EMS systems recommend the use of reflective cones instead of flares because of possible burns while lighting or using flares, the need to keep lighting new flares as old ones extinguish, the difficulty of keeping flares working in bad weather, and the possibility of toxins from the smoke. Follow local protocols.

The Patient Compartment

If you are part of an ambulance team, or if you assist other EMS providers, you face tremendous hazards every time you climb into the patient compartment.

It is normal and necessary to move around in the compartment as you treat the patient. However, too few rescuers remember to ensure their own safety. Using appropriate restraints and learning to position yourself properly can help prevent injury en route to the hospital.

Whenever you do not need to move around in the patient compartment, wear proper restraints, such as a safety harness.

Hanging On and Bracing

The principle of hanging on is one borrowed from rock climbers. You have four possible points of contact with the ambulance: two hands and two feet. At any one time, you must maintain at least a three-point contact for optimum safety and stability. In other words, you should never have more than one hand or one foot at a time off a stable surface in the patient compartment. Keep in mind that you do have a fifth possible point of contact—the seat of your pants. Follow these tips:

- To maintain the greatest stability, keep a wide base of support. Keep your feet about shoulder width apart. Do not place your hands too close together.
- If you need to reach for something, keep both feet planted firmly on the floor. Grasp a stable object, such as the overhead bar, with your free hand.
- If you need to walk—even a single step—hold on to a stable object with both hands. Slide your hands along as you walk instead of moving arm over arm. If you need to move equipment, try putting it down and sliding it.
- Even when you are sitting, hook your feet under the stretcher bar to give yourself increased stability.

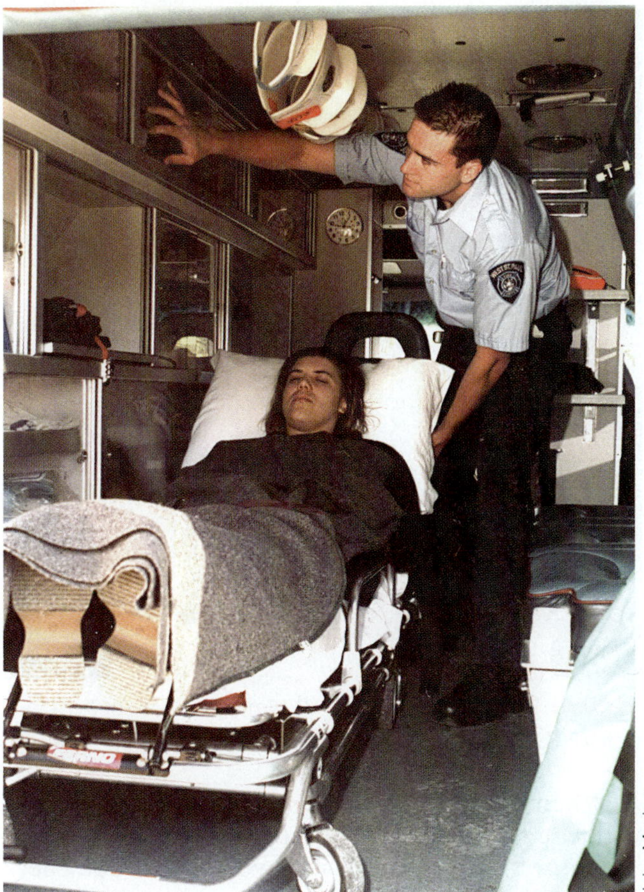

John Mackay

Figure 29–8 Hanging on and bracing help you achieve optimum safety and stability inside the patient compartment.

Bracing means to exert an opposing force against two parts of the ambulance with your body (Figure 29–8). It provides additional stability and protection. You can use your hands, feet, knees, or any combination of hip, shoulder, knees, and hands. You can brace yourself against any solid surface in the patient compartment, such as the squad bench or an interior wall. For greatest stability and safety, keep your centre of gravity low. For women, the centre of gravity is the hips. For men, it is the shoulders.

Securing the Patient

There are two reasons to secure the patient firmly in the compartment. First, you want to protect any patient from the risk of additional injury. Second, if the patient is hostile, you need to protect yourself and the patient from potential injury.

In the case of non-hostile patients, follow these guidelines:

- Secure anyone sitting on the squad bench with a seat belt.

- Place a pregnant woman in the jump seat since the lateral force from sudden stops is much less pronounced there than on the squad bench. Make sure she is wearing a seat belt.
- If the patient is on a stretcher, use snug but comfortable straps across the lower chest (but not over the arms) and just above the knees. Then secure the stretcher to the bar. If local protocol allows it, use additional straps. If the patient's medical condition allows, elevate the head of the stretcher slightly to ease the patient's anxiety during sudden stops.
- When transporting an infant or child, make use of his or her own car seat if you do not carry one in your unit.

In the case of hostile patients, follow these guidelines:

- Never apply restraints maliciously. Laws vary from one province to another about how and when restraints can be used. The use of restraints should always be a last-resort measure to protect your safety. If you do use restraints, document in your written report why you felt they were necessary.
- Once you restrain a patient, never remove the restraints, even if the patient calms down. The patient should stay restrained until you arrive at the hospital.
- Whenever possible, use soft restraints. A quick and easy one is made by folding a gauze bandage in half, slipping it over your hand, and turning it over on itself. You can then loop this over the patient's wrists and ankles. Secure the ends in a bow-tie knot far enough from the patient's hands that they cannot be untied. Combine regular strapping over the chest and knees with soft restraints at the ankles and wrists.
- If an extremely violent patient can break gauze bandages or leather straps, place him or her face down on a stretcher. Make sure to remove any pillows. If you are permitted, consider putting a scoop stretcher over the patient. Then, buckle the stretcher belts securely over the scoop. Be sure to tie the patient's arms down. This method allows for natural drainage and gives EMS personnel access for intravenous lines or blood pressure cuffs. Monitor the patient's ABCs with extreme care since he or she is at high risk of respiratory compromise. This method of restraint is the least advisable because of the potential detriment to the patient. Always try to have police accompany you if you must transport an extremely violent patient.

Securing Equipment

If an ambulance is involved in a crash—especially a rollover—any unsecured piece of equipment can become a projectile that could injure you and the patient. As part of the cleanup at the end of each ambulance run, secure all equipment (Figure 29–9). Stow equipment in appropriate storage areas and secure doors shut with latches. Clamp masks, oxygen equipment, and other heavy items to appropriate brackets. Use straps to secure portable gear. Devise hooks to keep bench tops closed.

Performing CPR in a Moving Ambulance

While you are performing CPR in an ambulance, you are in a risky position. You cannot maintain three-point contact. You cannot brace yourself adequately, and you cannot secure yourself in a seat belt. To improve your safety while performing CPR in a moving ambulance, follow these guidelines:

- Position your feet shoulder width apart for the best possible base.
- If you can, have someone secured by a seat belt sit on the squad bench and grasp the back of your belt. If the ambulance suddenly changes direction or accelerates, the person hanging onto you can keep you from catapulting.
- Try for as much bracing as you can. Bend your knees into the side of the stretcher, wedge your feet against the squad bench, or brace one knee against the stretcher and the other against the squad bench.

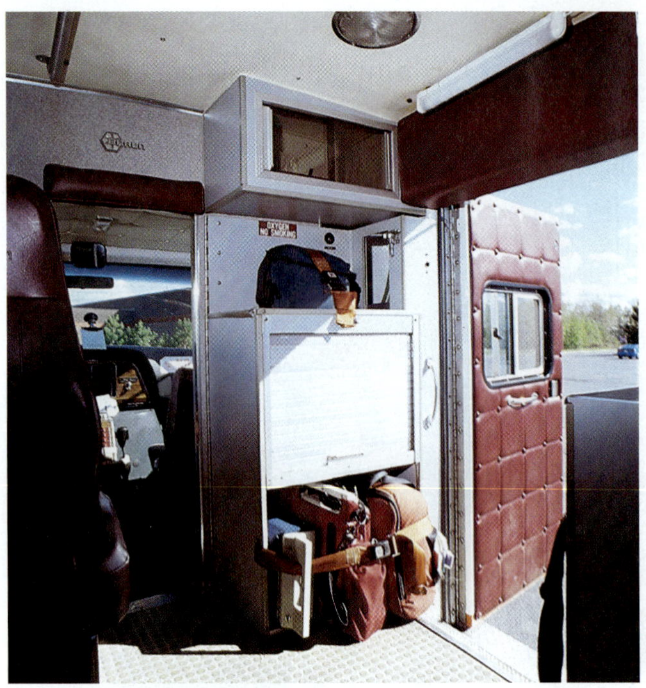

Figure 29–9 Make sure all equipment is secure before the emergency vehicle is in motion.

- When changing compressors, do so safely and advise the driver of your intent.
- Do not brace yourself with your head. Your neck will not withstand the pressure.

EMR FOCUS

The EMS adage "You can't help anyone if you don't get there" best describes the theme of this chapter. The time spent with a patient is perhaps the most notable and interesting part of being an EMR. However, without a safe response, adequate protection from danger, and fully stocked and prepared equipment, there would be no patient care at all. Never ignore the basic tasks that make it possible for you to perform your job as an EMR.

CASE STUDY FOLLOW-UP

At the beginning of this chapter, you read that EMRs had responded to the scene of an MVA. To see how the chapter skills apply to this emergency, read the following. It describes how the call was completed.

we continued to assess the scene for other hazards, put on our gloves, and approached the crash vehicles. We saw a driver in each of the two vehicles present. There were no passengers.

SCENE ASSESSMENT (Continued)

Since we arrived before the RCMP, we set up a pattern of flares and reflectors over 300 m in front of the crash scene to protect ourselves. We placed the EMR vehicle at the top of the grade so that it served as protection and extra warning. When we felt it to be safe, we exited our vehicle, watching our backs for traffic. Then

PRIMARY ASSESSMENT

Neither of the drivers wanted EMS, but we stuck around anyway until the paramedics arrived. Sometimes people realize they have been injured once they calm down. There wasn't much damage to the cars. It was a minor sideswipe. The mechanism of injury certainly didn't seem severe.

SECONDARY ASSESSMENT

We led the drivers over to the guard rail and out of traffic. They allowed us to check their vital signs, and we examined them for possible injuries. Neither had any complaints. The assessments turned up nothing.

PATIENT HISTORY

The drivers refused to answer any questions.

ONGOING ASSESSMENT

We observed the drivers until the paramedics arrived on the scene.

TRANSFER OF CARE

When the ambulance arrived, we told the crew what we had: vital signs and a rough description of the incident. Neither of the patients wanted to be transported. Both patients refused all emergency care.

Bill Cerby, the first RCMP officer on the scene, complimented us on the use of our reflectors and flares and the positioning of our vehicle. No one had to tell us about the possible danger. We'd all had too many calls to that location.

Most basic training programs for rescuers teach how to react safely to a variety of dangers. However, the most common threat to safety is likely to be something as simple as oncoming traffic or the way an emergency vehicle is driven. Be prepared. Have the knowledge, equipment, and skills that allow you to meet the standards set by your EMS system for each phase of an emergency response.

NOCPs

3.3 g Clean and disinfect equipment **S**
   h Clean and disinfect work environment **A**

7.1 a Conduct vehicle maintenance and safety check **S**
   b Recognize conditions requiring removal of vehicle from service **A**
   c Utilize all vehicle equipment and vehicle devices within ambulance **A**

7.2 a Utilize defensive driving techniques **A**
   b Utilize safe emergency driving techniques **A**
   c Drive in a manner that ensures patient comfort and a safe environment for all passengers **A**

REVIEW QUESTIONS

Page references where answers may be found or supported are provided at the end of each question.

SECTION 1

1. What non-medical equipment should all EMRs have on hand? (p. 434)

2. What medical equipment should all EMRs have on hand? (p. 434)

SECTION 2

3. What are the six basic phases of an EMS response? (p. 435)

4. When should you check, restock, clean, and maintain your supplies? (p. 435)

5. What information can you expect dispatch to give you when you are called to an emergency? (pp. 435–436)

6. What should you do upon arrival at a scene if it does not appear safe? (p. 436)

SECTION 3

7. Why is it recommended that EMRs travel in pairs? (p. 437)

8. Why should emergency lights be used during a daytime response? (p. 438)

9. What are some reasons why it is a good idea to turn off your lights and siren when you approach an emergency scene? (p. 438)

10. What method of exiting an emergency vehicle would give you the greatest protection? (p. 439)

11. What are the three goals of channelling traffic away from a scene? (p. 440)

12. What are the basic guidelines for setting up flares at the scene of a motor vehicle collision? (p. 440)

13. How many points of contact must you have in order to maintain optimum safety in the back of an ambulance? (p. 440)

30

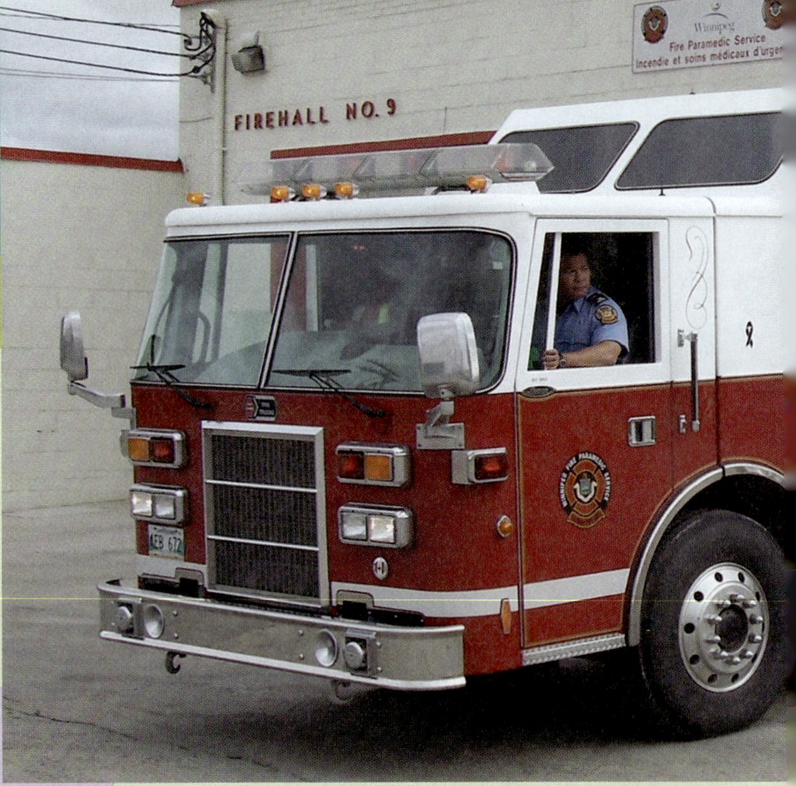

Pearson Education/PH College

Hazardous Material Incidents and Emergencies

OBJECTIVES

1. Define hazardous materials.

2. Identify the resources that may be called upon once a hazardous material incident is recognized.

3. Identify the four levels of training required to respond to a hazardous material emergency.

4. Discuss how to recognize the presence of a hazardous material at the scene of an emergency.

5. Describe what the EMR should do and the actions that need to be taken if there is reason to believe that there is a hazard at the scene, including identifying the hazardous material incident and the specific hazardous materials.

6. State the role the EMR should perform until appropriately trained personnel arrive at the scene of a hazardous material situation.

Note: The terms **hazardous materials** and **dangerous goods** are used synonymously throughout this chapter.

INTRODUCTION

Millions of tonnes of hazardous materials are made in Canada every year.

To manage the risk to the public, our government has developed specific regulations. They address nearly every aspect of the manufacturing, distribution, transportation, and use of such materials. Unfortunately, hazardous materials may still be spilled or released as a result of equipment failure, vehicle collisions, environmental conditions, and human error. The result can be the loss of life and property.

This chapter provides a brief overview of hazardous material emergencies. As an EMR, you are not required to deal with these materials unless you work as a firefighter. That takes specialized training and equipment. Instead, it is your job to recognize and report that a hazardous material emergency exists.

SECTION 1
IDENTIFYING HAZARDOUS MATERIALS

What Is a Hazardous Material?

Hazardous materials (HazMats) are those that in any quantity pose a threat or unreasonable risk to life, health, or property if not properly controlled. HazMats include chemicals, wastes, and other dangerous products. Any chemical, biological, radiological/nuclear, or explosive (CBRNE) incident should be considered a HazMat incident. The principal dangers they present are toxicity, flammability, and reactivity. The HazMats commonly shipped are as follows:

- Explosives
- Compressed and poisonous gases
- Flammable solids and liquids
- Oxidizers
- Corrosives
- Radioactive materials

Hazardous materials are often transported to the user. Although some travel by fixed pipeline (natural gas, for example), most go by rail or highway. That means that HazMats can be the cause of an emergency anywhere.

For example, is there a farm, business, or industry in your community that might have hazardous materials on the premises? Do you have a hospital in your area that has a nuclear medicine facility? Do you have a photo shop in town? If so, what chemicals are used to develop photos? Do you have any lawn and garden companies that stock fertilizers, insecticides, or pesticides? Do your grocery stores refrigerate their food stocks in freezers cooled by ammonia?

Placards and Shipping Papers

Transport Canada requires packages and containers to be marked with specific hazard labels. Placards are required on the outside of vehicles carrying HazMats. The driver of the vehicle must also have shipping papers that identify the exact substance and quantity being shipped, as well as its origin and destination.

A placard is usually a four-sided, diamond-shaped sign. Many are red or orange in colour. A few are white or green. Whatever the colour, the placards contain a number and a legend. They identify the material as flammable, radioactive, explosive, or poisonous.

Shipping papers are sometimes called manifests or waybills. If you can locate them, they are another important means of identifying HazMats. Shipping papers show the name of the substance, the danger it presents, and a four-digit identification number.

Note: Never endanger yourself or allow others to endanger themselves by trying to retrieve shipping papers. The benefit does *not* outweigh the risk.

Additionally, the National Fire Protection Association (NFPA) in the United States uses the NFPA 704 system (Figure 30–1 on p. 447). This system is generally used on fixed structures, such as buildings. Its diamond-shaped symbols identify danger by the use of colour and numbers. Blue indicates a health hazard, red indicates a fire hazard, and yellow, a reactivity hazard. White is used for information such as the need for protective equipment. Numbers used are 0 to 4. For example, 1 in a blue diamond and 4 in a red diamond mean the material presents a low health hazard but is highly flammable.

CASE STUDY

Dispatch

I was working security, patrolling the lower level of the mall, when I received a radio call: "Team A, respond to the lower entrance near the restaurant. Investigate a report of fumes and people with trouble breathing. Time out 22:03."

Scene Assessment

As I approached the scene, I slowed my pace. Ahead I could see dozens of people streaming out of the restaurant. Many were bent over, trying to catch their breath. Mike, the manager of the restaurant, ran over to me. He told me that the cleaning people were working in the kitchen. One of them had mixed bleach, ammonia, and green stuff together, which caused the problem.

Consider this situation as you read Chapter 30. What may be done to ensure scene safety? Are all these people injured? How can they be treated appropriately?

Available Resources

A special resource is the *2012 Emergency Response Guidebook* (Figure 30–2 on p. 447). Carry it in your vehicle at all times. It includes a table of commonly used Transport Canada labels and placards. That table is correlated with lists of chemicals. Each item in the lists is keyed to specific emergency action instructions.

Material safety data sheets (MSDSs) offer another resource. Under federal regulations, all employees working with hazardous materials have a right to know about the dangers of those materials. All manufacturers, therefore, are required to provide an MSDS on hazardous materials. These sheets generally name the substance and its physical properties as well as any fire, explosive, or health hazards. Emergency first aid is also usually listed.

The Canadian Transport Emergency Centre (CANUTEC) staff provide a 24-hour emergency advisory and regulatory service for accidents involving dangerous goods. They advise rescuers of the nature of a product and the steps that need to be taken to manage an incident. They may also contact the shipper, who will provide detailed information and field assistance. Other important resources are the regional poison control centre and your own system's medical control. They can guide you through decontamination and treatment.

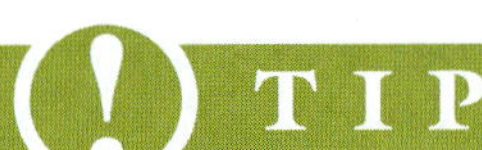

Transport Canada maintains a website that includes information on dangerous goods: www.tc.gc.ca/tdg/menu.htm.

Training Required by Law

People can get hurt or lose their lives at HazMat emergencies. The Occupational Safety and Health Administration (OSHA) in the United States has developed safety regulations. See the OSHA publication "29 CFR 1910.120—Hazardous Waste Operations and Emergency Response Standards (1989)."

Four levels of training are identified:

- *EMR Awareness.* This level of training is for those who are likely to witness or discover a HazMat emergency. They learn how to recognize a problem and how to call for the proper resources. No minimum training hours are required.
- *EMR Operations.* This level of training is for those who initially respond to a HazMat emergency in order to protect people, property, and the environment. They learn how to keep a safe distance

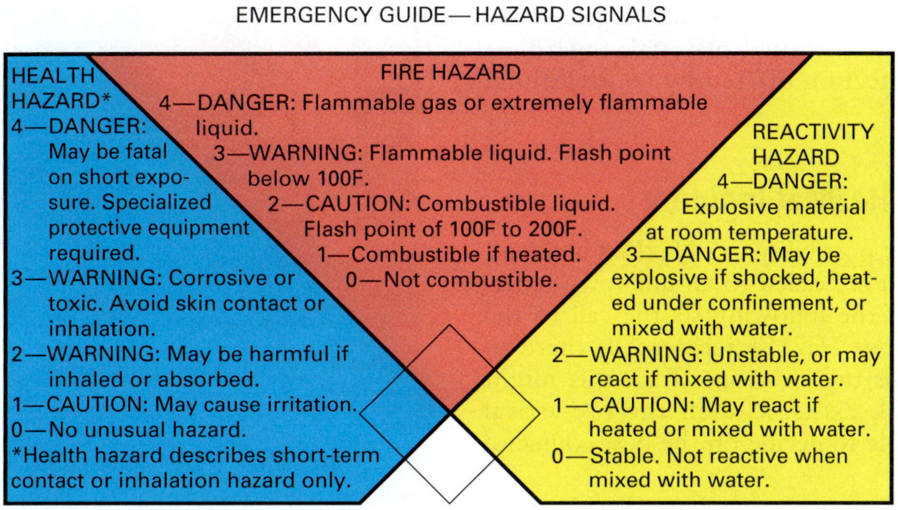

EMERGENCY GUIDE— HAZARD SIGNALS

Figure 30–1 The NFPA 704 system helps you identify health, reactivity, and fire hazards.

Reprinted with permission from NFPA 704-2012, System for the Identification of the Hazards of Materials for Emergency Response, Copyright © 2011, National Fire Protection Association. This reprinted material is not the complete and official position of the NFPA on the referenced subject, which is represented solely by the standard in its entirety. The classification of any particular material within this system is the sole responsibility of the user and not the NFPA. NFPA bears no responsibility for any determinations of any values for any particular material classified or represented using this system.

and how to stop the emergency from spreading. A minimum of eight hours of training is required.

- *Hazardous Materials Technician.* This level is for rescuers who actually plug, patch, or stop the release of a hazardous material. A minimum of 24 hours of training is required.
- *Hazardous Materials Specialist.* This level is for rescuers who want advanced knowledge and skills. They learn to provide command and support activities at the site of a HazMat emergency. A minimum of 24 hours of additional training is required.

Note that the NFPA has published Standard #473, which deals with competencies for EMS personnel at HazMat emergencies.

SECTION 2
GUIDELINES FOR A HAZARDOUS MATERIAL RESPONSE

Many HazMat incidents are dispatched as traffic accidents, poisonings, or unknown problem calls. Your initial actions build the crucial groundwork for the remainder of the incident. Your specific responsibilities include the following:

- Identifying the emergency as a HazMat incident
- Identifying the hazardous materials
- Establishing command and control zones
- Establishing a medical treatment sector

As always, your first priority is your own safety. *Never attempt a hazardous material rescue unless you are properly trained and equipped to do so.* If you have no training, radio immediately for help. While you are waiting, protect yourself and the

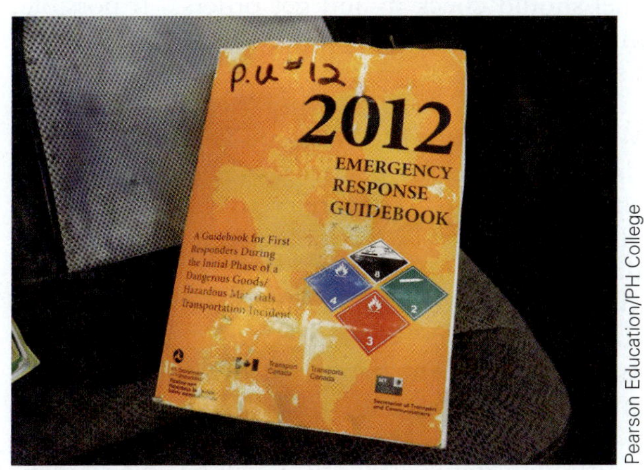

Pearson Education/PH College

Figure 30–2 *2012 Emergency Response Guidebook.*

bystanders by keeping away from the danger. Avoid contact with any unidentified material, regardless of the level of protection offered by your clothing and equipment.

Identifying the HazMat Incident

Always consider the possibility of a HazMat incident. For example, if you are called to an unknown emergency, ask yourself the following: Is the call to the location of a previous HazMat incident? Is there an emergency plan for the location? If so, this might indicate that a risk exists. Use all the pre-arrival information available to decide on the best course of action.

As you approach the scene, use binoculars to begin to assess the scene (Figure 30–3). Identify any placards on vehicles, buildings, or containers (Figure 30–4). Proceed, as always, with caution. Too many EMRs discover a HazMat incident only after they are in the middle of it. Use all your senses, coupled with a high index of suspicion. A number of visual clues can indicate a possible hazardous material:

- Smoking or self-igniting materials
- Extraordinary fire conditions
- Boiling or spattering of materials that have not been heated
- Wavy or unusual vapours over a container of liquid material
- Coloured vapour clouds
- Frost near a container leak (may indicate a liquid coolant)
- Unusual condition of containers (peeling or discoloration of finishes, unexpected deterioration, deformity, or unexpected operation of pressure-relief valves)

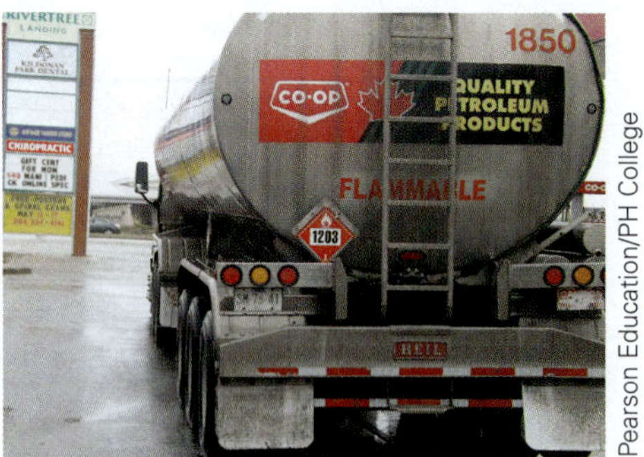

Figure 30–4 HazMat placards displayed on a truck.

Remember that you may not be able to see or smell a hazardous material. Some are odourless and colourless, while others have properties that can deaden your senses. Always assume that the area surrounding a spill or leak is dangerous.

Identifying the Hazardous Material

After you identify an emergency as a HazMat incident, station yourself uphill and upwind of the scene. This vantage point should prevent the vapours from overwhelming you. Once stationed, report your position and the situation to dispatch. Your report should include the following:

- The nature and exact location of the incident
- A description of the incident, including any potential for fire or explosion
- Number of patients involved
- Request for additional help, such as fire, police, EMS, and HazMat support

Also, suggest the best way for other EMS personnel to approach the scene. Include instructions for a staging area (the safe area where all EMS personnel should check in and get orders). If possible, identify the hazardous materials and the severity of the situation.

- What is the material? What are its properties and dangers? Look for placards, NFPA numbers, or shipping papers. Then refer to your *Emergency Response Guidebook* for the name, properties, and dangers of the material.
- What are the sizes, shapes, kinds, and conditions of the containers?
- Is there imminent danger of the contamination spreading?

Although the HazMat team will be able to identify an unknown substance, you will be expected to make an initial identification.

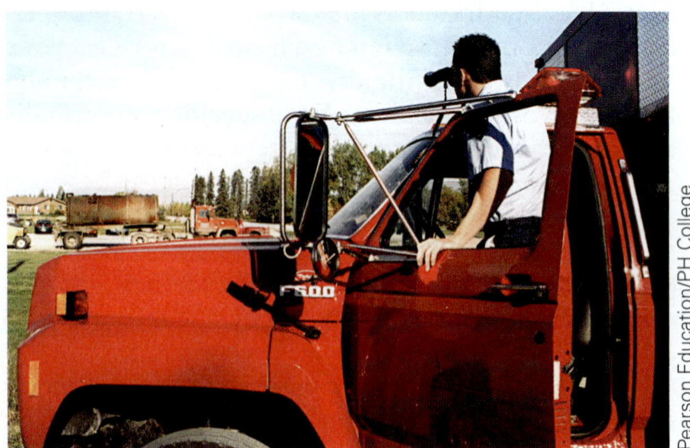

Figure 30–3 Use binoculars to identify HazMats from a distance.

Establishing Command

Your agency should have a plan ready in case of a HazMat incident. Before a HazMat emergency ever develops, all appropriate agencies need to know how the responding personnel will be mobilized to handle it. Generally, the plan addresses the worst possible scenario. That way, the community will be able to handle any emergency that arises. The following should be included in the plan:

- One command officer responsible for all rescue decisions at every stage of the incident (All rescuers should be aware of who the command officer is. If the command officer hands over the decision-making power to someone else, all rescuers must be notified of the change.)
- A clear chain of command from each rescuer to the command officer
- An established system of communications used throughout the emergency (It should be one that all rescuers are informed about, know how to use, and have access to.)
- Receiving facilities (Choose facilities that are capable of handling large numbers of patients, have surgical capability, and, if possible, have established decontamination procedures.)

As the EMR on the scene, activate the plan and establish command. Stay in command until you are relieved by someone higher in the chain of command. The incoming incident command officer will want to know the following:

- Nature of the problem
- Identification of the hazardous materials
- The kind and condition of the containers
- Existing weather conditions
- Whether or not there is any fire
- Time elapsed since the emergency occurred
- What has been done by the people on the scene
- The number of victims
- The danger of more people falling victim

Once the transfer of command has occurred, be prepared to care for decontaminated patients or to support rescue personnel as directed.

Creating Control Zones

To prevent a HazMat incident from becoming worse, the danger area must be identified and isolated. That is usually done by designating three zones (Figure 30–5):

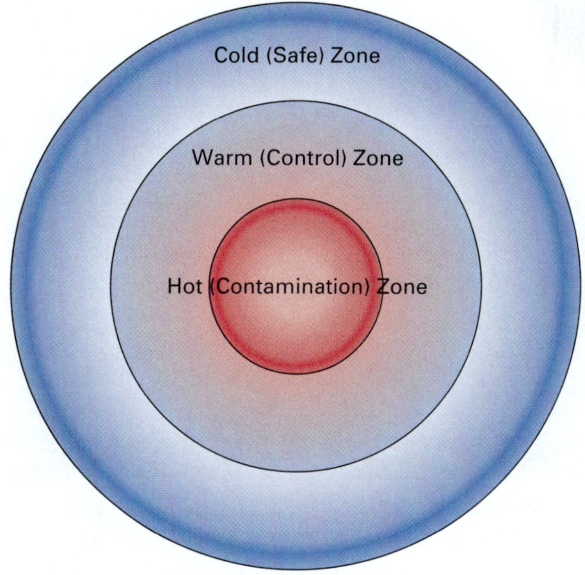

Hot (Contamination) Zone
Contamination actually present
Personnel must wear appropriate protective gear
Number of rescuers limited to those absolutely necessary
Bystanders never allowed

Warm (Control) Zone
Area surrounding the contamination zone
Vital to preventing spread of contamination
Personnel must wear appropriate protective gear
Life-saving emergency care performed

Cold (Safe) Zone
Normal triage, stabilization, and treatment performed
Rescuers must shed contaminated gear before entering the cold zone

Figure 30–5   Establish control zones.

- *Hot zone*—This is the most dangerous area. It can be entered only with the appropriate personal protective equipment. Initial or gross decontamination will be performed here.
- *Warm zone*—This is the area immediately outside the hot zone. The proper protective equipment must be worn here also (Figure 30–6). Once the immediate life threats to the patient are managed, complete decontamination of the patient is performed.
- *Cold zone*—This is the outer perimeter. All contaminated clothing and equipment should be removed before entering it.

Do not enter the warm zone unless you are trained and equipped to do so. Instead, patients should be brought to you for emergency medical treatment in the cold zone. Any people not necessary to the rescue should be kept away from the zoned areas.

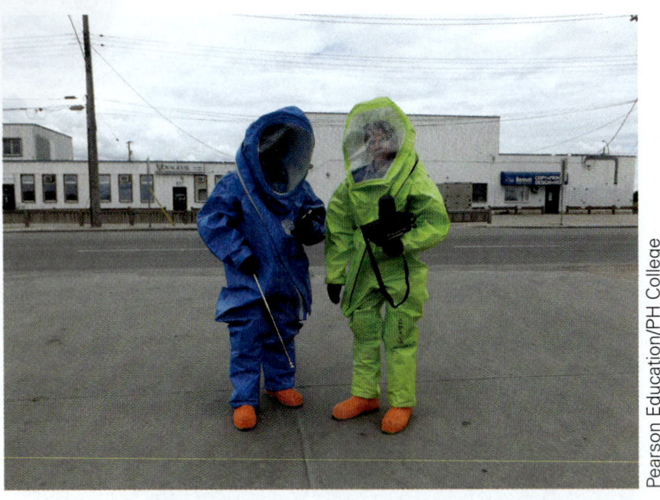

Figure 30–6 Rescuers in HazMat suits

Establishing a Medical Treatment Sector

All EMS personnel and equipment must be set up in the cold zone. The establishment of a definable perimeter cannot be overstressed. In even relatively small incidents, victims may scatter and spread the contamination. The result can be an ever-expanding scene that quickly becomes unmanageable. Anyone exiting the hot zone should be considered contaminated until proven otherwise.

If the hazardous materials can be identified, follow the treatment instructions given in your *Emergency Response Guidebook* or by the regional poison control centre.

EMR FOCUS

Understand that hazardous materials are everywhere. They can be found in more places than in tractor trailers with signs that warn of highly corrosive materials. Remember that even household cleaners can cause as deadly a reaction as most hazardous materials you can find on the highway.

The first step in staying safe from hazardous materials is to realize that you will encounter them sooner or later. Be prepared.

CASE STUDY FOLLOW-UP

At the beginning of this chapter, you read that an EMR was on the scene of a possible HazMat emergency. To see how the chapter skills apply, read the following. It describes how the call was completed.

SCENE ASSESSMENT *(Continued)*

I radioed communications immediately. "Team A, we have a possible hazardous material spill at the restaurant. Please begin the Chemical Incident Plan." Then I went on to report, "I will be incident command. Please have emergency services respond to my location at the lower entrance of the mall. Advise them that we have chemical fumes from a mixture of bleach, ammonia, and a green soap solution." Scanning the area quickly, I added, "We have about 26 people with trouble breathing. Medical assistance is needed immediately."

At this point, I realized I had a large number of people who could scatter, so I asked the other security guards to do several things.

First, we had to get all the injured people to go down the hall until help could arrive. Someone suggested that we ask them to wait outside, but I disagreed. I thought that if we let them outside, they would go to their cars and leave. That was where emergency services were setting up. With people leaving and EMS responding, I was also afraid things would get out of hand.

Second, I asked the other guards to set up a perimeter at least 30 m down the hall. I was amazed at the number of people who insisted that they had to get through to go shopping or get to work. Some even thought we were conducting a drill.

We were just getting things set up when the police arrived. I quickly explained what happened and what had been done. The fire chief joined us and declared a hazardous material incident. He requested the HazMat team. After consulting with poison control, the firefighters proceeded to treat the patients with high-flow oxygen and move them to a triage point where patient assessments could begin.

Several days after the incident, I was commended by my employer for quick thinking and decisive action at the scene of an emergency.

A hazardous material incident challenges the best in EMRs. Besides the usual patient care issues, there is the additional problem of safety. Be sure to learn and follow all your local protocols for such emergencies.

NOCPs

3.3 a Assess scene for safety **S**
 b Address potential occupational hazards **S**
 e Conduct procedures and operations consistent with Workplace Hazardous Materials Information System (WHMIS) and hazardous materials management requirements **A**

8.3 a Recognize indicators of agent exposure **A**
 b Possess knowledge of personal protective equipment (PPE) **A**
 c Perform CBRNE scene size-up **A**
 e Conduct decontamination procedures **A**
 f Provide care to patient involved in CBRNE incident **A**

REVIEW QUESTIONS

Page references where answers may be found or supported are provided at the end of each question.

SECTION 1

1. What is a hazardous material? (p. 445)

2. Explain what placards and shipping papers are. (p. 445)

3. What is the NFPA 704 system? (pp. 445, 448)

4. What are some of the resources available to EMS personnel on the scene of a HazMat incident? (p. 446)

5. What are the four levels of HazMat training described by OSHA? (pp. 446, 448)

SECTION 2

6. What is an EMR's first priority upon arrival at the scene of a HazMat incident? (p. 448)

7. What are some examples of visual clues that indicate a possible hazardous material? (p. 449)

8. After identifying an emergency as a hazardous material incident, what information should your report to EMS dispatch include? (p. 449)

9. When an incoming incident command officer takes over a HazMat scene from an EMR, what information will he or she need to know? (p. 450)

10. What are control zones? Briefly describe them. (p. 450)

11. In which zone should EMS personnel and equipment be set up? (p. 450)

31

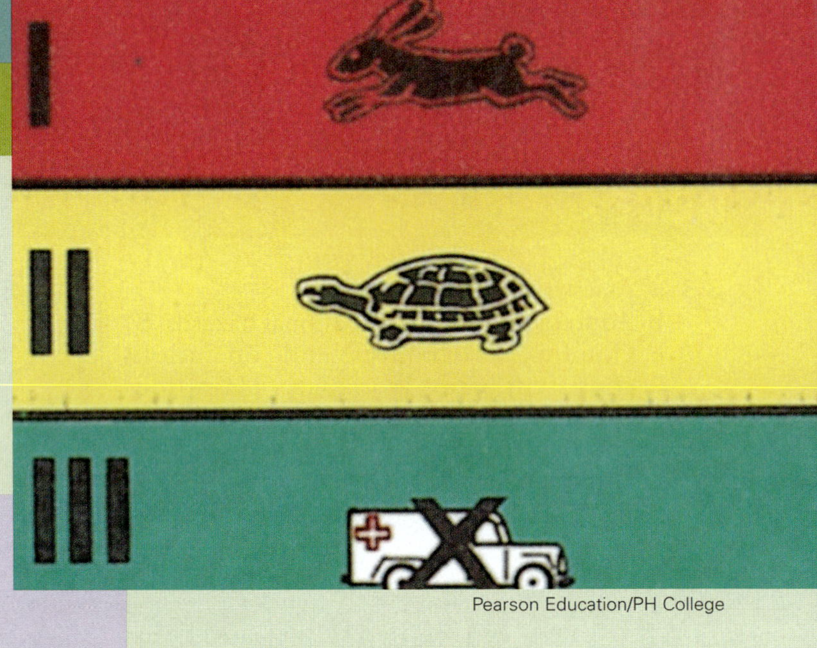

Pearson Education/PH College

Multiple-Casualty Incidents and Incident Command

OBJECTIVES

1. Describe the criteria for a multiple-casualty situation.
2. Describe the Incident Command System (ICS) and the role of command in a multiple-casualty incident.
3. Describe the functions of commonly used EMS sectors.
4. Discuss the role of the EMR in the multiple-casualty situation.
5. Explain the procedure for transferring command.
6. Discuss three-level and two-level triage systems.
7. Summarize how to conduct triage at a multiple-casualty incident, including using the START system.
8. Discuss ways to reduce the psychological impact of disasters on patients and rescuers.

INTRODUCTION

Multiple-casualty incidents range from an MVA to hurricanes, floods, earthquakes, and bombings. This chapter will introduce you to ways in which EMS systems respond to such emergencies. It will also give you an overview of your role as an EMR, including how you can provide the best emergency care to the greatest number of patients.

SECTION 1
INCIDENT COMMAND SYSTEM (ICS)

One of the most challenging situations for an EMR is a **multiple-casualty incident (MCI)**. An MCI is any event where three or more patients are involved. Most communities have a plan in place for handling an MCI. However, for any plan to be effective, it must be flexible enough to work with a three-person MVA (the most common MCI) as well as a large-scale disaster involving 15 or more patients, such as a CBRNE incident.

One widely used plan is the National Incident Management System's (NIMS) Incident Command System (ICS). Originating in California, it was designed to handle large-scale fires that involve multiple agencies. It now gives us a framework for all types of MCIs.

How resources are used is basic to the Incident Command System. Not every MCI will need every community resource. In fact, most MCIs use only limited resources. Sometimes this is referred to as the toolbox approach. Think of a community's resources as a toolbox. Instead of emptying it at every MCI, only the tools that are needed are used. This means that instead of calling for the police, fire service, EMS, HazMat teams, and all other rescuers just in case they may be needed, only the resources that are necessary are called for.

As an EMR, find out what your EMS system requires you to do in those first crucial minutes of an MCI. As the first medically trained rescuer on the scene, you will set the stage for how the incident will be handled.

EMS Sector Functions

The ICS establishes someone in command at all incidents (Figure 31–1). That person has command until it is transferred to someone else or until the incident comes to an end.

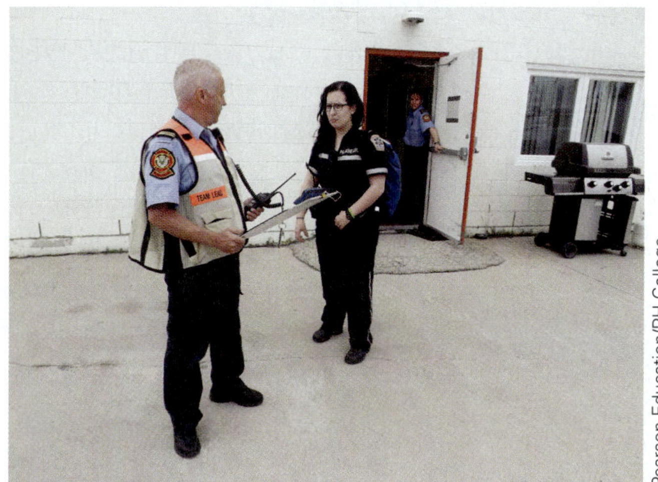

Figure 31–1 The incident commander directs the response and coordinates resources at an MCI.

If an incident is large or complex, command can designate sector officers to help (Figure 31–2). When needed, the EMS sector officers may include the following:

- *Triage officer.* This officer supervises patient assessment, tagging, and removal to a designated treatment area.
- *Treatment officer.* This officer sets up a treatment area and supervises treatment. Generally, one EMS rescuer is assigned to each patient. The treatment and transportation officers make sure that the most seriously injured patients are transported first.
- *Transportation officer.* This officer arranges for ambulances. He or she also tracks the priority, identity, and destination of all patients leaving the scene (Figure 31–3 on p. 456). The transportation and staging officers make sure resources are available as needed.
- *Staging officer.* This officer releases and distributes resources when they are needed. He or she also ensures that gridlock does not occur in the transportation area.
- *Safety officer.* This officer maintains scene safety. He or she identifies potential dangers and takes action to prevent them from causing injury to patients and rescuers.

CASE STUDY

Dispatch

Last week, while on duty for the fire department, I was assigned to the EMR unit. Shortly after checking out our equipment and supplies, my partner and I were dispatched to an explosion with fire at a small factory.

Scene Assessment

Our response time was five minutes. When we reached the scene, we were told where to park our vehicle. I was also told to establish EMS command and determine the number and extent of injuries. My partner and I immediately donned our identification vests. I wore the EMS command vest. She put on the triage sector vest.

A plant security guard told me that nine people were working in the area when the explosion occurred. Eight people escaped with their lives. One was still unaccounted for. I radioed this information to the incident commander.

Emotions were running high among the patients. I knew that many patients follow the lead of the rescuers. Therefore, calm was the rule.

> Consider this situation as you read Chapter 31. What can be done to ensure that all patients get timely and appropriate emergency medical care?

When there are many patients who need special rescue or extrication from wreckage, an extrication sector should be established.

In large-scale operations where a great many resources are used for long periods of time, a logistics officer may be needed. This officer makes certain that medical supplies, communications equipment, transportation units, food, and any other supplies are available when needed. This officer may also set up a rehabilitation sector where emergency personnel can go for evaluation and treatment as well as for food and water.

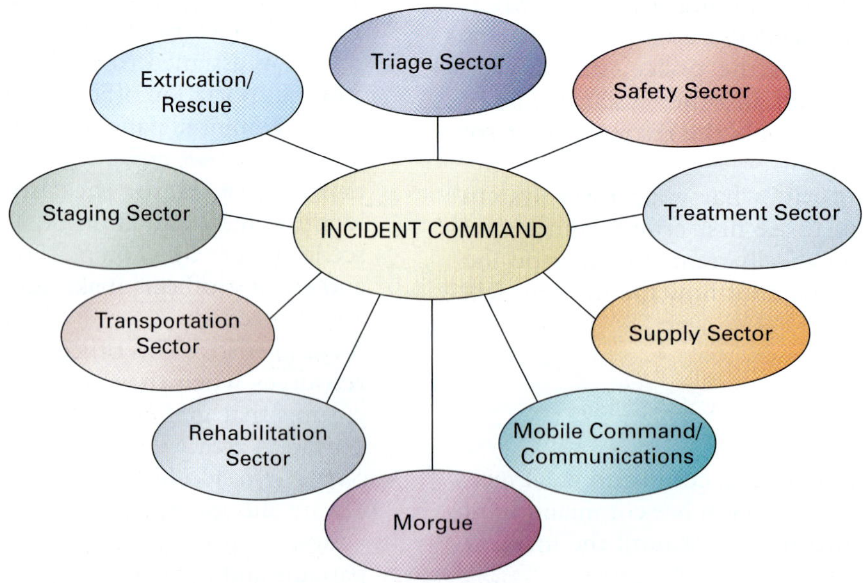

Figure 31–2 EMS sectors are established as needed.

THE COMMAND TOOLBOX

MULTICASUALTY RECORDER WORKSHEET

Ambulance Company	Ambulance ID Number	Patient Triage Tag Number	Patient Status	Hospital Destination	Off-Scene Time

Figure 31–3 Sample of a tracking sheet for the transportation officer at an MCI.

When there are deceased victims, a morgue may be set up. This sector should be overseen by the police along with a medical examiner or coroner.

EMR's Role

The most senior EMR arriving at an MCI is responsible for carrying out the MCI plan. Your major goals are then to do the following:

- Establish command
- Assess the scene
- Request additional resources
- Begin triage

Table 31–1 provides a summary of the command officer's responsibilities. Once you identify an incident as an MCI, resist the urge to jump in and provide treatment. Remember that patients with loud voices have open airways. Quiet patients may not be breathing.

During your scene assessment, identify the following:

- Scene safety
- Number of patients, including the walking wounded
- Needs for extrication
- Estimated number of ambulances needed
- Other factors affecting the scene and resources, such as weather or terrain
- Number of sectors needed
- Area to stage resources

Make an initial scene report to EMS dispatch. Keep it short and to the point. Be sure to give the information necessary for other rescuers to react to the MCI appropriately, as in the following example:

"Fire control, this is Engine 405. We are on the scene of a two-car collision with entrapment of three priority 1 red patients.

Dispatch a rescue unit and three ALS ambulances. Alert the trauma centre. I will now be called Central Avenue Command. Police are needed to assist with traffic and crowd control ASAP. Approach from the north. Staging is on Central between Kennedy and 67th Street."

TABLE 31–1
COMMAND OFFICER RESPONSIBILITIES

- Assume an effective command mode and position. Provide continuing command until relieved by a higher-ranking official.
- Transmit a brief preliminary report to EMS dispatch.
- Rapidly evaluate the situation.
- Request additional resources.
- Quickly develop a safe management strategy.
- Delegate authority.
- Review and evaluate effectiveness of sector operations through frequent progress reports from sector officers.
- Modify sector operations as required.
- As the incident winds down, return units to service and secure the incident when appropriate.

Some MCI plans call for the command vehicle to have two traffic cones on top of it. Whatever method you use, make sure command can be identified easily. Bibs or vests should be worn by command personnel and sector officers for easy recognition.

Communication is a key component of any MCI plan. Keep calm when making radio transmissions. Use plain English and common terms. Try to keep radio traffic to a minimum. Encourage face-to-face communication.

When you are relieved by someone higher in the chain of command, report the following to him or her:

- Nature of the problem
- Potential hazards
- Number of patients
- Time elapsed since the emergency occurred
- What has already been done

If you respond to an MCI where command is already established, report immediately to the command sector. Identify the incident commander. Introduce yourself and your level of training and ask for instructions. Be prepared to care for patients or to support rescue personnel as directed.

SECTION 2
TRIAGE AND EMERGENCY CARE

Triage is a French word defined as picking or sorting. It is a process of classifying sick and injured patients that was first used by the military. During the Korean and Vietnam Wars, it resulted in a dramatic improvement in survival rates of the injured. Today, triage is used to determine the order in which patients receive medical care and transport.

Triage Systems

In triage, the most critical but salvageable patients are treated and transported first. Different areas may have their own ways of performing triage, so know what your EMS system expects of you. Follow all local protocols.

Three-Level Triage Systems

Three-level triage systems are the most common (Figure 31–4). One that has proven very successful is START, which stands for simple triage and rapid treatment. START categories include the following:

- *Priority 1 Red.* This is the highest priority given to patients.
- *Priority 2 Yellow.* This is the second priority, or urgent care category.
- *Priority 3 Green.* This is the lowest priority, or delayed care category.

For the priority 1 red category, patients are given a red tag if they meet three criteria. First, their injuries must be life threatening and the risk of asphyxiation or shock is imminent or present. Second, they can be stabilized without constant care. Third, they have a very good chance of survival if treated and transported immediately. (Patients with catastrophic injuries to the head or chest are not included in this category. They have little chance of recovery.) This priority goes to patients with the following:

- Airway problems
- Respiratory arrest
- Severe uncontrolled bleeding
- Pneumothorax
- Respiratory tract burns
- Major or complicated burns
- Cervical spine injury
- Open abdominal wounds

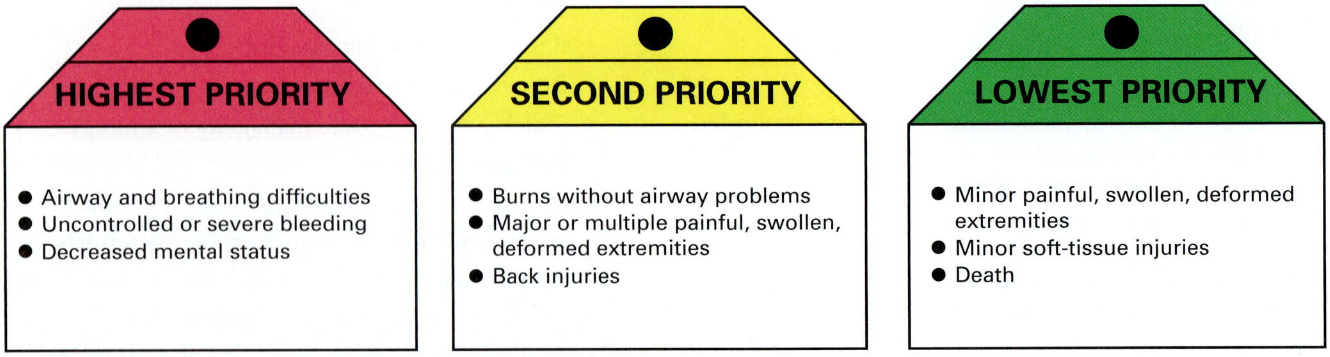

Figure 31–4 An example of a three-level triage system.

- Severe or impending shock
- Hyperthermia or hypothermia
- Unconsciousness without head injury
- Medical conditions, such as diabetes and poisoning
- Open—but not catastrophic—chest wounds and severe head injuries or head injuries accompanied by decreasing levels of consciousness

Priority 2 yellow patients are treated and transported next. They include patients with the following:

- Seizures
- Stable abdominal injuries
- Emergency childbirth
- Eye injuries
- Uncomplicated burns
- Major open wounds
- Multiple painful, swollen, deformed extremities

Priority 3 green is given to the patients who are not seriously injured, need minimal care, and can wait for treatment without getting worse. Their injuries include the following:

- Minor pain and swelling of extremities
- Minor burns
- Minor soft-tissue injuries such as small scrapes, cuts, and bruises that do not involve significant bleeding

A fourth category may be included in a START system. It is priority 0 black. This is the no care category. Black tags are given to individuals who are dead or who have injuries that would be fatal even if they receive treatment. Their injuries include the following:

- Catastrophic head or chest injuries
- Injuries certain to cause death, such as decapitation, severed trunk, and total incineration
- Unconsciousness and pulselessness

Cardiac arrest patients are treated as dead unless there are enough rescuers to care for them as well as for other injured patients. If rescuers are limited in number, these patients must be bypassed so that patients with better chances of survival can be treated.

Managing a cardiac arrest patient in triage is controversial. The decision to try to resuscitate depends on the number of patients involved and the resources available. However, when there are multiple victims of lightning strike, resuscitation efforts should be made. These patients tend to have a very good chance of survival.

Two-Level Triage Systems

A different system that can cut down on confusion uses only two categories: immediate and delayed. Patients in the immediate category have life-threatening injuries but can be saved if cared for immediately. They receive priority for treatment and transport.

Patients in the delayed category include all the rest of the patients on the scene. That includes patients with minor injuries, patients with injuries so critical that they will die even with aggressive treatment, and patients who are dead.

Triage Tags

After patients are assessed and sorted, they must be tagged for rapid identification. Triage tags come in a variety of sizes, shapes, and colours (Figure 31–5). Generally, use them only if more than 10 patients are involved in a single incident. Avoid tags that need a ballpoint pen or carbon paper. Avoid tags that are too detailed. Be sure there is a method of securing the tags so that they do not come loose or drop off.

Once a patient is given a tag, do not remove it. If the patient changes status before being treated, draw a bold line through the original tag, note the time, and put a new tag on the patient. This procedure helps rescuers know that the patient has had a change in status.

One of the most popular tags is the Mettag. It uses symbols instead of words for rapid identification. It is also highly visible. With perforated divisions, it contains a strip for each of the categories: red (rabbit) for the highest priority, yellow (turtle) for second priority, green (ambulance with X through it) for those not in need of transport, and black (shovel and cross) for the dead. Rescuers simply tear off the strips that are not needed so that the applicable strip is on the outside edge.

Conducting Triage

To perform triage at an MCI, you must assess each patient's condition, determine the urgency of the

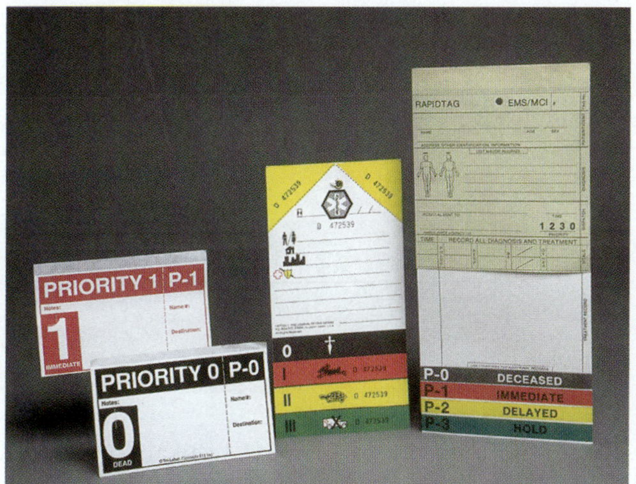

Figure 31–5 Commonly used triage tags.

condition, and assign a priority for treatment. In general, begin triage with a primary assessment, as follows:

- If the patient is alert and talking and has no major bleeding, reassure him or her and move on.
- If the patient is unconscious, open the airway as you check for a pulse. If there is no pulse, move on to the next patient.
- If the patient has severe bleeding, quickly apply a pressure dressing and elevation. Then, move on to the next patient.

In the START system, first tell all patients who can walk to get up and walk unassisted to a specified area. Give these patients—the walking wounded—a priority 3 green (delayed care). Then, turn your attention to the patients who were unable to walk away. Begin triage using the START system with a primary assessment as follows:

- Breathing
  - If breathing is faster than 30 breaths per minute, give the patient a priority 1 red.
  - If the patient is not breathing, quickly clear foreign matter from the mouth and open the airway. If breathing resumes, give the patient a priority 1 red. If breathing does not resume, tag with a priority 0 black.
  - If breathing is less than 30 breaths per minute, perform the next assessment.
- Circulation
  - If there is no carotid pulse, tag the patient as a priority 0 black.
  - If the carotid pulse is weak or irregular, give the patient a priority 1 red.
  - If the carotid pulse is strong, perform the next assessment.
- Mental status
  - If there is no response to a simple command such as "Close your eyes," give the patient a priority 1 red.
  - If the patient can respond to a simple command, give him or her a priority 2 yellow.

SECTION 3
PSYCHOLOGICAL IMPACT OF AN MCI

Psychological reactions to an MCI can also be severe. Almost all the people involved in an MCI experience fear. Many also feel shaky, perspire profusely,

and become confused, irritable, anxious, suspicious, moody, restless, and fatigued. Many will have sleep problems, concentration problems, depression, nausea, vomiting, and diarrhea. Survivors often experience anger, guilt, shock, denial, and feelings of isolation and vulnerability. All these reactions are normal.

The reactions of children depend on age, disposition, and family and community support. Generally, preschoolers cry, lose control of bowels and bladder, become confused, and suck their thumbs. Older children suffer from extreme fears about their safety. They may show confusion, depression, headache, inability to concentrate, withdrawal, poor performance, and a tendency to fight with peers. Older children and adolescents may show extreme aggression. Their stress may be severe enough to disrupt their lives.

Others at risk for severe reactions are older adults, those in poor physical or emotional health, people with disabilities, and those who have unresolved past losses or crises.

Rescuers also react. Often, they react in the same way their patients do. Common reactions are fear about personal safety, crying, anger, guilt, numbness, preoccupation with death, frustration, and fatigue. Most reactions peak within about one week and then diminish. About half of rescuers have dreams of the disaster for weeks or months afterwards. In some cases, rescuers suffer long-term reactions. A CISD is one of the best ways for the rescuers to deal with reactions to an MCI. (See Chapter 2 for details.)

General Guidelines for Rescuers

General guidelines for any type of MCI are as follows:

- Do not let yourself become overwhelmed by the size of the emergency. Learn your local MCI plans well. Follow them. They will help you stay calm and effective.
- Families of patients deserve accurate information. As soon as possible, assign several workers to provide it only to the properly authorized person. That is usually the chief town executive, the public relations officer, or the incident commander.
- Reunite the patients with their families as soon as possible. They will feel less stressed once they are together. Families can also provide medical histories that will increase your ability to care for patients. A separate area, away from the scene and patient care area, should be designated for bystanders and the press.
- If the MCI involves a large number of patients, group them with their families and neighbours. This will help reduce feelings of fear and isolation.

- Identify high-risk patients. Target them for immediate crisis intervention services.
- Provide structure. Tell the patients exactly what is happening.
- Work can be therapeutic. Encourage the walking wounded to do necessary tasks. Explain the tasks simply and clearly. Consider having the patients support each other until medical personnel are available.
- Help the patients confront the reality of the disaster. Encourage them to talk about it and what they feel. If you sense that they are not facing reality or that their expectations are much worse than reality, help them adjust their views. If you engage a patient in this type of talk, make sure you have time to listen and respond.
- Do not give false assurances. If you do, the patients may resist any further outside help. Appraise the situation honestly. Offer help where it is needed.
- Patients may refuse help. There are many reasons for this, including how they were brought up. Explain that accepting help is not an admission of weakness. Make sure they understand that help is only temporary and that as soon as things are under control, they can help someone else.
- Arrange for a group discussion where patients can share feelings as soon as physical needs are taken care of.
- Encourage all those involved—including rescuers—to get good follow-up care and support.

Also, consider using the help of the Canadian Red Cross or a similar organization. They may be able to assist with psychological counselling and other support services to patients and families. Such organizations should be identified in the disaster plan and alerted as soon as possible in the event of a large-scale MCI.

Reducing Stress in Rescuers

Once the rescue operation is underway, a new danger arises: the rescuers themselves may begin to suffer from stress. If measures are not taken immediately, rescue workers can become inefficient and, at worst, become victims themselves. To help reduce stress, the following guidelines may be useful:

- Make sure rescue workers are fully aware of their exact assignments. Well-defined limits help reduce stress.
- Assign rescue workers to tasks according to their skills and experience. If there are any questions, do not gamble. Give workers the tasks you are certain they can do.
- Tell the rescuers to rest at regular intervals away from the hub of the disaster. They should sit or lie down, have something to eat or drink, and relax as much as possible. Have counselling available for those who need defusing. If rest periods are effectively rotated, there will be enough workers to carry on disaster assistance.
- Have several workers circulate among the rescuers to watch for signs of physical exhaustion and stress. If one worker appears to be having problems, he or she should rest for a longer period than usual. After rest, give him or her a less stressful task. If appropriate, trained psychological support personnel can evaluate the workers if a high level of stress is suspected.
- Provide plenty of nourishing drinks and food. Encourage rescue workers to eat and drink to keep up their strength. Avoid foods high in fat, sugar, and caffeine.
- Encourage rescue workers to talk among themselves. Talking helps relieve stress. Discourage lighthearted conversation and joking. Some patients and workers may be offended, which can increase stress on the scene.
- Make sure that the rescuers have a chance to talk with trained counsellors after the incident. If your team has access to CISD, make sure all the rescuers who worked on the scene take advantage of it.

EMR FOCUS

Most people consider multiple-casualty incidents to be plane crashes and commuter train wrecks. While these certainly qualify, the most common MCIs are two cars that collide, each with three injured passengers. Most EMS systems would have to stretch resources to take care of these six patients. Alternatively, international disasters, like the tsunami that ravaged Southeast Asia in 2004, cannot be handled by even a group of local agencies. Learn what your EMS system expects of you.

In the first few minutes of an MCI, the most important task that the first trained person on the scene can perform is to plan, not rush in.

CASE STUDY FOLLOW-UP

At the beginning of this chapter, you read that EMRs were on the scene of an MCI. To see how the chapter skills apply to this emergency, read the following. It describes how the call was completed.

PRIMARY ASSESSMENT AND TRIAGE

My partner, Jan, started triage. When another EMR arrived, I assigned him to establish a transportation sector and gave him a staging vest. I reminded him to make sure that he identified a safe area where ambulances could enter and exit quickly and safely.

Jan soon reported that two patients were priority 1, three were priority 2, and three were priority 3. I updated the incident commander and requested seven ambulances, three of which were to be equipped for advanced life support. I also requested that he alert the trauma centre.

A minute or so later, it was confirmed that one patient was still inside the plant. We believed that patient to be a priority 0. At that moment, the paramedic EMS supervisor arrived. I provided a full report and turned the EMS command over to him. I was then assigned to assist in the treatment area.

Over the next half hour, all eight patients were transported to hospital. A police officer was assigned to guard the one dead body until the coroner arrived. Triage and transportation for the injured patients had taken 45 minutes.

When the EMS command was terminated, the incident commander told us that a CISD would be organized for all rescue personnel involved.

> For you to be an effective member of an EMS response to an MCI, you must learn your local plans and protocols. Review them often. Practise them whenever you are given the opportunity.

NOCPs

4.1 a Rapidly assess a scene based on the principles of a triage system **S**

    b Assume different roles in a mass-casualty incident **A**

    c Manage a multiple-patient incident **A**

8.1 d Utilize community support agencies as appropriate **A**

8.2 a Work collaboratively with other emergency response agencies **A**

    b Work within an incident management system (IMS) **A**

8.3 d Conduct triage at a CBRNE incident **A**

REVIEW QUESTIONS

Page references where answers may be found or supported are provided at the end of each question.

SECTION 1

1. What is a multiple-casualty incident? (p. 454)
2. What is the Incident Command System (ICS)? (p. 454)
3. What are some common EMS sector functions? (pp. 454–456)
4. What are the first critical steps that must be completed at an MCI? (p. 456)
5. What information must you report to EMS dispatch after your scene assessment? (pp. 456–457)

SECTION 2

6. What are the possible categories in two-level and three-level triage systems? (pp. 457–458)
7. How many patients should there be in a single incident before you use triage tags? (p. 458)

SECTION 3

8. Suggest several ways of reducing stress in rescuers at an MCI. (p. 460)

32

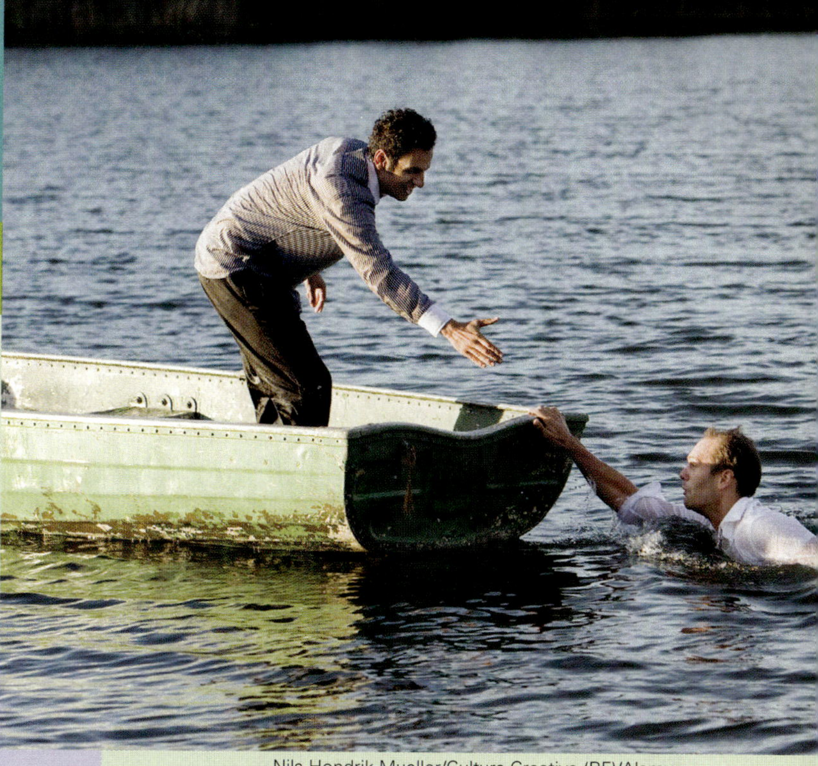

Nils Hendrik Mueller/Cultura Creative (RF)/Alamy

Water Emergencies

OBJECTIVES

1. Describe how drownings and near drownings occur.
2. Describe the three key components of scene assessment in a water emergency: patient condition, water condition, and resources at hand.
3. Discuss some of the difficulties in assessing a patient who is in the water.
4. Describe emergency care of near-drowning patients without injuries to the spine versus those with spinal injuries.
5. List the five hazards commonly associated with fast-moving water.
6. Discuss the differences between warm-water and cold-water rescues.
7. Describe the assessment and emergency medical care of a patient with a diving emergency, including air embolism and decompression sickness.

INTRODUCTION

Water is everywhere. Oceans, lakes, and streams are the most obvious sites of possible water emergencies, but numerous drownings occur in home pools and many industries have vats or pools large enough to drown several people. Even bathtubs and toilets can present a danger to small children.

This chapter offers an overview of water rescue. It introduces you to the challenges of providing emergency care in water and to some of the common hazards of water rescue.

SECTION 1
DROWNING AND NEAR DROWNING

Drowning is defined as death from suffocation due to submersion. It is one of the leading causes of preventable death in Canada. After MVAs, drowning is the most common preventable cause of death among children.

Drowning can be the result of cold, fatigue, injury, disorientation, intoxication, or limited swimming ability (Figure 32–1). Survival from a near drowning can depend on many factors, including whether or not the water is fresh or salty, warm or cold, clear or murky, still or moving.

Freshwater vs. Saltwater

In freshwater drowning, water passes through the patient's lungs into the bloodstream. There, it can cause hemodilution (thinning of the blood by excess water)

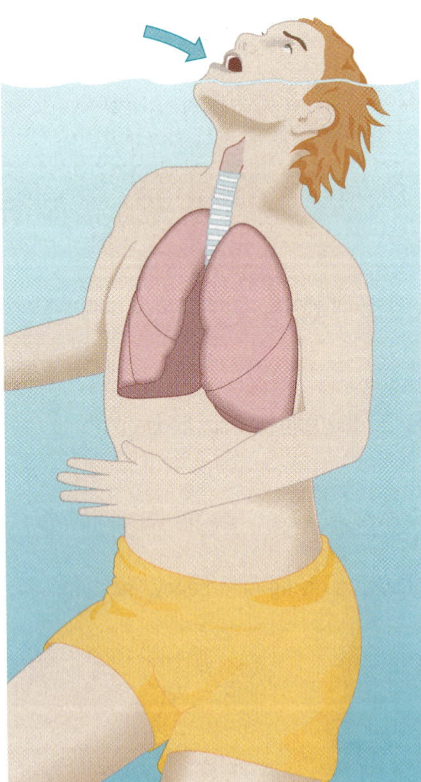

Drowning can be the result of cold, fatigue, injury, disorientation, intoxication, or limited swimming ability.

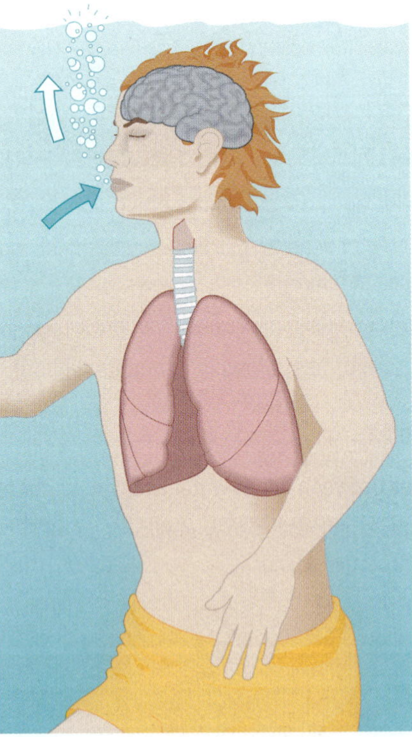

The drowning victim struggles to inhale air as long as possible. Eventually the victim inhales water or a muscle spasm of the larynx closes the airway.

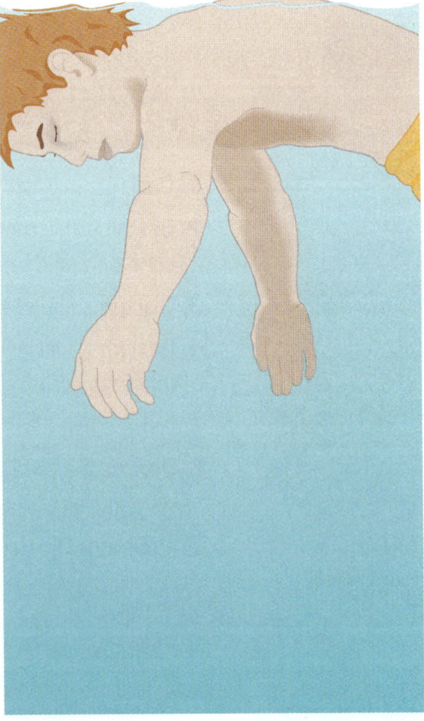

Loss of consciousness, convulsions, cardiac arrest, and death may follow.

Figure 32–1 Drowning.

CASE STUDY

Dispatch

I spend my summers working as a lifeguard at the town pool. I was on the scene when a water emergency occurred.

Scene Assessment

The pool was crowded that day. It was blindingly bright and very hot. I was on the stand watching some youngsters use the low diving board when I heard people start to yell. I looked toward the middle of the pool and saw a young male floating face down on the far side.

I knew him. It was Jimmy. I jumped in and swam over to him. Everyone was yelling. One bystander shouted that he had had a seizure.

I thought quickly. I didn't see him dive. I didn't know if he'd been in a fight. All I knew was that he appeared to be unconscious. I decided I'd better not move him from the water.

Consider this patient as you read Chapter 32. What should be done to assess and treat his condition?

and destruction of red blood cells. More commonly, simple asphyxia (suffocation) is the cause of death.

In saltwater drowning, aspirated water is saltier than body fluids. So, water leaves the blood and enters the lungs to help dilute the salt. The air in the lungs mixes with the fluids and forms a frothy foam, which acts as a barrier to oxygen exchange. The result can be death.

Wet vs. Dry Drowning

Wet drowning occurs when fluid is aspirated into the lungs. Dry drowning occurs when a severe muscle spasm of the larynx closes it, preventing aspiration and respiration. About 10 to 40 percent of all drownings are estimated to be dry. Autopsies reveal that only about 15 percent of drowning victims aspirate a significant amount of water.

Warm Water vs. Cold Water

There is a significant difference between warm-water and cold-water drowning. Unlike warm-water incidents, drownings that occur in cold water (below 20°C) have resulted in successful resuscitations, even up to 90 minutes after submersion.

Hypothermia and the diving reflex have something to do with this. Both slow down the body's metabolism and reduce the need for oxygen.

Muscles do not function properly when cold, so it becomes difficult for the patient to keep himself or herself afloat. The hypothermic patient may also be unable to follow directions or assist with the rescue. Cold water temperatures also affect rescuers.

SECTION 2
WATER RESCUE

General Guidelines for Emergency Care

Scene Assessment

In a water-related emergency, you obviously need to reach the patient. However, you must do so with the utmost concern for your own safety. Remember that water can conceal many hazards. Holes, sharp dropoffs, and underwater entanglements, such as fallen trees or wire fences, may not be visible from shore. The force of moving water can also be very deceptive. Do not walk into fast-moving water over knee depth. It is not safe. Moving water in streams, rivers, and even storm drains can push you over and hold you down.

Hazardous materials are also a concern in water emergencies. For example, a car in the water could leak oil and gas, which float on the surface. Such hazards pose a respiratory risk for both patients and rescuers. Floods can cause sewage to be released in normally safe waters. Risk of electrocution exists in flooded buildings or ground. Severe bleeding of the patient can also pose the risk of infection to other patients and rescuers.

When determining how to respond to a water emergency, take into account the patient's condition, water conditions, and the resources on hand:

- Patient condition
  - *Consciousness*—Is the patient conscious and able to assist in the rescue? If so, reaching out with a pole or throwing a rope may be the safest method of rescue.
  - *Injuries*—Does the patient have any obvious injuries? If the patient is unstable, you may have to extricate him or her from the water before beginning care.
  - *Location*—Is the patient on the surface of the water or submerged? The submerged patient may need basic life support immediately. He or she may also be difficult to locate.
- Water condition
  - *Visibility*—Can you see any potential hazards under the water? Can you see the patient and his or her injuries?
  - *Temperature*—For a cold-water drowning, you must continue resuscitation until the patient is rewarmed at the hospital. Note that even when the air is warm, the water may still be cold.
  - *Moving water*—Will the location of the victim change? Is it safe for you to enter it?
  - *Depth of the water*—Can your feet touch the bottom so that you can stand, or will additional equipment be needed?

- *Other hazards*—Are there hazardous materials present, such as oil, gas, or sewage? Is there any risk of electrocution?
- Resources on hand
  - *Rescuers*—How many rescuers are on the scene? Are they trained in water rescue? Can they all swim? Does each have a personal flotation device?
  - *Special resources*—Do you need any special rescue teams, such as a scuba diving team?

If a water emergency occurs in open, shallow water that has a stable, uniform bottom, attempt a rescue. However, never try a water rescue unless you meet all of the following criteria:

- You are a good swimmer.
- You are specially trained in water rescue.
- You are wearing a personal flotation device.
- You are accompanied by other rescuers.

If you meet all four criteria and your patient is conscious and close to shore, attempt a rescue. Use the "reach, throw, row, and go" strategy in the following order:

- *Reach*—Hold out an object for the patient to grab. Anything that will extend your reach will work. You can use a towel, shirt, backboard, or other strong object that will not break. Before holding out the object, make sure you have solid footing and will not slip into the water. Once the object has been grabbed, pull the patient to shore.
- *Throw*—If the patient is too far to reach, then throw an object that floats (Figure 32–2). Use anything that will float and is heavy enough to throw. A thermos jug, a picnic cooler, or capped

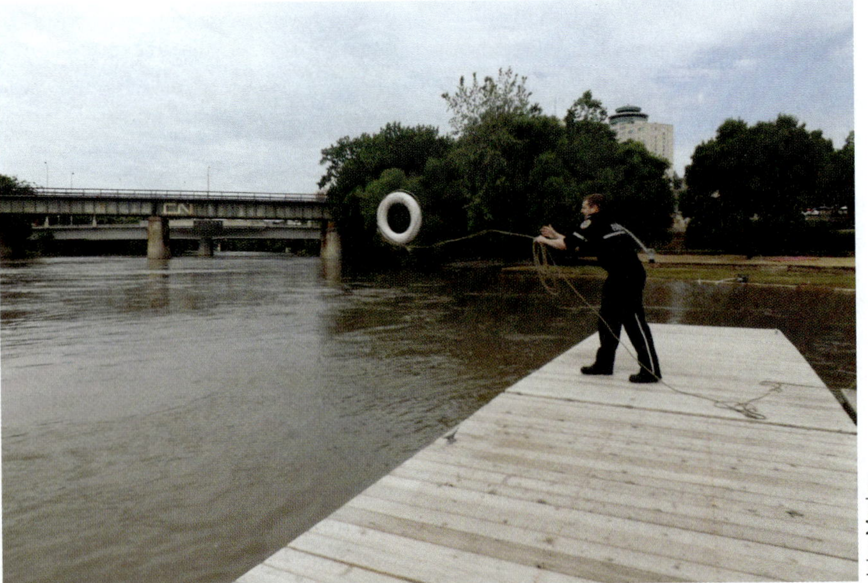

John Mackay

Figure 32–2 Tie a sturdy rope to an object that floats. Throw the object and pull the patient in.

empty milk jug will do. This will give the patient support and give you more time to make the rescue. If possible, tie a rope to the object you throw. Toss the object to the patient and pull on the rope to tow the patient in. Again, be sure of your own footing and stability.

- *Row*—If the patient is too far to reach or to throw an object to from shore, use a boat to get closer to the patient.
- *Go*—If reaching, throwing, and rowing are not possible, swim to the patient. However, do this only if you are a good swimmer, specially trained in water rescue, wearing a personal flotation device, and accompanied by other rescuers.

Patient Assessment

Any injury that can occur on land can also occur in water. However, it can be more difficult to detect and treat injuries in water.

Bleeding, for example, is easy to spot on land. In the water, any bleeding that occurs may be immediately diluted and dispersed. Therefore, it may not only be difficult to recognize that the patient is bleeding, it may also be difficult to judge how severe the bleeding is. In addition, if the patient is wearing a wet suit, a large amount of blood can pool inside it before bleeding is recognized.

Broken bones are also difficult to identify. The water may be murky or dark. The surface of water can also distort visual images. Limbs, for example, can appear angulated or straight when they are not. This occurs because of refraction. One way to deal with this problem is to assume fractures until proven otherwise in any unconscious patient.

If the emergency is the result of a diving accident, or if the patient has been struck by a boat, water skier, surfboard, or other object, suspect spinal injury. Also suspect spinal injury in any swimmer who is unconscious, especially one in shallow, warm water.

Emergency Medical Care

If the patient is conscious and you are sure there is no spinal injury, follow these guidelines:

1. Remove the patient from the water as quickly as you can by any safe method possible.
2. Complete the primary assessment. Administer high-flow oxygen if you are allowed to do so. Be prepared to suction.
3. Conserve the patient's body heat. Remove wet clothing. Place the patient on a blanket. Then, cover him or her with another blanket. If possible, move the patient to a warm environment. Do not allow him or her to walk.

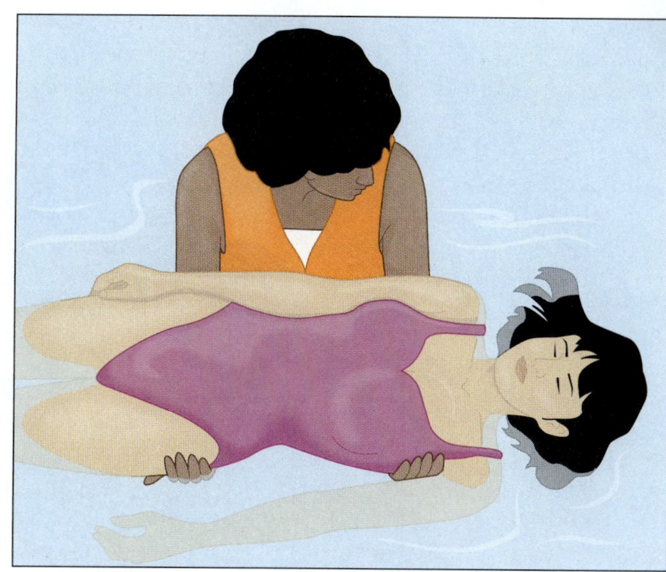

Figure 32–3   Hip and upper body support.

4. While you are waiting for the ambulance, perform a secondary assessment and gather a patient history.

If your patient is unconscious and in shallow, warm water, maintain the airway but do not move the patient. If the patient is breathing, keep him or her in a face-up position. Support the patient's back (Figure 32–3). If there is a second rescuer present, stabilize the patient's head and neck (Figure 32–4).

If you find the unconscious patient face down in shallow water, you must turn him or her face up. Perform the head-splint technique by following these steps (Figure 32–5 on pp. 467–468):

1. Get alongside the patient.
2. Extend the patient's arms straight up alongside the head. Press the arms against the patient's head to create a splint.
3. If necessary, move the patient forward to a horizontal position.
4. Rotate the patient by bringing the arm farthest away toward you and pushing the arm closest to you downward. As you rotate the patient, lower yourself in the water until the water is at shoulder level.
5. Maintain stabilization of the patient's head. Do this with one hand by holding the patient's head between his or her arms. With your other hand, support the patient's lower back until help arrives.

If the unconscious patient is in water that is unsafe (deep, cold, or moving), or if the patient needs CPR, qualified rescuers should position the patient on a backboard. Once immobilized, the patient should be removed from the water. Note that ventilations can start in the water. Chest compressions cannot. Patients who need CPR must be removed from the water first.

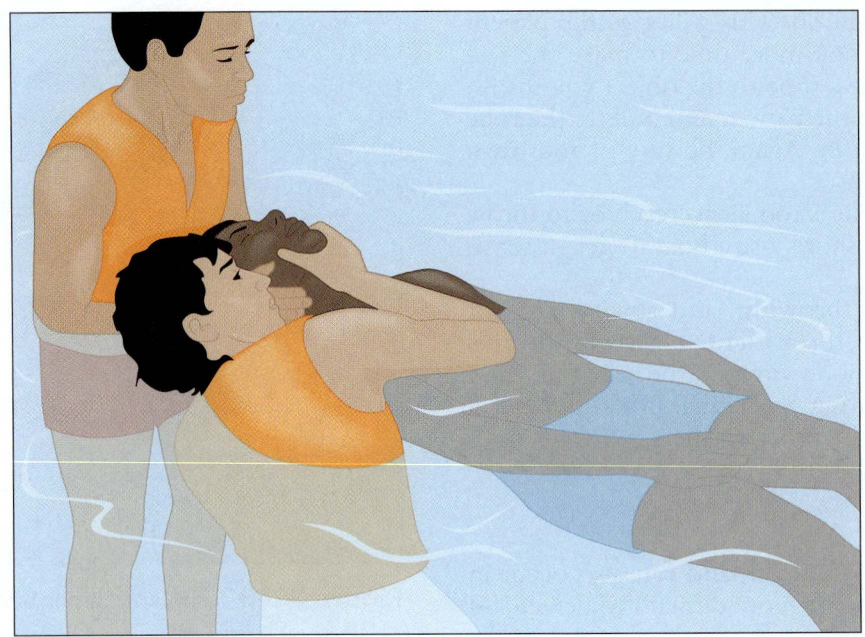

Figure 32–4 In-line head-chin stabilization with two rescuers.

HEAD-SPLINT TECHNIQUE

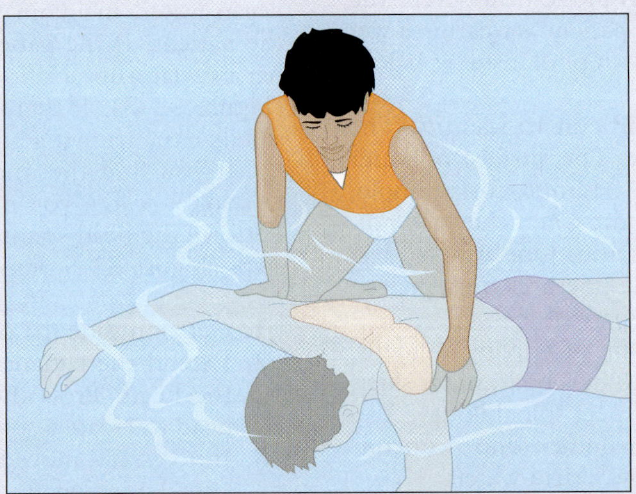

Figure 32–5a Position yourself alongside the patient.

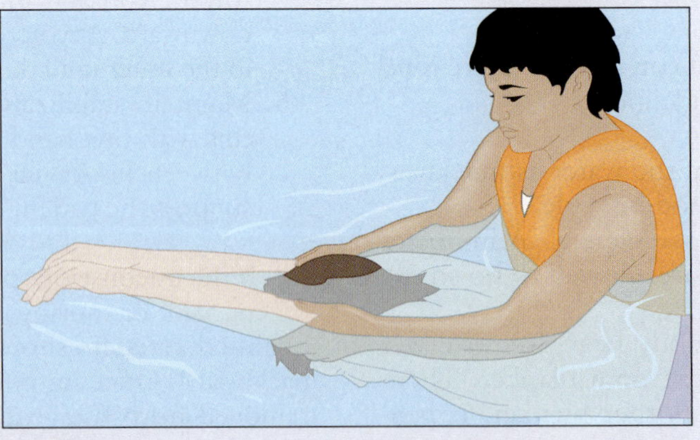

Figure 32–5b Extend the patient's arms straight up alongside his or her head to create a splint.

(continued)

HEAD-SPLINT TECHNIQUE *(continued)*

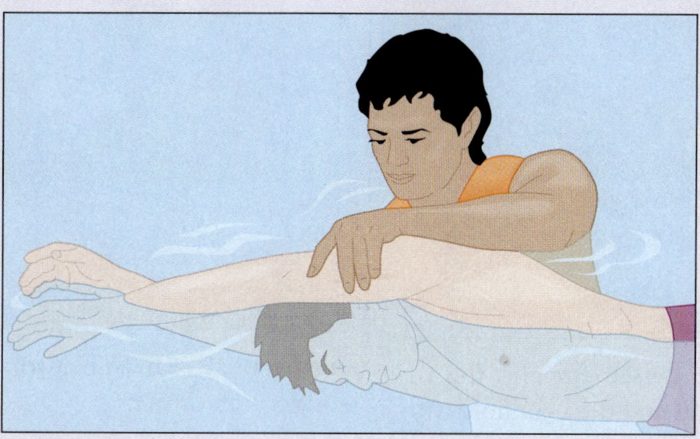

Figure 32–5c   Begin to rotate the patient toward you.

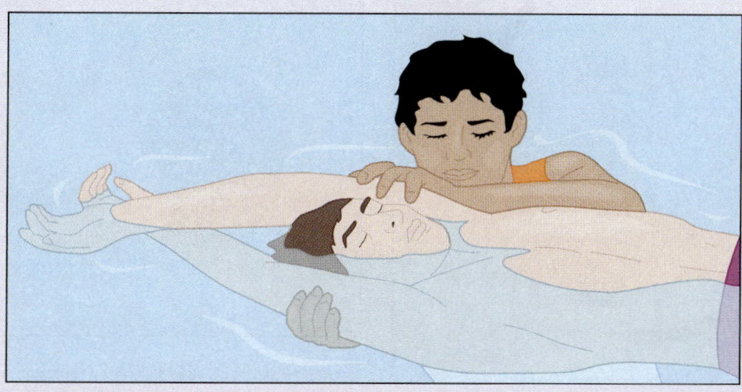

Figure 32–5d   As you rotate the patient, lower yourself in the water.

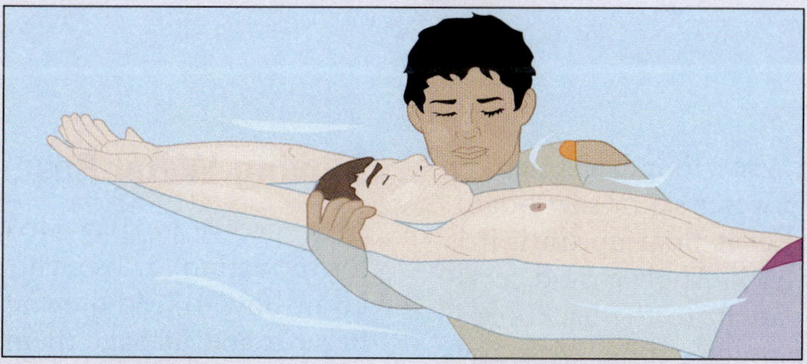

Figure 32–5e   Maintain stabilization by holding the patient's head between his or her arms.

To turn a patient to a face-up position in deep water, perform the head-chin support technique. Follow these steps (Figure 32–6 on p. 469):

1. Position yourself alongside the patient.
2. Position one arm along the patient's spine, supporting the patient's head with your hand. Place your other arm along the patient's chest in line with the sternum, supporting the mandible with your hand.
3. If necessary, move the patient forward to a horizontal position.
4. Then rotate the patient by ducking under his or her body while maintaining your hand positions.
5. Continue to maintain in-line stabilization until a backboard is used to immobilize the spine.

HEAD-CHIN SUPPORT TECHNIQUE

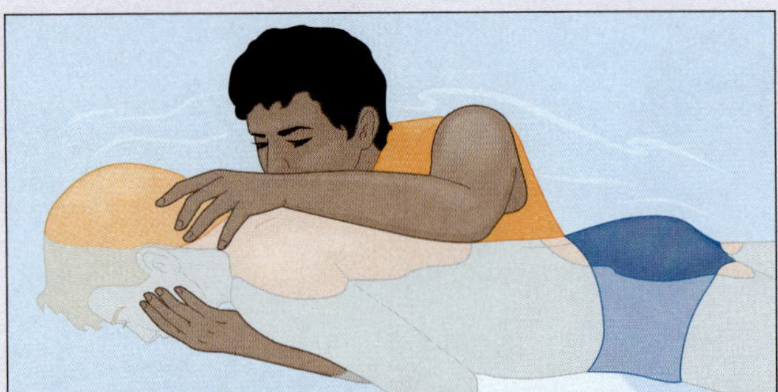

Figure 32–6a Position yourself. Support the patient's head with one hand and the mandible with the other.

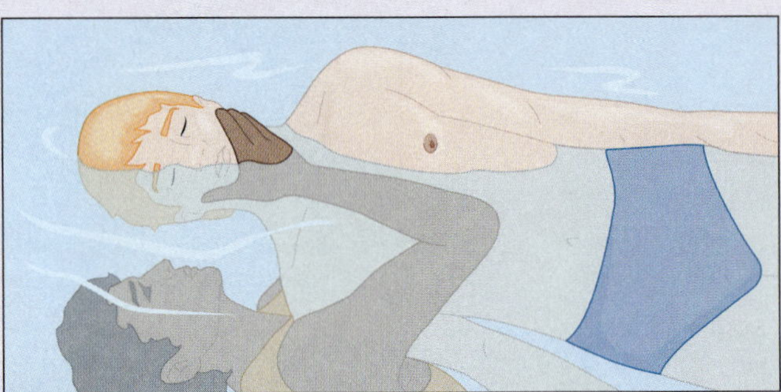

Figure 32–6b Then rotate the patient by ducking under him or her.

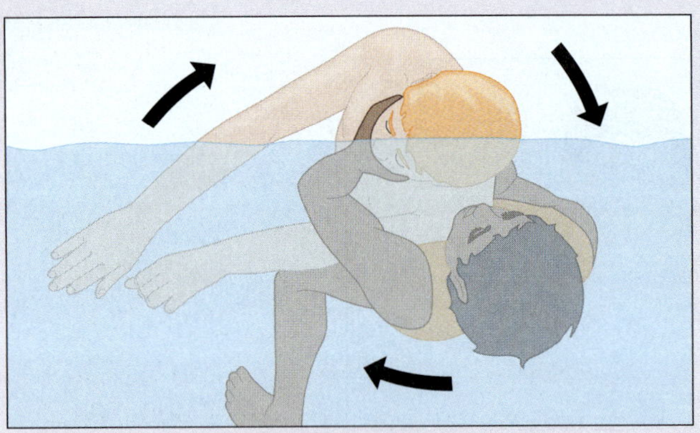

Figure 32–6c Continue to rotate until the patient is face up.

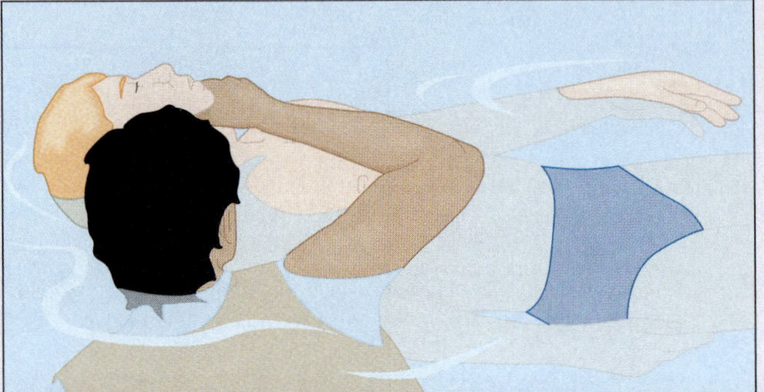

Figure 32–6d Maintain in-line stabilization until a backboard is used to immobilize the spine.

To immobilize a patient, use a long backboard or other rigid support such as a water ski or surf board. Slide it under the patient. Let it float up until it is snugly against the patient's back. Apply a rigid cervical collar. Then secure the patient to the backboard. Never try to support the patient's spine with anything that might bend or break, such as an air mattress or a Styrofoam float. As you are backboarding the patient, be sure to have enough rescuers helping. They need to make sure the patient's face does not become submerged. After immobilization, lift the patient head-first from the water. If the patient is wearing a lifejacket, leave it in place. Remember to pad under the patient's head to keep the spine in alignment.

Note: Always have a near-drowning patient taken to hospital, even if you believe the danger has passed. Complications can develop as long as 72 hours after the incident and may be fatal.

Moving-Water Rescue

Many people are drawn to moving water, or whitewater, for recreation. Those who are trained and experienced know how to read moving water. They understand the hazards and manage them. It is all part of their sport. Moving-water incidents usually occur when someone who is unaware of the dangers gets into the water. This is true of both victims and rescuers.

The force of moving water is measured by its depth, width, and velocity. For example, a river that is about 60 m wide, 1.25 m deep, and moving at 6 m/s will move about 450 cubic metres of water per second. That is roughly equal to 250 kg of force.

Fast-moving water is dangerous. Certain river features make it even more so. They include the following:

- *Strainers.* These are obstructions that allow water to pass through but catch people and other

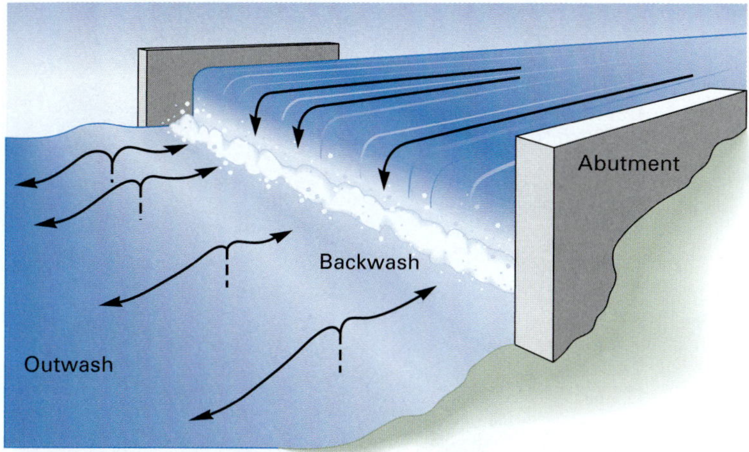

Figure 32–7a A low-head dam.

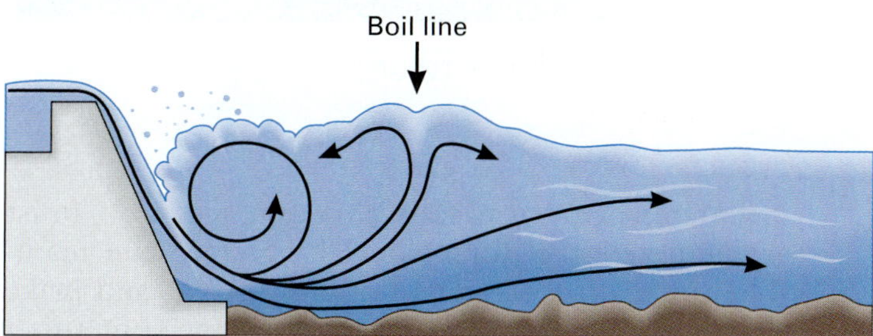

Figure 32–7b A hole formed by water flowing over a low-head dam.

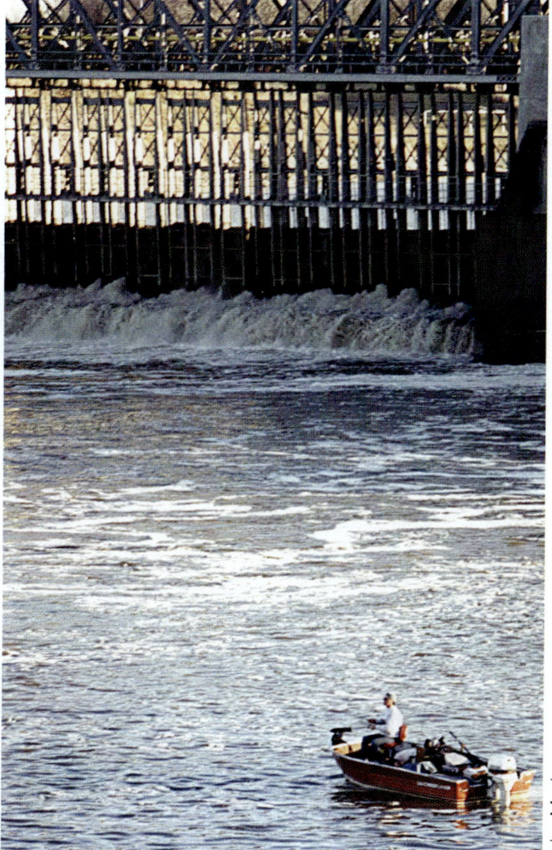

Figure 32–7c The Lockport Dam in Lockport, Manitoba, at the end of Duff's Ditch.

objects. Some of the most common objects are trees and branches. If a strainer catches a swimmer, the force of the water can hold the swimmer there until hypothermia sets in and he or she tires and drowns.

- *Obstructions.* Another problem is any type of obstruction in the river that a person can get pinned against, such as a bridge abutment. A person can easily become trapped against the object and be held there by the force of the moving water. Again, hypothermia can set in and he or she can tire and drown.
- *Holes.* Not all the water in a fast-moving river flows downstream. When water flows over a large object, a recirculating current, or hole, may form. When this happens, the current can keep recirculating a swimmer in its backwash until he or she tires and drowns. Holes are difficult to see from upstream. Large ones are very difficult to escape from.
- *Low-head dams* (Figure 32–7). These dams are only a few metres high. They are built from concrete and have vertical abutments on each side. They are very difficult to see from upstream and often tend

to be very wide. Water that flows over these dams can form a very large and uniform hole that extends across the river. If a boat gets too close to the boil line, it can get caught in the recirculating current and capsize. The boater and the boat can then get pushed to the bottom and back to the surface again and again.

- *Extremity traps* (Figure 32–8). Legs can get trapped between rocks or in other obstructions, especially in fast-moving water above a person's knees. Typically, this occurs to inexperienced people who fall out of a boat and try to stand up. When this happens, the best thing to do is a back stroke with feet pointed downstream. Note that when an extremity gets caught, it must be extracted in exactly the same orientation, but opposite direction, in which it went in.

The basic, time-honoured model for all water rescues is to reach, throw, row, and go. Remember, if you cannot easily effect a rescue using a simple shore-based technique (reach or throw), call for a team specializing in water rescue. Do not enter the water! Even special teams will attempt swimming or live

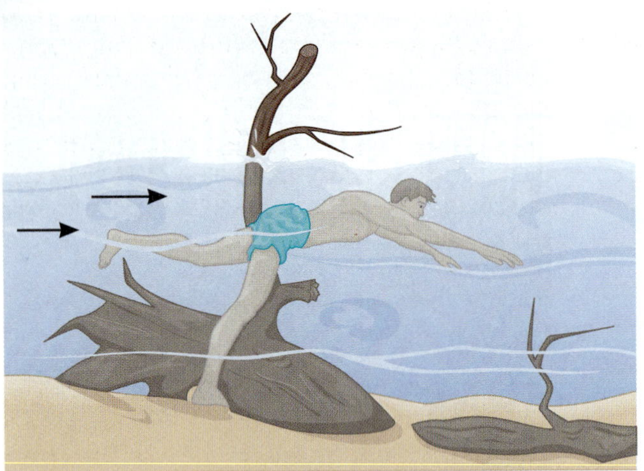

Figure 32–8   Entrapment in fast-moving water.

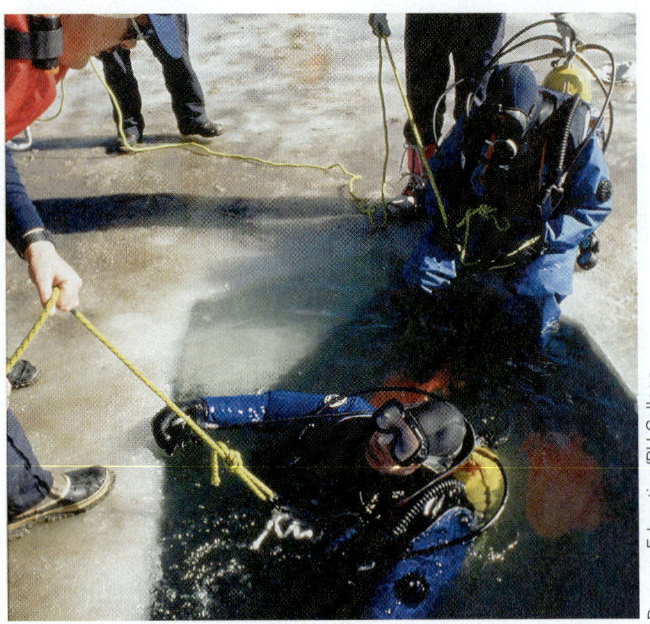

Figure 32–9   An ice rescue.

bait rescues (a rescuer swims to the rescue while attached to a secure line) only as a last resort.

Ice Rescue

Judging the thickness of ice and overall safety is very tricky. The old rule of thumb—"one inch, keep off; two inches, one may; three inches, small groups; four inches, okay"—is *not* accurate. Many factors can alter the thickness of ice over large and small areas. For example, underground springs cause water turbulence from beneath and thinner ice above. Decaying plant matter, schools of fish, and the like can also affect ice thickness.

The reach, throw, row, and go method is used for all water rescues, including ice rescue. However, there are some differences you should note:

- *Reach and throw.* As a drowning patient becomes more hypothermic, he or she will be less and less able to hold onto a rope. An alternative technique is to throw an inflated fire hose. By using modified end caps and air from a self-contained breathing apparatus tank, a fire hose can be inflated quickly and pushed out to the patient.
- *Row.* A conventional boat may not be able to break the ice as it moves unless the ice is very thin. An option may be to use a small inflatable craft with ropes to tether it and pull it from shore. Perhaps the best crafts for ice rescues are the air boat and hovercraft. Either can be manoeuvred over ice, water, or dry land.
- *Go.* When patients are too hypothermic to hang on, rescuers must go in to get them (Figure 32–9). This usually involves wearing a dry neoprene ice rescue suit, which is tethered to shore. The rescuer then crawls, shuffles, or swims out to grab and pull the patient in.

When a person falls through ice, you must immediately call for a special water rescue team. Then, put on a personal flotation device and make reasonable attempts to reach or throw something to the patient from shore. If you are successful, the team can be cancelled. If not, the team already on the way will have a chance to get to the scene in time to help the patient. Remember to prevent well-intentioned bystanders from going onto the ice. More people to save may lead to more lives being lost.

SECTION 3
BAROTRAUMA

The term *barotrauma* refers to several conditions. They occur when scuba or deep-water divers experience increasing underwater pressure or when they ascend in deep water improperly. Such patients may need both basic life support and transport to a treatment centre that specializes in diving injuries.

Note that patients with diving emergencies require specialized medical knowledge and care.

If needed, Duke University's Divers Alert Network (DAN) is a free medical consultation service for dive-related emergencies. Their 24-hour emergency hotline numbers are 1-919-684-8111 and 1-800-446-2671.

Air Embolism

An air embolism is one or more air bubbles that block a blood vessel. It occurs when a diver holds his or her breath during the ascent from a dive. Air in the lungs expands rapidly as a diver ascends and the pressure drops. If the air is not exhaled, the alveoli rupture and nearby blood vessels are damaged. As a result, air bubbles enter the bloodstream. The most dangerous places for air bubbles to lodge are in the heart, brain, or spinal cord.

The signs and symptoms have rapid onset. Within 15 minutes of surfacing, the diver may have any of the following:

- Difficulty breathing
- Blotching or itching skin
- Frothy blood in the nose and mouth
- Pain in the muscles and joints
- Chest pain or pain in the abdomen
- Swelling and a grating sound in the neck
- Numbness or tingling in the extremities
- General weakness, paralysis
- Possible convulsions
- Dizziness
- Vomiting
- Blurred or distorted vision
- Loss or distortion of memory
- Slurred speech, lack of coordination
- Unconsciousness
- Cardiac or respiratory arrest
- Behavioural changes (may be the only sign)

The patient needs recompression treatment at the hospital. Be sure to arrange for transport as soon as possible. To provide emergency care, treat all life threats first. Ensure an adequate airway and administer 100 percent oxygen. If there is no sign of spinal injury, position the patient on the left side, with the head and chest lower than the feet (Figure 32–10). Be prepared to provide ventilations or CPR.

Decompression Sickness

Decompression sickness, or the bends, usually occurs when a diver comes up too quickly from a deep, prolonged dive. It can happen to anyone who is exposed to increasing pressure while breathing compressed air. It can range from mild to severe. It is more common than an air embolism. The risk of decompression sickness increases if the diver flies in a plane within 12 hours after a dive.

Decompression sickness occurs when certain gases (usually nitrogen) are breathed in by the diver over time. When the diver ascends too quickly, the nitrogen turns into tiny bubbles that lodge in the tissues throughout the body and eventually enter the bloodstream. The worst injuries occur when the nitrogen bubbles lodge in the brain, lungs, heart, or spinal cord. A burst lung is the most dire injury associated with this condition.

The signs and symptoms are gradual in onset. They usually occur 12 to 24 hours after the dive

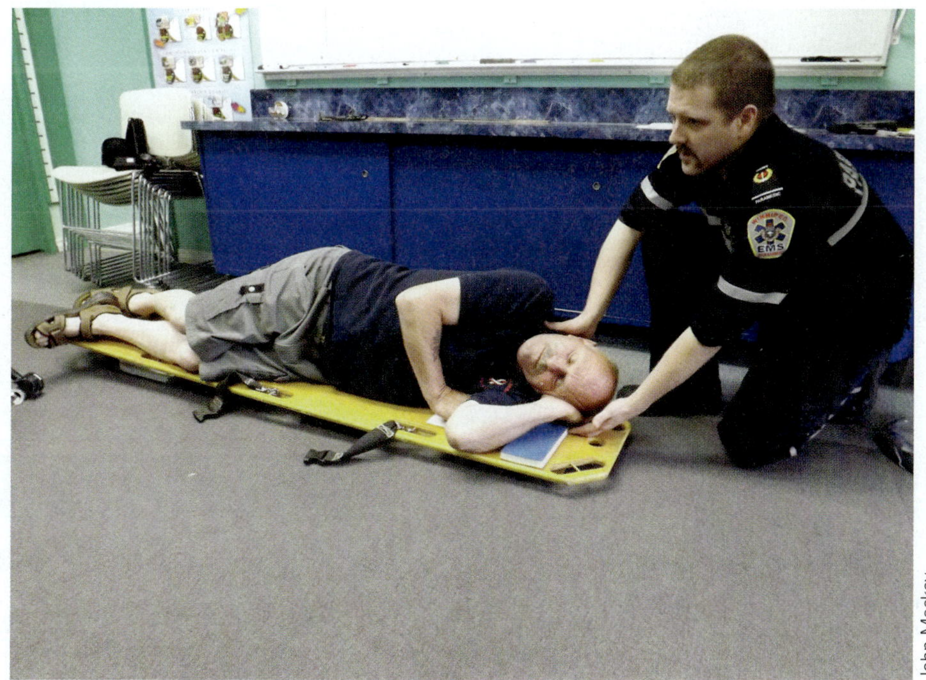

Figure 32–10 Proper positioning of a diving-accident patient.

but can occur up to 48 hours later. They include the following:

- Difficulty breathing, choking, or coughing
- Chest pain
- Itchy, mottled skin with a minor rash that can change in appearance
- Swelling of tissues, with pits in the swelling
- Severe, deep aching pain in the joints and muscles
- Nausea and vomiting with abdominal pain
- Fatigue, dizziness, collapse sometimes leading to unconsciousness
- Headache
- Blurred vision
- Hallucinations
- Ringing of the ears or partial deafness
- Staggering gait
- Numbness, paralysis
- Inability to urinate

The patient needs to be taken to a facility with a recompression chamber for rapid treatment. Arrange for transport immediately. To provide emergency care, treat life threats first. Ensure an adequate airway and administer 100 percent oxygen. Be prepared to provide CPR. If there is no sign of spinal injury, position the patient on the left side, with the head lower than the feet. Slant the patient's entire body about 15 degrees to help prevent gas bubbles from injuring the brain or lungs.

The Squeeze

The squeeze and the reverse squeeze can involve any part of the body that is filled with air. When divers descend or ascend, air pressure must be equalized to maintain proper pressure in the body's air cavities. If proper pressure is not maintained, injury to the tissues of the air cavities results. If there is an air pocket in a tooth due to decay or a defective filling, the tooth may rupture. Divers are at increased risk of the squeeze and reverse squeeze if they have an upper respiratory infection or an allergy that obstructs the sinuses.

The signs and symptoms include the following:

- Mild to severe pain in the affected area
- Blood or fluid discharge from the nose or ears
- Bleeding from the tiny blood vessels in the eyes
- Extreme dizziness, disorientation
- Nausea
- Ear pain (most common), ringing in the ears, possible deafness

The patient needs to be cared for immediately at a medical facility to prevent permanent blindness, deafness, dizziness, or the inability to dive in the future. Arrange for transport immediately. To provide emergency care, treat life threats first. Suction to ensure an adequate airway. Administer oxygen. Keep the patient calm while waiting for medical help to arrive.

EMR FOCUS

Water emergencies can be surprisingly dangerous, even for good swimmers. Many people do not realize that the currents or water temperatures affecting the victim will also affect them.

Television portrays water rescues as a simple matter of swimming out to the grateful victim and casually bringing him or her to shore. In real life, the victims are frantic. In their effort to save themselves, they can drown the rescuer.

This chapter presented several ways of conducting a water rescue from the safety of the shore. Do not attempt a rescue without the proper resources and a proper assessment of the dangers you will face.

CASE STUDY FOLLOW-UP

At the beginning of this chapter, you read that an EMR was on the scene of a possible drowning. To see how the chapter skills apply to this emergency, read the following. It describes how the call was completed.

PRIMARY ASSESSMENT

I moved to Jimmy's head and carefully turned him over without stressing his spine. Then I opened his airway and checked to see if he was breathing. He wasn't. But he had a pulse.

We were pretty close to the side of the pool. Two other lifeguards arrived just above us, and one was quick to open the first-aid kit and hand me a pocket mask. She jumped in to help while the other lifeguard went to call 9-1-1.

Even though I had never done it before on a real person, I put the face mask in place and started ventilations—one breath every five seconds. It felt as if we were working on him for a while, but I guess it was only a few minutes when he started to cough. He brought up a little water. All of a sudden there was an ambulance crew above us.

SECONDARY ASSESSMENT

The lifeguard who had jumped into the water to help did a visual inspection of the patient from head to toe. She reported that she found no signs of injury.

PATIENT HISTORY

I knew Jimmy had had seizures before. He had told me so. But I had never actually witnessed one.

ONGOING ASSESSMENT

The paramedics took over care before we had a chance to do anything other than provide basic life support.

TRANSFER OF CARE

Our hand-off report was brief. We told the crew chief that Jimmy was unconscious when we found him and that we had no evidence that he had hurt his neck or back. But since we didn't know for sure, we had maintained manual stabilization of his head and neck. We reported that Jimmy had a history of seizures and that, according to an unknown bystander, he may have experienced one.

The paramedics positioned a backboard under Jimmy, secured him, and lifted him from the water. He still wasn't wide awake, but we told him he was in good hands and that we'd contact his family.

> Water-related emergencies pose a special challenge to EMRs. Patients in such emergencies often need immediate life-saving care. However, the same hazards that caused the emergency can also endanger rescuers. Remember, your safety must come first. Do only what you are trained and equipped to do.

NOCPs

6.1 n Provide care to patient experiencing signs and symptoms due to exposure to adverse environments **S**

REVIEW QUESTIONS

Page references where answers may be found or supported are provided at the end of each question.

SECTION 1

1. What happens when a person drowns? Briefly describe freshwater, saltwater, wet, dry, and cold-water drowning. (pp. 463–464)

SECTION 2

2. What are some of the hazards a water emergency may pose for the rescuer? (pp. 464–465)

3. What determining factors should you consider when planning how to respond to a water emergency? (p. 465)

4. What criteria must you meet before you can attempt a water rescue? (p. 465)

5. What is the "reach, throw, row, and go" strategy for water rescue? (pp. 465–466)

6. What are the general guidelines for the emergency care of a near-drowning patient? (pp. 466–469)

7. What are the hazards commonly associated with fast-moving water? (pp. 469–470)

8. Why is it difficult to judge the thickness of ice before attempting a rescue? (p. 471)

SECTION 3

9. What are the general guidelines for the emergency care of a patient with a diving-related emergency, such as an air embolism or decompression sickness? (pp. 472–473)

33

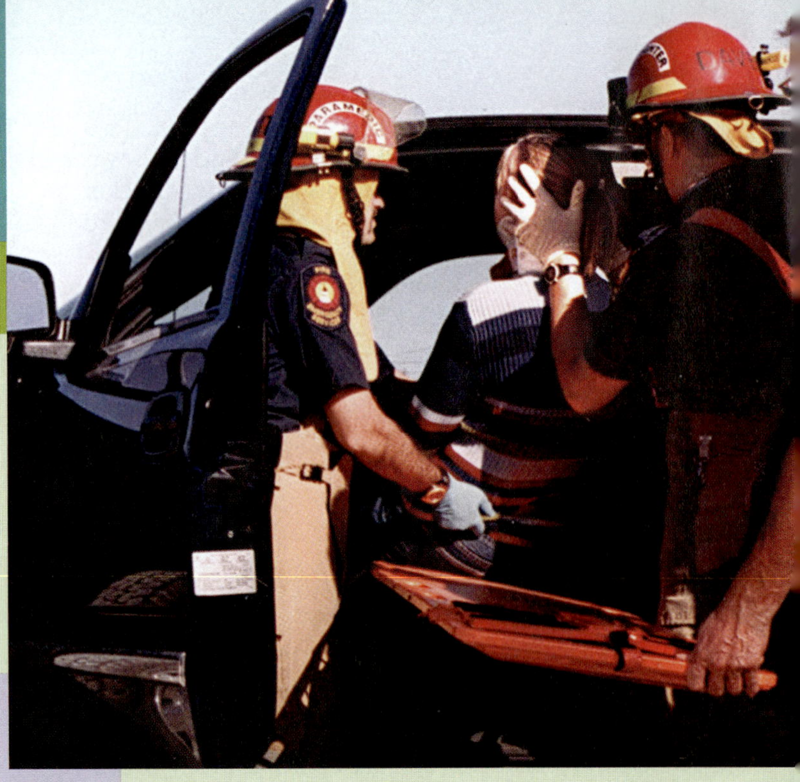

John Mackay

Vehicle Stabilization and Patient Extrication

OBJECTIVES

1. Describe the five types of personal protective equipment recommended for EMRs at the site of an MVA.
2. Discuss six ways to determine the number of patients at the scene of an MVA.
3. Describe the three basic goals of traffic control at the scene of an MVA.
4. State how a rescuer can recognize whether or not a vehicle is stable and describe the basic steps of stabilizing an upright vehicle and an overturned vehicle.
5. Discuss the role of the EMR in extrication and list various methods and tools for gaining single or complex access to the patient.

INTRODUCTION

Most of the time, you will find your patients in safe, easily accessible locations where gaining access is as easy as a knock on a door. However, there will be times when advanced rescue techniques must be used. By far the most common involve motor vehicle accidents (MVAs).

When you arrive at the scene of an MVA, you may find anything from an unhurt occupant and a stable vehicle to multiple vehicles with pinned occupants. This chapter provides an overview of how you can proceed safely and effectively. In practice, be sure to follow all local protocols.

SECTION 1
SCENE SAFETY

Personal Protective Equipment

All EMS responders working in or around a wrecked vehicle with an extrication in progress must wear the following:

- *Eye protection.* Goggles or safety glasses with side shields are best to prevent flying metal shards from penetrating the eyes. Safety glasses with side shields can also be used to protect you from blood-borne pathogens. The flip-down shield on a firefighter helmet is not adequate protection for the eyes.
- *Ear protection.* There are many brands of disposable ear plugs on the market. Generators for extrication equipment can damage your hearing, as can sirens on emergency vehicles. Always have a set available in a pocket or pouch.
- *Hand protection.* While firefighter gloves provide the best puncture protection, they allow for poor manual dexterity. Although they do not offer as much protection, a pair of snugly fitting leather work gloves is a good alternative.
- *Body protection.* In addition to wearing a helmet, a flame-retardant outer shell, such as firefighter turnout gear, brush fire garment, or jumpsuit, provides some protection from fire and limited protection from sharp objects. All garments should have reflective trim to improve night recognition.
- *Foot protection.* Wear turnout pants with either short rubber or leather boots with lug soles to prevent slippage. Boots should be above ankle height to prevent glass from dropping in.

Determine the Number of Patients

In an MVA—just as in every other type of emergency—assess personal safety. Then identify the mechanism of injury or nature of the illness, and determine necessary resources. To determine the resources you need on the scene, find out how many patients are involved. It may be difficult to locate all the patients at first, but it is critical that you do. Use a systematic approach:

- If it is safe to enter the scene, ask a conscious patient to tell you how many others were involved in the MVA.
- Question witnesses to see if any victims have walked away from the scene.
- In case of a high-impact crash, search the surrounding area carefully. Look in the ditches and tall weeds.
- Look for tracks in the earth or snow. A person who was able to get free from the wreckage may be wandering aimlessly.
- Carefully search the vehicle. A patient may be wedged under the dashboard.
- Look quickly for items that give clues to children who are unaccounted for, such as a lunch box, diaper bag, or extra jacket.

Combine this information with your evaluation of scene safety. Are there enough rescue personnel on the scene? If not, send for help immediately. Continue to evaluate the situation for the most efficient, safest way to help patients and protect rescue teams.

If a car is on fire, decide if you can remove the passengers quickly enough or if you should fight the fire. If the passengers are not trapped, move them first. If they cannot be extricated quickly, deal with the fire. This means to safely do what you can within your training and with the available equipment.

Control the Scene

The MVA scene can involve environmental hazards as well as a great deal of confusion. Call for law enforcement and fire services to help control the scene. While you wait for them to arrive, begin scene

CASE STUDY

Dispatch

My partner and I are police officers with EMR training. We were called to Taylor Road just north of Petersfield for an MVA involving multiple casualties. Time out was 10 p.m.

Scene Assessment

As we approached the scene, we saw a small red sports car sitting nose to nose with a large dump truck. The front of the little car was collapsed like an accordion under the front axle of the truck. The front bumper of the truck was even with the windshield of the car. We saw a driver and a passenger in the truck. Both appeared to be conscious. We also saw two motionless young people in the front seat of the car. There was a considerable amount of blood coming from multiple face wounds.

> Consider this emergency as you read Chapter 33. How would you proceed?

control. Quickly deal with bystanders by having them move out of the danger zone.

Spilled gasoline is often present at an MVA. Do not permit smoking on the scene. Turn off all vehicle ignitions. If possible, get a fire crew with hoses to stand by during rescue.

Control Traffic

The basic goals of traffic control at the scene of an MVA are as follows:

- To clear the scene so that emergency vehicles can get through quickly
- To regulate traffic around the scene so that no further crashes or injuries occur
- To regulate traffic so that passing vehicles have minimum inconvenience

Unless a distinct hazard justifies stopping all traffic, keep traffic moving. If the road is blocked, try to move traffic to an alternative route. Whatever you choose to do, make sure that motorists and pedestrians in the area know exactly what you want them to do. Keep rescue personnel well positioned along the roadway. Rescuers should wear reflective clothing so that they can be easily seen before and after dark. Use clear visual signals coupled with attention-getting devices such as flares or cones.

Flares should be set 3 to 5 m apart and extend 30 m toward traffic. The pattern of flares should lead traffic around the emergency. The danger zone includes at least a 15 m radius around the wrecked cars. When the crash occurs on a curve, consider the start of the curve as the edge of the danger zone. On a hill, one edge of the danger zone should be the crest of the hill. If the highway has two lanes, position flares in both directions. If heavy trucks travel the road, extend the flare string because trucks take much longer to stop than cars.

Vehicle Stabilization

After all possible outside hazards are controlled, make the rescue setting as safe as possible. Always suspect that a vehicle is unstable until you have made it stable. Assume the vehicle is not stable in the following circumstances:

- It is on a tilted surface, such as a hill.
- Part of it is stacked on top of another vehicle.
- It is on a slippery surface, such as ice, snow, or spilled oil.
- It is overturned.
- It rests on its side.

The basic premise of vehicle stabilization is cribbing (Figure 33–1). Cribbing is a system of wood or

STABILIZING WITH CRIBBING

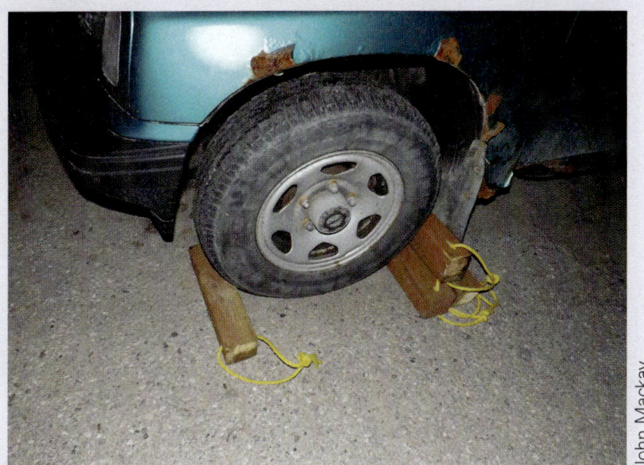

Figure 33–1a   Blocking a wheel.

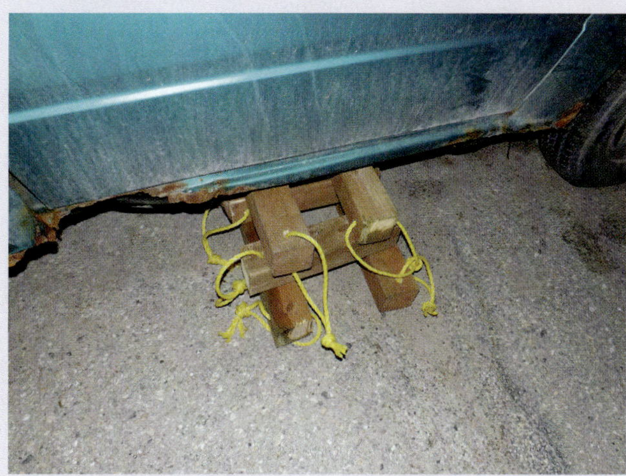

Figure 33–1b   Stacking cribbing for stability.

other supports used to prop up a vehicle. Wood is stacked in box-like squares and wedges to keep uniform pressure. To create a stable environment, the cribbing is arranged perpendicularly to the vehicle frame. Do not crib under wheels or tires because the vehicle will tend to roll. Never stack the cribbing higher than its own length. There should never be more than 5 cm between the cribbing and the vehicle.

Any vehicle that may move easily during extrication or patient care needs to be stabilized by the placement of cribbing or step blocks under the frame and by clipping the valve stems of the tires to let out the air. Excess movement of the vehicle could prove fatal to a patient with severe spinal injuries and may injure the rescue team. To stabilize vehicles, do the following:

- *Upright vehicles.* For a vehicle that rests on all four wheels, place the gear selector in park, or if it is a standard shift, into reverse. Use blocks or wedges at wheels to prevent unexpected rolling. Chock the wheels tightly against the curb when possible. To reduce the amount of movement, even when you are using power tools, cut the tire valve stems so that the car rests on the rims.
- *Overturned vehicles.* To stabilize an overturned vehicle, place a solid object between the roof and the roadway. Use an object such as a wheel chock, spare tire, cribbing, or timber. If necessary, use a bumper jack to angle the vehicle against the solid object until it is stable. Hook a chain to the vehicle's axle. Then loop the chain around a tree or post.

Emergency medical care is generally done before patient extrication, unless a delay would endanger the life of the patient or rescuer. The role of the EMR is to administer emergency medical care. The EMR must also ensure that the patient is removed in a way that minimizes further injury.

In certain circumstances, EMRs are required to take steps to gain access to the patient in a vehicle. Take only the steps you are trained to take. Call for additional assistance and rescue personnel if needed. In such cases, a chain of command should be established to ensure patient care priorities.

Gaining Access

There are two basic ways a rescuer can gain access to a patient. Simple access is access in which no tools are needed. Complex access is access that requires tools and specialized equipment.

Most emergencies do not present access problems. However, when you are confronted with one, quickly evaluate the situation and decide if simple or complex access is needed. If complex access is needed, call for rescuers who have the training and equipment. Remember, getting to the patient safely is critical. A lot of emotion can be involved at a crash scene. Do not allow that to hurry you into a setting that is not safe to enter. Enter the wreck to administer emergency care only when the vehicle is stabilized and safe.

Doors

A door is always the access of choice. This is because it is the largest uncomplicated opening in a vehicle. Always start by testing the door handles.

First try to open the door nearest the patient. If the doors are locked, try to open the lock by either having the patient in the car do it or by using a coat hanger or other device between the door frame and window. Routinely unlock all other doors to allow access for other rescuers. If the doors cannot be opened, determine the best point of entry and proceed accordingly.

Since 1983, cars have been made with a collision beam inside the door, which makes it tougher for a door to cave in. Be aware that the beam can buckle after impact and a sharp end may stick into the passenger compartment. As you try to gain access through a door, be sure that the angle of force does not propel the beam further into the vehicle.

If the frame of the vehicle has been bent on impact, it may not be possible to open a door by releasing the lock mechanism. A hydraulic set of jaws, or spreaders, may be needed to pop the door off its hinges (Figure 33–2). Only a trained technician who can ensure safety for the patient and all rescuers at the scene should carry out this form of extrication.

Windows

Car windows are usually made of tempered glass. Rear and side windows are designed to break into small granules. If you can, remove the window without breaking it. Fine particles of glass can stay unnoticed in a deep wound and cause damage after it closes. Cover the patient with a heavy safety blanket before breaking a window.

If fixed windows are installed in U-shaped black plastic or rubber, remove the rim. Insert the point of a linoleum knife, or similar tool, into the moulding at the midpoint of the glass. Keep the blade as flat against the glass as you can. Draw the knife across the top and down the side. Repeat on the other side. Soapy water will keep the blade moving easily. Work the end of a short pry bar behind the glass and pry it loose from the top. The window will pivot on its bottom edge.

If you must break a window, locate the window farthest from the patient. Give a quick hard thrust in the lower corner with a spring-loaded punch, screwdriver, or other sharp object (Figure 33–3). If you can, put strips of broad tape or a sheet of contact

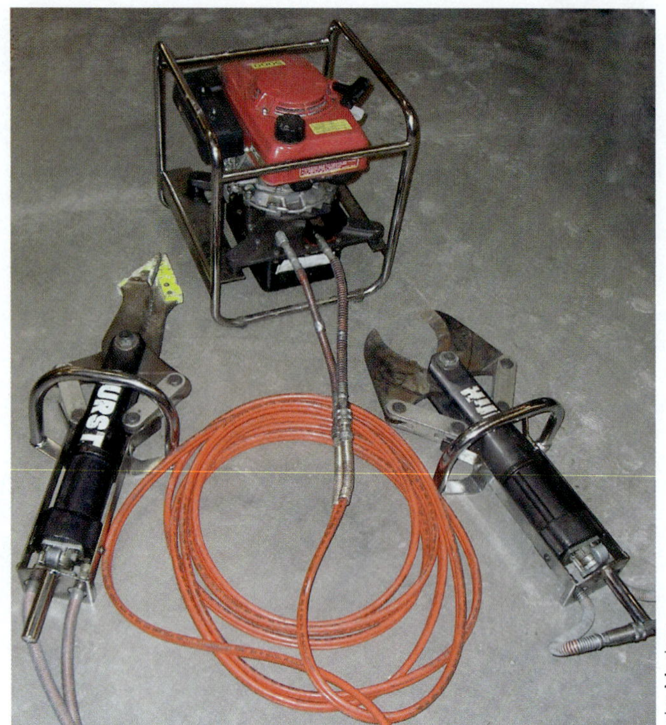

Figure 33–2 Jaws, or spreaders.

John Mackay

paper over the glass to prevent broken pieces from spraying onto the patient. Use your gloved hand to carefully pull the glass outside the vehicle. Clear all the glass away from the window opening. Reach in to open the door or roll down the window. If you must crawl in, drape a heavy tarp or blanket over the door edge and the interior of the car just below the window.

Windshield

Windshields are usually made of laminated safety glass, which cannot be safely broken. If the windshield is largely intact, pry up the chrome trim at the joints using a baling hook, pry bar, or screwdriver.

To remove the rubber seal that holds the windshield in the car, use a linoleum knife to slice the rubber bead. Drive the point into the channel and keep the blade flat against the glass. Then force a screwdriver behind the glass and simply pop out the windshield. For a Mastic-set windshield, remove the moulding. Then use a Mastic cutter to free the windshield. The Mastic cutter may be obtained from an auto parts store or an auto windshield business.

Removal of a broken Mastic-set windshield may cause a great deal of splintering. Therefore, as with any extrication, you and the patient must be properly protected. Cover the patient with a safety blanket. Make sure each rescuer has full facial protection and is wearing a long-sleeved shirt and heavy gloves.

BREAKING A CAR WINDOW

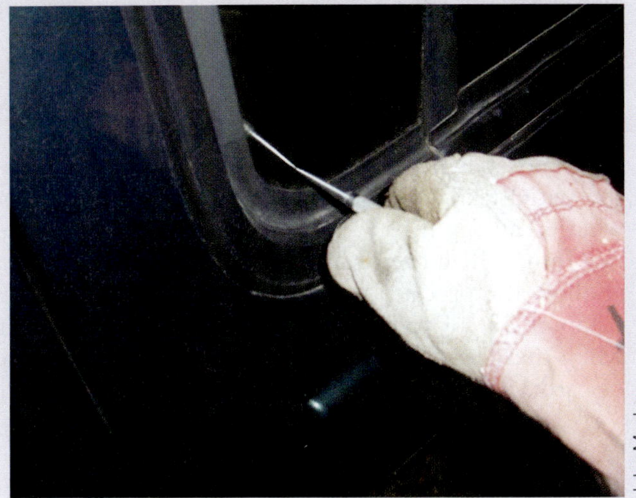

Figure 33–3a   Position a punch in the corner of the side window farthest away from the patient.

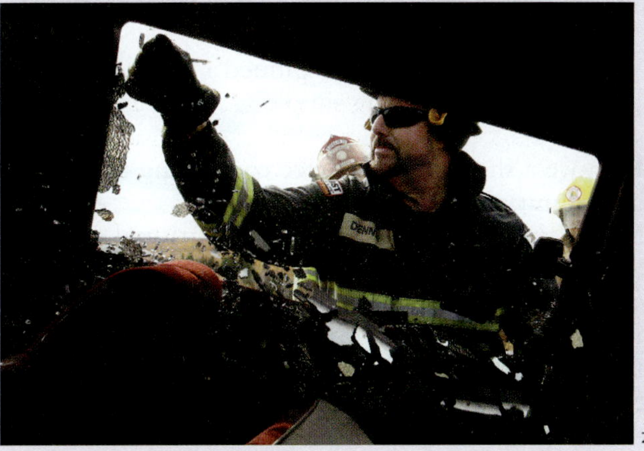

Figure 33–3b   Push in the shattered tempered glass, and reach in to open the door or roll down the window.

Always consider using an alternative entry method before breaking or cutting glass.

Airbags

If the airbag has been released, there may be some residue. This is not harmful and can be washed off. If the airbag (Figure 33–4) was not triggered by the crash, disconnect the negative side of the battery and the yellow airbag connector. Do not cut the connector or its wires; they keep the shorting bar activated, preventing accidental triggering. Some newer models have a passenger airbag shutoff switch. This is meant to protect small children in child seats, but can also be shut off when rescuers are attempting to extricate a patient.

Pinned Patients

Always summon a rescue unit when a patient is pinned beneath a vehicle. To raise a vehicle that has not completely overturned, use a sturdy jack. A pry bar and blocks may be used. A large group of bystanders can assist in lifting the vehicle off a patient. Be sure to shore up the vehicle so that it will not fall on the patient.

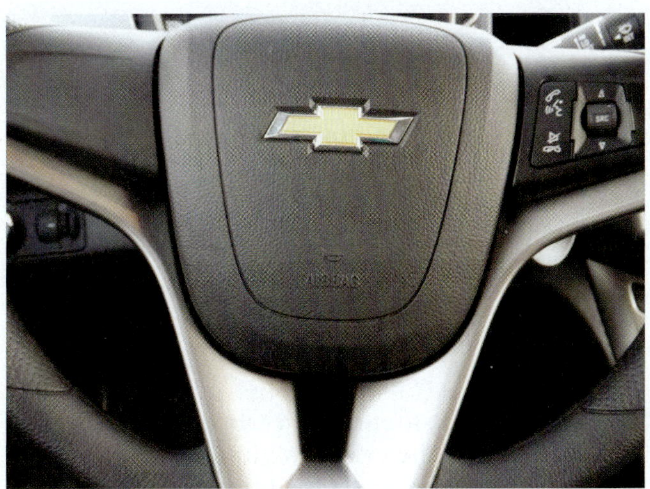

Figure 33–4a   Airbag compartment indicator.

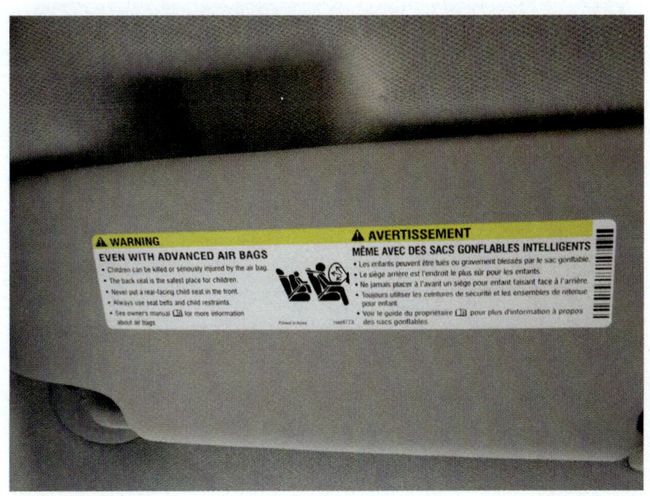

Figure 33–4b   Warning labels for airbags.

If a patient has a body part through a window, pad the extruded part well with bandaging material. Then, carefully use pliers or a knife to break or fold away the glass. Once the body part is freed, care for it.

If a patient is jammed or pinned inside the vehicle, consider the following simple procedures:

- Remove a shoe or other piece of clothing that may be pinning the patient.
- Move the front seat to give additional working space. It may be possible to lift the back seat entirely.
- Seat belts that will not open can be cut with shears or a knife. Support the dangling patient as you cut the belt.

Emergency Care of the Patient

As in any emergency, your first priority is always your own safety. (You cannot assist the patient if you become another casualty.) Be sure the scene is safe, the vehicle is stable, and you are wearing the appropriate personal protective equipment before you try to reach the patient.

After gaining safe access, provide the same care you would give to any trauma patient. Stabilize the head and neck. Complete a primary assessment. Provide critical interventions. Be sure you have called for the necessary resources.

Remain with the patient during a complex extrication. Continually monitor his or her condition. If it begins to deteriorate, advise the rescue crew. They may be able to change the approach to the incident and get the patient out more quickly. During the process, be sure to protect yourself and the patient from breaking glass and flying debris. Use heavy blankets, a tarp, or even a solid object like a backboard.

Try to keep the patient calm during the rescue. Even with altered mental status, the patient may become very frightened. Keep him or her informed about what is being done to help. For example, let the patient know when a loud noise will occur and what is causing it.

Immobilize the patient's spine during the rescue. (Follow the precautions and procedures described in Chapter 25.) The only exception to this rule occurs when there is an immediate threat to life, such as fire, or cardiac arrest and an emergency move is required.

Extrication Tools and Equipment

The majority of provinces in Canada have specially designed systems of patient extrication. The equipment is costly and requires special training. When possible and appropriate, contact the local rescue squad immediately after an MVA in which someone is trapped. They will be able to get to the patient quickly and safely.

It is important to be prepared in case a rescue squad is not available. Basic tools that can be used include hammers, screwdrivers, chisels, crowbars, pliers, linoleum knives, work gloves, goggles, shovels, tire irons, wrenches, knives, car jacks, and ropes or chains. Ingenuity can put these tools to work in a safe and effective way.

EMR FOCUS

Whether on or off duty, you will come across an MVA at some point in your career as an EMR. Most of the decisions you will make involving vehicle access and stabilization will be made during the scene assessment.

For your own safety, consider the following:

- Whether or not the vehicle is stable (Remember, unstable vehicles can shift and injure you.)
- Whether or not there are hazardous materials present (This includes transported substances and leaking gasoline.)

Patient care considerations include the following:

- Can access to the patient be gained?
- Can access be gained by simple or complex procedures?
- What is the priority of the patient? What are his or her injuries?
- Can the patient be removed from the vehicle while immobilized on a backboard? Will extrication require cutting or moving parts of the vehicle?

Careful consideration early in the call will help the rest of the call flow smoothly. It will also prevent unnecessary delays in patient access and transport.

CASE STUDY FOLLOW-UP

At the beginning of this chapter, you read that EMRs were on the scene of an MVA with multiple patients. To see how the chapter skills apply to this emergency, read the following. It describes how the call was completed.

SCENE ASSESSMENT *(Continued)*

This was a complex access situation. We immediately updated dispatch and requested specialized rescue crews and an ambulance for each patient. Then we positioned our vehicle about 40 m from the wreckage to give the rescue units space to pull in.

Once it was safe to approach, we saw that both vehicles had all four wheels on solid ground and appeared to be stable. We made sure that both engines were turned off and that the emergency brakes were on. We also looked for any smoke or leaks.

PRIMARY ASSESSMENT

Then we attempted to gain access to the patients and perform triage. From the open windows, we did as much of a primary assessment as we could on the patients in the sports car. The occupants of the truck did not appear to be seriously injured. They were alert with minor complaints. We instructed them to remain in their seats until more help arrived. Most of the damage and injuries were to the sports car and its occupants.

We were taking spinal precautions and attempting to maintain airways and control serious bleeding of the patients when the first ambulance arrived.

TRANSFER OF CARE

We reported the number of patients and our initial observations to the paramedics, including which patients we believed were a first priority.

While they proceeded to assess and care for the patients, we provided direction to the other responding units.

It took a while for the patients to be disentangled from the wreckage. We assisted in every way we could—from redirecting traffic to holding manual stabilization of a patient's head and neck during extrication.

After the patients were freed, we helped the paramedics quickly reassess them and move them into the ambulances.

> As in all emergency situations, remember that your first priority is your own safety. Do not enter the scene of an emergency until you have determined that it is safe. Do not attempt a complex rescue unless you are trained and equipped to do so. Follow your local protocols.

NOCPs

3.2 b Transfer patient from various positions using applicable equipment and/or techniques **S**

c Transfer patient using emergency evacuation techniques **S**

d Secure patient to applicable equipment **S**

3.3 a Assess scene for safety **S**

b Address potential occupational hazards **S**

c Conduct basic extrication **S**

REVIEW QUESTIONS

Page references where answers may be found or supported are provided at the end of each question.

SECTION 1

1. What are some types of personal protective equipment a rescuer should wear at the site of an MVA? (p. 476)

2. What are the basic goals of traffic control at the scene of an MVA? (p. 477)

3. How can a rescuer recognize whether or not a vehicle is stable? (p. 477)

4. What are some basic methods of stabilizing an upright vehicle? An overturned vehicle? (pp. 477–478)

5. In general, what is the role of the EMR in extrication? (p. 478)

SECTION 2

6. What is the difference between simple and complex access? (p. 478)

7. What is always the access of choice? Explain your answer. (p. 479)

8. If you must break a window to gain access to an entrapped patient, which window should you break? (p. 479)

9. What simple procedures should you consider if a patient is jammed or pinned inside a vehicle? (p. 480–481)

10. What are some basic guidelines for the emergency medical care of patients who are trapped in wreckage? (p. 481)

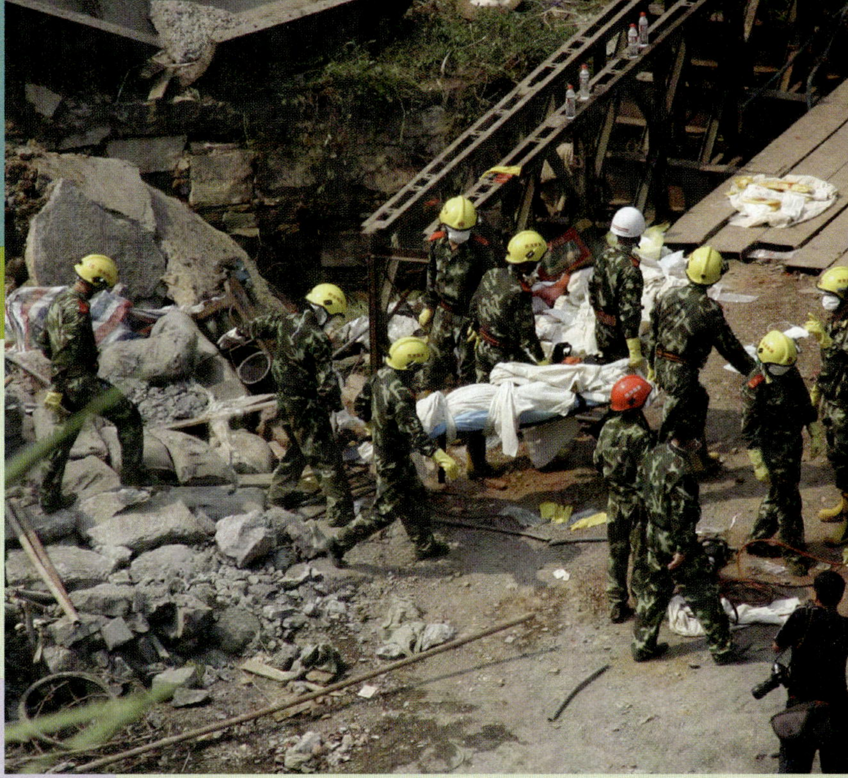

Special Rescue Situations

O B J E C T I V E S

1. Define a confined-space emergency and describe some of the inherent hazards for rescuers.
2. Identify the role of the EMR in a confined-space emergency.
3. Discuss the three general guidelines for performing safe litter carries over distances on rough terrain.
4. State the criteria for identifying a rescue as low angle or high angle.
5. Describe the basic capabilities of a helicopter in rescue operations.
6. List the characteristics of a safe helicopter landing zone and describe the procedure for safely approaching a helicopter that has just landed.

INTRODUCTION

People who are drawn to public safety and emergency work tend to be highly action oriented. They almost always prefer to do something rather than just stand and watch. The problem is that taking action in situations where you may be unaware of the hazards can result in serious injury or even death. This chapter will introduce you to some of the hazards of special rescue—hazards that could go unnoticed until it is too late.

SECTION 1
CONFINED-SPACE EMERGENCIES

Most of the time, we do not think about the air we breathe unless it has a bad odour or is irritating in some way. Unfortunately, not all hazards in the environment warn us with odours. Confined spaces can be especially dangerous to rescuers as well as to patients.

A confined space is defined as a place with limited access to get in and out that is not designed for human occupancy. Some examples of confined spaces are as follows:

- *Silos.* Silos are used in agriculture to store solid materials. Some are designed specifically to limit the presence of oxygen. Hazards include poisonous gases emitted during the natural fermentation of crops as well as engulfment and suffocation. Silos are perhaps the most common sites of confined-space emergencies.
- *Storage bins.* These include both grain bins and grain elevators. Like silos, they present the hazards of low oxygen levels and engulfment.
- *Underground vaults* (Figure 34–1). These include utility vaults for water, sewer, electrical power, telephone, and other communications cables. Hazards include poisonous gases and electrocution.
- *Wells, culverts, and cisterns.* These offer little oxygen and a high risk of drowning or entrapment.

A low oxygen level is a significant, common hazard in confined spaces. Also common are poisonous gases, such as hydrogen sulphide, carbon dioxide, carbon monoxide, and methane. Note that sometimes the atmosphere is explosive as well as poisonous.

Safety Precautions

The Occupational Health and Safety (OHS) regulations of Human Resources and Skills Development Canada take an aggressive approach to safety for workers in confined spaces. Among the rules are the following:

- The atmosphere must be properly ventilated and monitored for oxygen, carbon monoxide, and hydrogen sulphide.

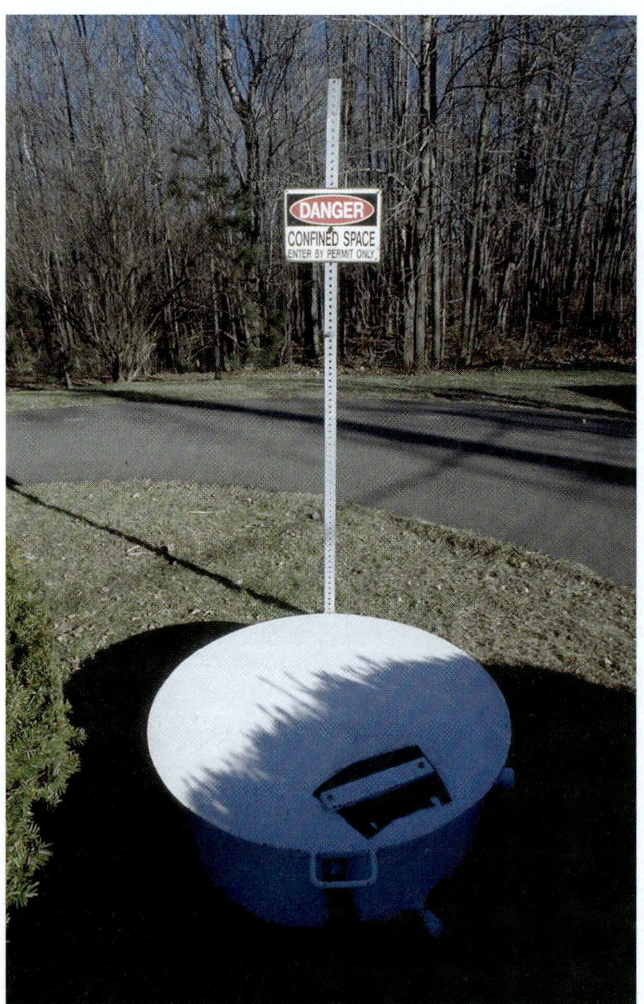

Pearson Education/PH College

Figure 34–1 Warning of a confined underground space.

CASE STUDY

Dispatch

My EMR unit was dispatched for an automobile crash on provincial road 402—the farthest part of our district. The report was that a car had left the road and rolled over.

Scene Assessment

We approached the scene. There were no signs of wires down, leaking gas, or hazardous materials. The car looked like it had been bounced around a lot but somehow ended up on its wheels. There was one passenger inside the vehicle. We put on our gear and gloves and approached. There was a star in the windshield where the driver had hit his head. The steering wheel was bent. We were unable to open the doors because the roof was pushed down on them. Rescue was notified.

> Consider this situation as you read Chapter 34. How would you proceed?

- Electrical systems must be locked and lagged out (discharged).
- Stored energy must be dissipated.
- Pipes must be disconnected or blanked out (blocked).
- A person who plans to enter a space must use the appropriate respiratory protection, such as a self-contained breathing apparatus.

A call to a confined-space emergency is usually for a fall, medical problem, asphyxia, explosion, or machinery entrapment. As an EMR, your responsibility is to recognize the emergency and to call for the proper help as soon as possible. Do not enter a scene unless you know that it is safe. Only members of specialized teams that are trained and equipped for the emergency should enter.

When you are called to a confined-space emergency, proceed with scene assessment as follows:

1. Determine the nature of the emergency.
   - Obtain a copy of the permit for the site and assess the type of work being done.
   - Determine how many workers are inside the confined space.
   - Without entering the space, determine what the hazards are.
2. Call for a specialized rescue team as well as for emergency medical personnel and transportation.
3. Establish a perimeter, and do not allow anyone to enter.
4. When they arrive, assist medical or rescue personnel if you are trained to do so and if you can do so safely.

Cave-Ins and Rescues from Trenches

OHS requires shoring in any trench that is deeper than 1.4 m with sides that are sloped at an angle of 45 degrees or more to the horizontal. They suggest that employers provide a system of steel plates and bracing from ground level to the bottom of the trench. Unfortunately, a contractor or a do-it-yourselfer sometimes does not use such shoring. Excavated soil may be too close to the top edge of a trench, and ground vibration, water seepage, or an intersecting trench could cause one of the walls to give way.

Most trench collapses occur at sites that are less than 2 m wide and 4 m deep. In most cases, a worker will have been inside the trench when the walls collapsed, burying the worker either partially or completely. If someone jumps into the trench to try to rescue the worker, a secondary collapse occurs and the rescuer also gets buried.

Soil weighs about 50 kg per cubic metre. This means that 60 cm of soil piled on top of a person's back or chest is equal to about 450 kg. Therefore, even if a person is only partially buried, the weight of the soil on his or her chest can cause respiratory difficulties. To safely rescue such a victim requires methodical and strenuous effort. It can be a slow process.

No matter how the cave-in occurred, if the trench is more than waist deep, a specialized trench rescue team is needed. As an EMR, your job is to secure the scene by establishing a perimeter. Do not allow anyone to enter the trench or its immediate area. Call for the rescue team as soon as possible. Remember, if a collapse has occurred, another one is very likely.

Suspension Injuries

Suspension injuries can occur when an individual's blood circulation is compromised while entangled and hanging. Often, the person is suspended in a rope or harness and the trauma is created as the body's own hanging weight impedes the circulation beyond the point of contact. EMRs dealing with suspension trauma must quickly recognize the need for appropriate scene assistance such as high-angle rescue teams.

Once a patient is brought down safely, typical suspension injuries must be considered. While these can include fractures, dislocations, strains, and sprains, the greatest concern is the lack of circulation that occurred while the patient was suspended. Because the entangling item can act as a tourniquet, impeding blood flow to and from a limb, compartment syndrome can occur. **Compartment syndrome** is a lack of blood and oxygen to tissues due to rising pressures in a restricted or isolated limb. When this happens, the region can become cyanotic as oxygen is consumed by the tissues. Pooling and clotting of blood can also occur. This, in turn, can cause further problems when clots and deoxygenated blood are released back into the central circulation.

Any musculoskeletal injury to the extremities, especially the forearm or leg, can potentially cause compartment syndrome. The following are signs and symptoms of compartment syndrome:

- Feeling of pressure within the limb
- Loss of sensation, particularly in the webs between fingers and toes
- Pain in the limb
- More severe condition than expected by the mechanism of injury
- Pain while trying to extend the limb
- Excessive time spent in suspension mechanism
- Decreased pulse in the extremity, distal to the injury

To treat a victim of suspension trauma, administer oxygen and maintain the patient in a sitting position. This is extremely important because laying a patient down could allow blood clots that have formed to block critical vessels. Also, a rush of deoxygenated blood back to the vital organs can create hypoxia in the patient.

If a spinal injury is suspected and immobilization is required, consider using an extrication vest. Place the patient in a semi-sitting position and administer high-flow oxygen via a non-rebreather mask. If you must use a long backboard, elevate the head of the board as best you can while considering the patient's condition. This will slow return circulation to the vital organs and give the blood a chance to oxygenate properly. Monitor vital signs. Advise incoming paramedic units of the patient's mechanism of injury and your suspicion of suspension trauma.

SECTION 2
ROUGH TERRAIN EVACUATIONS

More people are engaging in—and getting injured by—mountain biking, skiing, rock climbing, and other types of rough-terrain sports. As an EMR, you may be required to assist in the evacuation of these patients.

Litter Carries

It takes 10 to 12 people to carry a **litter**, or portable stretcher, for 1 km. Wheels may be attached to some types of portable stretchers, but they work well only on fairly flat terrain.

To perform a litter carry over rough terrain for some distance, follow these general guidelines:

- Select teams of four to six bearers each (Figure 34–2). Members of each team should be about equal in height.

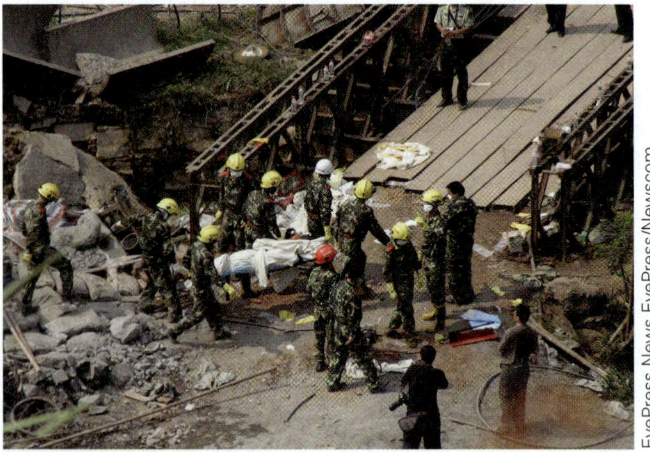

Figure 34–2   Litter carry over rough terrain.

- After a team carries the portable stretcher a short distance, team members should change positions and then sides.
- After another short distance, a fresh team should rotate into position and take over.

High-Angle and Low-Angle Rescues

When the angle of the terrain increases, the risk of falling and dropping a patient on a litter increases. One way to manage this risk is to use a rope system to lift or lower the stretcher while rescuers hold it and guide it (Figure 34–3).

In most cases, a high-angle rescue is obvious. It could involve moving up or down a cliff, gorge, or side of a building. If you have any doubt, a high-angle rescue team is needed under the following conditions:

- The slope forms more than a 40-degree angle.
- Slips or falls could result in serious injury or death due to the dangerous terrain below the slope.

- The terrain is so hazardous that it requires rappelling. (Rappelling is a special technique for getting down a cliff by means of a secured rope.)

Generally, a low-angle rescue does not need a rope system. You can identify a low-angle rescue by the following conditions:

- The slope forms less than a 40-degree angle.
- The rescuers' hands are not needed for balancing or scrambling.
- Slips or falls would not likely result in serious injury or death.

As soon as you recognize a low- or high-angle emergency, call immediately for specialized personnel to perform the rescue. Follow your local protocols.

A helicopter's ability to hover, land in small spaces, and carry people and equipment makes it a logical rescue method. Over the years, search and rescue operations have come to depend on helicopters (Figure 34–4). However, ground-based rescue efforts should never wait for air support. Weather conditions or other aircraft limitations can result in significant delays. Therefore, when calling for air support, make sure you have a backup plan in case air rescue is delayed or impossible. See Table 34–1 for guidelines on when to request air support.

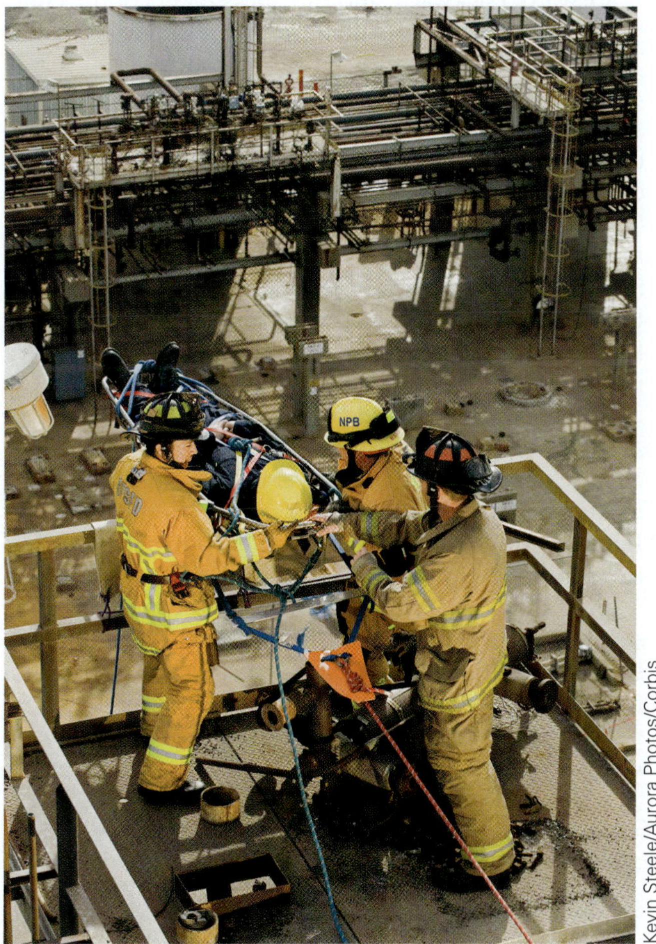

Figure 34–3 Rope system used for a high-angle rescue.

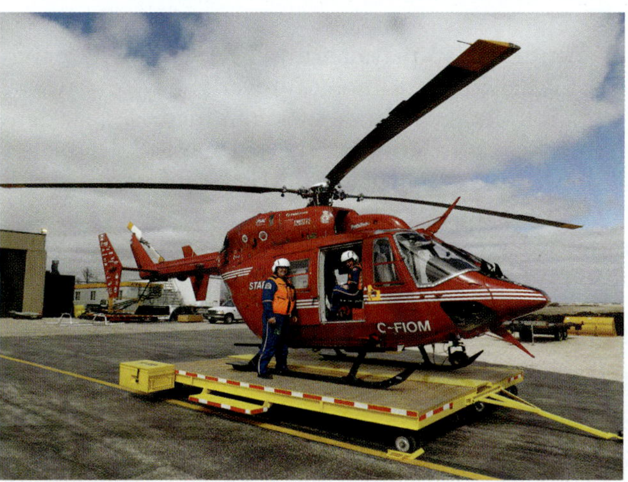

Figure 34–4 Helicopter rescue.

<table>
<tr><td colspan="2" align="center">TABLE 34–1
WHEN TO CALL FOR A HELICOPTER</td></tr>
<tr><td>Operational Reasons</td><td>Medical Reasons</td></tr>
<tr><td valign="top">

- Normal ground travel to the appropriate medical facility would take more than 30 minutes.
- Extrication will be prolonged.
- The location of the emergency is a remote site.
- The patient needs paramedic-level care.

</td><td valign="top">

- The patient has a life- or limb-threatening condition.
- The patient's condition is unstable (shock, head injury with altered mental status, chest trauma with respiratory distress, penetrating injuries to body cavity, amputations, burns over 15 percent of the body or to the face).
- There is a serious mechanism of injury (fall of 5 m or more, blow from a vehicle travelling over 30 km/h, ejection from vehicle, a rollover without restraints, major deformity to passenger compartment or to vehicle's front end, death of one of the car passengers).

</td></tr>
</table>

Helicopter Capabilities

Weather Limitations

An aircraft can take off and land either visually or by way of instruments. However, only instrument flight rules (IFR) are used to fly from one airport to another. Sometimes they are used to guide a pilot to safety when the weather suddenly turns bad.

Visibility is crucial to rescue operations. The pilot and crew must be able to see the ground team for flight instructions. An aircraft will not be able to launch if visibility is below minimum standards. A good rule of thumb to follow to estimate minimum flight conditions at the rescue site is as follows:

- *Day*—500 foot (approximately 150 m) cloud ceiling and 1 mile (1.6 km) of visibility
- *Night*—1000 foot (approximately 300 m) cloud ceiling and 3 miles (4.8 km) of visibility

Altitude also plays an important role. The ability of a helicopter to hold a hover is key to a rescue operation. As the altitude of a craft increases, air density decreases. In addition, the warmer the air, the less dense it is. As air density decreases, more power is needed for the aircraft to hover. At some point, altitude or air temperature may make it impossible to accomplish a rescue mission.

Control Systems

Piloting a helicopter is complex. The pilot must be able to operate three main control systems:

- The *collective* controls the angle of the main rotor blades. It also controls the vertical motion of the craft. By using the collective and a great deal of power, the aircraft can lift off the ground.
- The *cyclic* tilts the spinning rotors and produces the forward, backward, and side movements of the craft.
- The *rudder pedals* control the pitch of the tail rotor and the rotation of the aircraft.

During takeoff, the helicopter pilot must increase the power and rotor speed. Then he or she uses the collective to increase the angle of the rotor blades and lift off. The cyclic is moved forward to make the transition from vertical lift to forward flight. As the aircraft moves forward, additional air speed is needed for more lift. Once the craft is at the proper altitude, the need for power is reduced. Because of the engine power needed, takeoffs and landings are dangerous times.

The controls of the helicopter are very sensitive. A small movement of one of them can mean a major change in the altitude of the craft. To pilot a helicopter during a hover is especially strenuous and stressful. It has been compared to rubbing your belly, patting the top of your head, and reciting a poem all at once.

In addition, when in a hover, the pilot cannot see the target below. The crew chief watches the spot and verbally guides the pilot. The pilot also needs to spot a reference point. Normally, this is tricky. At night or in low-light conditions, it can be very difficult.

Space and Load

Some crafts are large enough to carry a whole squad of people. Others are small and cannot hold many more than a pilot, a patient, and one crew member. In general, helicopters are very weight sensitive.

When the capacity of a craft is listed, it usually does not take into account the fuel load, crew, equipment, altitude, and air temperature. All these factors have a major influence on the performance of the craft. If a craft is heavily weighted, for example, it may be able to land in a tight spot, but it may not be able to take off again without getting rid of unnecessary gear or crew.

Special Tactics

One of the main reasons to choose a helicopter for rescue is its ability to pick up and extract people without landing. That involves hoisting, rappelling, and flying with external loads. All these tactics are risky. Because of the danger and stress of hovering, special tactics are almost always aimed at reducing hover time.

Hoisting

Some aircraft are equipped with mechanical hoists. They are made to insert (or place) people onto or extract people off the ground. They are most commonly found on military craft and on some public safety aircraft.

Hoisting operations require hover time, which will vary depending on the speed of the hoist and the amount of cable out. Operations are also limited by the safe working load of the cable and by the number of duty cycles of the system.

If you work around helicopters that have hoists, become familiar with the ground safety procedures. One that applies to all hoist cables relates to static electricity. When a cable is lowered, it must touch the ground to allow its electrical charge to dissipate. If the cable is touched before that happens, the first person who touches it will get an electrical jolt.

SPIE Line

The use of a special insertion and extrication (SPIE) line is called the short-haul technique. It was developed by mountain rescue teams in Europe and by Parks Canada. It involves flying beneath the helicopter as an external load. It is commonly used with light-duty aircraft without hoists to both insert and extract rescuers and patients.

Generally, a weighted and backed-up rope system is attached to the cargo hook or belly band of a helicopter. At the other end of the rope, rescuers in flight helmets with communications and harnesses are clipped in. When the helicopter ascends, the rescuers dangle beneath the craft as they are flown to the target area and gently lowered to the ground. This is insertion.

To extract, the craft flies into position and the ground team clips the litter or patients into the SPIE line. They are then flown back to a staging area and gently lowered into position.

Both insertion and extraction are risky operations. They should only be undertaken by specialized rescue teams. Note that if an external load becomes destabilized during flight or if an emergency occurs in which the helicopter and crew are in jeopardy, an external load may be jettisoned.

Landing Zones

The helicopter landing zone should be at least 30 m by 30 m. The **landing zone (LZ)** should be flat or have no more than an eight-degree slope. The LZ should also have the following characteristics (Table 34–2):

- *Free of obstructions.* That includes wires, trees, buildings, and other obstructions. If it is surrounded by obstructions, the pilot will be forced into a vertical takeoff, which takes tremendous power and is very dangerous. If there are any obstructions near the LZ, inform the pilot by radio.
- *No loose objects.* Anything on the ground that is loose will blow around in the 160 km/h rotor wash of the helicopter. Stones, dirt, and other objects are easily picked up and blown into people and vehicles, causing both injury and property damage.
- *Scene lighting.* Keep emergency lights on to help the pilot locate the scene. Also, place markers on all four corners of the LZ. Chemical light sticks or small strobe lights work well. Avoid shining spotlights on the helicopter because they can blind the pilot.
- *Traffic control.* The LZ must be absolutely secure. There should be no traffic within 30 m of the aircraft.

Both the main and tail rotors on a helicopter are extremely dangerous. Do not approach the craft until the pilot or crew chief signals you to approach or escorts you to the craft. Never approach from the rear. The tail rotor spins so fast that it is nearly invisible, and it can kill. In addition, the main rotor may be

TABLE 34–2
LANDING ZONE GUIDELINES

- Approximately 30 m × 30 m area
- Free of all obstructions
- Clear of wires, towers, vehicles, people, and loose objects
- Firm ground with less than eight-degree slope
- Markers on all four corners
- All emergency red lights on
- No white lights, spotlights, or blue lights directed toward the helicopter or landing zone
- No smoking

lower than it appears to be. Depending on the grade of the LZ, the spinning blade may be no more than a couple of metres above the ground.

If you are signalled to approach the helicopter, maintain eye contact with the pilot or crew chief. Approach only from the front. Stay low. Avoid carrying anything above your head. Avoid wearing anything loose that can be blown away by the rotor wash.

SECTION 4
OTHER SPECIAL RESCUE SITUATIONS

Cold Environment Extrication

If the temperature is −30°C and a wind chill is present, the primary assessment is performed, but treatment and secondary assessment may have to wait until you can get the patient to a warmer environment. Oxygen adjuncts and BVM devices will not function well in extremely low temperatures. Remove the patient as quickly as possible to a more suitable environment. Be sure to handle an extremely cold patient with care because abrupt movement can cause the heart to fibrillate.

Aluminum stretchers and oxygen cylinders need very little exposure time to become cold enough to create a risk of frostbite to the patient or rescuer. When you hear the weather report on a cold winter day, organize appropriate clothing, including warm hand gear and footwear, before starting on a shift.

Elevator Rescue

Getting stuck in an elevator can be stressful. In everyday life, when the elevator doors close the occupants find themselves alone, or with strangers, in a confined space. Claustrophobia, a fear of confined spaces, can become a reality for elevator occupants during a stall. Elevators stall for one of three reasons: power failure, mechanical failure, and safety mechanisms overriding the system. It is beyond the scope of regular EMR duties to try to resolve elevator operational issues. While the majority of elevator stalls are corrected promptly and do not act as a catalyst for medical emergencies, an elevator that stops abruptly can cause trauma to its occupants.

When responding to an elevator emergency, have your dispatch confirm that the elevator service company has been notified. The elevator technician will likely respond and remedy a mechanical problem before a trained fire crew can conduct a rescue.

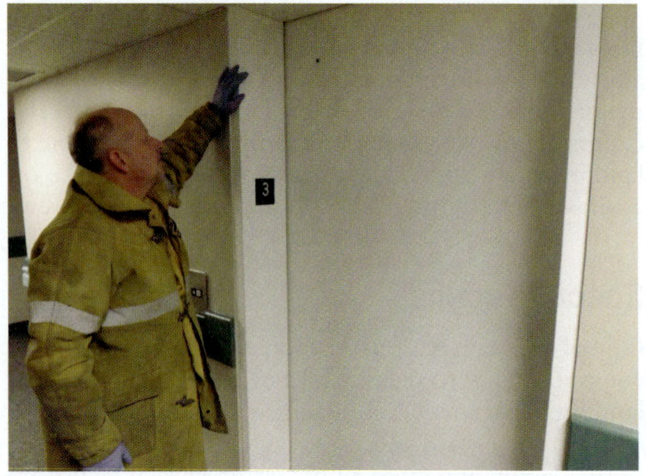

John Mackay

Figure 34–5 Elevator rescue.

Upon arrival at the scene, determine which floor the elevator is stalled at. Use the stairs to arrive at the floor closest to where the stall has occurred. Do not attempt to force the doors open if you have not been trained in elevator rescue, as you could further complicate accessibility and functioning of the elevator (Figure 34–5).

One EMR should establish communication with one occupant in order to help calm and reassure all occupants. The following are some points to consider as you await access:

- Tell them who you are and that you are a part of a coordinated effort to get them out safely as soon as possible.
- Assure them that there is no shortage of air and that they will be able to breathe comfortably. They should remain calm and not try to devise their own exit strategy.
- Confirm the number of occupants and ask if everyone is okay.
- If there are patients requiring medical attention before access is gained, discuss basic first aid techniques with your inside contact in order to help stabilize them.
- If there is no cellular phone service within the elevator, you may offer to have contact made with outside parties. This can alleviate the anxiety of feeling "trapped" and "incommunicado."
- Update the occupants of all progress being made in their regard. Knowledge is power and reassurance.

Ongoing communication will decrease anxiety, since the occupants will be aware that they have not been forgotten by those outside of the elevator. This will help time pass until the elevator technician arrives or the fire department plans a rescue.

When access is gained and secured, conduct your assessment and treatment outside of the elevator as you would with any patient.

Bariatric Emergencies

Any medical or trauma emergency can become a bariatric emergency if you encounter a patient who is larger or heavier than you can easily handle without additional resources.

If information about an extremely obese patient is not conveyed through your dispatch, you must advise incoming crews so that proper resources can be dispatched. Many EMS systems have developed a dedicated vehicle with special devices and paramedics trained for handling bariatric emergencies.

Both access and egress will have to be planned in advance. Many bariatric patients have not been out of their homes in a long time, so there may be physical impediments to getting equipment in and the patient out safely.

Assessment and treatment should be conducted as with any other patient. Bariatric patients can have a higher incidence of specific health concerns which can exist simultaneously. Cardiac and respiratory problems can be exacerbated by their bodies' increased metabolic demands. Musculoskeletal problems may be prevalent if joints are deteriorated. They can have poor circulation as well as integumentary issues such as skin breakdown and infections.

Do not let the patients' size intimidate you and do not allow personal or societal bias to be evident

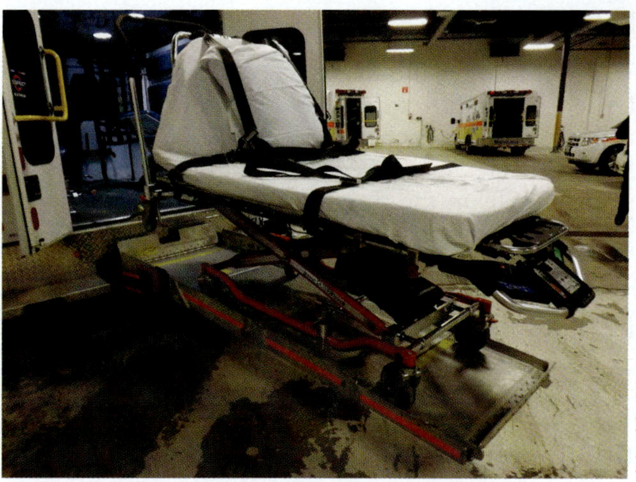

Figure 34–6   Bariatric emergency stretcher.

John Mackay

or to affect your care. Maintain your professionalism by communicating with the patient directly. Limit the number of responders that observe your assessment as you await the paramedics. The patient may be able to suggest the best way for you to assist him or her as you perform your history taking and assessments. Employ personal protective equipment as usual and utilize sufficient resources for personal and patient safety. Many hands, and the right equipment (Figure 34–6), make light work.

EMR FOCUS

One of the reasons you have decided to become an EMR may be the varied situations you will encounter. This chapter may have covered the most unusual. However, times change, and so have the situations in which people find themselves when in need of rescue.

Rescue technology and procedures have kept up with those changes. They have advanced dramatically in the past several years. It is now possible to safely rescue a person from a confined space or mountain slope and transport him or her to a trauma centre capable of handling the most complex and serious injuries.

Know the resources and special teams available in your area before you encounter a need to call them.

CASE STUDY FOLLOW-UP

At the beginning of this chapter, you read that EMRs were at the scene of an MVA. To see how the chapter skills apply to this emergency, read the following. It describes how the call was completed.

PRIMARY ASSESSMENT

The patient was moaning. He seemed to know who we were but he wasn't alert. He was moving air and

had no blood or other airway obstructions. We didn't see any obvious bleeding. The man's skin was pale and moist. My partner reached in through where the driver's side rear window used to be and stabilized his head, and I checked his pulse by reaching in through where his window had been. It was 110 and weak.

We were concerned about the mechanism of injury and the signs of shock. I radioed for the MedFlight helicopter. They were available and had an ETA of less than 20 minutes.

SECONDARY ASSESSMENT

We couldn't get the man out of the car, so we continued the stabilization. I began an assessment. He appeared to have a chest injury and a contusion to his forehead. His level of consciousness had diminished somewhat from the time we arrived. We had oxygen with us, so we applied it via a non-rebreather mask.

PATIENT HISTORY

We were unable to obtain a history.

ONGOING ASSESSMENT

We monitored the patient closely until the paramedics arrived.

TRANSFER OF CARE

After we reported what little we knew, the paramedics began emergency care. I went across the street to a level area and checked out a landing zone for the helicopter. I radioed dispatch with the exact location. There were wires on our side of the road, so I warned them that the pilot had to be careful.

Rescue had begun to extricate the patient. It didn't take that long to start once they got there. The helicopter arrived just as the paramedics, with help from my partner, performed a rapid extrication on the unstable patient. They turned him over to the crew from the helicopter. The travel time to the hospital was about 10 or 12 minutes. It would have been at least 30 minutes for us.

The patient survived—I called the hospital the next day to check. They said it had been close. He almost didn't make it to surgery. The helicopter saved time—and his life.

> Know the area you are assigned to. Find out how people live, work, and play there. Then, learn about the hazards common in your community and the resources available to handle them.

NOCPs

6.1 n Provide care to patient experiencing signs and symptoms due to exposure to adverse environments **S**

6.2 f Provide care to bariatric patient **A**

7.3 a Create safe landing zone for rotary-wing aircraft **A**

    b Safely approach stationary rotary-wing aircraft **A**

    c Safely approach stationary fixed-wing aircraft **A**

7.4 a Prepare patient for air medical transport **A**

REVIEW QUESTIONS

Page references where answers may be found or supported are provided at the end of each question.

SECTION 1

1. What are some of the hazards involved in the rescue of patients in confined-space emergencies? (p. 485)

2. What is the role of the EMR in a confined-space emergency? (p. 486)

3. How deep can a trench be before it is necessary to call a specialized trench rescue team? (p. 486)

4. Why might it be important to not lay a patient supine after he or she has experienced suspension trauma? (p. 487)

SECTION 2

5. What are the general guidelines for performing safe litter carries over distances on rough terrain? (pp. 487–488)

6. What are the criteria for identifying a rescue as a low-angle or high-angle rescue? (p. 488)

SECTION 3

7. What are the characteristics of a safe helicopter landing zone? (p. 490)

8. How should you approach a helicopter safely? (pp. 490–491)

SECTION 4

9. What complication might abrupt movement of an extremely cold patient cause? (p. 491)

Appendix

EMR Competencies

Level of competency:

N   Not applicable,
X   Basic awareness but no evaluation necessary,
A   Demonstrated understanding with evaluation,
S   Demonstrated proficiency in a simulated examination.

Appendix 4A (referenced below) may be viewed on pages 160–170 of the PAC's NOCP document at paramedic.ca/wp-content/uploads/2012/12/2011-10-31-Approved-NOCP-English-Master.pdf.

Area 1   PROFESSIONAL RESPONSIBILITIES

1) Function as a professional.

a) Maintain patient dignity. S	-Define "dignity." -Acknowledge cultural differences. -Acknowledge personal privacy. -Demonstrate empathy. -Demonstrate care appropriate to situation. -Demonstrate care appropriate to the needs of special populations.
b) Reflect professionalism through use of appropriate language. S	-Identify language appropriate for patients, peers, and other professions. -Choose language appropriate to situation. -Communicate verbally using appropriate language.
c) Dress appropriately and maintain personal hygiene. A	-Identify appropriate dress for situation and environment. -Identify characteristics of personal hygiene. -Acknowledge appearance and personal hygiene.
d) Maintain appropriate personal interaction with patients. A	-Describe appropriate personal interaction. -Describe inappropriate personal interaction. -Value appropriate professional relationships with patients.
e) Maintain patient confidentiality. A	-Describe legislative and regulatory requirements related to patient confidentiality. -Acknowledge conduct necessary to maintain patient confidentiality.
f) Participate in quality assurance and enhancement programs. A	-Describe common quality assurance and enhancement processes. -Acknowledge the relevance of quality assurance and enhancement programs to paramedic practice.
g) Promote awareness of emergency medical system and profession. A	-Describe the characteristics of local emergency medical services.
h) Participate in professional association. A	-Identify professional associations for paramedics in Canada. -Describe the role of professional associations. -Acknowledge the benefits of participation in professional association(s).

Area 1 PROFESSIONAL RESPONSIBILITIES (Continued)

i) Behave ethically. A	-Describe "ethical behaviour." -Value professional code of ethics and beliefs.
j) Function as patient advocate. A	-Discuss situations where patient advocacy is required. -Describe ways in which a practitioner can advocate for patients. -Value patient advocacy.

2) Participate in continuing education and professional development.

a) Develop personal plan for continuing professional development. X	-List professional development activities.
b) Self-evaluate and set goals for improvement, as related to professional practice. X	-Identify strategies for professional improvement.

3) Possess an understanding of the medicolegal aspects of the profession.

a) Comply with scope of practice. S	-Define "scope of practice." -Describe role of Medical Oversight. -Acknowledge importance of compliance with protocols. -Communicate scope of practice.
b) Recognize the rights of the patient and the implications on the role of the provider. A	-Identify legislative requirements. -Identify legal issues pertaining to patient rights -Value patient rights.
c. Include all pertinent and required information on reports and medical records. S	-Organize information for documentation. -Apply principles of correct documentation. -Acknowledge the importance of appropriate documentation. -Demonstrate proper documentation.

4) Recognize and comply with relevant provincial and federal legislation.

a) Function within relevant legislation, policies, and procedures. A	-Discuss legislation, policies, and procedures. -Acknowledge the rationale for policies and procedures.

5) Function effectively in a team environment.

a) Work collaboratively with a partner. S	-Acknowledge the impact of personal relationships between team members on patient care. -Describe characteristics of teamwork. -Demonstrate working cooperatively as a team member.
b) Accept and deliver constructive feedback. S	-Describe constructive feedback. -Receive constructive feedback. -Demonstrate providing constructive feedback within professional practice.

6) Make decisions effectively.

a) Employ reasonable and prudent judgement. S	-Describe reasonable and prudent judgement. -Value reasonable and prudent judgement. -Demonstrate reasonable and prudent judgement.
b) Practice effective problem solving. S	-Describe effective problem solving. -Apply effective problem solving. -Value the process of problem solving. -Demonstrate problem solving.

Area 1   PROFESSIONAL RESPONSIBILITIES (Continued)

c) Delegate tasks appropriately. S	-Describe appropriate task delegation. -Describe tasks delegated to non-healthcare professionals. -Value leadership. -Demonstrate task delegation.

7) Manage scenes with actual or potential forensic implications.

a) Collaborate with law enforcement agencies in the management of crime scenes. A	-Describe criminal law as it applies to paramedic practice. -Describe common characteristics of real or potential crime scenes. -Describe the benefits of note taking in real or potential crime scenes.
b) Comply with ethical and legal reporting requirements for situations of abuse. A	-Identify the requirements for reporting real or suspected situations of abuse.

Area 2   COMMUNICATION

1) Practice effective oral communication skills.

a) Deliver an organized, accurate, and relevant report utilizing telecommunication devices. S	-Identify relevant legislation and regulations. -List the components of effective telecommunication. -Describe the components of a telecommunication report. -Organize information for a telecommunication report. -Identify various telecommunication devices. -Demonstrate use of various telecommunication devices. -Demonstrate an organized, accurate, and relevant telecommunication report.
b) Deliver an organized, accurate, and relevant verbal report. S	-List the components of effective verbal communication. -Describe the components of a verbal report. -Organize information for a verbal report. -Demonstrate an organized, accurate, and relevant verbal report.
c) Deliver an organized, accurate, and relevant patient history. S	-List the components of a patient history. -Organize a patient history for the purposes of oral communication. -Communicate an organized, accurate, and relevant patient history.
d) Provide information to patient about their situation and how they will be cared for. S	-Identify information that should be communicated to the patient. -Evaluate patient comprehension. -Communicate to patient their situation and how they will be cared for.
e) Interact effectively with the patient, relatives, and bystanders who are in stressful situations. S	-List factors that contribute to stress in patient, relatives, and bystanders. -Identify verbal and non-verbal indicators of stress. -Describe techniques to maximize the effectiveness of communication. -Choose techniques to maximize the effectiveness of communication. -Demonstrate communication techniques during stressful situations.

Area 2 COMMUNICATION (Continued)

f) Speak in language appropriate to the listener. S	-Identify basic communication needs. -Describe common communication barriers. -Describe methods of meeting basic communication needs. -Adapt communication techniques effectively.
g) Use appropriate terminology. S	-Define common medical terminology. -Integrate medical and non-medical terminology.

2) Practice effective written communication skills.

a) Record organized, accurate, and relevant patient information. S	-Organize patient information for the purposes of a written report. -Communicate accurate, organized, and relevant documentation.

3) Practice effective non-verbal communication skills.

a) Employ effective non-verbal behaviour. A	-Describe non-verbal behaviours. -List examples of non-verbal behaviours that may impact others positively. -List examples of non-verbal behaviours that may impact others negatively. -Identify cultural factors that may affect non-verbal communication. -Acknowledge the relationship between positive non-verbal behaviour and personal feelings.
b) Practice active listening techniques. S	-Define "active listening." -Acknowledge the relationship between sincerity, genuine interest, and active listening. -Demonstrate active listening in interactions with colleagues, patients, and others.
c) Establish trust and rapport with patients and colleagues. A	-List behaviours that help establish trust. -List behaviours that help establish rapport. -Describe feedback that indicates that trust and rapport have been established.
d) Recognize and react appropriately to non-verbal behaviours. A	-Distinguish threatening and non-threatening behaviours.

4) Practice effective interpersonal relations.

a) Treat others with respect. S	-Define "respect." -List examples of ways to demonstrate respect. -Identify cultural differences that affect the demonstration of respect. -Value respect in patient care. -Demonstrate behaviour that is respectful to patients.
b) Employ empathy and compassion while providing care. S	-Define "empathy." -Define "compassion." -Define "sympathy." -Describe behaviours that convey empathy and compassion. -Value empathy and compassion. -Demonstrate empathy and compassion.

Area 2 COMMUNICATION (Continued)

c) Recognize and react appropriately to persons exhibiting emotional reactions. A	-List common emotional reactions exhibited by patient, relatives, bystanders, and paramedics. -List common coping mechanisms. -Describe positive and negative aspects of coping mechanisms. -Identify verbal means of supporting others displaying emotional reactions and coping mechanisms. -Identify non-verbal means of supporting others displaying emotional reactions and coping mechanisms. -Value the provision of emotional support. -Demonstrate behaviours that provide emotional support. -Identify community resources that may assist those in need.
d) Act in a confident manner. S	- Define "confidence." -Identify the impact of confidence on patient care. -Identify the risks associated with over confidence. -Choose behaviours that display confidence. -Adjust behaviour to exhibit an appropriate level of confidence.
e) Act assertively as required. S	-Discuss assertive behaviour. -Discuss aggressive behaviour. -Distinguish assertive and aggressive behaviour. -Describe techniques of assertive behaviour. -Choose assertive behaviour when appropriate. -Demonstrate appropriate assertive behaviour in interactions.
f) Employ diplomacy, tact, and discretion. S	-Define "diplomacy." -Define "tact." -Define "discretion." -Value diplomacy, tact, and discretion. -Demonstrate behaviour showing diplomacy, tact, and discretion.
g) Employ conflict resolution skills. S	-Define "conflict." -Identify situations of potential conflict. -Describe basic conflict resolution strategies. -Justify the use of basic conflict resolution skills. -Demonstrate basic conflict resolution skills.

Area 3 HEALTH AND SAFETY

1) Maintain good physical and mental health.

a) Maintain balance in your personal lifestyle. X	-List the components of a balanced, healthy lifestyle.
b) Develop and maintain an appropriate support system. X	-List personal support systems that promote the maintenance of physical and mental health.

Area 3   HEALTH AND SAFETY (Continued)

c) Manage your stress. X	-Define "stress." -Define "stress disorder." -List factors that typically contribute to personal stress. -List techniques to manage stress. -Describe the concept of critical incident stress management. -Recognize behaviours suggesting a negative response to stress.
d) Practice effective strategies to improve physical and mental health related to career. X	-List effects of shift work on physical and mental health. -List strategies to promote physical and mental health.
e) Exhibit physical strength and fitness consistent with the requirements of professional practice. S	-Describe the physical capabilities required of an EMS practitioner. -Describe strategies to develop and maintain physical strength and fitness. -Choose strategies to develop and maintain physical strength and fitness. -Demonstrate adequate strength and fitness.

2) Practice safe lifting and moving techniques.

a) Practice safe biomechanics. S	-Define "safe biomechanics." -Describe potential injuries common to EMS practitioners. -Describe strategies to reduce risk of injury. -Choose strategies to reduce the risk of injury. -Adapt proper lifting techniques.
b) Transfer patient from various positions using applicable equipment and/or techniques. S	-List equipment for patient transfer. -Describe indications for equipment use. -Identify specifications of the equipment to be used, including equipment for special patient populations. -Explain techniques of transfer using specified equipment. -Demonstrate patient transfers.
c) Transfer patient using emergency evacuation techniques. S	-Describe situations where emergency evacuation may be required. -Describe emergency lifting and moving techniques. -Describe alternative techniques and conditions for use. -Demonstrate emergency lifting and moving techniques.
d) Secure patient to applicable equipment. S	-Identify safe and secure methods. -Demonstrate safe and secure procedures for patient movement and transport.

3) Create and maintain a safe work environment.

a) Assess scene for safety. S	-Define "scene safety." -Describe factors contributing to scene safety. -Apply techniques for assessing scene safety. -Demonstrate techniques for the assessment of scene safety.
b) Address potential occupational hazards. S	-List potential occupational hazards. -Describe ways to manage occupational hazards. -Demonstrate techniques to manage occupational hazards.

Area 3   HEALTH AND SAFETY (Continued)

c) Conduct basic extrication. S	-Describe basic, non-mechanical patient extrication principles. -Apply basic, non-mechanical extrication principles. -Demonstrate basic, non-mechanical extrication principles.
d) Exhibit defusing and self-protection behaviours appropriate for use with patients and bystanders. S	-Describe methods of defusing. -Describe methods of self-protection. -Apply methods of defusing. -Apply methods of self-protection. -Choose methods of defusing and self-protection. -Apply safety precautions when dealing with patients suffering from psychiatric illnesses.
e) Conduct procedures and operations consistent with Workplace Hazardous Materials Information System (WHMIS) and hazardous materials management requirements. A	-Identify applicable legislation and regulations. -Apply regulations.
f) Practice infection control techniques. S	-Identify common routes for transmission of disease and infection. -Define "infection control precautions." -Apply infection control precautions. -Describe the appropriate procedures for the disposal of sharps and contaminated supplies. -Describe personal protective equipment utilized in practice. -Integrate infection control precautions and safe handling procedures. -Demonstrate proper use of personal protective equipment.
g) Clean and disinfect equipment. S	-List equipment and supplies used to clean/disinfect equipment. -List techniques to clean and disinfect equipment. -Demonstrate correct equipment cleaning and disinfecting techniques.
h) Clean and disinfect work environment. A	-List equipment and supplies required to clean and disinfect work environment. -Describe methods to clean and disinfect work environment.

Area 4   ASSESSMENT AND DIAGNOSTICS

1) Conduct triage in a multiple-patient incident.

a) Rapidly assess an incident based on the principles of a triage system. S	-Discuss triage. -Identify circumstances under which triage is required. -Apply the equipment and materials used to sort patients. -Perform targeted patient assessment based on a triage system. -Communicate with other responders.
b) Assume different roles in a multiple patient incident. A	-Identify the EMS practitioner roles involved when managing a multiple patient incident. -Describe the principal responsibilities of each role.

Area 4   ASSESSMENT AND DIAGNOSTICS (Continued)

c) Manage a multiple patient incident. A	-Apply management principles to a multiple patient incident. -Modify procedures to meet the needs of a specific incident.
2) Obtain patient history.	
a) Obtain list of patient's allergies. S	-List common examples of allergens. -Describe how an allergen can affect individuals. -Evaluate how information about an allergy will affect patient care. -Demonstrate the skill of obtaining information about allergies into history gathering procedures.
b) Obtain patient's medication profile. S	-Apply various methods of discovering a patient's medication profile. -Demonstrate the skill of obtaining a medication profile into history gathering procedures.
c) Obtain chief complaint and/or incident history from patient, family members, and/or bystanders. S	-List methods of discovering an incident history. -Describe common components of an incident history. -Demonstrate the skill of obtaining incident history in the overall patient assessment. -Adapt interview techniques to the incident history findings. -Integrate incident history information into patient care procedures.
d) Obtain information regarding a patient's past medical history. S	-List methods of discovering a patient's medical history. -Describe common components of a complete medical history. -Demonstrate the skill of obtaining medical history in the overall patient assessment. -Demonstrate interview techniques appropriate to the medical history findings. -Integrate medical history information into patient care procedures.
e) Obtain information about a patient's last oral intake. S	-List situations when information about a patient's last oral intake may be required. -List methods of discovering information regarding last oral intake. -Demonstrate the skill of obtaining information regarding last oral intake in the overall patient assessment.
f) Obtain information regarding incident through accurate and complete scene assessment. S	-List methods of discovering incident information. -Demonstrate the skill of obtaining incident information in the overall scene assessment. -Adapt scene management from information gathered during continuous scene assessment. -Integrate incident information into patient care procedures.
3) Conduct complete physical assessment demonstrating appropriate use of inspection, palpation, percussion, and auscultation.	
a) Conduct primary patient assessment and interpret findings. S	-Explain primary assessment. -Distinguish between trauma assessment and primary medical assessment. -Evaluate life threatening findings from primary assessment. -Apply appropriate sequential techniques for primary assessment. -Apply primary assessment to different age groups. -Demonstrate techniques for primary assessment. -Adapt assessment techniques to primary assessment findings. -Perform procedures to address problems found in the primary assessment.

Area 4 ASSESSMENT AND DIAGNOSTICS (Continued)

b) Conduct secondary patient assessment and interpret findings. S	-Explain secondary assessment. -Distinguish between trauma assessment and secondary medical assessment. -Evaluate life threatening findings from secondary assessment. -Apply appropriate sequential techniques for secondary assessment. -Apply secondary assessment to different age groups. -Demonstrate techniques for secondary assessment. -Adapt assessment techniques to secondary assessment findings. -Perform procedures to address problems found in the secondary assessment.
c) Conduct cardiovascular system assessment and interpret findings. S	-Describe the pathophysiology of specific cardiovascular illnesses and injuries listed in Appendix 4A. -Apply assessment techniques specific to the cardiovascular system. -Demonstrate assessment techniques for cardiovascular illnesses and injuries. -Adapt assessment techniques to cardiovascular history findings.
d) Conduct neurological system assessment and interpret findings. S	-Describe the pathophysiology of specific neurological illnesses and injuries listed in Appendix 4A. -Apply assessment techniques specific to the neurological system. -Demonstrate assessment techniques for neurological illnesses and injuries. -Adapt assessment techniques to neurological history findings.
e) Conduct respiratory system assessment and interpret findings. S	-Describe the pathophysiology of specific respiratory illnesses and injuries listed in Appendix 4A. -Apply assessment techniques specific to the respiratory system. -Demonstrate assessment techniques for respiratory illnesses and injuries. -Adapt assessment techniques to respiratory history findings.
f) Conduct obstetrical assessment and interpret findings. A	-Describe pathophysiology of specific illnesses and injuries to the female reproductive system listed in Appendix 4A. -Apply assessment techniques specific to the obstetrical patient.
g) Conduct gastrointestinal system assessment and interpret findings. S	-Describe the pathophysiology of specific gastrointestinal system illnesses and injuries listed in Appendix 4A. -Apply assessment techniques specific to the gastrointestinal system. -Demonstrate assessment techniques for gastrointestinal illnesses and injuries. -Adapt assessment techniques to gastrointestinal history findings.
h) Conduct genitourinary/reproductive system assessment and interpret findings. A	- Describe the pathophysiology of specific genitourinary/reproductive illnesses and injuries listed in Appendix 4A. -Apply assessment techniques specific to the genitourinary/reproductive system.
i) Conduct integumentary system assessment and interpret findings. S	-Describe the pathophysiology of specific integumentary illnesses and injuries listed in Appendix 4A. -Apply assessment techniques specific to the integumentary system. -Demonstrate assessment techniques for integumentary illnesses and injuries. -Adapt assessment techniques to integumentary history findings.

Area 4   ASSESSMENT AND DIAGNOSTICS (Continued)

j) Conduct musculoskeletal assessment and interpret findings. S	-Describe the pathophysiology of specific musculoskeletal illnesses and injuries listed in Appendix 4A. -Apply assessment techniques specific to the musculoskeletal system. -Demonstrate assessment techniques for musculoskeletal illnesses and injuries. -Adapt assessment techniques to musculoskeletal history findings.
k) Conduct assessment of the ears, eyes, nose, and throat, and interpret findings. S	-Describe the pathophysiology of specific illnesses and injuries to the ears, eyes, nose, and throat listed in Appendix 4A. -Apply assessment techniques specific to the ears, eyes, nose, and throat. -Demonstrate assessment techniques for illnesses and injuries to the ears, eyes, nose, and throat. -Adapt assessment techniques to ears, eyes, nose, and throat history findings.
l) Conduct neonatal assessment and interpret findings. A	-Define "neonatal patient." -Describe the pathophysiology of illnesses and injuries to the neonate listed in Appendix 4A. -Apply assessment techniques specific to the neonatal patient.
m) Conduct psychiatric assessment and interpret findings. S	-Distinguish between the "mentally well" and the "mentally unwell" person. -Describe the pathophysiology of the psychiatric disorders listed in Appendix 4A. -Apply assessment techniques specific to psychiatric disorders. -Evaluate psychiatric assessment findings. -Demonstrate assessment techniques for psychiatric disorders. -Adapt assessment techniques to psychiatric history findings. -Communicate appropriately with other health care providers when dealing with patients suffering from psychiatric disorders.
n) Conduct pediatric assessment and interpret findings. A	-Define "pediatric patient." -List developmental parameters. -List the anatomical and physiological differences between the pediatric and adult patient.
o) Conduct geriatric assessment and interpret findings. A	-Define "geriatric patient." -Describe the effects of the aging process. -List appropriate assessment techniques for the geriatric patient.
p) Conduct bariatric assessment and interpret findings. A	-Define "bariatric patient." -Describe the effects of obesity. -List appropriate assessment techniques for the bariatric patient.
4) Assess vital signs.	
a) Assess pulse. S	-Define "pulse." -Identify sites where a pulse may be found. -Modify pulse check to age of patient. -Evaluate arterial pulse rate, rhythm, and quality. -Distinguish between normal and abnormal findings. -Identify factors that influence the pulse rate. -Demonstrate pulse assessment. -Adapt techniques of obtaining pulse to patient situation.

Area 4   ASSESSMENT AND DIAGNOSTICS (Continued)

b) Assess respiration. S	-Describe the physiology of respiration. -Modify respiratory assessment to patient age. -Evaluate respiratory rate, effort, excursion, and symmetry. -Distinguish between adequate and inadequate respiratory effort. -List factors that influence the respiratory rate. -Demonstrate respiratory assessment. -Adapt techniques of obtaining respirations to patient situation.
c) Conduct non-invasive temperature monitoring. N	
d) Measure blood pressure by auscultation. S	-Describe the physiology of blood pressure. -Identify average blood pressure expectations for age. -Identify factors that may influence patient's blood pressure. -Demonstrate auscultated determination of blood pressure. -Adapt technique of auscultating blood pressure to patient situation.
e) Measure blood pressure by palpation. S	-Describe the physiology of pulse points. -Analyze the strengths and weaknesses of a palpated blood pressure. -Identify factors that may influence a palpated blood pressure. -Demonstrate palpated determination of blood pressure. -Adapt technique of palpating blood pressure to patient situation.
f) Measure blood pressure with non-invasive blood pressure monitor. N	
g) Assess skin condition. S	-List three parameters used to assess skin condition. -Identify the factors that affect skin temperature, colour, and moisture. -Distinguish between normal and abnormal findings when assessing skin colour. -Identify how to assess skin colour changes in different races. -Distinguish between normal and abnormal findings when assessing skin temperature. -Distinguish between normal and abnormal findings when assessing skin condition. -Demonstrate assessment of skin condition utilizing three parameters. -Adapt technique of skin assessment to patient age and race.
h) Assess pupils. S	-List the three parameters used to assess pupils. -Identify conditions that affect pupil size, symmetry, and reactivity. -Distinguish between normal and abnormal findings when assessing pupils for size, symmetry, and reactivity. -Demonstrate pupil assessment utilizing the three parameters. -Adapt technique of assessing pupils to patient situation.
i) Assess level of consciousness. S	-List factors that affect patient's mental status. -Apply methods of assessing level of consciousness. -Demonstrate assessment of level of consciousness. -Adapt technique of assessing level of consciousness to patient age.

Area 4 ASSESSMENT AND DIAGNOSTICS (Continued)

5) Utilize diagnostic tests.

a) Conduct oximetry testing and interpret findings. N	
b) Conduct end-tidal carbon dioxide monitoring and interpret findings. N	
c) Conduct glucometric testing and interpret findings. A	-Identify indications for glucometric testing. -Identify the factors that affect accuracy of glucometric testing. -Identify normal and abnormal findings when performing glucometric testing.

Area 5 THERAPEUTICS

1) Maintain patency of upper airway and trachea.

a) Use manual manoeuvres and positioning to maintain airway patency. S	-Define methods of relieving the symptoms of airway obstruction. -Describe the types of airway opening manoeuvres for various patients. -Describe the indication, contraindications, and precautions of performing airway manoeuvres. -Apply problem solving techniques required with various types of patients. -Demonstrate manoeuvres and positioning for head, neck, and jaw which improve airway patency. -Demonstrate manual airway manoeuvres under a variety of patient and environmental presentations. -Adjust to changes in patient's airway patency. -Demonstrate management of potential complications of airway manoeuvres.
b) Suction oropharynx. S	-Identify the purposes of and indications for oropharyngeal suctioning. -Describe suctioning equipment. -Explain established standards of maintenance for suctioning equipment. -Identify pressure limitations for suctioning various age groups. -Operate appropriate suctioning devices. -Demonstrate suctioning using safe technique. -Adjust suctioning techniques to changes in patient's condition. -List potential complications of suctioning. -Demonstrate how to clean and disinfect suctioning equipment.
c) Suction beyond oropharynx. N	

Area 5   THERAPEUTICS (Continued)

d) Utilize oropharyngeal airway. S	-Identify the purpose and indications for inserting an oropharyngeal airway. -Discuss oropharyngeal airway types and sizes. -Perform oropharyngeal airway sizing procedures. -Perform insertion of an oropharyngeal airway. -Adjust to changes in patient presentation.
e) Utilize nasopharyngeal airway. S	-Explain the purposes of and the indications for inserting a nasopharyngeal airway. -Perform nasopharyngeal airway sizing procedures. -Perform nasopharyngeal airway insertion. -Adjust to changes in patient presentation.
f) Utilize airway devices not requiring visualization of vocal cords and not introduced endotracheally. N	
g) Utilize airway devices not requiring visualization of vocal cords and introduced endotracheally. N	
h) Utilize airway devices requiring visualization of vocal cords and introduced endotracheally. N	
i) Remove airway foreign bodies (AFB). S	-Identify the indications for AFB removal. -Describe the methods of relieving airway obstructions. -Describe the differences in technique required for AFB removal in various age groups. -Perform AFB removal under a variety of presentations. -Adjust to changes in patient presentation. -Identify potential complications of AFB removal.

2) Prepare oxygen delivery devices.

a) Prepare oxygen delivery devices. A	-Identify indications for oxygen administration. -Identify the purpose of oxygen administration. -Identify oxygen administration complications. -Describe the safe handling of oxygen delivery systems. -Discuss oxygen administration precautions. -Identify different oxygen cylinder types and sizes. -Apply the formulas that determine oxygen cylinder factors, volume (or type), and maximum filling volumes and duration. -Identify various types of oxygen delivery systems. -Explain the difference between portable and fixed delivery systems.
b) Utilize portable oxygen delivery systems. S	-Describe the sequential steps for setting up oxygen delivery systems. -Operate oxygen delivery systems. -Demonstrate cleaning and disinfection of oxygen delivery systems.

Area 5   THEREPEUTICS (Continued)

3) Deliver oxygen and administer manual ventilation.

a) Administer oxygen using nasal cannula. S	-Identify the purposes of and indications for the use of a nasal cannula. -List the steps for administration of oxygen by nasal cannula. -Perform oxygen administration using a nasal cannula. -Adjust to changes in patient presentation.
b) Administer oxygen using low concentration mask. S	-Identify the purposes and indications for the use of a low concentration mask. -List the steps for administration of oxygen by a low concentration mask. -Adjust to changes in patient presentation.
c) Administer oxygen using controlled concentration mask. N	
d) Administer oxygen using high concentration mask. S	-Identify the purposes of and indications for the use of a high concentration mask. -List the steps for administration of oxygen by a high concentration mask. -Perform oxygen administration using a high concentration mask. -Adjust to changes in patient presentation.
e) Administer oxygen using pocket mask. S	-Identify the purposes of and indications for the use of a pocket mask. -List the steps for administration of oxygen by a pocket mask. -Adjust to changes in patient presentation.

4) Utilize ventilation equipment

a) Provide oxygenation and ventilation using manual positive pressure devices. S	-Identify the purposes of and indications for the use of a manual positive pressure device. -List the steps for oxygen administration by a manual positive pressure device. -Perform ventilation using a manual positive pressure device. -Distinguish between one person or two person application of a manual positive pressure device. -Adjust to changes in patient presentation.

5) Implement measures to maintain hemodynamic stability.

a) Conduct cardiopulmonary resuscitation (CPR). S	-Identify the purposes of and indications for CPR. -List the steps for CPR administration in a variety of presentations. -Perform CPR on various age groups. -Perform CPR while moving a patient from site of collapse. -Discuss potential complications of CPR. -Adapt to changes in patient presentation.
b) Control external hemorrhage through the use of direct pressure and patient positioning. S	-Identify the purposes of and indications for hemorrhage control through the use of direct pressure and patient positioning. -List the steps for hemorrhage control through the use of direct pressure and patient positioning. -Perform hemorrhage control through the use of direct pressure and patient positioning. -Discuss potential complications of hemorrhage control through the use of direct pressure and patient positioning. -Adapt to changes in patient presentation.

Area 5 THERAPEUTICS (Continued)

i) Conduct automated external defibrillation. S	-Define "defibrillation." -Describe the purposes of automated external defibrillation. -Discuss the indications for automated external defibrillation. -Identify the various types of automated external defibrillator. -List complications to the use of automated external defibrillation. -Apply the established standards of automated external defibrillation equipment maintenance. -Operate an automated external defibrillator. -Integrate CPR procedures and automated external defibrillation procedures. -Adapt procedures to patient presentation.
j) Conduct manual defibrillation. N	
6) Provide basic care for soft tissue injuries.	
a) Treat soft tissue injuries. S	-Identify the purposes of and indications for soft tissue dressing, bandaging, and immobilization. -Describe the various types of dressings and bandages. -Demonstrate appropriate dressing, bandaging, and immobilization procedures.
b) Treat burn. S	-Identify the purposes of and indications for dressing a burn. -Describe types of burn dressings. -Demonstrate application of burn dressing.
c) Treat eye injury. S	-Identify the purposes of and indications for an eye dressing. -Describe types of eye dressings. -Demonstrate application of eye dressing.
d) Treat penetration wound. S	-Identify the purposes of and indications for dressing a penetration wound. -Describe types of penetration wound dressings. -Demonstrate application of penetration wound dressing.
e) Treat local cold injury. S	-Describe methods for local cold injury assessment. -Identify the purposes of and indications for caring for local cold injury. -Identify the types of tissue damage that may result from local cold injury. -Demonstrate provision of care for local cold injury.
f) Provide routine wound care. N	
7) Immobilize actual and suspected fractures.	
a) Immobilize suspected fractures involving appendicular skeleton. S	-Identify signs and symptoms of a possible fracture not involving the spinal column. -Distinguish between open and closed fractures. -Modify splints to meet patient needs. -Demonstrate appropriate treatment of suspected fractures.
b) Immobilize suspected fractures involving axial skeleton. S	-Identify signs and symptoms of possible injury to the spinal column. -Modify immobilization devices to meet patient needs. -Demonstrate treatment of suspected fractures involving the axial skeleton.

Area 5 THERAPEUTICS (Continued)

8) Administer medications.

a) Not applicable to EMR N	-Recognize principles of pharmacology as applied to medications listed in Appendix 5.
b) Provide patient assist according to provincial list of medications. A	-Identify indications, relative and absolute contraindications, side effects, dosage parameters, and safe administration process for each medication.

Area 6 INTEGRATION

1) Utilize differential diagnosis skills, decision making skills, and psychomotor skills in providing care to patients.

a) Provide care to patient experiencing signs and symptoms involving cardiovascular system. S	-Describe the pathophysiology of specific cardiovascular conditions listed in Appendix 4A. -Describe the approach to a patient presenting with cardiovascular conditions. -Identify how patient history relates to patient presentation. -Demonstrate the ability to approach, assess, treat, and transport a patient. -Justify approach, assessment, care, and transport decisions.
b) Provide care to patient experiencing signs and symptoms involving neurological system. S	-Describe the pathophysiology of specific neurological conditions listed in Appendix 4A. -Describe the approach to a patient presenting with neurological conditions. -Identify how patient history relates to patient presentation. -Demonstrate the ability to approach, assess, treat, and transport a patient. -Justify approach, assessment, care, and transport decisions.
c) Provide care to patient experiencing signs and symptoms involving respiratory system. S	-Describe the pathophysiology of specific respiratory conditions listed in Appendix 4A. -Describe the approach to a patient presenting with respiratory conditions. -Identify how patient history relates to patient presentation. -Demonstrate the ability to approach, assess, treat, and transport a patient. -Justify approach, assessment, care, and transport decisions.
d) Provide care to patient experiencing signs and symptoms involving genitourinary/reproductive systems. S	-Describe the pathophysiology of specific genitourinary/reproductive conditions listed in Appendix 4A. -Describe the approach to a patient presenting with genitourinary/reproductive conditions. -Identify how patient history relates to patient presentation. -Demonstrate the ability to approach, assess, treat, and transport a patient. -Justify approach, assessment, care, and transport decisions.

Area 6   INTEGRATION (Continued)

e) Provide care to patient experiencing signs and symptoms involving gastrointestinal system. S	-Describe the pathophysiology of specific gastrointestinal system conditions listed in Appendix 4A. -Describe the approach to a patient presenting with gastrointestinal conditions. -Identify how patient history relates to patient presentation. -Demonstrate the ability to approach, assess, treat, and transport a patient. -Justify approach, assessment, care, and transport decisions.
f) Provide care to patient experiencing signs and symptoms involving integumentary system. S	-Describe the pathophysiology of specific integumentary conditions listed in Appendix 4A. -Describe the approach to a patient presenting with integumentary conditions. -Identify how patient history relates to patient presentation. -Demonstrate the ability to approach, assess, treat, and transport a patient. -Justify approach, assessment, care, and transport decisions.
g) Provide care to patient experiencing signs and symptoms involving musculoskeletal system. S	-Describe the pathophysiology of specific musculoskeletal conditions listed in Appendix 4A. -Describe the approach to a patient presenting with musculoskeletal conditions. -Identify how patient history relates to patient presentation. -Demonstrate the ability to approach, assess, treat, and transport a patient. -Justify approach, assessment, care, and transport decisions.
h) Provide care to patient experiencing signs and symptoms involving immunologic system. S	-Describe the pathophysiology of specific immunologic conditions listed in Appendix 4A. -Describe the approach to a patient presenting with immunologic conditions. -Identify how patient history relates to patient presentation. -Demonstrate the ability to approach, assess, treat, and transport a patient. -Justify approach, assessment, care, and transport decisions.
i) Provide care to patient experiencing signs and symptoms involving endocrine system. S	-Describe the pathophysiology of specific endocrine system conditions listed in Appendix 4A. -Describe the approach to a patient presenting with endocrine conditions. -Identify how patient history relates to patient presentation. -Demonstrate the ability to approach, assess, treat, and transport a patient. -Justify approach, assessment, care, and transport decisions.
j) Provide care to patient experiencing signs and symptoms involving the eyes, ears, nose, and throat. S	-Describe the pathophysiology of specific ear, eye, nose, and throat conditions listed in Appendix 4A. -Describe the approach to a patient presenting with ear, eye, nose, and throat conditions. -Identify how patient history relates to patient presentation. -Demonstrate the ability to approach, assess, treat, and transport a patient. -Justify approach, assessment, care, and transport decisions.

Area 6   INTEGRATION (Continued)

k) Provide care to patient experiencing toxicologic syndromes. S	-List the signs and symptoms of specific poisons and overdoses listed in Appendix 4A. -Describe the approach to a patient presenting with a toxicologic syndrome. -Identify how patient history relates to patient presentation. -Demonstrate the ability to approach, assess, treat, and transport a patient. -Justify approach, assessment, care, and transport decisions.
l) Provide care to patient experiencing non-urgent problem. S	-Describe the approach to a patient presenting with non-urgent problem. -Distinguish between urgent and non-urgent problems. -Identify how patient history relates to patient presentation. -Demonstrate the ability to approach, assess, treat, and refer a patient. -Justify approach, assessment, care, and transport decisions.
m) Provide care to a palliative patient. S	-Describe the approach to a palliative patient. -Identify disease processes that contribute to terminal illness. -Identify how patient history relates to patient presentation. -Demonstrate the ability to approach, assess, treat, and transport a patient. -Justify approach, assessment, care, and transport decisions.
n) Provide care to patient experiencing signs and symptoms due to exposure to adverse environments. S	-Describe the approach to a patient presenting with signs and symptoms due to exposure to adverse environments. -Identify conditions resulting from exposure to adverse environments. -Identify how patient history relates to patient presentation. -Demonstrate the ability to approach, assess, treat, and transport a patient. -Justify approach, assessment, care, and transport decisions.
o) Provide care to trauma patient. S	-List trauma indices (scores) for triage and transport decisions. -Demonstrate the ability to prioritize treatment and transport decisions. -Justify approach, assessment, care, and transport decisions.
p) Provide care to psychiatric patient. S	-Describe the approach to a patient presenting with psychiatric crisis. -Identify how patient history relates to patient presentation. -Demonstrate the ability to approach, assess, treat, and transport a patient. -Justify approach, assessment, care, and transport decisions.
q) Provide care to obstetrical patient. S	-Describe the approach to an obstetrical patient. -List complications of labour and delivery. -Identify how patient history relates to patient presentation. -List indications that suggest the need to prepare for imminent delivery. -Demonstrate the ability to manage an imminent delivery. -Demonstrate the ability to approach, assess, treat, and transport a patient. -Justify approach, assessment, care, and transport decisions.

Area 6   INTEGRATION (Continued)

2) Provide care to meet the needs of unique patient groups.

a) Provide care for neonatal patient. S	-List potential complications with neonatal patients. -Demonstrate the ability to approach, assess, treat, and transport a patient. -Justify approach, assessment, care, and transport decisions.
b) Provide care for pediatric patient. A	-Identify possible abuse or neglect. -Justify variations in approach, treatment, and transport decisions.
c) Provide care for geriatric patient. A	-Identify possible abuse or neglect. -Describe variations to the approach, treatment, and transport methods. -Justify variations in approach, treatment, and transport decisions.
d) Provide care for the physically impaired patient. A	-Define "physically impaired patient." -List common medical emergencies associated with physically impaired patients. -List common trauma emergencies associated with physically impaired patients. -Identify possible abuse or neglect of the physically impaired patient. -List appropriate assessment techniques for the physically impaired patient. -List the approach, treatment, and transport methods appropriate to the physically impaired patient. -Justify approach, assessment, care, and transport decisions.
e) Provide care for the mentally impaired patient. A	-Define "mentally impaired patient." -List common medical emergencies associated with mentally impaired patients. -List common trauma emergencies associated with mentally impaired patients. -Identify possible abuse or neglect of the mentally impaired patient. -List appropriate assessment techniques for the mentally impaired patient. -List the approach, treatment, and transport methods appropriate for the mentally impaired patient. -Justify approach, assessment, care, and transport decisions.
f) Provide care to bariatric patient. A	-Identify possible abuse or neglect. -Describe variations in approach, treatment, and transport methods. -Justify approach, treatment, and transport decisions.

3) Conduct ongoing assessments and provide care.

a) Conduct ongoing assessments based on patient presentation and interpret findings. S	-Demonstrate ongoing assessments based on patient presentation. -Evaluate results of ongoing assessments. -Integrate assessment and patient care procedures. -Justify ongoing assessment directions.
b) Redirect priorities based on assessment findings. S	-Demonstrate management priorities. -Communicate changes to patient, family, or primary caregiver(s). -Justify approach, assessment, care, and transport decisions.

Area 7   TRANSPORTATION

1) Prepare ambulance for service.

a) Conduct vehicle maintenance and safety check. S	-Identify components of a maintenance check. -Identify components of a safety check. -Demonstrate a maintenance check. -Demonstrate a safety check.
b) Recognize conditions requiring removal of vehicle from service. A	-List the conditions that require removal of a vehicle from service.
c) Utilize all vehicle equipment and vehicle devices within ambulance. A	-Describe the purpose of all vehicle equipment. -Describe the purpose of all vehicle devices.

2) Drive ambulance or emergency response vehicle.

a) Utilize defensive driving techniques. A	-Describe principles of defensive driving. -Apply techniques of defensive driving.
b) Utilize safe emergency driving techniques. A	-Distinguish between driving characteristics of an ambulance and a passenger vehicle. -Distinguish between emergency driving and driving under normal conditions. -Apply appropriate driving techniques. -Describe relevant legislative requirements regarding the operation of an emergency vehicle. -Discuss potential reactions from other drivers.
c) Drive in a manner that ensures patient comfort and a safe environment for all passengers. A	-Describe driving techniques for maximizing the safety of the working environment.

3) Transfer patient to air ambulance

a) Create safe landing zone for rotary wing aircraft. A	-List the required elements of a safe landing zone. -Describe procedure to create a safe landing zone.
b) Safely approach stationary rotary wing aircraft. A	-Describe the technique for safely approaching a rotary wing aircraft.
c) Safely approach stationary fixed wing aircraft. A	-Describe the technique for safely approaching a fixed wing aircraft.

4) Transport patient in air ambulance.

a) Prepare patient for air medical transport. A	-Identify the unique patient care principles for air transport. -Describe the preparation of patient for air medical transport.

Area 8 HEALTH PROMOTION AND PUBLIC SAFETY

1) Integrate professional practice into community care.

a and b not applicable to EMR a) Participate in health promotion activities and initiatives. N b) Participate in injury prevention and public safety activities and initiatives. N	
c) Work collaboratively with other members of the health care community. A	-List other members of the health community. -Describe the roles and relationship to other health care professionals. -Value working collaboratively with other health care professionals.
d) Utilize community support agencies as appropriate. A	-Identify common community support programs. -Describe situations that may require expertise of community support agencies. -Describe related legislative requirements. -Acknowledge the need for additional intervention. -Communicate options to patient.

2) Contribute to public safety through collaboration with other emergency response agencies.

a) Work collaboratively with other emergency response agencies. A	-List community emergency response agencies. -Describe the roles and relationship to other emergency response agencies. -Describe mutual assistance and tiered response. -Value collaborative work with other emergency response agencies.
b) Work within an incident management system (IMS). A	-Describe the principles of an IMS. -Identify the various participant roles in an IMS.

3) Participate in the management of a chemical, biological, radiological/nuclear, or explosive (CBRNE) incident.

a) Recognize indicators of agent exposure. A	-List common CBRNE agents. -List signs and symptoms due to agent exposure. -Identify potential dissemination devices.
b) Possess knowledge of personal protective equipment (PPE). A	-Discuss importance of PPE. -List levels of PPE. -Discuss limitations of PPE.
c) Perform CBRNE scene size up. A	-Describe how to safely perform CBRNE scene size up. -Describe agent/hazard avoidance techniques. -Describe how to define and establish inner and outer perimeters.
d) Conduct triage at CBRNE incident. A	-Describe the principles of triage specific to a CBRNE incident. -Control contaminated casualties.
e) Conduct decontamination procedures. A	-Conduct emergency decontamination procedures. -Assist with the decontamination process.
f) Provide care to patients involved in a CBRNE incident. A	-Discuss directed first aid and explain when its use is appropriate. -List chemical countermeasures. -Identify precautions to be taken when transporting patients. -Identify possible support requirements by hospitals. -Recognize psychological impact of CBRNE incidents on the community resources and first responders.

Glossary of Abbreviations

A

A/P: anterior/posterior
ABCs: airway, breathing, circulation
ACLS: advanced cardiac life support
ACP: advanced care paramedic
AED: automated external defibrillator
AIDS: acquired immune deficiency syndrome
ALS: advanced life support
ASA: acetylsalicylic acid
ATV: all-terrain vehicle
AVPU: alert, verbal, painful, unconscious

B

BSA: body surface area
BSI: body substance isolation
BVM: bag-valve-mask

C

CANUTEC: Canadian Transport Emergency Centre
CBRNE: chemical, biological, radiological/nuclear, or explosive
CCOHS: Canadian Centre for Occupational Health and Safety
CCP: critical care paramedic
CHF: congestive heart failure
CISD: critical incident stress debriefing
CNS: central nervous system
COPD: chronic obstructive pulmonary disease
CPR: cardiopulmonary resuscitation
CPS: *Compendium of Pharmaceuticals and Specialties*
CVA: cerebrovascular accident

D

DNR: do not resuscitate
DOTS: deformities, open injuries, tenderness, swelling

E

E-9-1-1: enhanced 9-1-1
E-PCR: electronic patient care report
ECG: electrocardiogram
EMD: emergency medical dispatcher
EMD: electro-mechanical disassociation
EMR: emergency medical responder
EMS: emergency medical services
ERT: emergency response team
ET: endotracheal
ETA: estimated time of arrival

F

FBAO: foreign body airway obstruction

H

HAINES: high arm in endangered spine
HazMat: hazardous material
HBIG: hepatitis B immunoglobulin
HBV: hepatitis B virus
HCD: health care directive
hep B: hepatitis B
HIV: human immunodeficiency virus
HRDC: Human Resources Development Canada
HSFC: Heart and Stroke Foundation of Canada

I

ICM: the National Incident Management System
ICS: Incident Command System
IM: intramuscular
IO: intraosseous
IV: intravenous

L

LCDC: Laboratory Centre for Disease Control
LZ: landing zone

M

MCI: multiple-casualty incident/mass-casualty incident
MRSA: methicillin-resistant *Staphylococcus aureus*
MSDS: material safety data sheet
MVA: motor vehicle accident

N

NFPA: National Fire Protection Association
NG: nasogastric

O

OB: obstetrical
OD: overdose
OG: orogastric
OHS: Occupational Health and Safety
OPQRRRST: onset, provocation, quality, region, radiation, relief, severity, time
OSHA: Occupational Safety and Health Administration

P

PAC: Paramedic Association of Canada
PAD: public access defibrillation
PCP: primary care paramedic
PEA: pulseless electrical activity
PO: per os (by mouth)
PPE: personal protective equipment
PSAP: public safety answering point
psi: pounds per square inch
PTO shaft: power takeoff shaft
PTSD: post-traumatic stress disorder

R

RCMP: Royal Canadian Mounted Police

S

SAED: semi-automated external defibrillator
SAMPLE: signs and symptoms, allergies, medications, past medical history, last oral intake, events
SARS: severe acute respiratory syndrome
SC, SQ, or SubQ: subcutaneous
SCBA: self-contained breathing apparatus
SIDS: sudden infant death syndrome
SL: sublingual
SPIE: special insertion and extraction
START system: simple triage and rapid treatment system

T

TB: tuberculosis
TIA: transient ischemic attack

Glossary of Terms

A

abandonment: a legal term referring to discontinuing emergency medical care without making sure that another health care professional with equal or better training has taken over.

abdominal cavity: the space below the diaphragm and continuous with the pelvic cavity.

abrasion: an open wound caused by scraping, rubbing, or shearing away of the epidermis.

abuse: improper or excessive action so as to injure or cause harm.

accessory muscles: additional muscles; in regard to breathing, these are the muscles of the neck and the muscles between the ribs.

acquired immune deficiency syndrome (AIDS): a terminal condition facilitated by HIV. *See* human immunodeficiency virus.

activated charcoal: a finely ground charcoal that is very absorbent and is sometimes used as an antidote to some ingested poisons.

Adult Chain of Survival: the steps of early intervention recommended for an adult having a heart attack.

advance directive: a patient's instructions, written in advance, regarding the kind of resuscitation efforts that should be made in a life-threatening emergency.

advanced cardiac life support (ACLS): emergency medical life-sustaining interventions such as defibrillation, airway management, and medications for patients experiencing a cardiac emergency.

advanced care paramedic (ACP): trained to the level above the primary care paramedic and the EMR.

advanced life support (ALS): emergency medical life-sustaining interventions such as defibrillation, airway management, and medications.

afterbirth: the placenta after it separates from the uterine wall and delivers.

agonal respirations: reflex gasping with no regular pattern or depth; a sign of impending cardiac or respiratory arrest.

airway adjunct: an artificial airway.

airway, breathing, circulation (ABCs): the three ordered considerations for basic life support.

alimentary tract: the food passageway that extends from the mouth to the anus.

all-terrain vehicles (ATVs): an open-air vehicle with three or more wheels used for off-road transportation.

altered mental status: a change in a patient's normal mental status.

alveoli: the air sacs of the lungs. *Singular* alveolus.

amniotic sac: a sac of fluid in which the fetus floats.

amputation: an open injury that occurs when a body part is severed from the body.

analgesic: a medication given to reduce pain.

anaphylactic shock: *See* anaphylaxis.

anaphylaxis: an acute allergic reaction with severe bronchospasm and vascular collapse that can be rapidly fatal.

anatomical position: the position in which the patient is standing erect with arms down at the sides, palms facing forward.

anatomical regions: the external landmarks of the body.

anatomy: structure of the body.

antecubital space: the hollow, or front, of the elbow.

anterior: a term of direction or position meaning toward the front. *Opposite of* posterior.

anticoagulant: medication that slows the clotting process.

apical pulse: a pulse point located under the left breast.

arterial bleeding: bright red blood spurting from an artery.

arteries: blood vessels that take blood away from the heart.

arterioles: the smallest arteries.

artifact: ECG rhythm interference of electrical or mechanical origin.

artificial ventilation: a method of assisting breathing by forcing air into a patient's lungs.

aspirate: to inhale material into the lungs.

atria: the two upper chambers of the heart. *Singular* atrium.

auscultation: a method of examination that involves listening for signs of injury or illness.

automated external defibrillator (AED): a device that monitors a patient's heart and can conduct an indicated shock as needed.

autonomic nervous system: the part of the nervous system that regulates involuntary activities.

AVPU: mnemonic for the four levels of consciousness used to classify patients: alert, verbal (response to stimuli), pain (response to stimuli), and unconscious.

avulsion: an open wound that is characterized by a torn flap of skin or soft tissue that is either still attached to the body or pulled off completely.

B

bag of waters: *See* amniotic sac.

bag-valve-mask (BVM): a handheld device used to conduct artificial respiration for a patient.

bariatric: pertaining to weight and excessively large patients.

barotrauma: an injury caused by a change in the atmospheric pressure between a closed space and the surrounding area.

behaviour: the way a person acts or performs.

behavioural emergency: a situation in which a patient exhibits behaviour that is unacceptable or intolerable to the patient, family, or community.

birth canal: a passage consisting of the cervix and vagina that a baby passes through during birth.

blanching: losing colour.

blood pressure: the amount of pressure the surging blood exerts against the arterial walls.

blood vessels: a closed system of tubes through which blood flows.

bloody show: the appearance of the mucous plug after it is discharged during labour.

blunt trauma: a sudden blow or force that has a crushing impact.

body armour: a garment made of a synthetic material that resists penetration by bullets.

body mechanics: the safest and most efficient methods of using the body to gain a mechanical advantage.

body substance isolation (BSI): a strict form of infection control based on the premise that all blood and body fluids are infectious.

body surface area (BSA): a calculated percentage of the body surface; can be determined by the rule of nines.

brachial pulse point: a pulse that can be felt on the inside of the arm between the elbow and the shoulder.

bracing: exerting an opposing force against two or more parts of a stable surface with your body; in EMS, it usually refers to a safety precaution taken while riding in an ambulance patient compartment.

brand name: a drug's proprietary name given by the manufacturer and most readily identified by consumers.

breach of duty: failure to act or act accordingly with one's training and scope of practice.

bronchi: the two main branches of the trachea that lead to the lungs. *Singular* bronchus.

bronchodilator: a medication, usually inhaled, that widens the bronchi, allowing for increased air exchange.

burnout: a state of exhaustion and irritability caused by the chronic stress of work-related problems in an emotionally charged environment.

C

capillaries: the smallest blood vessels through which the exchange of fluid, oxygen, and carbon dioxide takes place between the blood and tissue cells.

capillary bleeding: dark red blood that oozes slowly from capillaries.

capillary refill: the time it takes for capillaries that have been compressed to refill with blood.

capsules: gelatin shells containing medication for oral administration.

cardiac arrest: the sudden cessation of circulation.

cardiac muscle: one of three types of muscle; it makes up the walls of the heart.

cardiopulmonary resuscitation (CPR): the method of supplying artificial breathing and circulation in an attempt to restore life.

carotid pulse point: a pulse that can be felt on either side of the neck.

central nervous system (CNS): the brain and the spinal cord.

cerebrospinal fluid: a water cushion that helps protect the brain and spinal cord from trauma.

cerebrovascular accident (CVA): loss of brain function caused by a blocked or ruptured blood vessel in the brain. *Also called* stroke.

cervical spine: the neck, formed by the first seven vertebrae.

cervix: the neck of the uterus.

chemical name: describes the chemical and molecular structure of a drug.

chief complaint: the reason that EMS was called, stated in the patient's own words.

chronic obstructive pulmonary disease (COPD): a chronic lung condition that results in decreased air flow.

chronic stress: an ongoing state of psychological demand.

circulatory system: the system that transports blood to all parts of the body.

clamping injury: a soft-tissue injury usually caused by a body part being stuck in an area smaller than itself.

classification: with respect to drugs, the broad group to which a drug belongs.

clavicle: the collarbone.

cleaning: the process of washing a soiled object with soap and water. *See* disinfecting *and* sterilizing.

closed wound: an injury to the soft tissues beneath unbroken skin.

coccyx: the tail bone, formed by four fused vertebrae. *Also called* coccygeal spine.

compartment syndrome: increased pressure within a closed space resulting in circulatory compromise.

Compendium of Pharmaceuticals and Specialties (CPS): a reference book of information about drugs and pharmaceuticals.

competent adult: in EMS, a competent adult is one who is lucid and able to make an informed decision about medical care.

complete FBAO: total obstruction of the airway that prevents breathing.

complete lifts: a lift where the rescuers bear the full weight without mechanical aid or help from the patient.

complex access: the process of gaining access to a patient that requires the use of tools and specialized equipment.

consent: permission to provide emergency care. *See* expressed consent *and* implied consent.

constrict: get smaller.

contusion: a bruise; a type of closed soft-tissue injury.

cornea: the anterior part of a transparent coating that covers the iris and pupil.

cranium: the bones that form the top (including the forehead), back, and sides of the skull.

crepitus: the sound or feeling of bones grinding against each other.

cribbing: a system of wood or other materials used to support an object, often a vehicle or machinery.

critical care paramedic (CCP): the most highly trained paramedic in the EMS system.

critical incident: any situation that causes a rescuer to experience unusually strong emotions that interfere with the ability to function either during the incident or later.

critical incident stress debriefing (CISD): a session usually held within three days of a critical incident in which a team of peer counsellors and mental health professionals help rescuers work through the emotions that normally follow a critical incident.

cross contamination: the transfer of contaminants from one patient to another by a caregiver who fails to discard contaminated personal protective equipment or to properly clean medical equipment or surfaces.

cross-finger technique: a method of opening a patient's clenched jaw.

crowing: a sound made during respiration, similar to the cawing of a crow, that may mean the muscles around the larynx are in spasm.

crowning: the appearance of the baby's head at the opening of the birth canal.

crushing injury: an open or closed injury to soft tissues and underlying organs that is the result of blunt force that has a crushing impact.

cyanosis: a bluish discoloration of the skin and mucous membranes; a sign that body tissues are not receiving enough oxygen.

D

dangerous good: *See* hazardous material.

debriefing: a technique used to help rescuers work through their emotions within 24 to 72 hours of a critical incident.

deep: a term of position meaning remote or far from the surface. *Opposite of* superficial.

defibrillation: the process by which an electrical current is sent to the heart to correct fatal heart rhythms.

defusing: a short, informal type of debriefing held within hours of a critical incident.

dermis: the second layer of skin. *See* epidermis *and* subcutaneous tissue.

diabetes mellitus: a disease in which the normal relationship between glucose (sugar) and insulin is altered.

diaphragm: a muscle, located between the thoracic and abdominal cavities, that moves up and down during respiration.

diastolic pressure: the result of the relaxation of the heart between contractions. *See* systolic pressure.

digestive system: the system that functions to ingest food and excrete waste products.

dilate: enlarge.

direct medical control: refers to an EMS medical director or another physician giving orders to an EMS rescuer at the scene of an emergency via telephone, radio, or in person. *See* indirect medical control.

disinfecting: the process of cleaning plus using a disinfectant, such as alcohol or bleach, to kill microorganisms on an object. *See* cleaning *and* sterilizing.

distal: a term of direction or position meaning distant or far away from the point of reference, which is usually the torso. *Opposite of* proximal.

diving reflex: the body's natural response to submersion in cold water in which breathing is inhibited, heart rate decreases, and blood vessels constrict in order to maintain blood flow to the brain and heart. *Also called* mammalian diving reflex.

do not resuscitate (DNR) order: a document that relates the wish of a chronically or terminally ill patient not to be resuscitated. *See* advance directive.

dorsalis pedis pulse: a pulse point that can be felt at the top of the foot on the great toe side.

DOTS: a mnemonic for signs to look for during the physical assessment: deformities, open injuries, tenderness, and swelling.

downers: depressants that relax the central nervous system; a slang term for drugs that act as a sedative or depressant.

dressing: a covering for a wound.

drowning: death from suffocation due to submersion in water.

drug abuse: self-administration of one or more drugs in a way that is not in accordance with approved medical or social practice.

duty to act: the legal obligation to render care to a patient who requires it.

E

ecchymosis: black-and-blue discoloration.

elixirs: liquid medicines containing alcohol that have been sweetened for palatability.

emancipated minor: a minor who is married, pregnant, a parent, in the armed forces, or financially independent and living away from home with permission of the court.

emergency medical dispatching: the conveyance of critical information to a paramedic or EMR crew who must respond to an emergency.

emergency medical services (EMS) system: a network of resources that provide emergency care and transport to victims of illness or injury.

emergency move: a move made when there is immediate danger to the patient, usually performed by a single rescuer.

emergency medical responder (EMR): usually the first person on the scene with emergency medical care skills and typically trained to the most basic EMS level.

emulsions: suspensions of a drug in an oily solute or solvent.

endocrine system: the system that makes and secretes hormones to regulate other body systems.

enhanced 9-1-1 (E-9-1-1): a system that shows the dispatcher the street address and telephone number of the caller on a computer screen.

enteral: route of drug administration that involves the digestive tract.

epidermis: the outermost layer of skin. *See* dermis *and* subcutaneous tissue.

epiglottis: a leaf-shaped structure that prevents food from entering the trachea during swallowing.

epiglottitis: inflammation of the epiglottis caused by a bacterial infection.

esophagus: a passageway at the lower end of the pharynx that leads to the stomach.

estimated time of arrival (ETA): the time at which arrival at a destination is predicted.

evisceration: the protrusion of organs from an open wound, most commonly with abdominal wounds.

expiration: breathing out; exhaling.

expressed consent: permission that must be obtained from every conscious, competent adult patient before emergency medical care may be rendered.

external: a term of position meaning outside. *Opposite of* internal.

extremities: the limbs of the body.

extruded: pushed or forced out.

F

femoral pulse point: a pulse that can be felt in the area of the groin in the crease between the abdomen and the thigh.

femur: the bone in the thigh, or upper leg.

fibula: one of the bones of the lower leg.

finger sweep: a technique used to remove a foreign object from the mouth.

flail chest: a closed chest injury resulting in the chest wall becoming unstable due to fractures of the sternum, cartilage, or ribs.

flail segment: an area of chest wall between broken ribs that becomes free-floating.

foreign body airway obstruction (FBAO): can be complete or partial; limited or no breathing can take place because the airway is blocked. *See* complete FBAO *and* partial FBAO.

full-thickness burn: a burn that extends through all layers of skin and may involve muscles, organs, and bone.

G

gastric distention: inflation of the stomach.

generic name: a drug's non-proprietary name.

genitalia: external reproductive organs.

glucose: a type of sugar.

golden hour: the first 60 minutes after a patient suffers trauma. This is the time frame considered most critical for interventions that affect patient outcomes. Patients receiving care within the golden hour have a better chance of survival than those who do not.

grieving process: the process by which people cope with death.

guarding position: a position in which the patient is (a) on his or her side with knees drawn up toward the abdomen or (b) standing upright but bent over with arms crossed over the abdomen.

gurgling: sounds created as air or gas moves through a liquid medium.

H

HAINES position: the position in which a spine injury patient is lying on the left or right side. *Also called* lateral recumbent position.

hallucinogens: a group of mind altering drugs that can alter perception, feelings, and thoughts.

hand-off report: a report of the patient's condition and the care that was given, made to the EMS personnel who take over patient care.

hangman's fracture: broken vertebra in the upper neck.

hazardous material (HazMat): a substance that in any quantity poses a threat or unreasonable risk to life, health, or property if not properly controlled.

head-tilt/chin-lift manoeuvre: a manual technique used to open the airway of an uninjured patient. *See* jaw-thrust manoeuvre.

Heart and Stroke Foundation of Canada (HSFC): the Canadian division of an organization that promotes education and standards for cardiac and stroke care.

Heimlich manoeuvre: a technique used to dislodge and expel a foreign body that is causing airway obstruction. *Also called* subdiaphragmatic abdominal thrusts *and* abdominal thrusts.

hematoma: a collection of blood beneath the skin.

hemoglobin: a red blood cell protein that carries oxygen to the cells.

hemorrhage: profuse bleeding.

hepatitis B (hep B): a serious liver disease transferred by blood or body fluids that can last for months.

hepatitis B virus (HBV): a virus causing hepatitis, a disease of the liver.

high-pressure regulators: oxygen therapy regulators that can produce a higher rate of flow.

human immunodeficiency virus (HIV): the virus that causes AIDS.

humane restraints: padded soft leather or cloth straps used to tie a patient down in order to keep the patient from hurting himself or herself or others.

humerus: the bone that extends from the shoulder to the elbow.

hyperthermia: fever or raised body temperature.

hyperventilation: rapid breathing common to such diseases as asthma and pulmonary edema and to anxiety-induced states.

hypoglycemia: low blood sugar.

hypoperfusion: *See* shock.

hypothermia: the overall reduction of body temperature. *Also called* generalized cold emergency.

hypoxemia: a condition caused by a deficiency of oxygen in the blood.

hypoxia: decreased levels of oxygen in the blood.

hypoxic drive: a respiratory drive triggered and regulated by oxygen chemoreceptors rather than carbon dioxide chemoreceptors.

I

ilium: one of the bones that form the pelvis. *Plural* ilia.

immobilize: to make immovable, or incapable of movement.

impaled object: an object that is embedded in an open wound.

implied consent: the assumption that in an emergency, a patient who cannot give permission for emergency medical care would give it if he or she could.

incontinent: unable to retain, usually referring to urine or stool.

index of suspicion: an informal measure of anticipation that certain types of mechanisms produce specific types of injury.

indirect medical control: refers to EMS system design, protocols, and standing orders, education for EMS personnel, and quality management. *See* direct medical control.

infectious disease: a disease that can spread from one person to another.

inferior: a term of direction or position meaning toward or closer to the feet. *Opposite of* superior.

inspection: a method of examination that involves looking for signs of injury or illness.

inspiration: breathing in; inhaling.

insulin: a hormone secreted by the pancreas that is essential to the metabolism of blood sugar.

internal: a term of position meaning inside. *Opposite of* external.

internal bleeding: bleeding that occurs inside the body.

involuntary muscle: *See* smooth muscle.

ischium: the lower portion of the pelvis. *Plural* ischia.

J

jaw-thrust manoeuvre: a manual technique used to open the airway of an unconscious patient who is injured or any patient who has a suspected spine injury. *See* head-tilt/chin-lift manoeuvre.

K

kinematics of trauma: the science of analyzing mechanisms of injury.

kinetic energy: the total amount of energy contained in an object in motion.

L

Laboratory Centre for Disease Control (LCDC): a public organization that identifies and recommends modes of treatment and prevention of diseases.

labour: the process of childbirth.

laceration: an open wound of varying depth caused by a sharp object.

landing zone (LZ): the area required to safely land a helicopter.

larynx: the voice box.

lateral: a term of direction or position meaning to the left or right of the midline. *See* medial.

lateral recumbent position: the position in which a patient is lying on the left or right side. *Also called* HAINES position.

level of consciousness: mental status, usually characterized as alert, verbal, conscious to pain, or unconscious (AVPU).

ligaments: tissues that connect bone to bone.

litter: a portable stretcher or cot.

local cold injury: freezing or near freezing of a specific body part. *Also called* frostbite.

log roll: a method of rolling a supine patient onto his or her side and then back down without causing injury to his or her spine.

lumbar spine: the lower back, formed by five vertebrae.

M

mechanism of injury: how an injury occurs, including the force or forces that caused the injury.

meconium staining: a greenish or brownish colour to the amniotic fluid, which means the unborn infant had a bowel movement.

medial: a term of direction or position meaning toward the midline, or centre of the body. *Opposite of* lateral.

medical director: in EMS, this person is the physician legally responsible for the clinical and patient-care aspects of an EMS system.

medical patient: a patient who is ill, not injured.

minor: any person under the legally defined age of an adult, usually under the age of 18 or 21 years.

mouth-to-barrier device ventilation: a technique of artificial ventilation that involves the use of a barrier device, such as a face shield, to blow air into the mouth of a patient.

mouth-to-mask ventilation: a technique of artificial ventilation that involves the use of a pocket mask with one-way valve to blow air into the mouth of a patient.

mouth-to-mouth ventilation: a technique of artificial ventilation that involves blowing air directly from the rescuer's mouth into the mouth of a patient.

multiple-casualty incident (MCI): any emergency where three or more patients are involved.

musculoskeletal system: the system made up of the skeleton and muscles, which help give the body shape, protect the organs, and provide for movement.

N

narcotics: drugs that reduce pain and can alter mood and behaviour; they affect the nervous system and the body's activities.

nasal cannula: an oxygen-delivery device consisting of two soft plastic tips that are inserted a short distance into the nostrils.

nasopharyngeal airway: an artificial airway positioned in the nose and extending down to the larynx. *Also called* nasal airway.

nasopharynx: the nasal part of the pharynx.

nature of the illness: the type of medical condition or complaint a patient may be suffering.

neglect: insufficient attention or respect given to someone who has a claim to that attention and respect.

negligence: the act of deviating from the accepted standard of care through carelessness, inattention, disregard, inadvertence, or oversight that was accidental but avoidable.

nervous system: the system that controls the voluntary and involuntary activity of the body; includes the brain, spinal cord, and nerves.

neutral position: neither flexed nor extended from the anatomical position.

non-accidental trauma: such injuries as those caused by child abuse.

non-emergency move: a move made by several rescuers usually after a patient has been stabilized. *Also called* non-urgent move.

non-rebreather mask: an oxygen-delivery device consisting of an oxygen reservoir bag and a one-way valve.

O

occlude: block, close up, or obstruct.

occlusive dressing: a dressing that can form an air-tight and sometimes water-tight seal.

official name: the name for a medication used by hospital staff and pharmacists, listed in the CPS.

open injury: an injury to the soft tissues that results in breaking of the skin.

OPQRRRST: an acronym used for assessing pain.

oropharyngeal airway: an artificial airway positioned in the mouth and extending down to the larynx. *Also called* oral airway.

oropharynx: the central part of the pharynx.

out-of-hospital care: another term for pre-hospital care.

overdose (OD): an emergency that involves poisoning by drugs or alcohol.

P

package: refers to getting the patient ready to be moved and includes such procedures as stabilizing impaled objects and immobilizing injured limbs.

palmar surface method: a method used to estimate the percentage of body surface area (BSA) involved in a burn injury in which one of the patient's palms is estimated as one percent of BSA.

palpated systolic pressure: blood pressure measured by palpation; one cannot obtain a diastolic pressure by palpation.

palpation: a method of examination that involves feeling for signs of injury or illness.

paradoxical breathing: a segment of the chest moves in the opposite direction of the rest of the chest during respiration; typically seen with a flail segment.

parenteral: route of drug administration that does not involve the digestive tract.

partial FBAO: limited or restricted amount of breathing due to partial obstruction of the airway.

partial-thickness burn: a burn that involves both the epidermis and dermis.

patella: the knee cap.

patent airway: an airway that is open and clear of obstruction.

pathogen: an organism, usually a microorganism such as a bacterium or virus, that causes disease.

patient history: facts about the patient's medical history that are relevant to the patient's condition.

Pediatric Chain of Survival: the steps of early intervention recommended for a child in cardiac arrest, emphasizing the importance of prevention of arrest.

pediatric patients: patients who are infants or children.

pelvic cavity: the space bounded by the lower part of the spine, the hip bones, and the pubis.

pelvis: the bony structure that includes the hips.

penetration/puncture wound: an open wound that is the result of a sharp, pointed object being pushed or driven into soft tissues.

per os (PO): taken by mouth.

perfusion: refers to the circulation of blood throughout a body organ or structure.

peripheral nervous system: the portion of the nervous system that is located outside the brain and spinal cord; the nerves.

personal protective equipment (PPE): equipment used by a rescuer to protect against injury and the spread of infectious disease.

pharynx: the throat.

physiology: the study of the function of the body and the physical and chemical aspects involved in its activities.

pills: tablets or capsules that are ingested orally.

placenta: a disc-shaped organ on the inner lining of the uterus that provides nourishment and oxygen to a fetus.

posterior: a term of direction or position meaning toward the back. *Opposite of* anterior.

posterior tibial pulse: a pulse point that can be felt behind the medial ankle bone.

post-traumatic stress disorder (PTSD): a potentially debilitating condition following an intense physical or emotional event.

potential crime scene: a scene that may require police support or intervention.

powders: medications that can be mixed with liquid and taken orally.

power grip: a technique used to get maximum force from the hands while lifting and moving.

power lift: a technique used for lifting that is especially helpful to rescuers with weak knees or thighs.

pre-hospital care: emergency medical treatment in the field before arriving at a medical facility. *Also called* out-of-hospital care.

primary assessment: part of patient assessment, conducted directly after the scene assessment, in which the rescuer identifies and treats life-threatening conditions.

primary care paramedic (PCP): trained to the level above the EMR.

prone position: the position in which a patient is lying face down on his or her stomach. *Opposite of* supine.

protocol: a written order issued by the medical director that may be applied to patient care; a type of standing order.

proximal: a term of direction or position meaning close or near the point of reference, which is usually the torso. *Opposite of* distal.

pubis: the anterior portion of the pelvis.

public access defibrillation (PAD): a program that attempts to put life-saving defibrillators in the hands of the public.

public safety answering point (PSAP): the location at which a dispatcher receives a call and decides which emergency service to activate.

pulse: the wave of blood propelled through the arteries as a result of the pumping action of the heart.

pulse oximeter: a device that measures the heart rate and the saturation of the blood's hemoglobin.

pulse oximetry: the use of a device to measure the amount of oxygen in blood.

R

radial pulse point: a pulse that can be felt on the inside of the wrist.

radius: one of the bones of the forearm.

rape: sexual intercourse that is performed without consent and is imposed through force, threat, or fraud. In Canada, charges for rape are listed as assault.

rape trauma syndrome: a reaction to rape that involves four general stages: acute (impact) reaction, outward adjustment, depression, and acceptance and resolution.

reasonable force: the minimum amount of force needed to keep a patient from injuring himself or herself or others.

recovery position: lateral recumbent position; used to allow fluids to drain from the patient's mouth instead of into the airway.

relative skin temperature: an assessment of skin temperature obtained by touching the patient's skin.

reproductive system: the system responsible for reproduction.

respiration: the passage of air into and out of the lungs.

respiratory arrest: the cessation of spontaneous breathing.

respiratory distress: shortness of breath or a feeling of air hunger with laboured breathing.

respiratory system: the system involved in the interchange of gases between the body and the environment.

rule of nines: a method used to estimate the percentage of body surface area involved in a burn injury.

S

sacrum: the lower part of the spine, formed by five fused vertebrae.

SAMPLE: an acronym used for obtaining a patient history.

scapula: the shoulder blade. *Plural* scapulae.

scene assessment: an overall assessment of the emergency scene.

scope of practice: the actions and care legally allowed to be provided by a care provider.

seizure: a sudden and temporary change in mental status caused by massive electrical discharge in the brain.

self-contained breathing apparatus (SCBA): an enclosed breathing system worn by rescuers.

semi-automated external defibrillator (SAED): a device in which the operator must push a button to analyze a patient's heart rhythm and deliver the shock. *See* automated external defibrillator (AED).

septum: a wall that divides two cavities.

sexual assault: any touch that the victim did not initiate or agree to and that is imposed by coercion, threat, deception, or threats of physical violence.

shock: a life-threatening, progressive condition that results from the inadequate delivery of oxygenated blood throughout the body. *Also called* hypoperfusion.

shoulder girdle: bony structure that consists of the clavicles and scapulae.

sign: any injury or medical condition that can be observed in a patient.

simple access: the process of gaining access to a patient without the use of tools.

skeletal muscle: one of three types of muscle; it makes possible all deliberate acts, such as walking and chewing. *Also called* voluntary muscle.

skull: the bony structure that houses and protects the brain.

smooth muscle: one of three types of muscle; found in the walls of tubelike organs, ducts, and blood vessels. *Also called* involuntary muscle.

sniffing position: a position of a patient's head when the neck is flexed and the head is extended.

snoring: sounds created by a partially obstructed airway during respiration.

soft-tissue injuries: injuries to the skin, muscles, nerves, and blood vessels. *Also called* wounds.

solutions: liquid medications containing a dissolved substance.

sphygmomanometer: an instrument used to measure blood pressure. *Also called* blood pressure cuff.

spinal column: the column of bones, or vertebrae, that houses and protects the spinal cord.

spinal cord: the cord of nervous tissue extending from the brain to the second lumbar vertebrae within the spinal column.

spinal precautions: methods used to protect the spine from further injury; for EMRs, usually refers to the manual stabilization of the patient's head and neck until the patient is completely immobilized.

spirits: solutions of volatile drugs dissolved in alcohol.

splint: a device used to immobilize a body part.

spontaneous abortion: the miscarriage, or the loss of pregnancy, before the 20th week.

standard of care: the care that would be expected to be provided to the same patient under the same circumstances by another EMR who had received the same training.

standing orders: advance orders, rules, regulations, or step-by-step procedures to be taken under certain conditions; a type of indirect medical control.

status epilepticus: a seizure lasting longer than 10 minutes or seizures that occur consecutively without a period of consciousness between them.

sterile: free of all microorganisms and spores.

sterilizing: a process in which a chemical or other substance, such as superheated steam, is used to kill all microorganisms on an object. *See* cleaning *and* disinfecting.

sternum: the breastbone.

stethoscope: an instrument that aids in auscultation (listening) of sounds within the body.

stoma: a permanent surgically created opening that connects the trachea directly to the front of the neck.

street drugs: illegal drugs and chemicals classified as uppers, downers, narcotics, hallucinogens, and volatile chemicals.

stridor: a harsh, high-pitched sound made during inhalation that may mean the larynx is swollen and blocking the upper airway.

stroke: loss of brain function caused by a blocked or ruptured blood vessel in the brain. *Also called* cerebrovascular accident (CVA).

subcutaneous tissue: the layer of fat beneath the skin.

substance abuse: the use of substances such as drugs and alcohol for the purpose of intoxication.

sucking chest wound: an open wound to the chest that bubbles or makes a sucking noise.

suctioning: using negative pressure created by a commercial device to keep the patient's airway clear.

sudden infant death syndrome (SIDS): unexplained death of an infant. *Also called* crib death.

superficial: a term of position meaning near the surface. *Opposite of* deep.

superficial burn: a burn that involves only the epidermis.

superior: a term of direction or position meaning toward or closer to the head. *Opposite of* inferior.

supine position: the position in which a patient is lying face up on his or her back. *Opposite of* prone.

suppositories: a form of medication administered via the rectum or vagina.

suspensions: solutions of medication containing particles that do not dissolve.

symptom: any injury or medical condition that can only be described by the patient.

syrups: thick solutions of a drug dissolved in sugar and water.

syrup of ipecac: a drug used to induce vomiting, usually in a patient who has ingested poison.

systolic pressure: the result of a contraction of the heart, which forces blood through the arteries. *See* diastolic pressure.

T

tablets: powder medications compressed into a disc-like shape for oral administration.

Taser: acronym for Thomas A. Swift's Electric Rifle. An electrically wired projectile weapon used by police to subdue a suspect by interrupting neuromuscular function with electricity.

tendons: tissues that connect muscle to bone.

tension pneumothorax: a condition that is the result of a chest wound, in which a severe buildup of air outside one lung compresses the lungs and heart toward the uninjured side of the chest.

therapy regulators: an adjustable valve that controls the volume of oxygen being delivered.

thoracic cavity: the space above the diaphragm and within the walls of the thorax. *Also called* chest cavity.

thoracic spine: the upper back, formed by 12 vertebrae.

thorax: the chest. *Also called* rib cage.

tibia: one of the bones of the lower leg.

tinctures: oral solutions of medication that have been prepared by extraction with alcohol; some alcohol may remain in the solution.

tongue-jaw lift: a technique used to draw the tongue away from the back of the throat and away from a foreign body that may be lodged there.

topographic anatomy: detailed illustrations of body systems.

tort: a civil court action that may be used to determine if an individual's rights have been violated.

tourniquet: a constricting bandage used as a last resort on an extremity to apply pressure over an artery in order to control bleeding.

trachea: the windpipe.

trauma patient: a patient who is injured.

triage: the process of sorting patients to determine the order in which they will receive care.

tripod position: a position in which the patient is sitting upright and leaning forward while fighting to breathe.

tympanic: pertaining to the ear or ear canal.

tuberculosis (TB): an infectious disease of the lungs.

tympanic thermometer: a thermometer that takes a reading from the ear.

U

ulna: one of the bones of the forearm.

umbilical cord: an extension of the placenta through which the fetus receives nourishment while in the uterus.

unresponsive: not acting or moving in response to a stimulus.

uppers: slang term for a drug used to stimulate the central nervous system.

urinary system: the system that removes waste products from the blood and helps regulate body fluid volume and composition.

uterus: the organ that contains the developing fetus.

V

veins: blood vessels that carry blood back to the heart from the rest of the body.

velocity: the speed at which an object moves.

venous bleeding: dark red blood that flows steadily from a vein.

ventilation: a method of assisting breathing by forcing air into a patient's lungs.

ventricles: the two lower chambers of the heart.

venules: the smallest veins.

vertebrae: the 33 bone segments of the spinal column. *Singular* vertebra.

vital signs: signs of life; assessments related to breathing, pulse, skin, pupils, and blood pressure.

volatile chemicals: substances abused for the purpose of exciting and then depressing the central nervous system.

voluntary muscle: *See* skeletal muscle.

vomitus: material that has been vomited.

W

withdrawal: a syndrome that occurs after a period of abstinence from the drugs or alcohol to which a person's body has become accustomed.

wound: a soft-tissue injury.

X

xiphoid process: the lowest portion of the sternum.

Index

C